P9-CQN-153

Angiotensin II Receptor Antagonists

Angiotensin II Receptor Antagonists

Edited by

MURRAY EPSTEIN, MD, FACP
Professor of Medicine
University of Miami School of Medicine
Jackson Memorial Medical Center
Department of Veterans Affairs Medical Center
Miami, Florida

HANS R. BRUNNER, MD
Professor of Medicine
Head, Division of Hypertension and Vascular Medicine
Lausanne University
Centre Hospitalier Universitaire Vaudois
Lausanne, Switzerland

HANLEY & BELFUS, INC. / *Philadelphia*

Publisher: HANLEY & BELFUS, INC.
               Medical Publishers
               210 South 13th Street
               Philadelphia, PA 19107
               (215) 546-7293; 800-962-1892
               FAX (215) 790-9330
               Web site: http://www.hanleyandbelfus.com

Note to the reader: Although the information in this book has been carefully re-viewed for correctness of dosage and indications, neither the authors nor the editor nor the publisher can accept any legal responsibility for any errors or omissions that may be made. Neither the publisher nor the editor makes any warranty, expressed or implied, with respect to the material contained herein. Before prescribing any drug, the reader must review the manufacturer's current product information (package inserts) for accepted indications, absolute dosage recommendations, and other information pertinent to the safe and effective use of the product described. This is especially important when drugs are given in combination or as an adjunct to other forms of therapy.

Library of Congress Cataloging-in-Publication Data

Angiotensin II receptor antagonists / edited by Murray Epstein, Hans R. Brunner.
       p. ; cm.
     Includes bibliographical references and index.
     ISBN 1-56053-453-2 (alk. paper)
       1. Angiotensin II—Antagonists—Therapeutic use. 2. Renal
   hypertension—Chemotherapy. 3. Hypertension—Chemotherapy. I. Epstein, Murray,
   1937– II. Brunner, Hans R., 1937–
       [DNLM: 1. Angiotensin II—physiology. 2. Angiotensin II—antagonists & inhibitors.
   3. Receptors, Angiotensin—physiology. QU 68 A58775 2000]
   RC684.A52 A54 2001
   616.1'32061—dc21

                                                              00-040747

Angiotensin II Receptor Antagonists   ISBN 1-56053-453-2

© 2001 by Hanley & Belfus, Inc. All rights reserved. No part of this book may be reproduced, reused, republished, or transmitted in any form, or stored in a data base or retrieval system, without written permission of the publisher.

Last digit is the print number: 9   8   7   6   5   4   3   2   1

Table of Contents

Contributors

Ahmed G. Adam, M.D., Ph.D.
Research Fellow, Department of Nephrology and Hypertension, University of Minnesota Medical School, Minneapolis, Minnesota

Andrew M. Allen, Ph.D.
Research Fellow, The Howard Florey Institute of Experimental Physiology and Medicine, University of Melbourne, Victoria, Australia

Michael W. Brands, Ph.D.
Associate Professor of Physiology and Biophysics, University of Mississippi Medical Center, Jackson, Mississippi

Hans R. Brunner, M.D.
Professor of Medicine, and Head, Division of Hypertension and Vascular Medicine, Lausanne University, Centre Hospitalier Universitaire Vaudois, Lausanne, Switzerland

Hans Peter Brunner-La Rocca, M.D.
Division of Cardiology, University Hospital, Zurich, Switzerland

Michel Burnier, M.D.
Professor, Division of Hypertension and Vascular Medicine, Lausanne University, Lausanne, Switzerland

Duncan J. Campbell, M.D., Ph.D.
Senior Research Fellow, St. Vincent's Institute of Medical Research, Fitzroy, Victoria, Australia

Mark E. Cooper, M.D., Ph.D.
Associate Professor, Department of Medicine, University of Melbourne, Austin & Repatriation Medical Centre, Heidelberg, Australia

Lea M. D. Delbridge, B.Sc.(Hons.), Dip.Ed.(Tert.), Ph.D.
Lecturer, Department of Physiology, University of Melbourne, Melbourne, Australia

Dick de Zeeuw, M.D., Ph.D.
Professor of Clinical Pharmacology, University of Groningen, Groningen, The Netherlands

Janice G. Douglas, M.D.
Professor, Department of Medicine, Case Western Reserve University School of Medicine, Cleveland, Ohio

Murray Epstein, M.D., FACP
Professor of Medicine, University of Miami School of Medicine, Miami, Florida

Murray David Esler, M.D., Ph.D.
Professor of Medicine, Monash University; Associate Director, Baker Medical Research Institute, Melbourne, Australia

Maurice E. Fabiani, M.D.
Senior Research Fellow, Department of Medicine, University of Melbourne, Austin & Repatriation Medical Centre, Heidelberg, Australia

Ying-Hong Feng, M.D., Ph.D.
Instructor, Department of Medicine, Case Western Reserve University School of Medicine, Cleveland, Ohio

Frederik Fierens, M.Sc.
Ph.D. student, Department of Molecular and Biochemical Pharmacology, Free University of Brussels, Brussels, Belgium

Ronald T. Gansevoort, M.D., Ph.D.
Department of Nephrology, University Hospital, Groningen, The Netherlands

Haralambos Gavras, M.D., FRCP
Professor of Medicine, Boston University School of Medicine; Chief, Hypertension and Atherosclerosis, Boston Medical Center, Boston Massachusetts

Irene Gavras, M.D.
Clinical Professor of Medicine, Boston University School of Medicine; Attending Physician, Boston Medical Center, Boston, Massachusetts

Sharon L. Grant, Ph.D.
Postdoctoral Fellow, Department of Medicine, Division of Cardiology, Emory University School of Medicine, Atlanta, Georgia

Cory D. Griffiths, Ph.D.
Department of Physiology, University of Melbourne, Melbourne, Australia

Kathy K. Griendling, Ph.D.
Professor of Medicine, Department of Medicine, Division of Cardiology, Emory University School of Medicine, Atlanta, Georgia

John E. Hall, Ph.D.
Guyton Professor and Chairman, Department of Physiology and Biophysics, University of Mississippi Medical Center, Jackson, Mississippi

Raymond C. Harris, M.D.
Department of Medicine, Division of Nephrology, Vanderbilt University School of Medicine, Nashville, Tennessee

Lisa M. Harrison-Bernard, Ph.D.
Assistant Professor, Department of Physiology, Tulane University School of Medicine, New Orleans, Louisiana

Daniel Hayoz, M.D.
Division of Hypertension and Vascular Medicine, Centre Hospitalier Universitaire Vaudois, Lausanne, Switzerland

Norman K. Hollenberg, M.D., Ph.D.
Professor of Medicine, Director of Physiologic Research, Brigham and Women's Hospital and Harvard Medical School, Boston, Massachusetts

John D. Imig, Ph.D.
Assistant Professor, Department of Physiology, Tulane University School of Medicine, New Orleans, Louisiana

Areef Ishani, M.D.
Chief Resident, Department of Medicine, University of Minnesota Medical School, Minneapolis, Minnesota

Colin I. Johnston, M.D.
Professor of Medicine, University of Melbourne, Austin & Repatriation Medical Centre, Heidelberg, Australia

Bernard Jover, Ph.D.
University of Montpellier, Montpellier, France

Rahul Koushik, M.D.
Consultant in Nephrology, Maharashtra State Hospitals, India

Joohyung Lee, B.Sc.(Hons.)
Ph.D. student, The Howard Florey Institute of Experimental Physiology and Medicine, The University of Melbourne, Victoria, Australia

Lucia Mazzolai, M.D.
Division of Hypertension and Vascular Medicine, Lausanne University Centre Hospitalier Universitaire Vaudois, Lausanne, Switzerland

Michael J. McKinley, Ph.D., D.Sc.
Associate Director, Howard Florey Institute of Experimental Physiology and Medicine, University of Melbourne, Victoria, Australia

Frederick A.O. Mendelsohn, M.D., Ph.D., FRACP
Professor and Director, The Howard Florey Institute of Experimental Physiology and Medicine, University of Melbourne, Victoria, Australia

Albert Mimran, M.D., Ph.D.
Professor of Medicine, University of Montpellier, Montpellier, France

Kenneth D. Mitchell, Ph.D.
Associate Professor, Department of Physiology, Tulane University School of Medicine, New Orleans, Louisiana

Trefor O. Morgan, M.B.B.S., B.Sc.(Med.), M.D.
Professor, Department of Physiology, University of Melbourne, Parkville, Australia; Head, Hypertension Clinic, Austin & Repatriation Medical Centre, Heidelberg, Australia

L. Gabriel Navar, Ph.D.
Professor and Chairman, Department of Physiology, Tulane University School of Medicine, New Orleans, Louisiana

Jürg Nussberger, M.D.
Division of Hypertension and Vascular Medicine, Lausanne University, University Hospital, Lausanne, Switzerland

Leopoldo Raij, M.D.
Professor of Medicine, Department of Nephrology and Hypertension, University of Minnesota Medical School, Minneapolis; Chief, Department of Nephrology and Hypertension, VA Medical Center, Minneapolis, Minnesota

Ernesto L. Schiffrin, M.D., Ph.D., FRCPC, FACP
Professor of Medicine, University of Montreal; Director MRC Hypertension Group and Hypertension Clinic, Clinical Research Institute of Montreal (IRCM), Montreal, Quebec, Canada

Pieter B.M.W.M. Timmermans, Ph.D.
Vice President, Pharmacology and Preclinical Development, Tularik, Inc., South San Francisco, California

Patrick Vanderheyden, Ph.D.
Department of Molecular Biochemical Pharmacology, Free University of Brussels, St. Genesius-Rode, Belgium

Georges Vauquelin, Ph.D.
Assistant Professor, Molecular Biochemical Pharmacology, Free University of Brussels, St. Genesius-Rode, Belgium

Bernard Waeber, M.D.
Professor, Division of Pathophysiology, University Hospital, Centre Hospitalier Universitaire Vaudois, Lausanne, Switzerland

Alberto Zanchetti, M.D.
Professor of Medicine, Centro di Fisiologia Clinica e Ipertensione, University of Milano, Ospedale Maggiore and Istituto Auxologico Italiano, Milano, Italy

Preface

During the past three decades, much clinical and investigative attention has focused on blockade of the renin-angiotensin system (RAS). Blockade of the RAS with angiotensin-converting enzyme (ACE) inhibitors has proved a major advance in the treatment of hypertension and congestive heart failure. Despite their proven benefit, ACE inhibitors have several limitations that may restrict their therapeutic usefulness. Consequently, angiotensin-receptor antagonists were developed to overcome such limitations and to provide more specific and complete blockade of the RAS. They display great therapeutic potential as antihypertensive agents and are likely to become a mainstay in the battle against cardiovascular disease. Ongoing studies explore a wide range of potential therapeutic applications, including managing congestive heart failure and retarding the progression of renal disease. In this book invited experts review current knowledge of angiotensin II (Ang II) antagonists and survey the progress of their diverse applications.

In the first section, entitled *Angiotensins and Their Receptors*, the contributors examine a number of fundamental issues. Hollenberg marshals compelling evidence suggesting the involvement of a renin-dependent but ACE-independent pathway for Ang II generation. He raises the interesting hypothesis that non-ACE pathways become quantitatively more important in disease states. Campbell reviews what is known about angiotensin peptides other than Ang II. He demonstrates that Ang II, Ang IV, and Ang (1–7) are also bioactive; ongoing investigations should offer further insight into their roles. Feng and Douglas review the most recent progress in ligand recognition, activation, signal coupling, and desensitization related to Ang II receptors. Advances in these areas are likely to represent a major focus of research and development during the next several years. Harris reviews the array of signaling events and cellular effects of Ang II and considers the interaction of Ang II receptor subtypes in the mediation of its biologic effects. Nussberger reviews the important and evolving subject of circulating versus tissue Ang II.

In the second section, entitled *Blockade of the Renin-Angiotensin System*, Brunner and Gavras and Timmermans recount the development of and early experience with Ang II antagonists. Vauquelin, Fierens, and Vanderheyden examine the nature of the antagonist-AT_1 receptor complex and the distinction between surmountable and insurmountable antagonists.

In the third section, entitled *Experimental Studies of the Effects of Angiotensin II and AT_1 Receptor Blockade*, Esler and Brunner review the interactions between the RAS and sympathetic nervous system, and Allen, McKinley, Lee, and Mendelsohn review interactions with the central nervous system. Adam, Ishani,

Koushik, and Raij examine the major actions of angiotensin and AT_1 receptor blockers and their interactions with other vasoactive factors, including nitric oxide, endothelin, and bradykinin. Brands and Hall and Navar, Harrison-Bernard, Imig, and Mitchell provide complementary reviews of the effects of Ang II and AT_1 receptor blockade on the kidney. Gavras and Gavras review the available data about the cardiac effects of Ang II and AT_1 receptor blockade; Morgan, Griffiths, and Delbridge review the relative effects of wall stress and Ang II on left ventricular hypertrophy; and Grant and Griendling review the vascular effects of Ang II and AT_1 receptor blockade.

The fourth section, entitled *Clinical Experience with AT_1 Receptor Antagonists*, begins with an introductory overview by Epstein. Fabiani and Johnston provide a comprehensive review of the antihypertensive effects of AT_1 receptor antagonists. Schiffrin and Hayoz consider the role of AT_1 angiotensin receptors in vascular remodeling, concluding that treatment with AT_1 receptor antagonists may result in reversal of the structural and functional alterations of vessels, especially small arteries, in patients with hypertension. The next two chapters detail the pivotal effects of Ang II receptor antagonists on the kidney and the implications for renal protection. Gansevoort, Mimran, and de Zeeuw focus on nondiabetic renal disease, Cooper and Epstein on diabetes mellitus. Because the deleterious actions of Ang II are mediated by the AT_1 receptor, Ang II antagonists theoretically should offer renoprotective effects similar to ACE inhibitors. Waeber and Brunner discuss the combination of AT_1 receptor antagonists with other antihypertensive agents, and in the concluding chapter of this section Mazzolai and Brunner focus on their outstanding safety and tolerability profile.

In the fifth section, entitled *Ongoing Trials with AT_1 Receptor Antagonists*, Zanchetti focuses on major evolving morbidity and mortality trials in patients with hypertension.

In the concluding section, the editors summarize a number of unanswered questions and unmet challenges that should be addressed. Examples include the precise mechanisms of action of AT_1 receptor antagonists, to what extent the stimulation of the AT_2 receptor contributes to the observed effect, and whether angiotensin-independent actions play a role. Finally, to the extent that AT_1 receptor antagonists and ACE inhibitors exert their blockade at different levels of the enzymatic cascade, the clinical utility of combining these two classes of drugs should be defined.

We appreciate the cooperation of all of the contributors and hope that their rigorous reviews and critical insights will provide a platform for future basic and clinical investigations with AT_1 receptor antagonists.

Murray Epstein, M.D.   Hans Brunner, M.D.
Miami, Florida   Lausanne, Switzerland

CHAPTER 1

Species Variations in the Renin-Angiotensin System: Therapeutic Implications

NORMAN K. HOLLENBERG, M.D., Ph.D.

Over the past 40 years, there has been increasing recognition of substantial variation among species in the elements of the renin-angiotensin system. Differences among species in the structure of renin, angiotensin I (Ang I), and angiotensin II (Ang II) have been recognized for over 30 years.[1-3] In the case of Ang I and Ang II, the species variation in structure appears to have no functional implications. In the case of renin, the structural variations are more substantial and result in striking species specificity. As one example, the development of renin inhibitors was influenced strongly by species, because the target had to be primate renin.[4,5] As a consequence, all of the supporting laboratory studies had to be performed in primates, with the need to develop new models at substantial expense. Renin inhibitors have been developed for rats, primarily because so many of our useful models have been developed in rats.[6]

Although much less is known about the structure and function of the angiotensin receptor in different species, the available evidence concerning angiotensin II type 1 (AT$_1$) receptors and their response to AT$_1$ receptor antagonists suggests a similar series of mechanisms in small animals and humans.[3,7]

The most striking and important species differences emerge in the conversion of Ang I to Ang II. The differences appear to express themselves in two ways. First, reasonable evidence suggests that the mechanism through which angiotensin-converting enzyme (ACE) inhibitors influence the renal blood supply differs by species. In some species, the involvement of bradykinin accumulation appears to be substantial, whereas in other species it appears to be a minor theme. Perhaps more importantly, evidence indicates that non–ACE-dependent pathways for Ang II generation also differ by species. These findings have important implications for therapeutics.

■ Species Differences in the Contribution of Kinins, Prostaglandins, and Nitric Oxide to the Renal Vascular Response to Inhibition of Angiotensin-converting Enzyme

A series of impressive but mixed observations suggests a substantial contribution of kinins to the renal vascular response to ACE inhibition in animal models. The differences in these studies may reasonably be attributed to quantitatively important variations among species. ACE inhibition, for example, increases prostaglandin production in canine[8] but not rabbit[9] kidneys. This finding suggests that the renal vasodilatation that follows ACE inhibition involves different mechanisms in the two species. Is this hypothesis testable? Is the renal vasodilator response to ACE inhibition more dependent on reduction in Ang II formation in rabbits than in dogs? If so, an Ang II antagonist would be expected to blunt renal vasodilator responses to ACE inhibitors more in dogs than in rabbits. Indeed, in similar protocols a partial agonist-Ang II antagonist blunted the renal blood flow response to ACE inhibition in dogs and rats[10–12] but not in rabbits.[13] Moreover, bradykinin antagonists have a significant influence on the renal blood flow response to ACE inhibition in dogs and rats[8,14] but not in rabbits.[15,16] In rats, it is primarily medullary perfusion that is kinin-dependent.[17] Thus, apparent species differences may reflect the relative contribution of medullary perfusion to total renal blood flow. In this case, humans resemble rabbits far more than they resemble rats or dogs.[18,19] Whatever the explanation, one cannot extrapolate from studies of mechanisms by which the kidney responds to ACE inhibitors in animal models to the control of renal circulation in humans—even in health and much less when disease is superimposed.

■ Species Differences in Local Angiotensin II-forming Pathways

The vast majority of studies comparing the effectiveness of ACE inhibitors and AT_1 receptor antagonists have used rat models of cardiovascular disease. In rats, these inhibitors lower blood pressure and prevent cardiovascular remodeling to a similar degree. There are, however, important species differences in local Ang II-forming pathways in the cardiovascular system, due mainly to different characteristics of chymase.[20–25] Human and hamster chymases hydrolyze Ang I to form Ang II, whereas rat chymase does not hydrolyze Ang I to Ang II and in fact participates in the degradation of Ang II.[25] Thus, ACE inhibitors and Ang II antagonists are expected to induce a similar physiologic response in rats. Virtually all of the Ang II generation in rats occurs via the ACE pathway.

In accord with in vitro studies of chemical pathways, the physiologic evidence for alternative pathways first emerged from studies in hamsters.[26] Cornish et al. found that vasoconstriction induced by Ang I in the blood vessels of hamster cheek pouch was inhibited only partially by ACE inhibitors in high concentration but was completely inhibited by either an Ang II antagonist or an antiserum directed against Ang II. The character of the enzyme or enzymes responsible for conversion of Ang I to Ang II remained unclear.

In studies of blood vessels in humans, monkeys, and dogs between 1984 and 1990, Okunishi and coworkers described evidence for a unique enzyme that converts Ang I to Ang II but differs from ACE.[27–29] Their observation that the enzyme was inhibited by several serine-protease inhibitors, including chymostatin, provided a clue to its nature. Chymostatin in high concentration provided partial blockade of the conversion of Ang I to Ang II. Captopril or other ACE inhibitors also provided partial inhibition, but to a somewhat lesser degree. The combination of chymostatin and ACE inhibition led to total blockade of Ang II formation in primate and canine blood vessels.[20] Their primary experimental endpoint was the contractile response of isolated blood vessels to Ang I in vitro.

Okunishi and coworkers designated the newly found enzyme responsible for converting Ang I to Ang II as CAGE, an acronym for chymostatin-sensitive Ang II-generating enzyme. Evidence indicated that CAGE is a chymase derived from passenger mast cells located in the adventitia of the arterial segments studied in vitro, presumably a cellular passenger.[30] These unambiguous facts raised a major question: Is it likely that an enzyme derived from mast cells plays a role in normal physiology? A second concern was raised by the fact that in the in vitro experiment Ang I was injected into the tissue bath surrounding the artery. As a result, hormone concentrations were as high in the adventitia at the anteluminal surface as in the lumen near the media, where the contractile apparatus operates. If Ang I is generated in vivo primarily in the circulation rather than locally, its concentration in the adventitial interstitium may be too low for CAGE to make an important functional contribution.

Even more fundamentally, in a series of reports over the same interval other investigators were unable to confirm the findings of Okunishi et al.[31–33] Each study failed to demonstrate any evidence for the presence of non-ACE enzymatic pathways in the vasculature; the responses to Ang I were completely abolished by ACE inhibition. In view of the simplicity and wide use of the preparations, it seemed unlikely that technical factors were responsible.

In a more recent report, Okunishi et al.[20] accounted for the differences in an elegant study that raises crucial issues for future investigators. They noted that all of the studies which failed to confirm their original observations had been performed with rat or rabbit blood vessels. Their follow-up study is well described in the title of their report: "Marked Species Difference in the Vascular Angiotensin II-forming Pathways: Humans Versus Rodents." In isolated arteries, they demonstrated a marked difference in the pathways for Ang II formation among human, rat, and rabbit arteries. In human gastroepiploic arterial strips, treatment with captopril blocked only 30–40% of the conversion of Ang I to Ang II. Treatment with chymostatin blocked about 60% of Ang II generation. A combination of captopril and chymostatin was required to produce 100% blockade. In rabbit arteries, on the other hand, captopril induced over 90% inhibition, and chymostatin had little or no effect. One technical concern was that the smaller arteries from the rabbit would suffer more endothelial damage or loss, but Okunishi et al. provided both morphologic and functional evidence for the integrity of endothelium in all of their preparations. Of interest, they speculated that their observation may account for the disturbing inability of ACE inhibitors to prevent the arterial response to injury in primates,[34,35] despite their ability to prevent neointimal hyperplasia in rat injury models.[36,37] If their speculation is correct, the therapeutic implications of the alternative pathways are obvious.

■ Studies of the Intact Human Kidney: Evidence from Pharmacologic Interruption

During the past decade, pharmaceutical science has provided an alternative approach to this problem with the development of renin inhibitors and novel Ang II antagonists that are free of partial agonist activity.[4,5] Thus, the logic of our approach to exploring alternative pathways of Ang II formation was straightforward. If all of the Ang II acting on the intrarenal circulation was formed through the classic pathway, with conversion of Ang I to Ang II only in the transit of blood through the pulmonary circulation, ACE inhibition, renin inhibition, and Ang II antagonists would be expected to induce an identical increase in renal plasma flow. To facilitate comparison, we initiated studies in healthy young men who were in balance with a daily intake of 10 mEq sodium to activate the renin system. We chose renin inhibition as the initial pathway for exploring the control of renal perfusion for several reasons. First, the remarkable substrate specificity of the renin reaction made mechanistic specificity of the renin inhibitor very likely. Second, the fact that inhibition of both ACE and renin leads to a fall in plasma Ang II concentration facilitated comparison of the degree of blockade. Finally, the identification of multiple Ang II receptor subtypes[3] added another layer of complexity to the interpretation of studies that used Ang II antagonists to interrupt the system.

In our first study we anticipated that the renal hemodynamic response to ACE inhibition under these circumstances reflected not only the fall in local Ang II formation but also the reduction in kinin degradation. The result would be the accumulation of vasodilator products, including bradykinin, and kinin-dependent formation of prostaglandin or activation of endothelial nitric oxide release. To our surprise, the renal vasodilator response to the renin inhibitor, enalkiren, was remarkable, exceeding expectations from our experience with ACE inhibitors.[38] In a follow-up, three-arm study that compared placebo, captopril, and enalkiren, placebo had no effect, whereas both captopril and enalkiren led to renal vasodilation.[39] The response to enalkiren was larger than the response to captopril in 6 of 9 healthy men, confirming our early observation. The findings in two studies using enalkiren were supported by a third study that used zankiren as the renin inhibitor in the same model.[40]

Although renin is a fastidious enzyme with great substrate specificity, one possible interpretation of our findings was that the renin inhibitors had an effect unrelated to renin. Several lines of investigation make this interpretation unlikely. Administration of Ang II into the renal arteries in dogs completely reverses the diuresis and natriuresis induced by the renin inhibitor.[41] Moreover, in humans the renal vascular response to renin inhibition is blunted by a high-salt diet[38] and in instances of low renin hypertension.[39] Finally, the primary renal response to ACE and renin inhibition is vasodilation. Despite these considerations, the possibility remained that renin inhibition led to an overestimate of the contribution of the renin-angiotensin system to renal vascular tone because of a lack of specificity and reflected an action unrelated to renin.

In this context, the development of the Ang II antagonist class created the possibility of a tie-breaker. If the renin inhibitor acted via an alternative non–angiotensin-dependent mechanism, Ang II antagonists would be expected to provide a different renal vascular response under the conditions of our study. Conversely, if the renin inhibitor acted only through blockade of renin-dependent formation of Ang II, the response to the renin inhibitor and Ang II antagonist should be identical. We have studied three Ang II antagonists in this model: eprosartan, irbesartan, and candesartan. In each case we defined the relation between Ang II antagonist dose and response. At the top of the dose-response relationship, the Ang II antagonists induced a response that agreed with the response to renin inhibition.[42,43]

The most parsimonious interpretation of our finding—that multiple renin inhibitors and Ang II antagonists induce an almost identical renal vascular response in humans, which exceeds substantially the response to ACE inhibition—suggests the involvement of a renin-dependent but ACE-independent pathway for Ang II generation. From the blood flow ratios, one can calculate that in healthy human kidneys about two-thirds of Ang II formation stimulated by a low-salt diet occurs via the ACE pathway and about one-third via non–ACE-dependent pathways. Thus, the non–ACE-dependent pathway would be less than that in intact isolated human arteries.[20] At the moment, in light of the above studies, it is reasonable to attribute such responses to chymase or CAGE, a chymase-like enzyme.

Perhaps most importantly, these observations have implications for therapeutic applications. If Ang II is a toxin under some circumstances, the possibility that blocking the system by renin inhibition or Ang II antagonism provides greater efficacy than ACE inhibition requires exploration. Our studies in diabetes, moreover, raise the interesting possibility that non-ACE pathways become quantitatively more important under conditions of disease.[42] This possibility places an even higher priority on therapeutic trials with alternative blockers.

Acknowledgments

This work was supported in part by National Institutes of Health grants T32 HL-07609, NCRR GCRC M01RR026376, P01AC00059916, 1P50ML 53000-01, and 1R01DK54668-0.

References

1. Barajas L, Bing J, Boucher R, et al: Renin. In Page IH, McCubbin JW (eds): Renal Hypertension. Chicago, Year Book, 1969, pp 14–61.
2. Grutter MG, Rahuel J: Human renin: Biochemistry, crystal structure, and opportunities for development of specific inhibitors. In Laragh JH, Brenner BM (eds): Hypertension: Pathophysiology, Diagnosis and Management, 2nd ed. New York, Raven Press, 1995, pp 1607–1619.
3. de Gasparo M, Bottari S, Levens NR: Characteristics of angiotensin II receptors and their role in cell and organ physiology. In Laragh JH, Brenner BM (eds): Hypertension: Pathophysiology, Diagnosis and Management, 2nd ed. New York, Raven Press, 1995, pp 1695–1720.
4. Wood JM, Stanton JL, Hofbauer KG: Inhibitors of renin as potential therapeutic agents. J Enzyme Inhib 1:169–185, 1987.
5. Kleinert HD, Stein HH: Specific renin inhibitors: Concepts and prospects. In Laragh JH, Brenner BM (eds): Hypertension, Pathophysiology, Diagnosis, and Management, 2nd ed. New York, Raven Press, 1995, pp 3065–3077.
6. Allan DR, Hui KY, Coletti C, Hollenberg NK: Renin vs. angiotensin-converting enzyme inhibition in the rat: Consequences for plasma and renal tissue angiotensin. J Pharmacol Exper Ther 283:661–665, 1997.
7. Vanderheyden PML, Fierens FLP, De Backer JP, et al: Distinction between surmountable and insurmountable selective AT₁ receptor antagonists by use of CHO-K1 cells expressing human angiotensin II AT₁ receptors. Br J Pharmacol 126:1057–1065, 1999.
8. Oliver JA, Sciacca RR, Cannon PF: Renal vasodilatation by converting enzyme inhibition: Role of renal prostaglandins in hypertension. Hypertension 5:166–171, 1983.

9. Johns EJ, Murdock R, Singer B: The effect of angiotensin I-converting enzyme inhibitor (SO 20881) on the release of prostaglandins by rabbit kidney. Br J Pharmacol 60:573–581, 1977.

10. Wong PC, Zimmerman BG: Mechanism of captopril-induced renal vasodilatation in anesthetized dogs after nonhypotensive hemorrhage. J Pharmacol Exper Ther 215:104–109, 1980.

11. Johnston PA, Bernard DB, Perrin NS, et al: Control of rat renal vascular resistance during alterations in sodium balance. Circ Res 48:728–733, 1981.

12. Wong PC, Zimmerman BG, Kraft E, et al: Pharmacological evaluation in conscious dogs of factors involved in the renal vasodilator effect of captopril. J Pharmacol Exper Ther 219:646–650, 1981.

13. Hollenberg NK, Passan DR: Specificity of renal vasodilatation with captopril: Saralasin prevents the response in the DOCA-treated, salt-loaded rabbit. Life Sci 31:329–334, 1982.

14. Nakagawa M, Stewart JM, Vavrek RJ, Nasjletti A: Effect of a kinin antagonist on renal function in rats. Am J Physiol 258:F643–F648, 1990.

15. Hajj-Ali AF, Zimmerman BG: Kinin contribution to renal vasodilator effect of captopril in rabbit. Hypertension 17:504–509, 1991.

16. Chen KE, Zimmerman BG: Comparison of renal hemodynamic effect of ramiprilat to captopril: Possible role of kinins. J Pharmacol Exper Ther 270:491–497, 1994.

17. Roman RJ, Kaldunski ML, Scicli AG, Carretero OA: Influence of kinins and angiotensin II on the regulation of papillary blood flow. Am J Physiol 255:F690–F698, 1988.

18. Fourman J, Moffat DB: The vascular architecture of the human kidney. In Fourman J, Moffat DB (eds): The Blood Vessels of the Kidney. London, Blackwell Scientific Publications, 1971, pp 59–68.

19. Teitelbaum I, Kleeman CR, Berl T: The physiology of the renal concentrating and diluting mechanisms. In Narins RG (ed): Maxwell and Kleeman's Clinical Disorders of Fluid and Electrolyte Metabolism, 5th ed. New York, McGraw-Hill, 1994, pp 101–127.

20. Okunishi H, Oka Y, Shiota N, et al: Marked species difference in the vascular angiotensin II-forming pathways: Humans versus rodents. Jap J Pharmacol 62:207–210, 1993.

21. Balcells E, Meng QC, Johnson WH, et al: Angiotensin II formation from ACE and chymase in human and animal hearts: Methods and species considerations. Am J Physiol 273:H1769–H1774, 1997.

22. Akasu M, Urata H, Kinoshita A, et al: Differences in tissue angiotensin II-forming pathways by species and organs in vitro. Hypertension 32:514–520, 1998.

23. Takai S, Shiota N, Yamamoto D, et al: Purification and characterization of angiotensin II-generating chymase from hamster cheek pouch. Life Sci 58:591–597, 1996.

24. Urata H, Kinoshita A, Misono K, et al: Identification of a highly specific chymase as the major angiotensin II-forming enzyme in the human heart. J Biol Chem 265:22348–22357, 1990.

25. Le Trong H, Neurath H, Woodbury RG: Substrate specificity of the chymotrypsin-like protease in secretory granules isolated from rat mast cells. Proc Natl Acad Sci USA 84:364–367, 1987.

26. Cornish KG, Joyner WL, Gilmore JP: Direct evidence for the presence of a different converting enzyme in the hamster cheek pouch. Circ Res 44:540–544, 1979.

27. Okunishi H, Miyazaki M, Toda N: Evidence for a putatively new Ang II-generating enzyme in the vascular wall. J Hypertens 2:277–284, 1984.

28. Okunishi H, Miyazaki M, Okamura H, Toda N: Different distribution of two types of Ang II-generating enzymes in the aortic wall. Biochem Biophys Res Commun 149:1186–1192, 1987.

29. Okamura T, Okunishi H, Ayajiki K, Toda N: Conversion of angiotensin I to angiotensin II in rabbit aorta. Hypertension 6:216–221, 1984.

30. Wintroub BU, Schechter NB, Lazarus GS, et al: Angiotensin I conversion by human and rat chymotryptic proteinases. J Invest Dermatol 83:336–339, 1984.

31. Saye JA, Singer HA, Peach MJ: Role of endothelium in conversion of angiotensin I to angiotensin II in rabbit aorta. Hypertension 6:216–221, 1984.

32. Oliver JA, Sciacca RR: Local generation of angiotensin II as a mechanism of regulation of peripheral vascular tone in the rat. J Clin Invest 74:1247–1251, 1984.

33. Campbell DJ, Ziogas J, Kladis A: Metabolism of tetradecapeptide, angiotensinogen and angiotensin I and II by isolated perfused rat hindlimbs. J Clin Exp Pharmacol Physiol 17:335–350, 1990.

34. MERCATOR Study Group: Does the new angiotensin-converting enzyme inhibitor cilazepril prevent restenosis after percutaneous transluminal coronary angioplasty? Results of the MERCATOR Study: A multicenter, randomized, double-blind placebo-controlled trial. Circulation 86:100–110, 1992.

35. Hanson SR, Powell JS, Dodson T, et al: Effects of angiotensin converting enzyme inhibition with cilazapril on intimal hyperplasia in injured arteries and vascular grafts in the baboon. Hypertension 18:1170–1176, 1991.

36. Powell JS, Clozel JP, Muller RKM, et al: Inhibitors of angiotensin-converting enzyme prevent myointimal proliferation after vascular injury. Science 245:186–188, 1989.

37. Roux SP, Clozel JP, Kuhn H: Cilazapril inhibits wall thickening of vein bypass graft in the rat. Hypertension 18:S43–S46, 1991.
38. Cordero PL, Fisher NDL, Moore TJ, et al: Renal and endocrine response to a renin inhibitor, enalkiren, in normal renin humans. Hypertension 17:510–516, 1991.
39. Fisher NDL, Allan D, Kifor I, et al: Responses to converting enzyme and renin inhibition: Role of Ang II in humans. Hypertension 23:44–51, 1994.
40. Fisher NDL, Hollenberg NK: Renal vascular responses to renin inhibition with zankiren in men. Clin Pharmacol Ther 57:342–348, 1995.
41. Siragy HM, Lamb NE, Rose CE Jr, et al: Intrarenal renin inhibition increases renal function by an angiotensin II-dependent mechanism. Am J Physiol 363:F749–F754, 1988.
42. Price D, Porter L, DeOliveira J, et al: The paradox of the low-renin state: Hormonal and renal responses to an Ang II antagonist, irbesartan, in diabetic nephropathy. J Am Soc Nephrol 10:2382–2391, 1999.
43. Price DA, De'Oliveira JM, Fisher NDL, Hollenberg NK: Renal hemodynamic response to an ANG II antagonist, eprosartan, in healthy men. Hypertension 30:240–246, 1997.

CHAPTER 2

Bioactive Angiotensin Peptides Other Than Angiotensin II

DUNCAN J. CAMPBELL, M.D., Ph.D.

Angiotensin II (Ang II) is one of a family of bioactive angiotensin peptides. This chapter reviews the formation, physiology, and pathophysiology of angiotensin peptides other than Ang II: angiotensin-(2-8) [Ang III], angiotensin-(3-8) [Ang IV], and angiotensin-(1-7) [Ang-(1-7)]. Table 1 summarizes the nomenclature and sequences of angiotensin peptides discussed in this chapter. They are important because they mediate some of the effects of Ang II and contribute to the effects of angiotensin-converting enzyme (ACE) inhibitors and Ang II type 1 (AT_1) receptor antagonists. This chapter focuses on aspects of potential clinical relevance.

■ Formation of Angiotensin Peptides

All angiotensin peptides are derived from angiotensinogen. In addition to renin, enzymes that release Ang I from angiotensinogen include cathepsin D,[1,2] pepsin,[3] and other aspartyl peptidases[4-6] and renin-like enzymes.[7-10] Moreover, serine proteases, including tonin,[11] cathepsin G,[12] trypsin,[13] and kallikrein,[14] can release Ang II directly from angiotensinogen. Furthermore, enzymes other than ACE may convert Ang I to Ang II.[11,15-18] Figure 1 summarizes many of the enzymes that metabolize Ang I and Ang II; Figure 2 depicts the pathways of formation of bioactive angiotensin peptides.

■ Circulating Levels of Angiotensin Peptides

Using C-terminal-directed antisera in normal ambulant volunteers,[19] we found the following venous plasma levels (fmol/ml, mean ± SD, n = 29): 18.7 ± 10.7 for Ang I, 3.7 ± 2.1 for the nonapeptide Ang-(2-10), 10.7 ± 6.6 for Ang II, 2.4 ± 2.6 for Ang III, 1.0 ± 0.8 for Ang IV, and 1.5 ± 1.1 for the pentapeptide Ang-(4-8). These levels agree with those reported by Nussberger et al.[20] and with levels measured by N-terminal–directed radioimmunoassays[21] (Fig. 3). Shibasaki et al.[22] reported higher plasma levels of Ang II and Ang IV in normal subjects: 20.6 ± 2.4 fmol/ml for Ang II and 8.6 ±1.1 fmol/ml for Ang IV.

Table 1. Nomenclature and Sequence of Angiotensin Peptides

Trivial Name	Abbreviation	Systematic Name	Sequence									
			1	2	3	4	5	6	7	8	9	10
Angiotensin I	Ang I, Ang-(1-10)	Angiotensin-(1-10) decapeptide	Asp	Arg	Val	Tyr	Ile	His	Pro	Phe	His	Leu
	Ang-(2-10)	Angiotensin-(2-10) nonapeptide		Arg	Val	Tyr	Ile	His	Pro	Phe	His	Leu
Angiotensin II	Ang II, Ang-(1-8)	Angiotensin-(1-8) octapeptide	Asp	Arg	Val	Tyr	Ile	His	Pro	Phe		
Angiotensin III	Ang III, Ang-(2-8)	Angiotensin-(2-8) heptapeptide		Arg	Val	Tyr	Ile	His	Pro	Phe		
Angiotensin IV	Ang IV, Ang-(3-8)	Angiotensin-(3-8) hexapeptide			Val	Tyr	Ile	His	Pro	Phe		
	Ang-(4-8)	Angiotensin-(4-8) pentapeptide				Tyr	Ile	His	Pro	Phe		
	Ang-(1-7)	Angiotensin-(1-7) heptapeptide	Asp	Arg	Val	Tyr	Ile	His	Pro			
	Ang-(1-5)	Angiotensin-(1-5) pentapeptide	Asp	Arg	Val	Tyr	Ile					

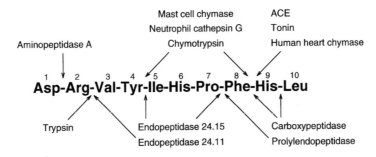

Figure 1. Metabolism of angiotensin I. ACE = angiotensin-converting enzyme.

■ *Methodology*

Accurate measurement of angiotensin peptides in blood and tissues requires adequate precaution to prevent angiotensin peptide generation and degradation during sample collection and processing and chromatographic procedures to separate peptides that cross-react in the radioimmunoassay.[20,23] It is customary to measure angiotensin peptides by radioimmunoassay after high-performance liquid chromatography.

Early reports of relatively high levels of Ang II and Ang-(1-7) in rat hypothalamus illustrate the importance of methodology.[24] Much lower levels of angiotensin peptides were measured when precautions were taken to prevent thawing of frozen tissue during processing.[25,26]

■ *Receptors for Bioactive Angiotensin Peptides*

Figure 4 summarizes bioactive peptides and their receptors. The importance of bioactive angiotensin peptides other than Ang II lies in part in the different effects

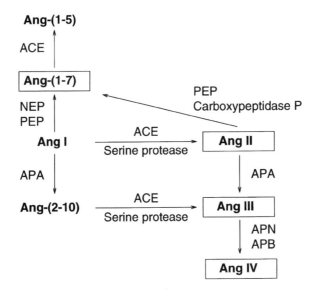

Figure 2. Pathways of formation of angiotensin-(1-7), angiotensin II, angiotensin III, and angiotensin IV. ACE = angiotensin-converting enzyme, APA = aminopeptidase A, APB = aminopeptidase B, APN = aminopeptidase N, NEP = neutral endopeptidase 24.11, PEP = prolylendopeptidase.

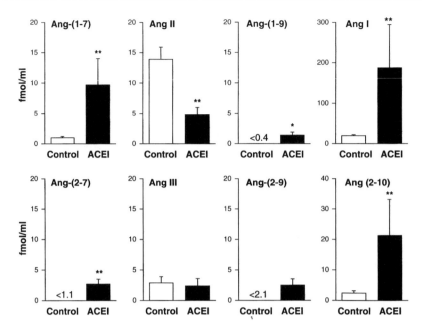

Figure 3.   Angiotensin peptide levels in cubital venous plasma of normal laboratory personnel (control) and subjects attending a hypertension clinic who were receiving angiotensin-converting enzyme inhibitor (ACE I) therapy. * $p < 0.05$, ** $p < 0.01$ in comparison with control subjects. Data from Lawrence et al.[21]

on their levels of ACE inhibition and AT_1 receptor antagonism (Figs. 5 and 6) and their possible role in mediating the therapeutic effects of ACE inhibitors and AT_1 receptor antagonists. The effect of ACE inhibition on angiotensin peptide levels depends on the responsiveness of renin secretion.[27] When renin shows little increase in response to ACE inhibition, the levels of Ang II and its metabolites decrease markedly with little change in the levels of Ang I and its metabolites. By contrast, a large increase in renin levels in response to ACE inhibition also increases the levels of Ang I and its metabolites. The increased levels of Ang I promote formation of Ang II by residual uninhibited ACE and by serine protease pathways of Ang I conversion, thereby buffering any decrease in Ang II levels during ACE inhibition.[28]

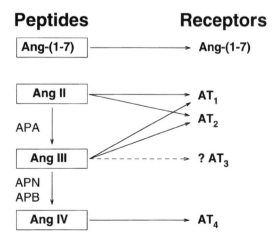

Figure 4.   Bioactive angiotensin peptides and their receptors. APA = aminopeptidase A, APB = aminopeptidase B, APN = aminopeptidase N.

ACE inhibition

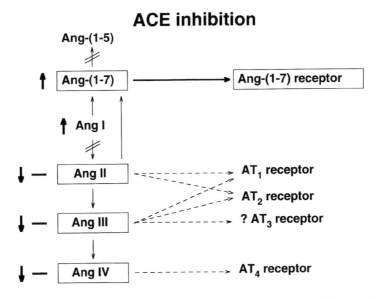

Figure 5. Effects of angiotensin-converting enzyme inhibition on angiotensin peptide levels.

ACE inhibition is accompanied by increased levels of Ang-(1-7) (see Figs. 3 and 5), in part because of the increase in levels of Ang I and its subsequent conversion to Ang-(1-7). Another mechanism for the increase in Ang-(1-7) levels is the inhibition of Ang-(1-7) metabolism by ACE, given that ACE is an important pathway of Ang-(1-7) metabolism.[29,30]

AT$_1$ receptor antagonism increases the levels of all angiotensin peptides (see Fig. 6). Whereas blockade of the AT$_1$ receptor may prevent its stimulation by the elevated levels of Ang II, other receptors are exposed to increased levels of angiotensin peptides. Shibasaki et al.[22] reported that AT$_1$ receptor antagonism causes marked increases in levels of both Ang II and Ang IV. We observed marked

AT$_1$ receptor antagonism

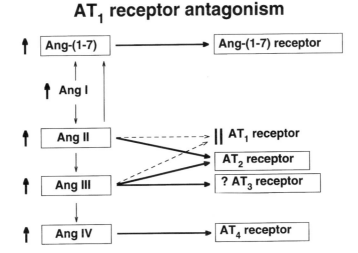

Figure 6. Effects of AT$_1$ receptor antagonism on angiotensin peptide levels.

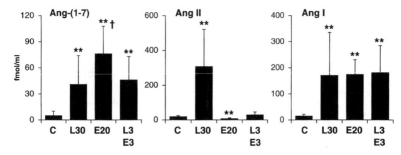

Figure 7.   Effects of losartan (30 mg/kg, L30), enalapril (20 mg/kg, E20) and their combination (losartan 3 mg/kg, enalapril 3 mg/kg, L3E3) on plasma levels of angiotensin-(1-7), angiotensin II, and angiotensin I in spontaneously hypertensive rats. The drugs were administered for 14 days. C = control rats, ** $p < 0.01$ in comparison with control; † $p < 0.05$ in comparison with L30 rats. Whereas all three drug regimens caused similar increases in plasma angiotensin I levels, losartan alone increased angiotensin II levels and enalapril alone suppressed angiotensin II levels. All three drug regimens increased plasma levels of angiotensin I and angiotensin-(1-7), but the increase in angiotensin-(1-7) levels seen with enalapril alone was higher than that seen with losartan alone, possibly because of inhibition of angiotensin-(1-7) metabolism by enalapril. Data from Ménard et al.[31]

increases in levels of Ang-(1-7) in response to AT_1 receptor antagonism in rats[31,32] (Fig. 7). Of note, the combination of ACE inhibition and AT_1 receptor antagonism prevented the increase in Ang II levels in response to AT_1 receptor antagonism but did not modify the increase in levels of Ang I and Ang-(1-7) (see Fig. 7).

■ Compartmentalization

The renin-angiotensin system operates in many different compartments, each with compartment-specific pathways of angiotensin peptide generation and metabolism. For example, we found that levels of Ang-(1-7) in hypophysial portal blood of sheep was higher than systemic levels.[33] Moreover, in studies in rats we found differences between the relative abundance of angiotensin peptides in plasma and tissues.[34] Whereas plasma levels of Ang II were similar to or less than plasma levels of Ang I, tissue levels of Ang II were much greater than tissue levels of Ang I.[34] Moreover, we found higher representation of aminopeptidase metabolites of Ang II and Ang I in rat kidney than in rat plasma.[34]

Angiotensin peptides respond differently to ACE inhibition and AT_1 receptor antagonism in different tissues.[32,34–36] The effects of these agents on angiotensin peptide levels suggest that, of all tissues examined, angiotensin-mediated processes in the kidney were most sensitive to inhibition by ACE inhibition and AT_1 receptor antagonism.[36] Renal levels of Ang II were reduced by lower doses of ACE inhibitor than those required to reduce Ang II levels in other tissues. Moreover, the kidney showed the smallest increase in Ang II levels in response to AT_1 receptor antagonism.[32,35,36]

Many questions about angiotensin peptide levels in discrete tissue compartments remain unanswered. For example, at sites of inflammation or coagulation where kallikrein and/or cathepsin G may be activated, Ang II may be formed by processes independent of renin.

■ Angiotensin III

Ang II and Ang III have similar affinities for the AT_{1B} and AT_2 receptors,[37,38] but Ang III has a lower affinity than Ang II for the AT_{1A} receptor.[39,40] Ang III reproduces all of the effects of Ang II, although usually with lower potency. For example, the pressor effect of Ang III in humans was approximately 20% of the pressor effect of Ang II,[41–43] although Ang III was either equipotent[41,42] or less potent than Ang II[43] in the stimulation of aldosterone secretion. Carey et al.[43] found that sodium deprivation sensitized the adrenal cortex more markedly to Ang III than to Ang II, with differing dose-response curves. This finding suggests that Ang III and Ang II may act at different receptor sites. Moreover, Devynck et al.[44] provided evidence that, in addition to the classic Ang II-binding site with lower affinity for Ang III, rat adrenal contains a high-affinity binding site with greater affinity for Ang III than for Ang II. These observations may be explained in part by the greater proportion of AT_{1B} receptors in adrenal cortex.[45]

Recently Zini et al.[46] published data suggesting the existence of specific Ang III receptors that do not respond to Ang II. The authors studied the effects of specific inhibitors of aminopeptidase A and aminopeptidase M on the stimulation of vasopressin release by intracerebroventricular injections of Ang II and Ang III (Fig. 8). The stimulation of vasopressin release by Ang II was blocked by aminopeptidase A inhibition, whereas the stimulation of vasopressin release by Ang III was potentiated by aminopeptidase N inhibition. Thus, Ang II itself was inactive, requiring aminopeptidase A-mediated conversion to Ang III before stimulation of vasopressin secretion occurred.

■ *Angiotensin IV*

Specific Ang IV-binding sites (presumptive AT_4 receptors) occur widely in the brain and peripheral tissues, including blood vessels, endothelial cells, heart, adrenal, and kidney.[47–54] Ang IV-binding sites are found in the cortex and outer medulla of the kidney[55] and have been localized to the cell body and apical membrane of the convoluted and straight proximal tubules in the cortex of the outer stripe of the outer medulla of the rat[56] and to collecting duct cells in humans.[57] Ang IV-binding sites are also present on mesangial cells, although binding could not be demonstrated in freshly isolated glomeruli.[58] As reviewed

Stimulation of AVP release in mice

Peptide given icv	Enzyme inhibited	AVP response
Ang II ⟶ Ang III		↑
Ang II —//→ Ang III	APA	—
Ang III ⟶ Ang IV		↑
Ang III —//→ Ang IV	APN	↑ ↑
	APA	—
	APN	↑

Figure 8.   Effects of inhibitors of aminopeptidase A (APA) and aminopeptidase N (APN) on stimulation of arginine vasopressin (AVP) release in mice by angiotensin II and angiotensin III. This study by Zini et al.[46] showed that stimulation of vasopressin secretion by angiotensin II was dependent on conversion of angiotensin II to angiotensin III. Moreover, angiotensin III acted through a mechanism or receptor unresponsive to angiotensin II.

Table 2.   Actions of Angiotensin IV

	References
Nervous system	
Learning, memory, exploratory behavior	47, 71–74
Inhibition of neurite outgrowth of sympathetic neurons	75
Cardiovascular system	
Activation of endothelial eNOS and cGMP content	54
Endothelium-dependent vasodilatation	54
Increase in endothelial PAI-1 mRNA levels	63
Stimulation of hypertrophy/hyperplasia of cardiac fibroblasts	66
Antagonism of Ang II-induced increase in mRNA and protein in chick heart cells	129
Dilatation of cerebral vessels	64, 65
Kidney	
Increase in renal cortical blood flow	55

by Zhuo et al.,[48] high levels of AT_4 receptors in the brain are found in many cholinergic nuclei and their terminals. A high density of AT_4 receptors also is found in several motor nuclei, some sensory nuclei, and several hypothalamic nuclei.[48]

In high concentrations, Ang IV activates AT_1 receptors, and many of the cardiovascular effects of Ang IV are inhibited by AT_1 receptor antagonists. Ang IV has approximately 0.2% of the pressor activity of Ang II and weak aldosterone-stimulating action in humans.[59] Ang IV has similar relative pressor potency in the rat, which is blocked by AT_1 receptor antagonism.[60] Moreover, Ang IV produces vasoconstriction in the renal and mesenteric vascular beds and pulmonary circulation—effects that are blocked by AT_1 receptor antagonism.[60,61] Similar findings were obtained for the isolated human saphenous vein.[62]

Many actions of Ang IV differ from those of Ang II, are mediated by specific AT_4 receptors, and are not modified by AT_1 or AT_2 receptor antagonism[47] (Table 2). Ang IV stimulates expression of plasminogen-activator inhibitor-1 (PAI-1) in endothelial cells.[63] Moreover, the stimulation of endothelial PAI-1 expression by Ang II and Ang III depends on their conversion to Ang IV. Figure 9 summarizes the studies by Kerins et al.[63] Using a similar strategy, Haberl et al.[64] found evidence suggesting that dilatation of rabbit cerebral resistance

Stimulation of PAI-1 mRNA in bovine aortic endothelial cells

Peptide	Control	Dup753	PD123177	WSU1291	Amastatin
Ang II	↑	↑	↑		—
Ang III	↑				—
Ang IV	↑	↑	↑	—	↑
Ang-(4-8)	—				

Figure 9.   Effects of AT_1 receptor antagonist (Dup753), AT_2 receptor antagonist (PD123177), AT_4 receptor antagonist (WSU1291), and aminopeptidase A inhibitor (amastatin) on stimulation of plasminogen activator inhibitor 1 (PAI-1) mRNA levels by Ang II, Ang III, and Ang IV. This study by Kerins et al.[63] showed that stimulation of PAI-1 expression by Ang II was not mediated by either the AT_1 or AT_2 receptor but was dependent on conversion of Ang II to Ang IV, with Ang IV acting through the AT_4 receptor.

vessels in response to Ang II and Ang III depends on their aminopeptidase-mediated metabolism to Ang IV, which, together with L-arginine, produces endothelium-dependent dilatation. In porcine arterial endothelial cells, Ang IV increased cyclic guanosine monophosphate (GMP) content and constitutive nitric oxide synthase activity, but not nitric oxide synthase protein, and caused endothelium-dependent relaxation of pulmonary artery rings.[54] Ang IV also exerted a vasodilatory effect on cerebral arteries in rats,[65] stimulated DNA and RNA synthesis in cultured rabbit cardiac fibroblasts,[66] and increased renal cortical blood flow in anesthetized rats. The last effect was blocked by inhibition of nitric oxide synthase, suggesting that Ang IV-induced renal vasodilatation is mediated by nitric oxide.[55] Moreover, Ang IV inhibited transcellular sodium transport in rat proximal tubules, possibly by inhibition of an ouabain-sensitive component of sodium-potassium-adenosine triphosphatase (Na^+-K^+-ATPase) activity.[56] In addition, Ang IV stimulated cytosolic calcium concentration of rat mesangial cells[58] and opossum kidney cells.[67]

Any receptor may respond to multiple ligands; the challenge is to identify the endogenous ligands for a specific receptor, particularly for the Ang IV receptor in the brain. The distribution of AT_4 receptors in the brain does not correspond with the major components of the renin-angiotensin system, including angiotensinogen, ACE, or Ang II immunoreactivity, and does not overlap the distribution of AT_1 and AT_2 receptors.[48] There are no published reports of Ang IV levels in the brain, although unpublished data from my laboratory indicate that Ang IV levels in brain are much lower than the levels of Ang II in this tissue.[25] Thus, it is possible that Ang IV is not the endogenous ligand for AT_4 receptors in the brain. LVV-hemorphin-7, a decapeptide recently isolated from brain, displays high affinity and specificity for AT_4 receptors and may function as the endogenous ligand for brain AT_4 receptors.[68] Because AT_4 receptors occur predominantly in the cholinergic, motor, and sensory processing nuclei, Ang IV and LVV-hemorphin-7 may modulate central motor and sensory activities and memory.[68–70] Ang IV has been shown to facilitate memory and to stimulate exploratory locomotor behavior.[47,71–74] Ang IV also inhibited neurite outgrowth in cultured embryonic chicken sympathetic neurones.[75]

Although many studies suggest that administration of exogenous Ang IV may have effects mediated by specific AT_4 receptors, as yet little evidence indicates that these effects are mediated by endogenous Ang IV. As noted above, Ang IV levels are much lower than Ang II levels in plasma. Levels of endogenous Ang IV may have a discernible role during AT_1 receptor antagonism when increased Ang IV levels may influence PAI-1 levels. Brown et al. discuss the complexities of regulation of PAI-1 levels.[76] Whereas Ang IV increases expression of PAI-1 in cultured endothelial cells via AT_4 receptors, Ang II increases PAI-1 expression in vascular smooth muscle cells via AT_1 receptors.[63,77] ACE inhibitors and AT_1 receptor antagonists would be expected to have different effects on the component of endothelial expression of PAI-1 mediated by Ang IV. ACE inhibition would be expected to reduce Ang IV levels and therefore endothelial expression of PAI-1, whereas AT_1 receptor antagonism would be expected to increase Ang IV levels and therefore expression of PAI-1 (see Figs. 5 and 6). ACE inhibiton is reported to reduce plasma levels of PAI-1 antigen and activity in normal subjects on a low-salt diet and in patients after myocardial infarction,[76,78–82] although this effect was not confirmed in other studies.[83,84] AT_1 receptor antagonism did not modify plasma levels of PAI-1 antigen or activity in patients with essential hypertension.[85] However, conflicting results were obtained in two studies that directly compared ACE inhibition and AT_1 receptor antagonism. Brown et al.[76] found that ACE inhibition, but not AT_1 receptor antagonism, reduced plasma levels of PAI-1 antigen and activity in normal subjects on a low-salt diet, whereas Goodfield et al.[86] found the opposite result in patients with congestive cardiac failure.

■ *Angiotensin-(1-7)*

Ang-(1-7) has less than 0.028% of the pressor activity of Ang II, does not increase plasma aldosterone levels in humans,[87] and does not stimulate drinking in experimental animals.[88] For many years Ang-(1-7) was thought to have no biologic role. However, the biologic effects of Ang-(1-7) are now under active investigation. Despite many years of intense effort, it has been difficult to demonstrate Ang-(1-7)-binding sites in tissues where this peptide has its effects. Before the development of specific Ang-(1-7) antagonists, evidence for Ang-(1-7) receptors was based on actions of Ang-(1-7) that were not modified by specific AT_1 or AT_2 receptor antagonists but were blocked by nonspecific Ang II antagonists such as Sar^1-Ile^8-Ang II. Recently, a specific high-affinity Ang-(1-7)-binding site was identified on bovine endothelial cells[89] and on the endothelium of dog coronary arteries.[90] Sar^1-Ile^8-Ang II and D-Ala^7-Ang-(1-7)—but not the AT_1 receptor antagonist losartan or the AT_2 receptor antagonist PD 123319—competed for the binding of ^{125}I-Ang-(1-7).[89] Moreover, inhibition of the effects of Ang-(1-7) by specific Ang-(1-7) antagonists such as D-Ala^7-Ang-(1-7) and A-779 support the existence of specific Ang-(1-7) receptors, although these binding sites are yet to be identified in many tissues.

Ang-(1-7) has many actions in many tissues (Table 3) that can be divided into three main groups: (1) actions similar to but much less potent than those of Ang II, such as the pressor effect; (2) actions similar to and approximately equipotent to those of Ang II; and (3) actions different from those of Ang II. Many aspects of Ang-(1-7) physiology and pathophysiology remain to be defined. A critical issue concerns the nature of the receptors that mediate the effects of Ang-(1-7). At least four different scenarios have been described:

1. Ang II and Ang-(1-7) have similar actions with similar potencies that are blocked by AT_1 receptor antagonism[91] and also may be blocked by AT_2 receptor antagonism.[92] Although the ability of AT_1 receptor antagonism to block the effects of both Ang II and Ang-(1-7) suggests that the effects of both peptides are mediated by AT_1 receptors, these AT_1 receptors must be atypical, given their responsiveness to Ang-(1-7). An alternative possibility is that AT_1 antagonists may block a subtype of Ang-(1-7) receptor.[93]

2. Ang II and Ang-(1-7) have similar actions with similar potencies; the effects of Ang II but not of Ang-(1-7) are blocked by AT_1 receptor antagonism, whereas the effects of Ang-(1-7) but not of Ang II are blocked by Ang-(1-7) receptor antagonism.[94-96] In this context, it is likely that Ang II activates AT_1 receptors and Ang-(1-7) activates Ang-(1-7) receptors.

3. Ang-(1-7) has actions different from Ang II, but these actions are blocked by both AT_1 receptor and Ang-(1-7) receptor antagonism.[97] Santos et al.[98] suggested that Ang-(1-7) acts through at least two different Ang-(1-7) receptor subtypes—one that is not blocked by AT_1 receptor antagonists and one that is blocked by AT_1 and, to a variable extent, AT_2 receptor antagonists.

Table 3. Actions of Angiotensin-(1-7).

	References
Actions similar to and approximately equipotent to those of angiotensin II	
General	
Stimulation of prostaglandin production in rabbit isolated vasa deferentia, rat smooth muscle cells, human astrocytes, and C6 glioma cells	121, 130–132
Nervous system	
Stimulation of vasopressin release	88, 89
Stimulation of substance P release from rat hypothalamus	133
Dilatation of piglet pial arterioles	134
Stimulation of psychotropic activity	135
Cardiovascular system	
Cardiovascular effects of microinjection into the medulla of rats	136, 141
Stimulation of proliferation of human cardiac fibroblasts	142
Coronary vasoconstriction and facilitation of reperfusion arrhythmias	143, 144
Stimulation of ^{3}H-noradrenaline release from rat atria	91, 145
Stimulation of nitric oxide production by dog coronary vessels	92
Kidney	
Stimulation of phospholipase activity and transcellular sodium flux in renal proximal tubule cells	146
Actions different from those of angiotensin II	
Cardiovascular system	
Hypotension	101–103
Endothelium-dependent vasodilatation	104–106
Potentiation of the hypotensive effects of bradykinin	107, 108
Inhibition of rat aortic smooth muscle cell growth	147, 148
Increased baroreflex control of heart rate	149, 150
Kidney	
Antidiuresis in water-loaded rats	97, 114
Natriuresis, diuresis, and increase in glomerular filtration rate in isolated perfused rat kidney, in spontaneously hypertensive rats, and in anesthetized Wistar rats	103, 115, 117

4. Ang-(1-7) has actions different from Ang II that are blocked by specific Ang-(1-7) receptor antagonism and not by AT_1 receptor antagonism.[95] In this context, Ang-(1-7) probably acts through specific Ang-(1-7) receptors, although a subtype of these receptors may be blocked by AT_2 receptor antagonists.[85]

Further understanding of the role of Ang-(1-7) must await clarification of the mechanisms by which this peptide exerts its effects.

One of the earliest reported effects of Ang-(1-7) was the stimulation of arginine vasopressin release from rat hypothalamoneurohypophysial explants with a potency equal to that of Ang II.[99] However, Ang-(1-7) was much less potent than Ang II in the stimulation of vasopressin secretion after intracerebroventricular administration to conscious rats—an effect that was prevented by AT_1 receptor antagonism.[88]

In support of its role in the brain, Ang-(1-7) was demonstrated by immunocytochemistry in the rat forebrain,[100] and relatively high levels of Ang-(1-7) were measured in rat brain.[24] However, subsequent studies using more rigorous methodology found very low levels of Ang-(1-7) in rat and sheep brain, including hypothalamus and pituitary.[25,26] Lawrence et al.[33] found increased Ang-(1-7) in hypophysial-portal blood of sheep. The levels of Ang-(1-7) in median eminence were very low, however, and the increased Ang-(1-7) levels in hypophysial-portal blood were attributed to endopeptidase-mediated conversion of Ang I to Ang-(1-7) in the median eminence vasculature.

Many actions of Ang-(1-7) are contrary to those of Ang II (see Table 3), and Ang-(1-7) has been proposed to function as a counter-regulatory hormone in blood pressure control and in other cardiovascular actions of Ang II. Ang-(1-7) reduces blood pressure and produces endothelium-dependent vasodilatation,[101-106] actions that may be due in part to potentiation by Ang-(1-7) of the hypotensive effects of bradykinin[107,108] and/or to stimulation of vascular prostaglandin production.[101,107] In support of a role for bradykinin-mediated nitric oxide production in the vasodilator effects of Ang-(1-7), Ang-(1-7)-induced vasodilatation and hypotension were attenuated by inhibition of nitric oxide synthase,[104,109] and antagonism of bradykinin type 2 (B_2)[104,108-110] and AT_2 receptors.[109] Moreover, Ang-(1-7)-induced stimulation of nitric oxide release from coronary vessels was blocked by B_2 receptor antagonism.[92]

High concentrations of Ang-(1-7) inhibit ACE. Li et al.[111] suggested that Ang-(1-7) potentiates the effects of bradykinin through ACE inhibition. However, the IC_{50} for Ang-(1-7) inhibition of ACE was 650 nmol/L, and it is unlikely that endogenous Ang-(1-7) levels would be sufficient to produce this effect. Deddish et al.[112] found that Ang-(1-7), like other ACE inhibitors, can potentiate the actions of a B_2 receptor agonist indirectly by a mechanism independent of blocking bradykinin hydrolysis—possibly by sensitization of the B_2 receptor.[113] However, it is unlikely that this is the mechanism of the potentiation by Ang-(1-7) of bradykinin-induced hypotension because micromolar concentrations of Ang-(1-7) were required to produce the effect.[112]

Reports of the effects of Ang-(1-7) on renal function are conflicting. Santos and Baracho[114] found a profound antidiuretic response to Ang-(1-7) in water-loaded rats with a potency similar to that of vasopressin—an effect that was blocked by both A-779 and the AT_1 receptor antagonist losartan.[97] By contrast, other authors reported that Ang-(1-7) produced diuresis and natriuresis in denervated[115] and intact kidneys[103,116] as well as in isolated perfused kidney,[117] and increased glomerular filtration rate.[116,117] These effects were not modified by AT_1 receptor antagonism, but were blocked by D-Ala^7-Ang-(1-7).[116] These effects of Ang-(1-7) were accompanied by increased secretion of prostaglandin and reduced by concomitant administration of indomethacin.[103,118]

Several effects of Ang-(1-7) on renal tubular function have been reported, including the inhibition of an ouabain-sensitive Na^+-K^+-ATPase exit step in proximal tubular transport of cellular sodium[115] and a fourfold increase in the hydraulic conductivity of inner medullary collecting ducts.[98] Vallon et al.[119] reported that intratubular application of Ang-(1-7) did not alter tubular reabsorption in the proximal convoluted or distal tubule or tubuloglomerular feedback. However, intratubular Ang-(1-7) at 10 nmol/L increased fluid, K^+, and Na^+ reabsorption in Henle's loop, an effect that was prevented by AT_1 receptor antagonism.[119] By contrast, Garcia and Garvin[120] reported that Ang-(1-7) had a biphasic effect when perfused through isolated proximal straight tubules. Fluid absorption was increased at picomolar concentrations of Ang-(1-7) and decreased at concentrations of 10 nmol/L. Both effects were prevented by AT_1 receptor antagonism.

The complexity of the effects of Ang-(1-7) on renal function is illustrated by the report that losartan blocks the stimulation of prostaglandin E_2 release by

Ang-(1-7) but not the stimulation of prostacyclin release. The release of both prostaglandins was blocked by Sar^1,Thr^8-Ang II.[121]

Several reported effects of administration of Ang-(1-7) antagonists support a role for endogenous levels of Ang-(1-7). These effects include the production of diuresis and natriuresis in rats,[98,116,122] which suggests that endogenous Ang-(1-7) levels have antidiuretic and antinatriuretic actions.[116] Microinjection of A-779 into the rostral ventrolateral medulla of the rat caused hypotension.[96] In addition, intracerebroventricular injection of A-779 attenuated the baroreflex sensitivity in rats and also counteracted the improvement in baroreflex sensitivity caused by enalapril in rats with renal hypertension.[123] Together, these studies support a role for endogenous brain Ang-(1-7) in cardiovascular control. However, these effects of Ang-(1-7) antagonists should be interpreted with caution. In the kidney, levels of Ang-(1-7) (~ 30 fmol/gm) are one-third the levels of Ang II; in brain and other tissues, however, Ang-(1-7) levels are very low,[25,26,35,124] and Ang-(1-7) receptors have yet to be identified.

As discussed above, both ACE inhibition and AT_1 receptor antagonism are associated with increased plasma levels of Ang-(1-7). Various approaches have been used to demonstrate a role for endogenous Ang-(1-7) in mediating the hypotensive effects of ACE inhibition and AT_1 receptor antagonism. Iyer et al.[125,126] showed that administration of either a specific monoclonal Ang-(1-7) antibody or a neutral endopeptidase inhibitor, which reduces plasma levels of Ang-(1-7),[127,128] increased blood pressure in spontaneously hypertensive rats treated with combined ACE inhibition and AT_1 receptor antagonism. This effect was not modified by B_2 receptor antagonism. The authors proposed that the increased Ang-(1-7) levels that accompany ACE inhibition and AT_1 receptor antagonism mediate in part the hypotensive effects of ACE inhibitors and AT_1 receptor antagonists. The plasma Ang-(1-7) levels in rats treated with combined ACE inhibition and AT_1 receptor antagonism, however, were at least 20-fold higher than the Ang-(1-7) concentrations in patients treated with ACE inhibition (see Fig. 3). Whether these mechanisms operate in humans remains to be seen.

■ *Conclusion*

In addition to Ang II, the truncated angiotensin peptides Ang III, Ang IV, and Ang-(1-7) are also bioactive, but their role in normal physiology and in disease states is unclear. It is uncertain whether the endogenous levels of these peptides are sufficient to exert effects in vivo, and the nature of AT_3, AT_4, and Ang-(1-7) receptors also remains unclear. One must keep an open mind about the possible role of alternative endogenous ligands for these receptors. Nevertheless, the potential contribution of Ang III, Ang IV, and Ang-(1-7) to the effects of ACE inhibition and AT_1 receptor antagonism cannot be ignored. Active investigation should offer further insight into the role of these peptides in the near future.

References

1. Dorer FE, Lentz KE, Kahn JR, et al: A comparison of the substrate specificities of cathepsin D and pseudorenin. J Biol Chem 253:3140–3142, 1978.
2. Hackenthal E, Hackenthal R, Hilgenfeldt U: Isorenin, pseudorenin, cathepsin D and renin: A comparative enzymatic study of angiotensin-forming enzymes. Biochim Biophys Acta 522:574–588, 1978.
3. Franze de Fernandez MT, Paladini AC, Delius AE: Isolation and identification of a pepsitensin. Biochem J 97:540–546, 1965.

4. Haas E, Lewis LV, Scipione P, et al: Angiotensin-producing enzyme I of serum: Formation by immunization with renin. J Hypertens 2:131–140, 1984.

5. Haas E, Lewis LV, Scipione P, et al: Angiotensin-producing serum enzyme II. Formation by inhibitor removal and proenzyme activation. Hypertension 7:938–947, 1985.

6. Husain A, Smeby RR, Wilk D, et al: Biochemical and immunological properties of dog brain isorenin. Endocrinology 114:2210–2215, 1984.

7. Deboben A, Inagami T, Ganten D: Tissue renin. In Genest J, Kuchel O, Hamet P, Cantin M (eds): Hypertension, 2nd ed. New York, McGraw-Hill, 1983, pp 194–209.

8. Haber E, Slater EE: Purification of renin: A review. Circ Res 40(Suppl I):I-36–I-40, 1977.

9. Menard J, Galen FX, Devaux C, et al: Immunochemical differences between angiotensin I-forming enzymes in man. Clin Sci 59(Suppl 6):41s–44s, 1980.

10. Dzau VJ, Brenner A, Emmett N, Haber E: Identification of renin and renin-like enzymes in rat brain by a renin-specific antibody. Clin Sci 59(Suppl 6):45s–47s, 1980.

11. Boucher R, Demassieux S, Garcia R, Genest J: Tonin, angiotensin II system. A review. Circ Res 41(Suppl II):II-25–II-29, 1977.

12. Tonnesen MG, Klempner MS, Austen KF, Wintroub BU: Identification of a human neutrophil angiotensin II generating protease as cathepsin G. J Clin Invest 69:25–30, 1982.

13. Arakawa K, Yuki M, Ikeda M: Chemical identity of tryptensin with angiotensin. Biochem J 187:647–653, 1980.

14. Maruta H, Arakawa K: Confirmation of direct angiotensin formation by kallikrein. Biochem J 213:193–200, 1983.

15. Okunishi H, Miyazaki M, Toda N: Evidence for a putatively new angiotensin II-generating enzyme in the vascular wall. J Hypertens 2:227–284, 1984.

16. Reilly CF, Tewksbury DA, Schechter NM, Travis J: Rapid conversion of angiotensin I to angiotensin II by neutrophil and mast cell proteinases. J Biol Chem 257:8619–8622, 1982.

17. Urata H, Konoshita A, Misono KS, et al: identification of a highly specific chymase as the major angiotensin II-forming enzyme in the human heart. J Biol Chem 265:22348–22357, 1990.

18. Padmanabhan N, Jardine AG, McGrath JC, Connell JM: Angiotensin-converting enzyme-independent contraction to angiotensin I in human resistance arteries. Circulation 99:2914–2920, 1999.

19. Campbell DJ, Kladis A: Simultaneous radioimmunoassay of six angiotensin peptides in arterial and venous plasma of man. J Hypertens 8:165–172, 1990.

20. Nussberger J, Brunner DB, Waeber B, Brunner HR: Specific measurement of angiotensin metabolites and in vitro generated angiotensin II in plasma. Hypertension 8:476–482, 1986.

21. Lawrence AC, Evin G, Kladis A, Campbell DJ: An alternative strategy for the radioimmunoassay of angiotensin peptides using amino-terminal-directed antisera: Measurement of eight angiotensin peptides in human plasma. J Hypertens 8:715–724, 1990.

22. Shibasaki Y, Mori Y, Tsutumi Y, et al: Differential kinetics of circulating angiotensin IV and II after treatment with angiotensin II type 1 receptor antagonist and their plasma levels in patients with chronic renal failure. Clin Nephrol 51:83–91, 1999.

23. Campbell DJ, Lawrence AC, Kladis A, Duncan A-M: Strategies for measurement of angiotensin and bradykinin peptides and their metabolites in central nervous system and other tissues. Meth Neurosci 23:328–343, 1995.

24. Chappell MC, Brosnihan KB, Diz DI, Ferrario CM: Identification of angiotensin-(1-7) in rat brain: Evidence for differential processing of angiotensin peptides. J Biol Chem 264:16518–16523, 1989.

25. Lawrence AC, Clarke IJ, Campbell DJ: Angiotensin peptides in brain and pituitary of rat and sheep. J Neuroendocrinol 4:237–244, 1992.

26. Senanayake PD, Moriguchi A, Kumagai H, et al: Increased expression of angiotensin peptides in the brain and transgenic hypertensive rats. Peptides 15:919–926, 1994.

27. Mooser V, Nussberger J, Juillerat L, et al: Reactive hyperreninemia is a major determinant of plasma angiotensin II during ACE inhibition. J Cardiovasc Pharmacol 15:276–282, 1990.

28. Juillerat L, Nussberger J, Ménard J, et al: Determinants of angiotensin II generation during converting enzyme inhibition. Hypertension 16:564–572, 1990.

29. Chappell MC, Pirro NT, Sykes A, Ferrario CM: Metabolism of angiotensin-(1-7) by angiotensin-converting enzyme. Hypertension 31:362–367, 1998.

30. Yamada K, Iyer SN, Chappell MC, et al: Converting enzyme determines plasma clearance of angiotensin-(1-7). Hypertension 32:496–502, 1998.

31. Ménard J, Campbell DJ, Azizi M, Gonzales M-F: Synergistic effects of ACE inhibition and Ang II antagonism on blood pressure, cardiac weight, and renin in spontaneously hypertensive rats. Circulation 96:3072–3078, 1997.

32. Campbell DJ, Kladis A, Valentijn AJ: Effects of losartan on angiotensin and bradykinin peptides, and angiotensin converting enzyme. J Cardiovasc Pharmacol 26:233–240, 1995.

33. Lawrence AC, Clarke IJ, Campbell DJ: Increased angiotensin-(1-7) in hypophysial-portal plasma of conscious sheep. Neuroendocrinology 55:105–110, 1992.

34. Campbell DJ, Lawrence AC , Towrie A, et al: Differential regulation of angiotensin peptide levels in plasma and kidney of the rat. Hypertension 18:763–773, 1991.

35. Campbell DJ, Kladis A, Duncan A-M: Effects of converting enzyme inhibitors on angiotensin and bradykinin peptides. Hypertension 23:439–449, 1994.

36. Campbell DJ: Endogenous angiotensin II levels and the mechanism of action of angiotensin-converting enzyme inhibitors and angiotensin receptor type 1 antagonists. Clin Exp Pharmacol Physiol Suppl 3:S125–S131, 1996.

37. Sandberg K, Ji H, Clark AJL, et al: Cloning and expression of a novel angiotensin II receptor subtype. J Biol Chem 267:9455–9458, 1992.

38. Kambayashi Y, Bardhan S, Takahashi K, et al: Molecular cloning of a novel angiotensin II receptor isoform involved in phosphotyrosine phosphatase inhibition. J Biol Chem 268:24543–24546, 1993.

39. Sasaki K, Yamano Y, Bardhan S, et al: Cloning and expression of a complementary DNA encoding a bovine adrenal angiotensin II type-1 receptor. Nature 351:230–233, 1991.

40. Murphy TJ, Alexander RW, Griendling KK, et al: Isolation of a cDNA encoding the vascular type-1 angiotensin II receptor. Nature 351:233–236, 1991.

41. Kono T, Oseko F, Shimpo S, et al: Biological activity of des-asp^1-angiotensin II (angiotensin III) in man. J Clin Endocrinol Metab 41:1174–1177, 1975.

42. Blair-West JR, Coghlan JP, Denton DA, et al: The effect of the heptapeptide (2-8) and hexapeptide (3-8) fragments of angiotensin II on aldosterone secretion. J Clin Endocrinol Metab 32:575– 578, 1971.

43. Carey RM, Vaughan ED Jr, Peach MJ, Ayers CR: Activity of (des-Aspartyll)-angiotensin II and angiotensin II in man. Differences in blood pressure and adrenocortical response during normal and low sodium intake. J Clin Invest 61:20–31, 1978.

44. Devynck M-A, Pernollet M-G, Mathews PG, et al: Specific receptors for des-Asp^1-angiotensin II ("angiotensin III") in rat adrenals. Proc Natl Acad Sci USA 74:4029–4032, 1977.

45. Inagami T: Molecular biology and signaling of angiotensin receptors: An overview. J Am Soc Nephrol 10(Suppl 11):S2–S7, 1999.

46. Zini S, Fournie-Zaluski MC, Chauvel E, et al: Identification of metabolic pathways of brain angiotensin II and III using specific aminopeptidase inhibitors: Predominant role of angiotensin III in the control of vasopressin release. Proc Natl Acad Sci USA 93:11968–11973, 1996.

47. Wright JW, Krebs LT, Stobb JW, Harding JW: The angiotensin IV system: Functional implications. Frontiers Neuroendocrinol 16:23–52, 1995.

48. Zhuo J, Moeller I, Jenkins T, et al: Mapping tissue angiotensin-converting enzyme and angiotensin AT1, AT2 and AT4 receptors. J Hypertens 16:2027–2037, 1998.

49. Briand SI, Bellemare JM, Bernier SG, Guillemette G: Study on the functionality and molecular properties of the AT4 receptor. Endocr Res 24:315–323, 1998.

50. Zhang JH, Stobb JW, Hanesworth JM, et al: Characterization and purification of the bovine adrenal angiotensin IV receptor (AT$_4$) using [^{125}I]benzoylphenylalanine-angiotensin IV as a specific photolabel. J Pharmacol Exp Ther 287:416–424, 1998.

51. Swanson GN, Hanesworth JM, Sardinia MF, et al: Discovery of a distinct binding site for angiotensin II (3-8), a putative angiotensin IV receptor. Regul Pept 40:409–419, 1992.

52. Jarvis MF, Gessner GW, Ly CQ: The angiotensin hexapeptide 3-8 fragment potently inhibits [^{125}I]angiotensin II binding to non-AT$_1$ or -AT$_2$ recognition sites in bovine adrenal cortex. Eur J Pharmacol 219:319–322, 1992.

53. Hanesworth JM, Sardinia MF, Krebs LT, et al: Elucidation of a specific binding site for angiotensin II(3-8), angiotensin IV, in mammalian heart membranes. J Pharmacol Exp Ther 266:1036–1042, 1993.

54. Patel JM, Martens JR, Li YD, et al: Angiotensin IV receptor-mediated activation of lung endothelial NOS is associated with vasorelaxation. Am J Physiol 275:L1061–1068, 1998.

55. Coleman JKM, Krebs LT, Hamilton TA, et al: Autoradiographic identification of kidney angiotensin IV binding sites and angiotensin IV-induced renal cortical blood flow changes in rats. Peptides 19:269–277, 1998.

56. Qadri F, Wolf A, Waldmann T, et al: Sensitivity of hypothalamic paraventricular nucleus to *C*- and *N*-terminal angiotensin fragments: Vasopressin release and drinking. J Neuroendocrinol 10:275–281, 1998.

57. Czekalski S, Chansel D, Vandermeersch S, et al: Evidence for angiotensin IV receptors in human collecting duct cells. Kidney Int 50:1125–1131, 1996.

58. Chansel D, Czekalski S, Vandermeersch S, et al: Characterization of angiotensin IV-degrading enzymes and receptors on rat mesangial cells. Am J Physiol 275:F535–542, 1998.

59. Kono T, Ikeda F, Oseko F, et al: Biological activity of des-asp^1-,des-arg^2-angiotensin II in man. Acta Endocrinol (Copenh) 99:577-584, 1982.

60. Champion HC, Czapla MA, Kadowitz PJ: Responses to angiotensin peptides are mediated by AT$_1$ receptors in the rat. Am J Physiol 274:E115–E123, 1998.

61. Nossaman BD, Feng CJ, Kaye AD, Kadowitz PJ: Analysis of responses to ANG IV: Effects of PD-123319 and DuP-753 in the pulmonary circulation of the rat. Am J Physiol 268:L302–L308, 1995.

62. Li Q, Feenstra M, Pfaffendorf M, et al: Comparative vasoconstrictor effects of angiotensin II, III, and IV in human isolated saphenous vein. J Cardiovasc Pharmacol 29:451–456, 1997.

63. Kerins DM, Hao Q, Vaughan DE: Angiotensin induction of PAI-1 expression in endothelial cells is mediated by the hexapeptide angiotensin IV. J Clin Invest 96:2515–2520, 1995.

64. Haberl RL, Decker PJ, Einhäupl KM: Angiotensin degradation products mediate endothelium-dependent dilation of rabbit brain arterioles. Circ Res 68:1621–1627, 1991.

65. Naveri L, Stromberg C, Saavedra JM: Angiotensin IV reverses the acute cerebral blood flow reduction after experimental subarachnoid hemorrhage in the rat. J Cereb Blood Flow Metab 14:1096–1099, 1994.

66. Wang L, Eberhard M, Erne P: Stimulation of DNA and RNA synthesis in cultured rabbit cardiac fibroblasts by angiotensin IV. Clin Sci 88:557–562, 1995.

67. Dulin N, Madhun ZT, Chang CH, et al: Angiotensin IV receptors and signaling in opossum kidney cells. Am J Physiol 269:F644–F652, 1995.

68. Moeller I, Lew RA, Mendelsohn FA, et al: The globin fragment LVV-hemorphin-7 is an endogenous ligand for the AT4 receptor in the brain. J Neurochem 68:2530–2537, 1997.

69. Moeller I, Chai SY, Oldfield BJ, et al: Localization of angiotensin IV binding sites to motor and sensory neurons in the sheep spinal cord and hindbrain. Brain Res 701:301–306, 1995.

70. Moeller I, Paxinos G, Mendelsohn FA, et al: Distribution of AT4 receptors in the Macaca fascicularis brain. Brain Res 712:307–324, 1996.

71. Wright JW, Miller-Wing AV, Shaffer MJ, et al: Angiotensin II(3-8) (ANG IV) hippocampal binding: Potential role in the facilitation of memory. Brain Res Bull 32:497–502, 1993.

72. Braszko JJ, Kupryszewski G, Witczuk B, Wisniewski K: Angiotensin II-(3-8)-hexapeptide affects motor activity, performance of passive avoidance and a conditioned avoidance response in rats. Neuroscience 27:777–783, 1988.

73. Wright JW, Clemens JA, Panetta JA, et al: Effects of LY231617 and angiotensin IV on ischemia-induced deficits in circular water maze and passive avoidance performance in rats. Brain Res 717:1–11, 1996.

74. Wright JW, Harding JW: Important roles for angiotensin III and IV in the brain renin-angiotensin system. Brain Res Rev 25:96–124, 1997.

75. Moeller I, Small DH, Reed G, et al: Angiotensin IV inhibits neurite outgrowth in cultured embryonic chicken sympathetic neurones. Brain Res 725:61–66, 1996.

76. Brown NJ, Agirbasli M, Vaughan DE: Comparative effect of antiogensin-converting enzyme inhibition and angiotensin II type 1 receptor antagonism on plasma fibrolytic balance in humans. Hypertension, 34:285–290, 1999.

77. Van Leeuwen RTJ, Kol A, Andreotti F, et al: Angiotensin II increases plasminogen activator inhibitor type 1 and tissue-type plasminogen activator messenger RNA in cultured rat aortic smooth muscle cells. Circulation 90:362–368, 1994.

78. Wright RA, Flapan AD, Alberti KGMM, et al: Effects of captopril therapy on endogenous fibrinolysis in men with recent, uncomplicated myocardial infarction. J Am Coll Cardiol 24:67–73, 1994.

79. Vaughan DE, Rouleau JL, Ridker PM, et al: Effects of ramipril on plasma fibrinolytic balance in patients with acute anterior myocardial infarction. Circulation 96:442–447, 1997.

80. Oshima S, Ogawa H, Mizuno Y, et al: The effects of the angiotensin-converting enzyme inhibitor imidapril on plasma plasminogen activator inhibitor activity in patients with acute myocardial infarction. Am Heart J 134:961–966, 1997.

81. Brown NJ, Agirbasli MA, Williams GH, Litchfield WR, Vaughan DE: Effect of activation and inhibition of the renin-angiotensin system on plasma PAI-1. Hypertension 32:965–971, 1998.

82. Moriyama Y, Ogawa H, Oshima S, et al: Captopril reduced plasminogen activator inhibitor activity in patients with acute myocardial infarction. Jpn Circ J 61:308–314, 1997.

83. Zehetgruber M, Beckmann R, Gabriel H, et al: The ACE-inhibitor lisinopril affects plasma insulin levels but not fibrinolytic parameters. Thromb Res 83:143–152, 1996.

84. Pedersen OD, Gram J, Jeunemaitre X, et al: Does long-term angiotensin converting enzyme inhibition affect the concentration of tissue-type plasminogen activator inhibitor-1 in the blood of patients with a previous myocardial infarction? Coronary Artery Dis 8:283–291, 1997.

85. Seljeflot I, Moan A, Kjeldsen S, et al: Effect of angiotensin II receptor blockade on fibrinolysis during acute hyperinsulinemia in patients with essential hypertension. Hypertension 27:1229–1304, 1996.

86. Goodfield NE, Newby DE, Ludlam CA, Flapan AD: Effects of acute angiotensin II type 1 receptor antagonism and angiotensin converting enzyme inhibition on plasma fibrinolytic parameters in patients with heart failure. Circulation 99:2983–2985, 1999.

87. Kono T, Taniguchi A, Imura H, et al: Biological activities of angiotensin II-(1-6)-hexapeptide and angiotensin II-(1-7)-heptapeptide in man. Life Sci 38:1515–1519, 1986.

88. Qadri F, Wolf A, Waldmann T, et al: Sensitivity of hypothalamic paraventricular nucleus to *C*-and *N*-terminal angiotensin fragments: Vasopressin release and drinking. J Neuroendocrinol 10:275–281, 1998.

89. Tallant EA, Lu XW, Weiss RB, et al: Bovine aortic endothelial cells contain an angiotensin-(1-7) receptor. Hypertension 29:388–393, 1997.

90. Brosnihan KB, Li P, Tallant EA, Ferrario CM: Angiotensin-(1-7): A novel vasodilator of the coronary circulation. Biol Res 31:227–234, 1998.

91. Gironacci MM, Adler-Graschinsky E, Peña C, Enero MA: Effects of angiotensin II and angiotensin-(1-7) on the release of [³H]norepinephrine from rat atria. Hypertension 24:457–460, 1994.

92. Longobardi G, Ferrara N, Leosco D, et al: Failure of protective effect of captopril and enalapril on exercise and dipyridamole-induced myocardial ischemia. Am J Cardiol 76:225–258, 1995.

93. Simoes-e-Silva AC, Baracho NC, Passaglio KT, Santos RA: Renal actions of angiotensin-(1-7). Braz J Med Biol Res 30:503–513, 1997.

94. Ambühl P, Felix D, Khosla MC: [7-D-ALA]-angiotensin-(1-7): Selective antagonism of angiotensin-(1-7) in the rat paraventricular nucleus. Brain Res Bull 35:289–291, 1994.

95. Santos RAS, Campagnole-Santos MJ, Baracho NCV, et al: Characterization of a new angiotensin antagonist selective for angiotensin-(1-7): Evidence that the actions of angiotensin-(1-7) are mediated by specific angiotensin receptors. Brain Res Bull 35:293–298, 1994.

96. Fontes MAP, Silva LCS, Campagnole-Santos MJ, et al: Evidence that angiotensin-(1-7) plays a role in the central control of blood pressure at the ventro-lateral medulla acting through specific receptors. Brain Res 665:175–180, 1994.

97. Baracho NC, Simoes-e-Silva AC, Khosla MC, Santos RA: Effect of selective angiotensin antagonists on the antidiuresis produced by angiotensin-(1-7) in water-loaded rats. Braz J Med Biol Res 31:1221–1227, 1998.

98. Santos RAS, Silva ACSE, Magaldi AJ, et al: Evidence for a physiological role of angiotensin-(1-7) in the control of hydroelectrolyte balance. Hypertension 27:875–884, 1996.

99. Schiavone MT, Santos RAS, Brosnihan KB, et al: Release of vasopressin from the rat hypothalamo-neurohypophysial system by angiotensin-(1-7) heptapeptide. Proc Natl Acad Sci USA 85:4095–4098, 1988.

100. Block CH, Santos RAS, Brosnihan KB, Ferrario CM: Immunocytochemical localization of angiotensin-(1-7) in the rat forebrain. Peptides 9:1395–1401, 1988.

101. Benter IF, Diz DI, Ferrario CM: Cardiovascular actions of angiotensin-(1-7). Peptides 14:679–684, 1993.

102. Nakamoto H, Ferrario CM, Fuller SB, et al: Angiotensin-(1-7) and nitric oxide interaction in renovascular hypertension. Hypertension 25:796–802, 1995.

103. Benter IF, Ferrario CM, Morris M, Diz DI: Antihypertensive actions of angiotensin-(1-7) in spontaneously hypertensive rats. Am J Physiol 269:H313–H319, 1995.

104. Pörsti I, Bara AT, Busse R, Hecker M: Release of nitric oxide by angiotensin-(1-7) from porcine coronary endothelium: Implications for a novel angiotensin receptor. Br J Pharmacol 111:652–654, 1994.

105. Brosnihan KB, Li P, Ferrario CM: Angiotensin-(1-7) dilates canine coronary arteries through kinins and nitric oxide. Hypertension 27:523–528, 1996.

106. Le Tran Y, Forster C: Angiotensin-(1-7) and the rat aorta: Modulation by the endothelium. J Cardiovasc Pharmacol 30:676–682, 1997.

107. Paula RD, Lima CV, Khosla MC, Santos RAS: Angiotensin-(1-7) potentiates the hypotensive effect of bradykinin in conscious rats. Hypertension 26:1154–1159, 1995.

108. Lima CV, Paula RD, Resende FL, et al: Potentiation of the hypotensive effect of bradykinin by short-term infusion of angiotensin-(1-7) in normotensive and hypertensive rats. Hypertension 30:542–548, 1997.

109. Gorelik G, Carbini LA, Scicli AG: Angiotensin-(1-7) induces bradykinin-mediated relaxation in porcine coronary artery. J Pharmacol Exp Ther 286:403–410, 1998.

110. Abbas A, Gorelik G, Carbini LA, Scicli AG: Angiotensin-(1-7) induces bradykinin-mediated hypotensive responses in anesthetized rats. Hypertension 30:217–221, 1997.

111. Li P, Chappell MC, Ferrario CM, Brosnihan KB: Angiotensin-(1-7) augments bradykinin-induced vasodilation by competing with ACE and releasing nitric oxide. Hypertension 29:394–400, 1997.

112. Deddish PA, Marcic B, Jackman HL, et al: N-domain-specific substrate and C-domain inhibitors of angiotensin-converting enzyme angiotensin-(1-7) and Keto-ACE. Hypertension 31:912–917, 1998.

113. Marcic B, Deddish PA, Jackman HL, Erdos EG: Enhancement of bradykinin and resensitization of its B2 receptor. Hypertension 33:835–843, 1999.
114. Santos RA, Baracho NC: Angiotensin-(1-7) is a potent antidiuretic peptide in rats. Braz J Med Biol Res 25:651–654, 1992.
115. Handa RK, Ferrario CM, Strandhoy JW: Renal actions of angiotensin-(1-7): In vivo and in vitro studies. Am J Physiol 270:F141–F147, 1996.
116. Vallon V, Heyne N, Richter K, et al: [7-D-ALA]-angiotensin-(1-7) blocks renal actions of angiotensin-(1-7) in the anesthetized rat. J Cardiovasc Pharmacol 32:164–167, 1998.
117. DelliPizzi A, Hilchey SD, Bell-Quilley CP: Natriuretic action of angiotensin-(1-7). Br J Pharmacol 111:1–3, 1994.
118. Hilchey SD, Bell-Quilley CP: Association between the natriuretic action of angiotensin-(1-7) and selective stimulation of renal prostaglandin I_2 release. Hypertension 25:1238–1244, 1995.
119. Vallon V, Richter K, Heyne N, Osswald H: Effect of intratubular application of angiotensin-(1-7) on nephron function. Kidney Blood Press Res 20:233–239, 1997.
120. Garcia NH, Garvin JL: Angiotensin-(1-7) has a biphasic effect on fluid absorption in the proximal straight tubule. J Am Soc Nephrol 5:1133–1138, 1994.
121. Jaiswal N, Diz DI, Tallant EA, Khosla MC, Ferrario CM: Characterization of angiotensin receptors mediating prostaglandin synthesis in C6 glioma cells. Am J Physiol 260:R1000–R1006, 1991.
122. Silva ACSE, Bello APC, Baracho NCV, et al: Diuresis and natriuresis produced by long term administration of a selective angiotensin-(1-7) antagonist in normotensive and hypertensive rats. Regul Pept 74:177–184, 1998.
123. Britto RR, Santos RAS, Fagundes-Moura CR, et al: Role of angiotensin-(1-7) in the modulation of the baroreflex in renovascular hypertensive rats. Hypertension 30:549–556, 1997.
124. Campbell DJ, Kladis A, Duncan A-M: Nephrectomy, converting enzyme inhibition and angiotensin peptides. Hypertension 22:513–522, 1993.
125. Iyer SN, Chappell MC, Averill DB, et al: Vasodepressor actions of angiotensin-(1-7) unmasked during combined treatment with lisinopril and losartan. Hypertension 31:699–705, 1998.
126. Iyer SN, Ferrario CM, Chappell MC: Angiotensin-(1-7) contributes to the antihypertensive effects of blockade of the renin-angiotensin system. Hypertension 31:356–361, 1998.
127. Yamamoto K, Chappell MC, Brosnihan KB, Ferrario CM: In vivo metabolism of angiotensin I by neutral endopeptidase (EC 3.4.24.11) in spontaneously hypertensive rats. Hypertension 19:692–696, 1992.
128. Duncan AM, James GM, Anastasopoulos F, et al: Interaction between neutral endopeptidase and angiotensin converting enzyme inhibition in rats with myocardial infarction: Effects on cardiac hypertrophy and angiotensin and bradykinin peptide levels. J Pharmacol Exp Ther 289:295–303, 1999.
129. Baker KM, Aceto JF: Angiotensin II stimulation of protein synthesis and cell growth in chick heart cells. Am J Physiol 259:H610–H618, 1990.
130. Trachte GJ, Meixner K, Ferrario CM, Khosla MC: Prostaglandin production in response to angiotensin-(1-7) in rabbit isolated vasa deferentia. Prostaglandins 39:385–394, 1990.
131. Jaiswal N, Jaiswal RK, Tallant EA, et al: Alterations in prostaglandin production in spontaneously hypertensive rat smooth muscle cells. Hypertension 21:900–905, 1993.
132. Tallant EA, Jaiswal N, Diz DI, Ferrario CM: Human astrocytes contain two distinct angiotensin receptor subtypes. Hypertension 18:32–39, 1991.
133. Diz DI, Pirro NT: Differential actions of angiotensin II and angiotensin-(1-7) on transmitter release. Hypertension 19(Suppl II):II-41–II-48, 1992.
134. Meng W, Busija DW: Comparative effects of angiotensin-(1-7) and angiotensin II on piglet pial arterioles. Stroke 24:2041–2044, 1993.
135. Holy Z, Braszko J, Kupryszewski G, et al: Angiotensin II-derived peptides devoid of phenylalanine in position 8 have full psychotropic activity of the parent hormone. J Physiol Pharmacol 43:183–192, 1992.
136. Campagnole-Santos MJ, Diz DI, Santos RAS, et al: Cardiovascular effects of angiotensin-(1-7) injected into the dorsal medulla of rats. Am J Physiol 257:H324–H329, 1989.
137. Ferrario CM, Barnes KL, Block CH, et al: Pathways of angiotensin formation and function in the brain. Hypertension 15(Suppl I):I-13–I-19, 1990.
138. Campagnole-Santos MJ, Diz DI, Ferrario CM: Actions of angiotensin peptides after partial denervation of the solitary tract nucleus. Hypertension 15(Suppl I):I-34–I-39, 1990.
139. Barnes KL, Knowles WD, Ferrario CM: Angiotensin II and angiotensin-(1-7) excite neurons in the canine medulla in vitro. Brain Res Bull 24:275–280, 1990.
140. Fontes MAP, Pinge MCM, Naves V, et al: Cardiovascular effects produced by microinjection of angiotensins and angiotensin antagonists into the ventrolateral medulla of freely moving rats. Brain Res 750:305–310, 1997.

141. Silva LCS, Fontes MAP, Campagnole-Santos MJ, et al: Cardiovascular effects produced by micro-injection of angiotensin-(1-7) on vasopressor and vasodepressor sites of the ventrolateral medulla. Brain Res 613:321–325, 1993.

142. Neuss M, Regitz-Zagrosek V, Hildebrandt A, Fleck E: Human cardiac fibroblasts express an angiotensin receptor with unusual binding characteristics which is coupled to cellular proliferation. Biochem Biophys Res Commun 204:1334–1339, 1994.

143. Kumagai H, Khosla M, Ferrario C, Fouad-Tarazi FM: Biological activity of angiotensin-(1-7) heptapeptide in the hamster heart. Hypertension 15(Suppl I):I-29–I-33, 1990.

144. Neves LA, Almeida AP, Khosla MC, et al: Effect of angiotensin-(1-7) on reperfusion arrhythmias in isolated rat hearts. Braz J Med Biol Res 30:801–809, 1997.

145. Gironacci MM, Lorenzo PS, Adler-Graschinsky E: Possible participation of nitric oxide in the increase of norepinephrine release caused by angiotensin peptides in rat atria. Hypertension 29:1344–1350, 1997.

146. Andreatta-van Leyen S, Romero MF, Khosla MC, Douglas JG: Modulation of phospholipase A_2 activity and sodium transport by angiotensin-(1-7). Kidney Int 44:932–936, 1993.

147. Freeman EJ, Chisolm GM, Ferrario CM, Tallant EA: Angiotensin-(1-7) inhibits vascular smooth muscle cell growth. Hypertension 28:104–108, 1996.

148. Strawn WB, Ferrario CM, Tallant EA: Angiotensin-(1-7) reduces smooth muscle growth after vascular injury. Hypertension 33:207–211, 1999.

149. Campagnole-Santos MJ, Heringer SB, Batista EN, et al: Differential baroreceptor reflex modulation by centrally infused angiotensin peptides. Am J Physiol 263:R89–R94, 1992.

150. Benter IF, Diz DI, Ferrario CM: Pressor and reflex sensitivity is altered in spontaneously hypertensive rats treated with angiotensin-(1-7). Hypertension 26:1138–1144, 1995.

CHAPTER 3

Angiotensin Receptors: An Overview

YING-HONG FENG, M.D., Ph.D.
JANICE G. DOUGLAS, M.D.

Over 100 years after the discovery of renin, the first component of the renin-angiotensin system to be identified, knowledge about the angiotensin receptors continues to emerge. Among the four major biologically active peptides in this cascade, the octapeptide angiotensin II (Ang II, Asp^1-Arg^2-Val^3-Tyr^4-Ile^5-His^6-Pro^7-Phe^8) has received the most intense investigation for many decades. Ang II regulates body fluid homeostasis, blood pressure, cell growth, and neuronal activities. The discovery and the successful clinical administration of Ang II-converting enzyme (ACE) inhibitors (e.g., captopril), to avert cardiovascular and renal complications with excessive mortality have greatly encouraged many investigators from various disciplines to conduct research on Ang II receptors. The recent success with clinical use of the nonpeptide Ang II type 1 receptor blockers has provided additional impetus. This chapter reviews the most recent progress in ligand recognition, activation, signal coupling, and desensitization related to Ang II receptors. Advances in these areas are likely to represent a major focus of research and development during the twenty-first century in biology, medicine, and therapeutic intervention.

The major biologically active hormones of the renin-angiotensin system in addition to Ang II include Ang III [des-Asp^1-Ang II or Arg^2-Val^3-Tyr^4-Ile^5-His^6-Pro^7-Phe^8], Ang IV [Ang-(3-8) or Val^3-Tyr^4-Ile^5-His^6-Pro^7-Phe^8], and Ang II-(1-7) [Asp^1-Arg^2-Val^3-Tyr^4-Ile^5-His^6-Pro^7]. Both Ang II type 1 (AT_1) and type 2 (AT_2) receptors recognize Ang III, which appears to utilize Ang II receptors for function. Receptors for Ang IV and Ang-(1-7) have been characterized pharmacologically but not yet cloned.

This chapter concentrates mainly on recent studies. Readers are directed to a number of excellent reviews that cover earlier studies or other aspects of the renin-angiotensin system.[1–14]

■ *AT₁ Receptor*

Pharmacologic studies using the thiol-reducing agent dithiothreitol (DTT)[14,15] and subtype-specific antagonists[14–17] were the first to unveil the presence of two distinct classes of receptors, now designated as AT_1 and AT_2. DTT treatment potentiates the binding of Ang II to AT_2 receptors and inactivates the binding of Ang II to AT_1 receptors. This sharp contrast forms the hallmark for distinguishing the two classes of receptors (Fig. 1). The binding of Ang II to AT_1 receptors, but not to AT_2 receptors, can be blocked by losartan, an AT_1 receptor-specific

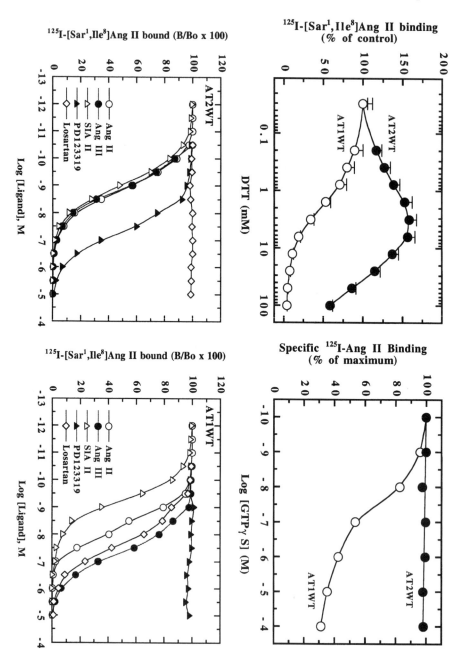

Figure 1. Ligand-binding properties of angiotensin II AT_1 and AT_2 receptors expressed in COS-1 cells by transient transfection. DTT = dithiothreitol; GTPγS = guanosine 5'-O-(3-thio)triphosphate; SIA II = [Sar^1,Ile^8]Ang II.

antagonist. Likewise, the binding of Ang II to AT_2 receptors, but not to AT_1 receptors, can be blocked by PD123319, the AT_2 receptor-specific antagonist (see Fig. 1). Consistent with these earlier observations, recent studies[18–27] in receptor gene cloning and recombinant gene expression have revealed that both AT_1 and AT_2 receptors belong to the type A family of the G protein-coupled receptor (GPCR) superfamily.

AT_1 Receptor Subtypes

Shortly after the initial description of the rat and bovine AT_1 receptor,[18–19] the cDNA was cloned from human and mouse tissues.[20–22] Of interest, a second AT_1 receptor in the rat and mouse was also cloned within 1 year.[21–24] Rodents are unique in that they have two AT_1 receptor genes, whereas both cows and humans express only a single AT_1 receptor protein. The second rodent AT_1 receptor protein has been designated AT_{1B}, whereas the original molecule is called AT_{1A}. All identified mammalian AT_1 receptors are single polypeptides consisting of 359 amino acids.

Of interest, an Ang II receptor cloned from *Xenopus laevis* binds Ang II with high affinity but does not recognize any nonpeptide antagonist specific for the mammalian AT_1 or AT_2 receptor. Like the AT_2 receptor, this Ang II receptor consists of 363 amino acids. Nevertheless, based on conservation of structural features and motifs and similarity in signal coupling mechanisms, this *Xenopus* Ang II receptor was termed the amphibian counterpart of the mammalian AT_1 receptor rather than the AT_2 receptor.[27]

In rats and mice, the AT_{1A} and AT_{1B} receptor-coding regions are 95% homologous in protein sequence and appear to be located on two different chromosomes. The rat AT_{1B} subtype is the predominant form in adrenal cortex and pituitary, whereas the AT_{1A} receptor is the primary subtype expressed in vascular smooth muscle cells, liver, kidney, heart, aorta, lung, and testis.[28] Both subtypes of the AT_1 receptor bind Ang II with similar affinity and couple to the same G proteins. No subtype-specific antagonist can distinguish between AT_1 receptor subtypes.[29] Despite the difference in tissue distribution, no functional significance in ligand binding, activation, signal coupling, and desensitization has been detected.[29] A recent study[30] in mice lacking both AT_{1A} and AT_{1B} receptors indicates that both subtypes promote somatic growth and maintenance of normal blood pressure and kidney structure. Either subtype can compensate in varying degrees for the absence of the other subtype.[30]

Ligand Recognition

Like other members of the GPCR superfamily, AT_1 receptors are single polypeptides consisting of seven hydrophobic transmembrane (TM) helix domains, an N-terminal domain on the extracellular side, a C-terminal domain on the intracellular side, and three loop domains on either side of the membrane (Fig. 2). AT_1 receptors also preserve most structural features of the GPCR superfamily, including (1) an aspartic acid located in the middle of the TM helix two; (2) a disulfide bond formed between Cys in the beginning of the third TM and Cys in the second exoloop (extracellular loop); (3) an Asp-Arg-Tyr (DRY) motif at the end of TM3; (4) various sites for glycosylation; and (5) other residues conserved in more than 90% of GPCR members (see Fig. 2).

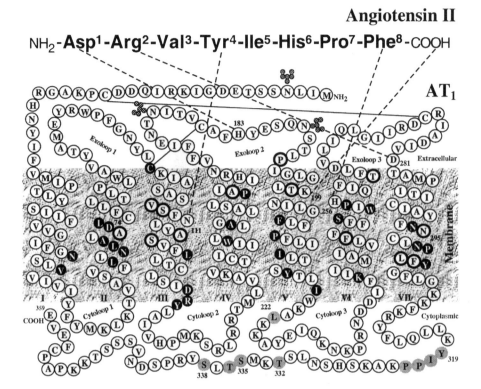

Figure 2. A secondary structure model of human AT_1 receptor and angiotensin II. Three potential glycosylation sites are shown. Residues and motifs in closed black circles are highly conserved in more than 90% GPCR members. Solid lines show two disulfide bonds. Dashed lines show five interactions between peptide angiotensin II and the AT_1 receptor. Thirteen residues in bold circles are involved in binding to the nonpeptide antagonist losartan. Shaded residues are involved in signal coupling and desensitization. The membrane interface boundaries for all seven transmembrane helices are tentative.

GPCR domains involved in ligand binding are nearly as diverse as the chemical structures of the known agonists. Low-molecular-weight ligands (e.g., photon, biogenic amines, nucleosides, eicosanoids, and moieties of lipids) bind to sites within the hydrophobic core formed by the TM α-helices. Binding sites for peptides and protein agonists often include various combinations of the N-terminus, hydrophilic exoloops, and TM core. Consistent with these findings from other members of the peptide (< 40 amino acids) GPCR subfamily,[31] studies using site-directed mutagenesis and side-chain replacement of Ang II have shown that both TM core and exoloops are involved in Ang II binding.[12,32–41] These studies have identified five pairs of interactions between the AT_1 receptor and Ang II (see Fig. 2). Lys[199] and Asp[281] previously were shown to form a salt-bridge interaction with the α-COO-group of Phe[8] and the guanidium group of Arg[2] of Ang II, respectively.[34–36] Asn[111] and His[256] interact directly with Tyr[4] and Phe[8] of Ang II, respectively.[35–37] His[183] residue of the AT_1 receptor has been proposed to interact with Asp[1] of Ang II.[12,38] For binding of the nonpeptide AT_1 receptor-specific antagonist losartan, only the TM core is involved.[12,40–42] Taking the advantage of the *Xenopus* AT_1 receptor, which lacks a losartan-binding pocket, these studies used mutational analysis to identify the 13 residues that significantly influence binding of losartan. The involvement of these residues in binding of losartan was substantiated by a gain-of-function mutant in which the residues crucial to formation of a losartan-binding site in a mammalian AT_1 receptor were transferred to a previously unresponsive *Xenopus* AT_1 receptor. This observation, however, does not encompass residues conserved between both mammalian and amphibian AT_1 receptors (e.g., Lys^{199}).[35] It is now suggested that the binding pockets for the native Ang II and the peptide analogs are different from those of the nonpeptide antagonist. However, the site Lys^{199} in the AT_1 receptor is shared by both peptide and nonpeptide ligands.[35]

Active Conformational State

Elucidation of the mechanisms of GPCR activation upon agonist binding represents an area of active investigation. This research addresses a fundamental question about the nature of conformational changes in the receptor that link agonist binding to transducer activation (e.g., G protein activation). Recent models of receptor activation suggest that the receptor exists in an equilibrium of two functionally distinct states: inactive (**R**) and active (**R***). Conversion from the **R** to the **R*** state does not require the hormone agonist. The agonist preferentially selects the **R*** state, and the inverse agonist preferentially selects the **R** state, thereby shifting the equilibrium toward **R*** and **R** states, respectively. Neutral competitive antagonists have equal affinity for **R** and **R*** and do not displace the equilibrium but can competitively antagonize the effects of both agonists and inverse agonists. In the absence of agonists, **R** state is the dominant form, maintaining a minimal level of basal receptor activity. In the presence of agonists, **R*** state becomes the dominant form because the selective binding of agonists leads to receptor activation. This "selection" model is perhaps the most widely accepted model. It explains the mode of action of inverse agonists in both native and overexpressed receptors.[43–45]

Constitutive activation caused by several mutations, some occurring naturally and some generated through mutagenesis, suggests a constrained basal state of the GPCR. Intramolecular constraint is proposed to control the equilibrium between the **R** and **R*** states. Breakage of these intramolecular interactions is required for receptor activation. This evidence challenges the selection model and supports an induction model.[37,46,47] The induction model emphasizes that the **R*** state of the receptor is induced by removal of the intramolecular constraint (e.g., by agonist binding or certain mutations). In the AT_1 receptor, breakage of intramolecular interaction by replacement of Asn^{111} with Gly or replacement of TM III helix with the corresponding fragment from the AT_2 receptor resulted in an intermediate transition state of receptor conformation, leading to 50% constitutive activity. Of particular importance is the fact that this constitutively active mutant N111G can be activated fully with an agonism-defective Ang II analog ([Sar^1,Ile^4,Ile^8]Ang II) and also can be inactivated by an inverse agonist, EXP3174. This result indicates that agonist binding not only stabilizes the **R*** state but also induces an intermediate active (**R'**) state or the **R*** state conformation. Failure of this agonism-defective Ang II analog in activation of wild type AT_1 receptor but not in binding further supports the central role of the agonist in induction of active conformation.

In addition, residues Asp[74], Tyr[292], Asn[295], and the Asn[298] in a highly conserved NPxxY sequence have been reported to play important roles in AT_1 receptor activation.[48–51] It has been suggested that disruption of interactions between Asn[111] and Tyr[292] by Ang II binding can release Tyr[292], which in turn interacts with Asp[74] and leads to receptor activation.[52] An interaction between Asn[111] and Asn[295] also has been proposed.[50] However, our study found no key evidence to support this mechanism of activation in Tyr[292] and Asn[295] mutant receptors.[46]

Homo- or heterodimerization is a documented essential mechanism for stimulation of the intrinsic catalytic activity and autophosphorylation of growth factor receptors. For GPCR, dimerization is a new concept. Accumulating evidence (e.g., from the β2-adrenergic receptor, δ-opioid receptor, muscarinic receptor, dopamine receptor, and gamma-aminobutyric acid-B [GABA-B] receptor) suggests that GPCR also undergoes dimerization, raising the possibility that dimerization may be part of the activation process.[45,53] Observations using these receptors further support the GPCR dimerization hypothesis first proposed by Rodbell in 1992.[54] However, our knowledge about GPCR dimerization remains rudimentary, and the functional significance has as yet not been explored. In the case of the AT_1 receptors, coexpression of two binding-defective mutants, K102A and K199A, was demonstrated to rescue ligand binding, whereas their individual expression in COS-7 cells did not result in a functional receptor. These observations strongly suggest that intermolecular complementation may have occurred for gain of Ang II-binding function from two functionally defective mutants,[55] thereby supporting the hypothesis of dimerization.

Inverse Agonism of the AT_1 Receptor Antagonist

Elucidation of receptor activation mechanisms has important implications for therapeutic interventions and should facilitate our understanding of the pharmacologic mechanisms of the full agonist (native agonist or agonist with potency equivalent to the native agonist [e.g., Ang II]), partial agonist (less potent than the native agonist, such as [Sar[1],Ile[8]]Ang II[37,46]), neutral antagonist (as defined earlier in the discussion of active conformation state), and inverse agonist. The concept of inverse agonists and the related explanatory framework, although not new, have not been widely accepted, perhaps because the concept did not seem relevant to the majority of pharmacologic and clinical experience. Recently, evidence for the existence of inverse agonists became available when the β2-adrenoceptor ligand ICI-118,551 functioned as an inverse agonist in the transgenic mouse model, in which the constitutively **R*** state was present because of marked myocardial overexpression of the receptors.[56] Moreover, the inverse agonism of the H_2 receptor antagonists, cimetidine and ranitidine, was found to be responsible for receptor upregulation, whereas burimamide, a neutral antagonist, did not induce receptor upregulation after long-term exposure. This finding provides a plausible explanation for the observed development of tolerance after prolonged clinical use.[56] The AT_1 receptor antagonists losartan, LF7-0156, and LF8-0129 and the losartan metabolite EXP3174 possess the property of inverse agonism.[37,52] These antagonists were able to inhibit the constitutive production of inositol triphosphate (IP_3) in the AT_1 mutant N111G receptor. The inverse agonism of losartan is rather weak and was not able to suppress the constitutive activity in the AT_1 N111G mutant receptor (Feng and Karnik, unpublished data). This observation contradicts the work of a French group.[52] Thus, it is not clear whether losartan is an inverse agonist or neutral antagonist.

Although currently no convincing data indicate that prolonged use of an AT_1 inverse agonist, including losartan, can upregulate AT_1 receptor expression, the possibility needs to be addressed systematically. Such an experiment may not be straightforward. Treatment with losartan results in increased plasma levels of Ang II because of blockade of Ang II inhibition of renin release (comparable to suppression of renin release by sodium loading). The increased Ang II can then upregulate the AT_1 receptor.[57] Another interesting question is how inverse agonists influence receptor desensitization and internalization.

Signal Coupling

Although the extracellular and TM domains clearly are involved in ligand binding, domains critical for interactions with G proteins as well as non-G protein molecules are believed to be the intracellular loops and the C-terminus. However, it remains unclear how these intracellular domains regulate coupling of multiple transducer molecules with diverse structures. It is known that AT_1 receptors can generate at least three lines of signals (Fig. 3): G protein pathways, non-G protein SHP-2/Jak2 pathways, and desensitization/internalization pathways.

Stimulation of the AT_1 receptor induces production of IP_3 through activation of the $G\alpha_{q11}$ or $G\alpha_{13}\beta_1\gamma_3$ heterotrimer[58,59] (see Fig. 3). As expected, all structural determinants identified as critical for AT_1 receptor signaling by various methods are located within the intracellular domains. Using AT_1/ AT_2 chimeric receptors, Wang et al. demonstrated that both N-terminal and C-terminal portions of the cytoloop 3, especially the seven amino acids 219–225 in the N-terminal portion, are important in determining $G\alpha_q$ coupling.[60] This region encompasses a conserved apolar residue Leu^{222}, which Catt et al. earlier had shown was crucial in AT_1 receptor activation.[61] Using a synthetic peptide approach, Kai et al. have shown that all cytoloop 2, cytoloop 3, and C-terminal regions can interact with G proteins, indicating that multiple contacts with these receptor domains may be important for binding and activation of the G proteins.[62] Studies from other groups consistently have shown that the polar residues in these three regions and the structure of the C-terminal fragment 300-320 of the AT_1 receptor are relevant to G-protein coupling.[63,64] Experiments by Griendling et al. in vascular smooth muscle cells first demonstrated that activation of phospholipase D by stimulation of the AT_1 receptor is mediated by $G_{\beta\gamma}$ subunits[65] (see Fig. 3).

A recent advance in signaling mechanisms of GPCR is development of the novel concept that GPCR can also transduce signals through a variety of discrete signaling molecules originally attributed to other receptor superfamilies. The AT_1 receptor can transactivate receptors for epidermal growth factor and platelet-derived growth factor and also activate the Jak2/Stat pathway.[66–68] Activation of the Jak2/Stat pathway requires physical association of Jak2 with the AT_1 receptor, but the involvement of G proteins in this process remains unknown (see Fig. 3). Further studies have identified a YIPP motif (see Fig. 2) in the C-terminal of the AT_1 receptor that is responsible for coupling of both SHP-2/Jak2 and phospholipase (PL)C_γ1.[69,70] This finding shows that GPCR can also couple to non-G protein transducers. At present, however, the mode of interaction between the AT_1 receptor and SHP-2/Jak2 or PLC_γ1 that leads to Jak2 and PLC_γ1 activation is not

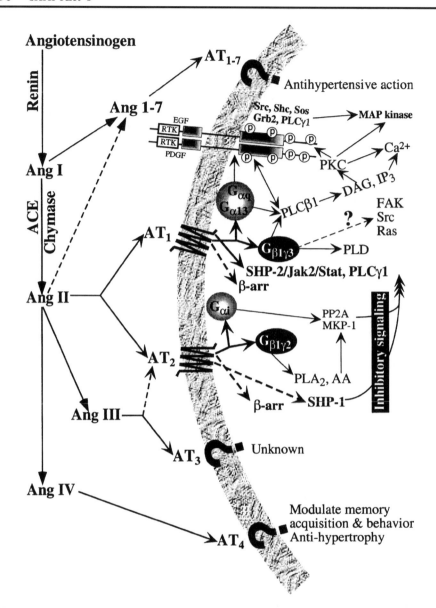

Figure 3.   Summary of angiotensin receptors and three forms of signal coupling mechanisms for each angiotensin II receptor (AT_1 and AT_2) involving (1) G proteins, (2) non-G protein molecules, and (3) β-arrestins. Dashed lines and question marks mean poorly established or unknown. ACE = angiotensin II converting enzyme; RTK = receptor tyrosine kinase; Src = sarcoma virus-transforming gene products; SH2 = Src homology sequence-2; Shc = Src homologous and collagen; Sos = son-of-sevenless; Grb2 = growth factor receptor binding protein-2; PLCγ1 = phospholipase C-γ1; PLCβ1 = phospholipase C-β1; MAP kinase = mitogen-activated protein kinase; PKC = protein kinase C; DAG = diacylglycerol; IP_3 = inositol triphosphate; PLD = phospholipase D; SHP-2 = SH2 domain-containing protein tyrosine phosphatase 2; SHP-1 = SH2 domain-containing protein tyrosine phosphatase 1; Jak2 = Janus kinase-2; Stat = signal transducer and activator of transcription; FAK = focal adhesion kinase; Ras = homologous oncogene products of Harvey and Kirsten murine sarcoma viruses originally isolated in rat genetic sequences with molecular weight of 21,000 dalton; β-arr = β-arrestin; PP2A = serine/threonine phosphatase 2A; AA = arachidonic acid; MKP-1 = MAP kinase phosphatase-1; EGF = epidermal growth factor; PDGF = platelet-derived growth factor.

clear. If tyrosine phosphorylation of the YIPP motif is required for AT_1 receptor association with the SH2 domains of these molecules, which tyrosine kinase is the primary force? How do AT_1 receptor-associated Jak2 and $PLC_\gamma1$ function on their target molecules? These and many other questions certainly deserve more detailed investigation.

Among the many forms of GPCR regulation (e.g., transcriptional, translational, and various forms of modifications on the GPCR proteins), receptor phosphorylation and desensitization appear to be the most important with respect to the rapid control (seconds to minutes as opposed to hours or days) of receptor function. Three families of regulatory molecules have been found to participate in GPCR desensitization/internalization: (1) second-messenger kinases (e.g., protein kinase A [PKA] and protein kinase C [PKC]; (2) G protein-coupled receptor kinases (GPKs); and (3) β-arrestins (see Fig. 3). Of great interest is the recent discovery that these desensitization and internalization processes are required not only for signal termination or attenuation but also for signal activation. In other words, this new information indicates that receptor signaling and desensitization/internalization are in reality two intimately linked aspects of receptor function and that mechanisms previously viewed as "desensitizing" with respect to one signaling pathway may be "activating" with respect to another.[71] For example, agonist stimulation of β2-adrenergic receptor activates $G_{\alpha s}$ and adenylyl cyclase, leading to PKA activation. PKA phosphorylation of the receptor uncouples it from $G_{\alpha s}$ and facilitates its coupling to $G_{\alpha i}$, which inhibits adenylyl cyclase. Moreover, GRK phosphorylation of the receptor and subsequent binding further desensitize the receptor. Then, the β-arrestin–mediated internalization of the receptor via clathrin-coated pits and vesicles participates in activation of mitogen-activated protein (MAP) kinase. Stimulation of β2-adrenergic receptor fails to activate MAP kinase when the β-arrestin-mediated internalization is blocked on several levels.[71]

AT_1 receptors undergo rapid phosphorylation, desensitization, and internalization upon Ang II stimulation.[72–76] Residues Thr^{332}, Ser^{335}, Thr^{336}, and Ser^{338} in the serine/threonine-rich region (Thr^{332} to Ser^{338}) of the C-terminal play a central role in this process.[72–76] It is also documented that PKC and GRK2, 3, and 5 are required for AT_1 receptor phosphorylation.[77] These findings suggest that mechanisms employed by the $β_2$-adrenergic receptor may be applicable to the AT_1 receptor for desensitization and signaling. Surprisingly, agonist-induced AT_1 receptor internalization does not require dynamin and β-arrestin,[78] indicating an as-yet unidentified dynamin/β-arrestin–independent mechanism. Elucidation of this dynamin/β-arrestin–independent mechanism and its role in mediating AT_1 receptor signaling is certainly an exciting challenge for many investigators.

■ *AT₂ Receptor*

The distinct DTT potentiation property in ligand binding and the discovery of the highly selective nonpeptidic ligand PD123319 and peptidic ligand CGP42112A have led to the identification of a second major receptor of Ang II, the AT_2 receptor[14–17] (see Fig. 1). Since its genetic cloning in 1993,[25,26] this receptor has been an area of intense research in many disciplines related to angiotensin and its receptors. Although many questions have been answered, the unresolved original issues and new questions generated in the process of research remain an exciting challenge to investigators. In contrast to the well-studied AT_1 receptor, which mediates most known stimulatory actions of Ang II, emerging evidence indicates that the adult AT_2 receptor mediates inhibitory actions that appear to antagonize the AT_1 receptor. These inhibitory actions include pressure natriuresis, antigrowth, antiproliferation, and proapoptosis.[9,10,13]

AT_2 Receptor Subtypes and Tissue Distribution

The wide and abundant tissue distribution of the AT_2 receptor in many mesenchymal tissues of developing fetus and embryonic brain constrasts sharply with its low abundance in adult tissues, such as the adrenal gland, kidney, brain, uterus, ovary, and heart. The ubiquitous expression of the AT_2 receptor in the developing fetus disappears within days after birth, and the AT_2 receptor is restricted to tissues subject to periodic stress and remodeling (e.g., uterus, ventricle, arterial smooth muscle cells).[5,9,13,14,17,25,26] The characteristic patterns of expression of the AT_2 receptor suggest a potentially important role in tissue differentiation, development, and embryonic maturation. However, knockout mice for the AT_2 receptor gene develop and thrive.[79,80] Thus, either the hypothesis is wrong or the knockout mice compensate for the lack of AT_2 receptor expression with other known or unknown genes that influence protein expression and physiologic responses. Of interest, the expression of this AT_2 receptor can be up-regulated after dietary sodium depletion[30] and re-activated in pathologic states such as wound healing, heart failure, and vascular injury.[9,10] In addition, treatment with AT_1 receptor antagonists causes a marked elevation of plasma Ang II, which selectively binds to AT_2 receptors and exerts as yet unidentified effects.[9,10]

The AT_2 receptor exists in only one isoform because its single gene copy contains no intron in its coding region.[81–83] However, the existence of other AT_2 receptor subtypes, currently indistinguishable by the AT_2 receptor-selective ligands such as PD123319 and CGP42112A or by other biochemical properties such as DTT sensitivity, is still possible. Indeed, earlier studies by Douglas et al.[84,85] and two other groups[86,87] suggest the existence of an AT_2 receptor subtype distinct from the cloned conventional AT_2 receptor in rabbit proximal tubular epithelial (RTE) cells,[84] in rat adrenal tissue,[86] and in the ventral thalamic and medial geniculate nuclei and locus coeruleus of the rat brain.[87] Identification of this AT_2 receptor subtype, called the AT_{2B} receptor,[85,87] was based mainly on AT_1 receptor-like DTT sensitivity, reduced affinity for CGP42112A, sensitivity to GTPγS and PTX treatment, and ability to induce production of arachidonic acid. However, more direct evidence is lacking because the presence of native AT_1 receptors in proximal tubular epithelial cells and rat tissues may complicate the situation. Recently, we cloned an 800 bp fragment from the rabbit proximal tubular epithelial cells corresponding to residues from Val^{64} to Ser^{311} (Fig. 4; Feng and

---

Figure 4 *(Facing page, broadside).* A secondary structure model of human AT_2 receptor. Five potential glycosylation sites are shown. The lines show two disulfide bonds. Residues and motifs in bold circles are highly conserved in more than 90% of members of the G protein-coupled receptor superfamily. Shaded residues are conserved between human AT_1 and AT_2 receptors. Four numbered residues at positions 127, 215, 273, and 297 are the conserved residues identified in the AT_1 receptor essential for angiotensin II binding and activation. The site of His^{273} is shifted one residue toward the C-terminal of the AT_2 receptor. The six numbered residues in closed black circles are nonconserved unique residues at which sites substitutions have been identified in the rabbit AT_2 receptor cloned from RTE cells (Leu^{94} and Glu^{188} are also conserved in the AT_1 receptors). The membrane interface boundaries for all seven transmembrane helices are tentative.

Douglas, unpublished results). This fragment covers most critical functional domains of a GPCR, including all exoloops and cytoloops and five transmembrane domains (see Fig. 4). When aligned with human, rat, and mouse AT$_2$ genes, 6 of 11 residues have been identified as nonconserved unique residues that probably are not attributable to species differences: Y106H, E188D, and I293T in exoloops

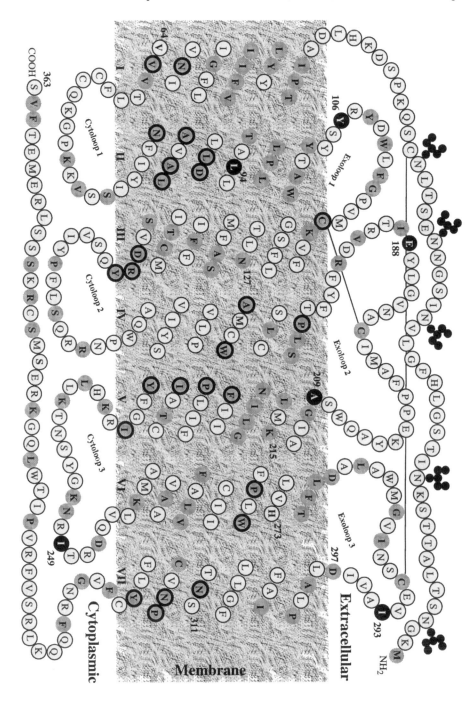

(50%), L94V and A209V in TM regions (33%), and I249V in cytoloop 3 (17%) (see Fig. 4). Of these six residues, Leu[94] and Glu[188] are conserved residues in the AT$_1$ receptor. This finding adds important information to our knowledge about the AT$_2$ receptor, although more solid evidence is needed to justify the existence of an AT$_{2B}$ receptor subtype.

Ligand Recognition

The AT$_2$ receptor is a single polypeptide of 363 residues consisting of 7 hydrophobic transmembrane α-helical segments that are connected by three loop regions on both the cytoplasmic and extracellular sides of the embedding membrane[25,26] (see Fig. 4). It conserves major structural features common to all members of GPCR superfamily, including *N*-glycosylation sites.[88] AT$_2$ and AT$_1$ receptors share the lowest sequence homology (about 30%) among GPCR subtypes[89] (Fig. 5). Consistent with the low sequence identity, recent evidence from two laboratories indicates that the Ang II-binding site of the AT$_2$ receptor is quite distinct from that of the AT$_1$ receptor.[39,91] Karnik et al.[39] reported that the AT$_2$ receptor is "relaxed" in conformation so that no single interaction is critical for Ang II binding (much like the constitutively active N111G mutant AT$_1$ receptor).[37,46,47] On the other hand, Pulakat[92] and Bouley[93] documented that the role of the C-terminal of Ang II is similar for binding to both receptors. Several residues of the AT$_1$ receptor, identified as critical for Ang II binding, also are conserved in the AT$_2$ receptor (see Figs. 4 and 5). Of these, Lys[215] of the AT$_2$ receptor and Lys[199] in the AT$_1$ receptor have been found to play equivalent roles in Ang II binding.[92] The roles of residues Asn[127], His[273], and Asp[297] in Ang II binding are not clear at present. However, indirect evidence[91,93] from studies using photolabile angiotensin analogs does not support similar roles for Asn[127] and Asp[297] in Ang II binding.

```
AT1  =----ILNSS TED------- =IKRI--QDD CP---KAGRH NYIFVM==== =S====V=IF   44
AT2  MKGNSTLATT SKNITSGLHF GLVNISGNNE STLNCSQKPS DKHLDAIPTL YYIIFVIGFL   60
                                                             I
AT1  G=SL==IVIY FYMKL=T=A= VFLL===L== =CF=L===== =V=TAME=R= P==NYL==IA  104
AT2  VNIVVVTLFC CQKGPKKVSS IYIFNLAVAD LLLLATLPLW ATYYSYRYDW LFGPVMCKVF  120
                  II
AT1  SASVSF=LY= =V=LL==L=I ===LAIVH=M K=RL=RTMLV AKVTCIII=L L=G=A===AI  164
AT2  GSFLTLNMFA SIFFITCMSV DRYQSVIYPF LSQRRNPWQA SYIV-PLVWC MACLSSLPTF  179
          III                                      IV
AT1  IH=N=FF==N TNITV=AFHY ESQN-STLPI =LG=T===== =LF=FLI=L= S=TL=W=A=K  223
AT2  YFRDVRTIEY LGVNACIMAF PPEKYAQWSA GIALMKNILG FIIPLIFIAT CYFGIRKHLL  239
                                                    V
AT1  =AYEIQ==KP RN=DIF=IIM =I===F=FFS= I=HQIF==== V=IQL=I=RD =RIADIV=T= 283
AT2  KTNSYGKNRI TRDQVLKMAA AVVLAFIICW LPFHVLTFLD ALAWMGVINS CEVIAVIDLA  299
                                    VI
                                          ****
AT1  M=IT=CIAYF =N=L===LF=G =L=KK=KRYF LQLLKYI=PK AKSHSN=ST= MSTL=Y=P=D 343
AT2  LPFAILLGFT NSCVNPFLYC FVGNRFQQKL RSVFR-VP-- ---ITWLQGK RESMSCRKSS  350
          VII
AT1  NVSSSTKKPA PC=E=E                                                  359
AT2  SL-----REM ETF-VS                                                  363
```

Figure 5. Aligned amino acid sequences of human AT$_1$ and AT$_2$ receptors deduced from the nucleotide sequences of isolated cDNA. Amino acids are designated using the single-letter code. Gaps are automatically introduced to optimize alignment by Geneworks program. Putative transmembrane segments determined using the HRG algorithm[90] are indicated by the Roman numerals and solid lines. * indicates the site for PLCγ1 and SHP-2/Jak2 binding in the AT$_1$ receptor. = indicates the residues conserved in the AT$_2$ receptor.

Both AT_1 and AT_2 receptors are sensitive to reduction by thiol agents.[14,15,94,95] Upon DTT treatment the functional potentiation of the AT_2 receptor contrasts sharply with the inactivation of the AT_1 receptor, forming a hallmark basis for distinguishing the two receptors. Like the AT_1 receptor, the AT_2 receptor has one cysteine (Cys) residue in each of four extracellular domains, and these Cys residues are believed to form two disulfide bonds. One disulfide bond linking the second and third exoloop domains is highly conserved in the entire GPCR superfamily. Of four Cys residues, only the first in the N-terminus is not conserved at the identical position in the two receptors (see Fig. 5). Experiments by Karnik et al.[95] suggest that the two disulfide bonds of the AT_2 receptor are formed between Cys^{117} and Cys^{195} and between Cys^{35} and Cys^{290}, respectively (see Fig. 4). This pattern is similar to that of the AT_1 receptor.[94] However, several striking differences have been observed between the two receptors[94,95]:

1. The disulfide bond Cys^{117}-Cys^{195} is highly resistant to DTT, whereas the Cys^{35}-Cys^{290} bond is highly sensitive.

2. The Cys^{117}-Cys^{195} disulfide bond alone is sufficient for the formation and stabilization of functional conformation of the AT_2 receptor.

3. Reduction of the Cys^{35}-Cys^{290} disulfide bond attributes to the hallmark property of DTT-potentiation in ligand binding.

4. Both C35A (Ala mutation of Cys^{35}) and C290A single-mutant AT_2 receptor, but not C35A-C290A double-mutant receptor, produce an inactive population of mutant receptors.

5. The defect of the inactive population of the C35A or C290A mutant receptor can be fully rectified by DTT treatment, indicating disulfide exchange with another as-yet unidentified Cys residue.

6. Molecular modeling of the AT_2 receptor and the characterization of six AT_1/AT_2 chimera receptors suggest that disulfide bond exchange between the Cys^{117}-Cys^{195} disulfide and the free-SH group of the C35A or C290A mutant receptor may be responsible for the inactive population.

Given that redox potential also can serve as an important regulation mechanism for many proteins, the distinct DTT property of the AT_2 receptor may provide an alternative mechanism for rapid regulation of receptor function under pathologic states in which redox potential is often subject to change. This intriguing biologic issue certainly deserves more investigation.

Active Conformational State

How the active conformational state of the AT_2 receptor is generated remains unknown. The inability to detect any AT_2 receptor-mediated second-messenger signal in surrogate cell systems has hampered research efforts. Tyr^4 and Phe^8 of Ang II specify the agonistic property for the AT_1 receptor,[37,46,47] whereas the remaining residues of Ang II specify exclusively the binding property.[37,46,47] It is not clear whether the agonism-specifying side chains of Ang II are identical for the AT_2 receptor. It is likely that Ang II uses similar mechanisms to induce the AT_2 receptor **R*** state because the active state-switch residue Asn^{111} in the AT_1 receptor is conserved (see Figs. 4 and 5). This asumption, however, requires experimental proof.

At least three reports have suggested that the wild type AT_2 receptor is constitutively active. In an AT_2/AT_1 chimera receptor with the cytoloop 3 domain of the AT_2 receptor replaced by the corresponding region from the AT_1 receptor, movement of calcium was observed in the absence of Ang II stimulation.[60] The AT_2 receptor residue at position 311 is a Ser (see Fig. 5) because mutation of the corresponding residue Asn[295] in the AT_1 receptor (N295S mutant) was found to be constitutively active, just like the N111S mutant.[50] Karnik et al., however, failed to reproduce the constitutive activity of the N295S mutant receptor.[46] Finally, the Ang II-binding profile has shown that, in sharp contrast to the wild type AT_1 receptor but in agreement with the constitutively active mutant N111G AT_1 receptor,[37,46] the AT_2 receptor is insensitive to modification of Ang II side chains at any position.[39] This observation recalls comparison of the binding affinity of Ang III for AT_1 and AT_2 receptors (see Fig. 1) and also offers a possible explanation of how Ang III may act as an AT_2 receptor agonist (see Fig. 3).

GPCR can couple to multiple signal transduction pathways and may use different active conformations for differential activation of these signal pathways.[96] It is possible that the AT_2 receptor constitutively activates one signal but requires occupancy of Ang II for activation of another signal. This theory may explain the lack of direct evidence in support of the constitutive activity of the AT_2 receptor. The current inability to establish a constitutively active AT_2 receptor makes it impossible to characterize the inverse agonism property for AT_2 receptor antagonists.

Signal Coupling

Unlike the AT_1 receptor, stimulation of the AT_2 receptor with Ang II in various systems failed to elicit any of the intracellular second-messenger responses, including IP_3, intracellular calcium, cyclic adenosine monophosphate (cAMP), and cyclic guanosine monophosphate (cGMP).[9,10,13,25] The Ang II displacement curve of the receptor is generally not affected by guanylnucleotide analogs (e.g., GTPS or Gpp(NH)p[9,10,13,25]) (see Fig. 1). Based on these observations, it was originally suggested that the AT_2 receptor is not a G protein-coupled receptor, although the sequence suggests G protein interactions.

Consistent with the inhibitory actions of the AT_2 receptor, the corresponding signal transduction pathways as yet identified for this receptor are mainly inhibitory.[8–11,95–97] Of particular note is the fact that phosphatases MKP-1, PP2A, and SHP-1 have been found to be activated upon AT_2 receptor stimulation.[97–99] In PC12W cells, pretreatment with antisense oligonucleotide of MKP-1 inhibited the AT_2 receptor-mediated proapoptotic effect.[97] In primary neurons of newborn rats, both AT_2- and arachidonic acid-mediated increases in delayed-rectifier potassium current were abolished by specific inhibition of PP2A.[98] In N1E-115 neuroblastoma cells expressing endogenous AT_2 receptors and in Chinese hamster ovary (CHO) cells expressing recombinant human AT_2 receptors, Ang II rapidly stimulates the activity of SHP-1, a soluble protein tyrosine phosphatase (PTPase) essential for termination of signaling by cytokine and growth factor receptors.[99] This SHP-1 activation is insensitive to pertussis toxin (PTX). In addition, nitric oxide, cGMP, and prostaglandin E_2 also have been implicated in renal AT_2 receptor signaling.[8–11] At the transducer level, several lines of evidence suggest that both PTX-sensitive $G_{\alpha i}$,[98,100,101] and PTX-insensitive proteins[99,102,103] are involved in AT_2 receptor signaling. Zhang,[100] using various anti-G protein antibodies in rat fetus membrane preparation, and Hayashida,[101] using the peptide transfer approach in vascular smooth muscle cells, found that $G_{\alpha i}$ protein isoforms are involved in AT_2-mediated signal transduction. Of particular interest is the fact that we have documented a novel mechanism in kidney proximal tubular epithelial cells by which $G_{\beta 1\gamma 2}$ subunits mediate AT_2 receptor-initiated release of arachidonic acid.[103] These observations indicate that the AT_2 receptor is indeed a G protein-coupled receptor.

The AT_2 receptor also activates SHP-1 in a PTX-insensitive manner.[99] How to activate SHP-1 and whether SHP-1 directly couples to the AT_2 receptor for activation remain unknown. As shown in Figure 3, it is not impossible that SHP-1 can be directly activated by AT_2 receptor, since only PTX-sensitive $G_{\alpha i}$ protein isoforms are capable of coupling to the AT_2 receptor.[100,101]

It has been reported that the AT_2 receptor does not undergo internalization,[91,104] and how the AT_2 receptor desensitizes is unclear. Thus, information about the third signaling pathway (see Fig. 3) is lacking at present.

■ *AT₃ Receptor*

Ang III is a physiologic effector of the renin-angiotensin system. It has been suggested for a long time that Ang III also plays a physiological role in vasopressin release and aldosterone biosynthesis.[105–108] Recent evidence suggests that Ang III behaves as one of the main effector peptides of the brain renin-angiotensin system in the presence of EC27 [(S)-2-amino-pentan-1,5-dithiol], which inhibits aminopeptidase N (APN), the enzyme responsible for the N-terminal cleavage of Ang III.[105] This observation agrees with the previous suggestion that Ang II must be converted into Ang III to exert its physiologic action in the brain.[108] Because no specific receptor for Ang III has been identified and, of greater importance, because both Ang II receptors, particularly the AT_2 receptor, recognize Ang III, a specific AT_3 receptor does not appear to exist. AT_1 and AT_2 receptors serve as AT_3 receptors.

■ *AT₄ Receptor*

Recently it was discovered that Ang II fragments smaller than the heptapeptide (2-8) fragment (Ang III) also mediate biologic actions. The C-terminal 3-8 hexapeptide fragment of Ang II, designated as Ang IV, has been shown to possess a biologic activity in many different tissues by interacting with a unique high-affinity binding site .[108–112] Most recent studies using biochemical approaches suggest that the AT_4 receptor is a 186-kDa integral membrane glycoprotein with a large extracellular domain. The functionality and mechanism of action of the AT_4 receptor was assessed in bovine aortic endothelial cells (BAEC). The results revealed that none of the classic second messengers (i.e., cAMP, calcium, inositol phosphates, nitric oxide, or arachidonic acid derivatives) was modified significantly during acute (less than 1 hour) stimulation of cells with Ang IV. Under normal culture conditions, BAEC efficiently internalizes ^{125}I-Ang IV. After 2 hours of incubation at 37 C°, acid-resistant binding corresponded to about 50% of total cell-associated radioactivity. This rapid internalization process also suggests that the AT_4 receptor is a functional protein. A photoaffinity-labeling approach suggests that the AT_4 receptor bears some properties that are consistent with those of growth factor or cytokine receptors.[109,110] These observations may be confirmed when the sequence identity of the AT_4 receptor becomes available.

■ *AT₁₋₇ Receptor*

Like Ang II and Ang III, Ang-(1-7) is a primary èffector product of the angiotensin system (see Fig. 3). It has been known for more than a decade that Ang-(1-7) is biologically active and able to counterbalance the antihypertensive and antigrowth actions of Ang II.[113,114] Earlier work by Douglas et al. also demonstrated that Ang-(1-7) can modulate PLA2 activity and sodium transport,[115] an ability also shared with the AT_2 receptor.[103] However, evidence in support of an Ang-(1-7)-specific receptor (AT_{1-7}) is not conclusive at present. In cultured rat renal mesangial cells, Douglas et al. observed that Ang-(1-7) binds to an AT_2 receptor with 35-nM affinity, 40-fold higher than its affinity for the AT_1 receptor (1,400-nM).[116] On the other hand, indirect evidence suggestive of the existence of an Ang-(1-7)-specific receptor AT_{1-7} also has been documented.[113] Results from Bouley et al. indicate that Ang-(1-7) binds poorly to AT_1 and AT_2 receptors in human myometrium membranes.[93]

Molecular confirmation of an AT_{1-7} receptor is somewhat controversial, and solid evidence in support of a unique AT_{1-7} receptor is currently lacking. Unfortunately, little progress has been made toward identifying and cloning the AT_{1-7} receptor.

REFERENCES

1. Bumpus FM, Khosla MC: Angiotensin analogs as determinants of the physiological role of angiotensin and its metabolit. In Genest J, Koiw E, Kuchel O (eds): Hypertension: Physiology and Treatment. New York, McGraw-Hill, 1997, pp 183–201.
2. Peach MJ: Molecular actions of angiotensin. Biochem Pharmacol 30:2745–2751, 1981.
3. Timmermans PBMW, Wong PC, Chiu AT, et al: Angiotensin II receptors and angiotensin II receptor antagonists. Pharmacol Rev 45:205–251, 1993.
4. Sayeski PP, Ali MS, Semeniuk DJ, et al: Angiotensin II signal transduction pathways. Regul Pept 78:19–29, 1998.
5. Catt KJ: Angiotensin II receptors. In Robertson JIS, Nicholls MG (eds): The Renin-Angiotensin System. London, Gower Medical Publishing, 1994, pp 12.1–12.14.
6. Bernstein KE, Berk BC: The biology of angiotensin II receptors. Am J Kidney Dis 22:745–754, 1993.
7. Douglas JG, Hopfer U: Novel aspect of angiotensin receptors and signal transduction in the kidney. Annu Rev Physiol 56:649–669, 1994.
8. Gelband CH, Sumners C, Lu D, Raizada MK: Angiotensin receptors and norepinephine neuromodulation: Implications of functional coupling. Regul Pept 73:141–147, 1998.
9. Matsubara H: Pathophysiological role of angiotensin II type 2 receptor in cardiovascular and renal diseases. Circ Res 83:1182–1191, 1998.
10. Horiuchi M, Akishita M, Dzau VJ: Recent progress in angiotensin II type 2 receptor research in the cardiovascular system. Hypertension 33:613–621, 1999.
11. Inagami T, Eguchi S, Numaguchi K, et al: Cross-talk between angiotensin II receptors and the tyrosine kinases and phosphatases. J Am Soc Nephrol 10:S57–S61, 1999.
12. Hunyady L, Balla T, Catt KJ: The ligand binding site of the angiotensin AT1 receptor. TiPS 17:135–140, 1996.
13. Nahmias C, Strosberg AD: The angiotensin AT2 receptor: Searching for signal-transduction pathways and physiological function. Tips 16:223–225, 1995.
14. Douglas JG: Angiotensin receptor subtypes of the kidney cortex. Am J Physiol 253:F1–F7, 1987.
15. Chiu AT, McCall DE, Nguyen TT, et al: Discrimination of angiotensin II receptor subtypes by dithiothreitol. Euro J Pharmacol 170:117–118, 1989.
16. Dudley DT, Panek RL, Major TC, et al: Subclasses of angiotensin II binding sites and their functional significance. Mol Pharmacol 38:370–377, 1990.
17. Pucell AG, Hodges JC, Sen I, et al: Biochemical properties of the ovarian granulosa cell type 2-angiotensin II receptor. Endocrinology 128:1947–1959, 1991.
18. Murphy TJ, Alexander RW, Runger MS, Bernstein KE: Isolation of a cDNA encoding the vascular type-1 angiotensin II receptor. Nature 351:233–236, 1991.

19. Sasaki K, Yamano Y, Murray JJ, et al: Cloning and expression of a complementary DNA encoding a bovine adrenal angiotensin II type-1 receptor. Nature 351:230–233, 1991.
20. Furuta H, Guo DF, Inagami T: Molecular cloning and sequencing of the gene encoding human angiotensin II type 1 receptor. Biochem Biophys Res Commun 183:8–13, 1992.
21. Yoshida H, Kakuchi J, Guo D, et al: Analysis of the evolution of angiotensin II type 1 receptor gene in mammals (mouse, rat, bovine and human). Biochem Biophys Res Commun 186: 1042–1049, 1992.
22. Sasamura H, Hein L, Krieger JE, et al: Cloning, characterization, and expression of two angiotensin receptor (AT-1) isoforms from the mouse genome. Biochem Biophys Res Commun 185: 253–259, 1992.
23. Kakar SS, Sellers JC, Devor DC, et al: Angiotensin II type 1 receptor subtype cDNAa: differential tissue expression and hormonal regulation. Biochem Biophys Res Commun 183:1090–1096, 1992.
24. Sandberg K, Ji H, Clark AJL, et al: Cloning and expression of a novel angiotensin II receptor subtype. J Biol Chem 267:9455–9458, 1992.
25. Mukoyama M, Nakajima M, Horiuchi M, et al: Expression cloning of type 2 angiotensin II receptor reveals a unique class of seven-transmembrane receptors. J Biol Chem 268:24539–24542, 1993.
26. Kambayashi Y, Bardhan S, Takahashi K, et al: Molecular cloning of a novel angiotensin II receptor isoform involved in phosphotyrosine phosphatase inhibition. J Biol Chem 268:24543–24546, 1993.
27. Bergsma DJ, Ellis C, Nuthulaganti PR, et al: Isolation and expression of a novel angiotensin II receptor from xenopus laevis heart. Mol Pharmacol 44:277–284, 1993.
28. Kitami Y, Okura T, Marumoto K, et al: Differential gene expression and regulation of type 1 angiotensin Ii receptor subtypes in the rat. Biochem Biophys Res Commun 188:446–452, 1993.
29. Chiu AT, Dunscomb J, Kosierowski J, et al: The ligand binding signatures of the rat AT1A, AT1B, and the human AT1 receptors are essentially identical. Biochem Biophys Res Commun 197:440–449, 1993.
30. Oliverio MI, Kim HS, Ito M, et al: Reduced growth, abnormal kidney structure, and type 2 (AT2) angiotensin receptor-mediated blood pressure regulation in mice lacking both AT1A and AT1B receptors for angiotensin II. Proc Natl Acad Sci USA 95:15496–15501, 1998.
31. Ji TH, Grossmann M, Ji I: G protein-coupled receptors: I. Diversity of receptor-ligand interactions. J Biol Chem 273:17299–17302, 1998.
32. Yamano Y, Ohyama K, Chaki S, et al: Identification of amino acid residues of rat angiotensin II receptor for ligand binding by site directed mutagenesis. Biochem Biophys Res Commun 187:1426–1431, 1992.
33. Hjorth SA, Schambye HT, Greenlee WJ, Schwartz TW: Identification of peptide binding residues in the extracellular domains of the AT1 receptor. J Biol Chem 269:30953–30959, 1994.
34. Feng YH, Noda K, Saad Y, et al: The docking of Arg2 of angiotensin II with Asp281 of AT1 receptor is essential for full agonism. J Biol Chem 270:12846–12850, 1995.
35. Noda K, Saad Y, Husain A, Karnik SS: Tetrazol and carboxylate groups of angiotensin receptor antagonists bind to the same subsite by different mechanisms. J Biol Chem 270:2284–2289, 1995.
36. Noda K, Saad Y, Karnik SS: Interaction of Phe8 of angiotensin II with Lys199 and His256 of AT1 receptor in agonist activation. J Biol Chem 270:28511–28514, 1995.
37. Noda K, Feng YH, Liu XP, et al: The active state of the AT1 angiotensin receptor is generated by angiotensin II induction. Biochemistry 35:16435–16442, 1996.
38. Carini DJ, Duncia JV, Aldrich PE, et al: Nonpeptide angiotensin II receptor antagonists: The discovery of a series of N-(biphenylyl-methyl) imidazoles as potent, orally active antihypertensives. J Med Chem 34:2525–2547, 1991.
39. Miura SI, Karnik SS: Angiotensin II type 1 and type 2 receptors bind angiotensin II through different types of epitope recognition. J Hypertension 17:397–404, 1999.
40. Karnik SS, Husain A, Graham RM: Molecular determinants of peptide and nonpeptide binding to the AT1 receptor. Clin Exp Pharmacol Physiol S3:S58–S66, 1996.
41. Schambye HT, Hjorth SA, Bergsma DJ, et al: Differentiation between binding sites for angiotensin II and nonpeptide antagonists on the angiotensin II type 1 receptors. Proc Natl Acad Sci USA 91:7046–7050, 1994.
42. Ji H, Zheng W, Zhang Y, et al: Genetic transfer of a nonpeptide antagonist binding site to a previously unresponsive angiotensin receptor. Proc Natl Acad Sci USA 92:9240–9244, 1995.
43. Black JW, Shankley NP: Drug receptors. Inverse agonists exposed. Nature 374:214–215, 1995.
44. Samama P, Cotecchia S, Costa T, Lefkowitz RJ: A mutation-induced activated state of the beta 2-adrenergic receptor. Extending the ternary complex model. J Biol Chem 268:4625–4636, 1993.

45. Gether U, Kobilka BK: G protein-coupled receptors: II. Mechanism of agonist activation. J Biol Chem 273:17979–17982, 1998.

46. Feng YH, Miura SI, Husain A, Karnik SS: Mechanism of constitutive activation of the AT1 receptor: Influence of size of the agonist switch binding residue Asn[111]. Biochemistry 37:15791–15798, 1998.

47. Miura SI, Feng YH, Husain A, Karnik SS: Mechanism of angiotensin II-dependent activation of the AT1 receptor: Role of aromaticity of agonist switch residues. J Biol Chem 274: 7103–7110, 1999.

48. Bihoreau C, Monnot C, Davies E, et al: Mutation of Asp74 of the rat angiotensin II receptor confers changes in antagonist affinities and abolishes G-protein coupling. Proc Natl Acad Sci USA 90:5133–5137, 1993.

49. Marie J, Maigret B, Joseph MP, et al: Tyr292 in the seventh transmembrane domain of the AT1A angiotensin II receptor is essential for its coupling to phospholipase C. J Biol Chem 269: 20815–20818, 1994.

50. Balmforth AJ, Lee LJ, Warburton P, et al: The conformational change responsible for AT1 receptor activation is dependent upon two juxtaposed asparagine residues on transmembrane helices III and VII. J Biol Chem 272:4245–4251, 1997.

51. Hunyady L, Bor M, Baukal AJ, et al: A conserved NPLFY sequence contributes to agonist binding and signal transduction but is not an internalization signal for the type 1 angiotensin II receptor. J Biol Chem 270:16602–16609, 1995.

52. Groblewski T, Maigret B, Larguier R, et al: Mutation of Asn111 in the third transmembrane domain of the AT1A angiotensin II receptor induces its constitutive activation. J Biol Chem 272:1822–1826, 1997.

53. Bockaert J, Pin JP: Molecular tinkering of G protein-coupled receptors: An evolutionary success. EMBO J 18:1723–1729, 1999.

54. Rodbell M: The role of GTP-binding proteins in signal transduction: from the sublimely simple to the conceptually complex. Curr Top Cell Regul 32:1–47, 1992.

55. Monnot C, Bihoreau C, Conchon C, et al: Polar residues in the transmembrane domains of the type I angiotensin II receptor are required for binding and coupling: reconstitution of the binding site by co-expression of two deficient mutants. J Biol Chem 271:1507–1513, 1996.

56. Milligan G, Bond RA: Inverse agonism and the regulation of receptor number. TiPS 18:468–474, 1997.

57. Cheng HF, Becker BN, Burns KD, Harris RC: Angiotensin II upregulates type-1 angiotensin II receptors in renal proximal tubule. J Clin Invest 95:2012–2019, 1995.

58. Gutowski S, Smrcka A, Nowak L, et al: Antibodies to the alpha q subfamily of guanine nucleotide-binding regulatory protein alpha subunits attenuate activation of phosphatidylinositol 4,5-bisphosphate hydrolysis by hormones. J Biol Chem 266:20519–20524, 1991.

59. Macrez-Lepretre N, Kalkbrenner F, Morel JL, et al: G protein heterotrimer $G_{\alpha13\beta1\gamma3}$ couples the angiotensin AT1A receptor to increases in cytoplasmic Ca^{2+} in rat portal vein myocytes. J Biol Chem 272:10095–10102, 1997.

60. Wang C, Jayadev S, Escobedo JA: Identification of a domain in the angiotensin II type 1 receptor determining Gq coupling by the use of receptor chimeras. J Biol Chem 270:16677–16682, 1995.

61. Hunyady L, Zhang M, Jagadeesh G, et al: Dependence of agonist activation on a conserved apolar residue in the third intracellular loop of the AT1 angiotensin receptor. Proc Natl Acad Sci U S A 93:10040–10045, 1996.

62. Kai H, Alexander RW, Ushio-Fukai M, et al: G-Protein binding domains of the angiotensin II AT1A receptors mapped with synthetic peptides selected from the receptor sequence. Biochem J 332(Pt 3):781–787, 1998.

63. Franzoni L, Nicastro G, Pertinhez TA, et al: Structure of the C-terminal fragment 300-320 of the rat angiotensin II AT1A receptor and its relevance with respect to G-protein coupling. J Biol Chem 272:9734–9741, 1997.

64. Ohyama K, Yamano Y, Chaki S, et al: Domains for G-protein coupling in angiotensin II receptor type I: studies by site-directed mutagenesis. Biochem Biophys Res Commun 189:677–683, 1992.

65. Ushio-Fukai M, Alexander RW, Akers M, et al: Angiotensin II receptor coupling to phospholipase D is mediated by the betagamma subunits of heterotrimeric G proteins in vascular smooth muscle cells. Mol Pharmacol 55:142–149, 1999.

66. Linseman DA, Benjamin CW, Jones DA: Convergence of angiotensin II and platelet-derived growth factor receptor signaling cascades in vascular smooth muscle cells. J Biol Chem 270:12563–12568, 1995.

67. Hackel PO, Zwick E, Prenzel N, Ullrich A: Epidermal growth factor receptors: critical mediators of multiple receptor pathways. Curr Opin Cell Biol 11:184–189, 1999.

68. Marrero MB, Schieffer B, Paxton WG, et al: Direct stimulation of Jak/STAT pathway by the angiotensin II AT1 receptor. Nature 375:247–250, 1995.
69. Ali MS, Sayeski PP, Dirksen LB, et al: Dependence on the motif YIPP for the physical association of Jak2 kinase with the intracellular carboxyl tail of the angiotensin II AT1 receptor. J Biol Chem 272:23382–23388, 1997.
70. Venema RC, Ju H, Venema VJ, et al: Angiotensin II-induced association of phospholipase Cgamma1 with the G-protein-coupled AT1 receptor. J Biol Chem 273:7703–7708, 1998.
71. Lefkowitz RJ: G protein-coupled receptors: III. New roles for receptor kinases and b-arrestins in receptor signaling and desensitization. J Biol Chem 273:18677–18680, 1998.
72. Hunyady L, Bor M, Balla T, Catt KJ: Identification of a cytoplasmic Ser-Thr-Leu motif that determines agonist-induced internalization of the AT1 angiotensin receptor. J Biol Chem 269:31378–31382, 1994.
73. Thomas WG, Baker KM, Motel TJ, Thekkumkara TJ: Angiotensin II receptor endocytosis involves two distinct regions of the cytoplasmic tail. A role for residues on the hydrophobic face of a putative amphipathic helix. J Biol Chem 270:22153–22159, 1995.
74. Thomas WG, Motel TJ, Kule CE, et al: Phosphorylation of the angiotensin II (AT1A) receptor carboxyl terminus: a role in receptor endocytosis. Mol Endocrinol 12:1513–1524, 1998.
75. Smith RD, Hunyady L, Olivares-Reyes JA, et al: Agonist-induced phosphorylation of the angiotensin AT1a receptor is localized to a serine/threonine-rich region of its cytoplasmic tail. Mol Pharmacol 54:935–941, 1998.
76. Tang H, Guo DF, Porter JP, et al: Role of cytoplasmic tail of the type 1A angiotensin II receptor in agonist- and phorbol ester-induced desensitization. Circ Res 82:523–531, 1998.
77. Oppermann M, Freedman NJ, Alexander RW, Lefkowitz RJ: Phosphorylation of the type 1A angiotensin II receptor by G protein-coupled receptor kinases and protein kinase C. J Biol Chem 271:13266–13272, 1996.
78. Zhang J, Ferguson SSG, Barak LS, et al: Dynamin and beta-arrestin reveal distinct mechanisms for G protein-coupled receptor internalization. J Biol Chem 271:18302–18305, 1996.
79. Hein L, Barsh GS, Pratt RE, et al: Behavioural and cardiovascular effects of disrupting the angiotensin II type-2 receptor in mice. Nature 377:744–747, 1995.
80. Ichiki T, Labosky PA, Shiota C, et al: Effects on blood pressure and exploratory behaviour of mice lacking angiotensin II type-2 receptor. Nature 377:748–750, 1995.
81. Lazard D, Briend-Sutren MM, Villageois P, et al: Molecular characterization and chromosome localization of a human angiotensin II AT2 receptor gene highly expressed in fetal tissues. Recept Chann 2:271–280, 1994.
82. Tsuzuki S, Ichiki T, Nakakubo H, et al: Molecular cloning and expression of the gene encoding human angiotensin II type 2 receptor. Biochem Biophys Res Commun 200:1449–1454, 1994.
83. Nakajima M, Mukoyama M, Pratt RE, et al: Cloning of cDNA and analysis of the gene for mouse angiotensin II type 2 receptor. Biochem Biophys Res Commun 197:393–399, 1993.
84. Dulin NO, Ernsberger P, Suciu DJ, Douglas JG: Rabbit renal epithelial angiotensin II receptors. Am J Physiol 267:F776–F782, 1994.
85. Ernsberger P, Douglas JG: Rabbit renal epithelial angiotensin II receptors. Am J Physiol 267:F776–F782, 1994.
86. Speth RC: [125I]CGP 42112 binding reveals differences between rat brain and adrenal AT2 receptor binding sites. Regul Pept 44:189–197, 1993.
87. Tsutsumi K, Saavedra JM: Heterogeneity of angiotensin II AT2 receptors in the rat brain. Mol Pharmacol 41:290–297, 1992.
88. Servant G, Guillemette G: Analysis of the role of N-glycosylation in cell-surface expression and binding properties of angiotensin II type-2 receptor of rat pheochromocytoma cells. Biochem J 313:297–304, 1996.
89. Stadel JM, Wilson S, Bergsma DJ: Orphan G protein-coupled receptors: a neglected opportunity for pioneer drug discovery. Tips 18:430–437, 1997.
90. Riek RP, Handschumacher MK, Sung S, et al: Evolutionary conservation of both the hydrophilic and hydrophobic nature of transmembrane residues. J Theoret Biol 172:245–258, 1995.
91. Servant G, Laporte SA, Leduc R, Guillemette G: Identification of angiotensin II-binding domains in the rat AT2 receptor with photolabile angiotensin analogs. J Biol Chem 272:8653–8659, 1997.
92. Pulakat L, Tadesee AS, Dittus JJ, Gavini N: Role of Lys215 located in the fifth transmembrane domain of the AT2 receptor in ligand-receptor interaction. Redul Pept 73:51–57, 1998.
93. Bouley R, Perodin J, Plante H, et al: N- and C-terminal structure-activity study of angiotensin II on the angiotensin AT2 receptor. Euro J Pharmacol 343:323–331, 1998.
94. Ohyama K, Yamano Y, Sano T, et al: Disulfide bridges in extracellular domains of angiotensin II receptor type IA. Regul Pept 57:141–147, 1995.

95. Feng YH, Karnik SS: Rectification of defective AT2 angiotensin mutant receptors induced by cysteine-disulfide bond exchange. J Biol Chem [in press].

96. Perez DM, Hwa J, Brown F, Graham RM: Constitutive activation of a single effector pathway: evidence for multiple activation states of a G protein-coupled receptor. Mol Pharmacol 49:112–122, 1996.

97. Horiuchi M, Hayashida W, Kambe T, et al: Angiotensin type 2 receptor dephosphorylates Bcl-2 by activating mitogen-activated protein kinase phosphatase-1 and induces apoptosis. J Biol Chem 272:19022–19026, 1997.

98. Zhu MY, Gelband CH, Moore JM, et al: Angiotensin II type 2 receptor stimulation of neuronal delayed-rectifier potassium current involves phospholipase A2 and arachidonic acid. J Neurosci 18:679–686, 1998.

99. Bedecs K, Elbaz N, Sutren M, et al: Angiotensin II type 2 receptors mediate inhibition of mitogen-activated protein kinase cascade and functional activation of SHP-1 tyrosine phosphatase. Biochem J 325:449–454, 1997.

100. Zhang J, Pratt RE: The AT2 receptor selectively associates with Gia_2 and Gia_3 in the rat fetus. J Biol Chem 271:15026–15033, 1996.

101. Hayashida W, Horiuchi M, Dzau VJ: Intracellular third loop domain of angiotensin II type-2 receptor. Role in mediating signal transduction and cellular function. J Biol Chem 271:21985–21992, 1996.

102. Jacobs LS, Douglas JG: Angiotensin II type 2 receptor subtype mediates phospholipase A2-dependent signaling in rabbit proximal tubular epithelial cells. Hypertension 28:663–668, 1996.

103. Haithcock D, Jiao HY, Cui XL, et al: Renal proximal tubular AT2 receptor: signaling and transport. J Am Soc Nephrol 10:S69, 1999.

104. Hein L, Meinel L, Pratt RE, et al: Intracellular trafficking of angiotensin II and its AT1 and AT2 receptors: evidence for selective sorting of receptor and ligand. Mol Endocrinol 11:1266–1277, 1997.

105. Llorens-Cortes C: Identification of metabolic pathways of brain angiotensin II and angiotensin III: Predominant role of angiotensin III in the control of vasopressin secretion. C R Seances Soc Biol Fil 192:607–618, 1998.

106. Reaux A, de Mota N, Zini S, et al: PC18, a specific aminopeptidase N inhibitor, induces vasopressin release by increasing the half-life of brain angiotensin III. Neuroendocrinology 69:370–376, 1999.

107. Douglas JG, Bartley P, Kondo T, Catt K: Formation of Des-Asp1-Angiotensin II is not an obligatory step in steroidogenic action of angiotensin II in the canine adrenal. Endocrinology 102:1921–1924, 1978.

108. Wright JW, Harding JW: Important role for angiotensin III and IV in the brain renin-angiotensin system. Brain Res Rev 25:96–124, 1997.

109. Briand SI, Bellemare JM, Bernier SG, Guillemette G: Study on the functionality and molecular properties of the AT4 receptor. Endocr Res 24:315–323, 1998.

110. Bernier SG, Bellemare JM, Escher E, Guillemette G: Characterization of AT4 receptor from bovine aortic endothelium with photosensitive analogues of angiotensin IV. Biochemistry 37:4280–4287, 1998.

111. Handa RK, Krebs LT, Harding JW, Handa SE: Angiotensin IV AT4-receptor system in the rat kidney. Am J Physiol 274(2 Pt 2):F290–F299, 1998.

112. Dulin N, Madhun ZT, Chang CH, et al: Angiotensin IV receptors and signaling in opossum kidney cells. Am J Physiol 269(5 Pt 2):F644–F652, 1995.

113. Ferrario CM, Iyer SN: Angiotensin-(1-7): A bioactive fragment of the renin-angiotensin system. Regul Pept 78:13–18, 1998.

114. Strawn WB, Ferrario CM, Tallant EA: Angiotensin-(1-7) reduces smooth muscle growth after vascular injury. Hypertension 33(1 Pt 2):207–211, 1999.

115. Andreatta-van Leyen S, Romero MF, Khosla MC, Douglas JG: Modulation of phospholipase A2 activity and sodium transport by angiotensin-(1-7). Kidney Int 44:932–936, 1993.

116. Ernsberger P, Zhou J, Damon TH, Douglas JG: Angiotensin II receptor subtypes in cultured rat renal mesangial cells. Am J Physiol. 263(3 Pt 2):F411–F416, 1992.

CHAPTER 4

Signaling and Cellular Effects of Angiotensin II

RAYMOND C. HARRIS, M.D.

Angiotensin II is a multifunctional hormone that mediates contraction of vascular smooth muscle cells and cardiac myocytes, and regulates epithelial cell function and growth responses of vascular and epithelial cells through a complex series of intracellular signaling events initiated by the interaction with its receptors. Two receptors, type 1 (AT_1) and type 2 (AT_2) have been identified. These receptors use distinct signaling pathways and mediate dramatically divergent physiologic responses.

■ AT_1 Receptors

G-Protein Coupling

The predominant physiologic effects of angiotensin II (Ang II) appear to be mediated through AT_1 receptors, which are members of the seven-transmembrane G-protein–coupled receptor (GPCR) superfamily.[1,2] AT_2 receptors are also G-protein– coupled receptors.[3,4] Over 1000 GPCRs are encoded in the human genome, of which approximately 50% have been cloned to date. As their name implies, GPCRs associate with heterotrimeric G proteins, which mediate transduction of extracellular signals into the intracellular milieu after receptor activation.[5]

Heterotrimeric G proteins are members of the guanosine triphosphatase (GTPase) superfamily of proteins, identified by their ability to hydrolyze guanosine triphosphate (GTP). They are membrane-bound proteins composed of alpha, beta, and gamma subunits. The molecular weight of alpha (α) subunits is 39–52 kDa; of beta (β) subunits, 36 kDa; and of gamma (γ) subunits, 6–8 kDa, depending on the subtype. The four major types of alpha subunits—$G\alpha_s$, $G\alpha_{i/o}$, $G\alpha_{q/11}$ and $G\alpha_{12/13}$—couple to different signaling pathways. Multiple isoforms of each subunit have been identified; at least 23 α, 6 β and 11 γ isoforms have been identified so far. Although this diversity presents the possibility for a bewildering number of combinatorial events, it appears that expression of the different isoforms is cell-specific, with ordered rather than random association. In addition, ordering and limitation determine which trimers associate with a specific GPCR.[5]

When heterotrimeric G proteins are inactive, guanidine diphosphate (GDP) is bound to the α, β, γ trimer via the α subunit. Ligand binding to the receptor is followed by association of the heterotrimeric G protein with the GPCR, release of GDP, binding of GTP and magnesium (Mg^{2+}) to the α subunit, and dissociation of $\beta\gamma$ subunits. Both the $G\alpha$-GTP and the $\beta\gamma$ subunits then activate downstream effector proteins. Signaling is terminated by hydrolysis of GTP to GDP and reassociation of α and $\beta\gamma$ subunits. Desensitization of GPCRs leads to uncoupling from G proteins, which is associated with receptor phosphorylation, followed by internalization and recycling. The receptor phosphorylation is mediated at least in part by G-protein receptor kinases (GRKs), a family of serine/threonine kinases that phosphorylate the receptor and desensitize it to further activation.[6]

Of the $G\alpha$ subtypes, $G\alpha_s$ (stimulatory) activates adenylate cyclase and increases cyclic adenosine monophosphate (cAMP), whereas $G\alpha_{i/o}$ (inhibitory) inhibits adenylate cyclase activity and decreases cAMP. $G\alpha_{q/11}$ activates phospholipase C-β, which hydrolyses a minor plasma membrane phospholipid, phosphatidylinositol 1,4-bisphosphate (PIP_2), to inositol triphosphate (IP_3) and diacylglycerol (DAG). IP_3 binds to specific receptors in endoplasmic reticulum, which results in opening of calcium (Ca^{2+})-permeable channels that allow release of sequestered calcium into the cytoplasm In contrast, in certain tissues the release of intracellular calcium stores may be secondary to entry of extracellular calcium via L-type calcium channels, which subsequently induces Ca^{2+}-activated release of intracellular calcium stores. Evidence suggests G protein-mediated regulation of L-type calcium channels.[7-9] Diacylglycerol is a potent activator of the family of serine/threonine kinases, protein kinase C. In addition, other signaling pathways are activated by different $G\alpha$ subunits in certain cells and tissues. Although the classic paradigm for heterotrimeric G protein signaling suggested that the activated signal pathways were defined entirely by the identity of the α subunit, more recent studies have identified $\beta\gamma$ subunits as signal transducers.[10]

AT_1 receptors are expressed in many different types of cells and can mediate a broad array of responses. Therefore, a discussion of AT_1 receptor signaling may define certain general principles but cannot review all of the specifics of AT_1-mediated cell signaling.

Current evidence suggests that signaling pathways mediated by AT_1 receptors are linked predominantly to the $G\alpha_{q/11}$, $G\alpha_{12/13}$, and $G\alpha_{i/o}$ classes of G proteins.[8,9,11] G proteins couple to the AT_1 receptor at the second and third cytoplasmic loop ($G\alpha_{i/o}$ and $G\alpha_q$)[12-14] and in the proximal carboxyl terminal tail ($G\alpha_q$).[15] In addition, AT_1 receptor phosphorylation and desensitization are mediated by GRKs,[16,17] as well as possibly by protein kinase C.[17-20]

In vascular smooth muscle, the early and primary signal involved in Ang II-mediated contraction is the increase in intracellular calcium. The subsequent activation of calmodulin and myosin-light chain kinase initiates actin-myosin interactions, resulting in hydrolysis of adenosine triphosphate (ATP) with cross-bridge formation and force generation.[21] The sensitivity to calcium can be modified by other signaling pathways, including mitogen-activated protein (MAP) kinase–dependent phosphorylation of thin filament proteins (caldesmon and calponin)[22] and myosin phosphatase activity.[23] There appears to be heterogeneity among vessels relating to the nature of the calcium response to Ang II; in

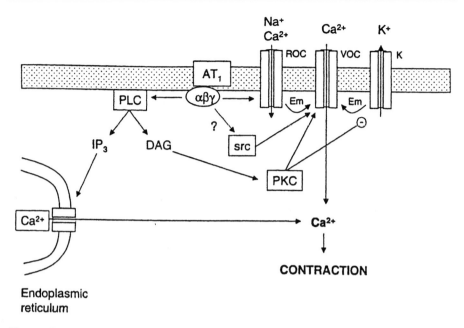

Figure 1. Signaling pathways involved in AT$_1$ receptor-mediated vasoconstriction. αβγ = heterotrimeric G protein, PLC = phospholipase C, PKC = protein kinase C, VOC = L-type calcium channel, ROC = cation channel, K = K channels, IP$_3$ = inositol, 1,4,5-trisphosphate, DAG = diacylglycerol. (From Hughes AD: Molecular and cellular mechanisms of action of angiotensin II (AT$_1$) receptors in vascular smooth muscle cells. J Hum Hypertens 12:275–281, 1998, with permission.)

smaller arteries, calcium release from intracellular stores may be less important than calcium influx in mediating the initial contraction events.[8,24,25]

In cultured vascular smooth muscle and glomerular mesangial cells, binding of Ang II to AT$_1$ receptors induces activation of phospholipase C, leading to DAG-mediated stimulation of PKC and to IP$_3$-mediated release of calcium from intracellular stores (Fig. 1). AT$_1$-mediated increases in cytoplasmic calcium have been shown to be mediated predominantly by Gα$_q$,[8,9,11,26] but in rat portal myocytes, Gα$_{13}$ also has been shown to be involved.[10] In cardiac fibroblasts, Ang II-induced activation of Ras/extracellular signal-regulated kinases (ERKs) is also activated by Gα$_q$-coupled Ca^{2+}/calmodulin signaling.[27]

Although the AT$_1$-mediated release of calcium from intracellular stores is activated by increases in IP$_3$, increased calcium influx into vascular smooth muscle also has been shown to depend on βγ-mediated activation of L-type Ca^{2+} channels. Angiotensin II also may directly activate receptor-operated channels,[28] which are dihydropyridine-insensitive; this insensitivity indicates that they are not L-type channels. It has been suggested that increased intracellular Ca^{2+} influx from these channels depolarizes the cells, leading to activation of voltage-activated Ca^{2+} channels. Evidence also suggests that Ang II can modulate the activity of three types of potassium (K$^+$) channels: delayed rectifier, calcium-activated and ATP-dependent,[29–32] as well as increase chloride conductance via activation of calcium-activated chloride channels.[33–35]

Although the predominant mediator of AT$_1$-activated vascular contraction is the increased intracellular calcium, a role for protein kinase C (PKC) also has been determined. PKCs are serine/threonine kinases. They are classified as "classical" because they are phosphatidylserine-, Ca^{2+}- and DAG- or phorbol ester-dependent (α, $\beta1$, $\beta2$, and γ); as "novel" because they are calcium-independent (ε, η, δ and θ); and as "atypical" because they require neither Ca^{2+} nor DAG for activation (ζ and τ).[36,37] As noted above, phospholipase C hydrolysis of PIP_2 increases DAG. In addition, evidence suggests that AT_1 receptor-mediated activation of phospholipase D (PLD) may be a major source of DAG.[38,39] $G\beta\gamma$ and $G\alpha_{12}$ subunits mediate coupling of AT_1 receptors to activation of tonic PLD via a $pp60^{c-src}$-dependent mechanisms.[40] Each cell type has its own component of PKC isoforms, and it is assumed that each PKC has specific downstream targets. One signaling pathway mediated by PKC involves activation of cRaf, which then leads to activation of the MAP kinases, p44/p42 ERKs.[41] MAP kinases act as a point of convergence for multiple signaling pathways and may mediate a variety of immediate and long-term cellular responses. As mentioned above, MAP kinases may act to modify contractile response. In addition to MAP kinase activation, PKC may directly phosphorylate calcium channels.[42]

Although the predominant effects on intracellular calcium are mediated by $G\alpha_q$ and $G\alpha_{13}$ in vascular tissue, an important role for AT_1-mediated $G\alpha_i$ activation has been demonstrated in both vascular and nonvascular tissue.[43–45] In renal proximal tubule, Ang II-mediated AT_1 activation is the single most important hormonally regulated pathway of fluid, sodium (Na^+) and bicarbonate (HCO_3^-) reabsorption. Ang II can regulate up to 50% of the Na^+ and water transport of the proximal convoluted tubule.[46,47] Furthermore, in combination with similar but smaller effects on the straight segment, it has been estimated that Ang II can modulate 15% or more of all Na^+ reabsorbed by the kidney.[46] Ang II also markedly stimulates HCO_3^- reabsorption in the proximal tubule,[48] affecting 60% of the acidification capacity of this segment and thus potentially controlling up to 30% of all renal acidification.[46,49] The stimulatory effects of Ang II are associated with a significant decrease in proximal tubule cAMP levels and are inhibited by pertussis toxin pretreatment,[48] indicating coupling of proximal tubule AT_1 receptors to $G\alpha_i$. Partial inhibition of adenylate cyclase activity also has been observed in rabbit proximal tubule cells, in which intracellular cAMP levels were decreased by 22% and 34% by Ang II 10^{-11} M and 10^{-9} M, respectively.[50] Cyclic cAMP has been shown to inhibit brush-border membrane Na^+/H^+ exchange (NHE_3) through a protein kinase A-dependent phosphorylation.[51] Activation of AT_1 receptors also stimulates basolateral Na^+,K^+-ATPase activity via pentoxyfylline-sensitive, G protein-linked inhibition of the adenylyl cyclase pathway.[52,53] Ruiz et al. have shown that stimulation of the basolateral Na^+/HCO_3^- cotransport activity by angiotensin II is mediated by both $G\alpha_i$ and $G\alpha_q$.[54] Functional AT_1 receptors are found on both apical and basolateral membranes of proximal tubules, and evidence suggests $G\alpha_i$ coupling of receptors on both membranes.[55–57] In bovine adrenal glomerulosa cells activation of Ras/Raf signaling also depends on G_i.[58]

A role also has been suggested for PKC activation in mediating the effects of Ang II on proximal tubule Na^+/H^+ exchange. Karim et al. have shown that angiotensin II activates both alpha and epsilon isoforms of protein kinase C in rat proximal tubule.[59] Wang and Chan demonstrated that the stimulatory effect of Ang II (10^{-11} M) on volume and HCO_3^- transport in the rat proximal tubule was inhibited by H-7.[60] Liu and Cogan also found that PKC inhibition attenuated the stimulatory effect of Ang II on proximal tubule transport.[61] Although they are relatively specific, the PKC inhibitors used in these studies may inhibit other kinases. In the proximal tubule, low concentrations of Ang II (10^{-12}–10^{-9} M) inhibit and higher concentrations (10^{-8}–10^{-5} M) inhibit transport and net fluid reabsorption.[47,62,63] From these studies, it is difficult to define with certainty the mechanisms of the biphasic effect of Ang II on transport in the proximal tubule. According to one theory, suggested by Wang and Chan,[60] low concentrations of Ang II inhibit adenylate cyclase and activate PKC, leading to stimulation of Na^+/H^+ exchange. Higher concentrations additionally raise cytosolic calcium and inhibit the antiporter, perhaps by activation of calcium/calmodulin-dependent protein kinase II and by phospholipase A_2/cytochrome P450-mediated metabolites.[64] The effects of stimulation of PKC in the proximal tubule are complex. Phorbol ester was found either to stimulate or to inhibit HCO_3^- and fluid reabsorption in the rat proximal tubule, depending on the dose and time of administration.[60]

Tyrosine Kinases

An important regulatory mechanism of many proteins is phosphorylation/dephosphorylation. Protein phosphorylation is mediated by protein kinases, which are classified as either serine/threonine or tyrosine, depending on which residues they selectively phosphorylate. Most phosphoproteins are phosphorylated on serine or threonine residues; phosphotyrosine residues represent < 0.1% of all phosphorylated proteins but are important for cell signaling.

The signal transduction of many peptide growth factors, such as epidermal growth factor (EGF) and platelet-derived growth factor (PDGF), has long been recognized to be mediated by tyrosine kinase-mediated phosphorylation of selected target proteins, many of which are themselves involved in signal transduction. The activation of tyrosine kinase cascades by growth factors is regulated by the intrinsic tyrosine kinase activity of the growth factor receptors (receptor tyrosine kinases [RTKs]). However, after the identification of the signaling actions of RTKs, it was appreciated that other growth factors, such as interferon gamma, also signaled through tyrosine kinase-mediated pathways, although their receptors do not contain intrinsic tyrosine kinase activity.[65] More recently, there has been an increasing awareness that many GPCRs, which also lack intrinsic tyrosine kinase activity, also activate tyrosine kinase cascades that are integral to the signal transduction of these receptors.

Increasing evidence suggests that AT_1 receptor activation initiates tyrosine kinase cascades that may be involved in mediation of the physiologic actions of Ang II, including smooth muscle contraction.[66–69] Studies in smooth muscle cells and mesangial cells have shown that AT_1 activation leads to tyrosine phosphorylation of Grb2,[70] Shc,[71] focal adhesion kinase,[72,73] paxillin,[73–75] Jak_2 and STAT-1,[76] PLCγ,[77,78] IRS-1,[79] and tyrosine phosphatases,[79–82] among other proteins.

GPCR-mediated tyrosine phosphorylation is regulated by different families of tyrosine kinases; for AT_1 receptors, at least five tryosine kinase families have been shown to be activated: Src, Jak/STAT, FAK, calcium-dependent tyrosine kinases (Pyk2 and CADTK),[83–85] and receptor tyrosine kinases (EGFR and PDGR).[86,87]

A central role for Src and Src-like kinases has been demonstrated in the activation of Ang II-activated tyrosine kinase cascades.[76,88–90] These tyrosine kinases (of which nine have been described to date) are cytosolic proteins with a molecular weight of 55–62 kDa. All of them have amino terminal myristoylation that is important for membrane targeting, an SH2 (Src homology domain) and an SH3 domain, and a tyrosine kinase domain. The SH2 domain mediates association of Src-like tyrosine kinases with proteins. Of the nine members of the Src tyrosine kinase family, only three—*pp60^{src}*, *fyn* and *yes* are found in nonhematopoietic cells. Binding of Ang II to the AT_1 receptor activates Src and Src-like tyrosine kinases,[79,80,89–95] which mediate downstream signaling. The mechanisms by which AT_1 receptor activation leads to increased Src kinase activity are still under investigation, although recent evidence in rat vascular smooth muscle cells indicates that *pp60^{src}* is tyrosine phosphorylated and activated by another non–receptor-mediated tyrosine kinase, PYK2, which may be activated by increased cytosolic calcium.[83]

In cultured rat vascular smooth muscle cells and mesangial cells, Ang II-induced stimulation of inositol phosphate hydrolysis by PLC, release of IP_3-dependent intracellular Ca^{2+} stores, and activation of Ca^{2+}-dependent chloride (Cl^-) channels have been shown to be partially dependent on the tyrosine phosphorylation of PLC-γ.[96,97] Unlike PLC-β, which is activated by $G\alpha_q$ (see above), PLC-γ is activated by tyrosine phosphorylation and can associate with the tyrosine-phosphorylated AT_1 receptor at the YIPP motif in the cytosolic tail of the receptor by binding of SH2 domains contained in PLC-γ.[78,92] The demonstration that initial increases in IP_3 secondary to AT_1 receptor activation are mediated by PLC-β[98] and that subsequent, more sustained increases are mediated by PLCγ reconciles the conflicting findings about PLC isoform activation[99] (Fig. 2).

In addition to phospholipase C activation, Src family kinase activation is required for Ang II stimulation of MAP kinase signaling pathways.[90] PLD activation also may depend partially on both calcium- and tyrosine kinase-mediated pathways.[100,101] In smooth muscle and cardiac muscle cells, activation of c-Src and fyn have been shown to activate p21Ras by the Shc-Grb$_2$-Sos pathway, which activates the MAP kinases, ERK1/2.[102–105] In addition, in proximal tubule

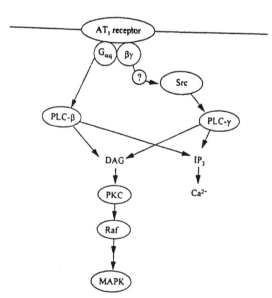

Figure 2. Coupling of AT_1 receptor to downstream effectors. After ligand binding, the AT_1 receptor activates PLC-β via the $G\alpha q$ subunit. PLC-γ becomes tyrosine phosphorylated and activated by src kinase. Activation of both PLC isozymes leads to IP_3 and DAG formation and the activation of PKC and MAP kinase. (From van Bilsen M: Signal transduction revisited: Recent developments in angiotensin II signaling in the cardiovascular system. Cardiovasc Res 36:310–322, 1997, with permission.)

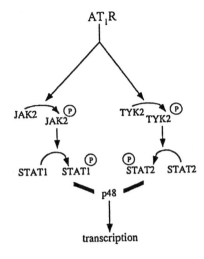

Figure 3. Stimulation of the Jak/STAT pathway by AT$_1$ receptor. Both Jak2 and Tyk2 are activated by tyrosine phosphorylation, and these activated kinases then phosphorylate STATs, which associate with p48 to form an active transcriptional complex. (From Griendling KK, Ushio-Fukai M, Lassegue B, Alexander RW: Angiotensin II signaling in vascular smooth muscle. New concepts. Hypertension 29:366–373, 1997, with permission.)

cells, c-Src is required for angiotensin II-induced increases in Na^+/H^+ exchanger (NHE$_3$) activity.[106]

AT$_1$ receptors also rapidly tyrosine phosphorylate and activate the Janus kinase (Jak) family of nonreceptor tyrosine kinases, Jak$_1$, Jak$_2$, Jak$_3$, and Tyk$_2$, all of which have a molecular weight of approximately 130 kDa.[76] This family of kinases were named after the Roman god Janus, who looks both forward and backward, because initially they were thought to contain two kinase domains. Subsequent study, however, has determined that the N-terminal domain is a nonactive pseudokinase.[107] After activation, Jaks tyrosine phosphorylate cytosolic proteins called signal transducers and activators of transcription (STATs) translocate to the nucleus and activate gene transcription by binding to specific promoter elements, especially in early response genes such as c-fos.[108] In vascular smooth muscle cells and cardiac myocytes, AT$_1$ has been shown to activate Jak$_2$ and Tyk$_2$, leading to increased phosphorylation of STATs 1–3.[76,109,110] Recent evidence indicates that under certain conditions Src activation may mediate Jak activation[111] (Fig. 3). The carboxyl-terminal cytoplasmic tail of the AT$_1$ receptor physically associates with Jak$_2$ as well as STAT-1 and -3.[110,112] Mutational analysis indicates that this association depends on the receptor motif, YIPP (tyrosine-isoleucine-proline-proline) in the AT$_1$ receptor, which has characteristics of an SH$_2$ binding domain.[113] However, because Jaks do not contain either SH$_2$- or SH$_3$-binding domains, other binding proteins also may be involved in their association with AT$_1$ receptors.

AT$_1$ receptors also activate the tyrosine kinase, focal adhesion kinase (FAK).[72,114] After activation and autophosphorylation, FAK translocates and is associated with focal adhesions; phosphorylates other substrates in the focal adhesion plaque, including paxillin[74] and p130Cas; and promotes cytoskeletal rearrangement. Evidence also suggests an association of phosphorylated FAK and c-Src. In this regard, AT$_1$ may activate FAK by both autophosphorylation and Src-mediated tyrosine phosphorylation. Tyrosine phosphorylation of p130Cas by Ang II depends on Src, intracellular Ca^{2+}, and PKC signaling pathways.[105,115]

The tyrosine kinase-mediated signaling pathways activated by AT$_1$ and other GPCRs have targets similar to those of the RTKs. Recently, it has been found that activation of AT_1 and other GPCRs leads to rapid tyrosine phosphorylation of RTKs, such as PDGF,[71] EGF,[91,116,117] and IGF-1 receptors.[91] Receptor tyrosine phosphorylation occurs in the absence of the RTK ligands. Phosphorylated RTKs provide docking sites for the upstream activators of the Src family of tyrosine kinases and the downstream adaptor proteins,[116] with formation of a Shc/Grb$_2$/SOS complex that leads to Ras activation.[94] The protein p21Ras is a low-molecular-weight GTP-binding protein that is known to activate c-Raf, which is upstream of MAP kinase activation. This "scaffolding" function of the intrinsic tyrosine kinase receptors is a necessary step in the mediation of AT_1 activation of MAPK.[91]

Phospholipase A_2

Angiotensin II activates phospholipase A_2 (PLA$_2$) to release the fatty acid, arachidonic acid, which normally is bound to membrane phospholipids in the sn-2 position.[118] MAP kinase phosphorylates and activates cytosolic PLA$_2$ (cPLA$_2$).[119] In addition, activation of PLD also increases free arachidonic acid levels.[120] Arachidonic acid then serves as substrate for metabolism to biologically active compounds by cyclooxygenases, lipoxygenases and cP450 epoxygenases, and omega/omega-1 hydroxylases.[121] The synthesis of vasodilatory prostaglandins (PGE$_2$ and PGI$_2$) acts as a negative feedback loop to antagonize the contractile actions of angiotensin II. Inhibition of prostaglandin synthesis with nonsteroidal antiinflammatory drugs (NSAIDs) enhances the constrictor actions of Ang II on the vasculature of the kidney and the glomerulus.[122]

In the renal proximal tubule, Ang II activation of PLA$_2$ by luminal receptors may be an important step in the regulation of sodium reabsorption.[123,124] Because proximal tubule contains abundant cP450 activity but minimal cyclooxygenase or lipoxygenase activity, it has been proposed that cP450-derived arachidonic acid metabolites—epoxyeicosatrienoic acids (EET), especially 5,6-EET[64,125] and HETEs—may be involved in Ang II-mediated responses.[126,127] Both micropuncture and in vitro microperfusion studies indicate a biphasic effect of Ang II in the proximal tubule. Low doses (10^{-12}–10^{-10} M) stimulate and high doses (10^{-7}–10^{-5} M) inhibit proximal tubule Na^+ and water reabsorption.[47,62,128,129] PLA$_2$-mediated release of arachidonic acid has been implicated in regulation of both stimulatory and inhibitory responses of apical receptors in the proximal tubule.[130] Cytochrome P450 arachidonic acid metabolites, EETs and/or 20 HETEs,[64,125] may regulate the inhibitory effect of high concentrations of Ang II by increased calcium influx and inhibition of Na^+ transport, as mediated by both direct inhibition of apical membrane Na^+/H^+ exchange and basolateral membrane Na^+/K^+ ATPase.[53]

Reactive Oxygen Species

Cellular responses to angiotensin II are multiphasic, involving stimulation within seconds of phospholipase C and Ca^{2+} mobilization; activation within minutes of tyrosine kinases, PLD, PLA$_2$, protein kinase C, and MAP kinases; and stimulation after a period of hours of gene transcription. Recent evidence suggests an important role for reactive oxygen species as mediators of both early and more delayed AT_1 receptor signaling.[70,131] Ang II produces increased intracellular H_2O_2 and a rapid phosphorylation of both p42/44MAPK and p38MAPK

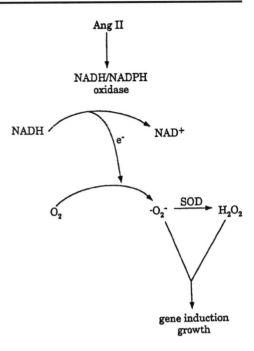

Figure 4. Stimulation of the NADPH/NADH oxidase pathway by angiotensin II. Angiotensin II activates a membrane NADPH/NADH oxidase to produce O_2^-, which is converted by superoxide dismutase (SOD) to H_2O_2. Both of these species have been implicated in gene induction and cell growth. (From Griendling KK, Ushio-Fukai M, Lassegue B, Alexander RW: Angiotensin II signaling in vascular smooth muscle. New concepts. Hypertension 29:366–373, 1997, with permission.)

and induces oxidant stress-dependent hypertrophy in cultured vascular smooth muscle cells.[131] AT_1 activation leads to increases in reduced nictotinamide adenine dinucleotide (NADH)/NADH phosphate oxidase, the source of the intracellularly generated reactive oxygen species, as well as an increase in p22phox mRNA[132] (Fig. 4).

Intracellular Receptors

The classic paradigm for receptor activation implicates plasma membrane receptors that are activated by extracellular ligands and initiate cytoplasmic signaling cascades from the plasma membrane. The AT_1 receptor surely fits this model; clearly its signaling results primarily from plasma membrane signaling. However, studies also have suggested that some components of the signaling cascade, such as increased DAG accumulation, MAP kinase activation, and calcium influx, may require receptor internalization, whereas other early signals, such as PLC activation, do not.[133,134]

For many G-protein–coupled receptors, endocytosis motifs are recognized by adaptor proteins that mediate ligand-bound receptors that aggregate into clathrin-coated pits; in vascular smooth muscle cells, there is evidence for AT_1 receptors in clathrin-coated vesicles.[135] AT_1 receptors, however, may not use clathrin-associated endocytosis exclusively. Dynamin and β-arrestin are key components of the clathrin-mediated internalization machinery, but AT_1 receptor internalization was not impaired in dynamin-deficient or β-arrestin–deficient cells, although internalization of another GPCR, β2-adrenergic receptor, was significantly inhibited. Such results suggest that AT_1 receptors may use other mechanisms, such as caveolae or non–clathrin-coated vesicles.[136] In certain tissues, the caveolar pathway of internalization may be important for AT_1, as recently documented in vascular smooth muscle cells.[137] Caveolae contain many components of intracellular signaling, including G proteins, phospholipases, protein kinases, and calcium channels. Therefore, AT_1 internalized in caveolae may continue to transduce intracellular signals.

The endocytic behavior of AT_1 receptors may play an important role in the physiologic functions of the receptor. In cultured proximal tubule cells, inhibition of endocytosis decreased apical, but not basolateral, Ang II-stimulated generation of IP_3 and Ang II-induced Na^+ flux.[138,139] Therefore, the endocytic movement of proximal tubule AT_1 receptors may serve not only as a mechanism for regulating receptor number at the cell surface but also as a means for mediating the cellular effects of Ang II.

Certain tissues, such as adrenal gland, with high concentrations of AT_1, appear to sequester Ang II from circulation and to stimulate intracellular AT_1.[140] AT_1 internalization appears to be a major means by which Ang II enters cells.[141,142] Of interest, the kidney can accumulate concentrations of Ang II that are higher than circulating levels, and the half-life of Ang II is significantly longer in kidney than in blood.[140,143] AT_1 endocytosis, therefore, may be important for accumulation of intracellular Ang II, which may activate putative cytoplasmic and nuclear receptors.[144–150] Translocation of cell surface AT_1 receptors to the nucleus has been suggested.[151] In smooth muscle cells, microinjected fluorescently tagged Ang II concentrated in submembranous domains and the perinuclear area induced increases in calcium influx in both cytosol and nucleus, mediated by IP_3.[152] This effect was blocked by simultaneous microinjection of an AT_1 antagonist, suggesting a possible physiologic role for nuclear receptors. It has been suggested that IP_3-linked events, such as steroidogenesis in adrenal glomerulosa, do not require receptor internalization, but protein kinase C activation does.[153] This process may be mediated in part by PLD-dependent increases in DAG.[133,154]

Long-term Effects

Signaling responses to AT_1 activation regulate vascular tone and ion transport; in addition, longer-term effects mediate gene regulation and tissue remodeling. The most evident example of AT_1 mediation of gene regulation is in the adrenal glomerulosa, in which Ang II induces production of aldosterone. Numerous studies, however, demonstrate that AT_1 activation induces increased expression of immediate early genes, such as c-fos and egr-1[155,156]; matrix proteins, such as collagen[157] and fibronectin[117,158]; and numerous other genes related to cellular growth. The delayed cellular responses to Ang II are mediated both directly by receptor signaling and indirectly by Ang II-mediated induction of growth factors, such as PDGF[159,160] and TGF-β.[161–163]

Angiotensin II is now viewed as a growth factor for vascular tissue.[95,165,166] Growth can involve an increase in cell number (hyperplasia), an increase in cell size (hypertrophy), or a change in structure without alterations in cell number or size (remodeling). In various organs in either physiologic or pathophysiologic conditions, Ang II has been implicated as a mediator of all types of growth.[167–169] PKC may be necessary for growth of vascular smooth muscle cells.[84–87] Ang II also has direct effects on proximal tubule cell growth.[170–172] The hypertrophy of renal proximal tubular cells occurs as an adaptive response to a variety of stimuli and may be involved with the progression of renal disease. Ang II acting alone or in combination with other growth factors has been implicated in this process.[173]

AT_1 activation may induce the cyclin-dependent kinase inhibitor p27Kip1 in renal epithelial cells, which prevents completion of the cell cycle and results in hypertrophy.[174] Activation of p27Kip1 appears to depend on generation of reactive oxygen species.[175]

■ *AT_2 Receptors*

AT_2 receptors are expressed in the vasculature during later stages of development and in neonates.[176,177] AT_2 receptors also are expressed in high levels in the metanephros during embryonic kidney development; expression has been localized in the metanephric kidney to uninduced mesenchyme and differentiating epithelia.[178,179] AT_2 receptor expression in kidney and vasculature declines rapidly after birth, although detectable expression and functional responses have been reported (Fig. 5).

Striking cellular responses mediated by AT_2 receptors include growth inhibition and/or programmed cell death (apoptosis). The AT_2-specific antagonist, PD123319, prevented the decline in aortic DNA synthesis that normally occurs late in embryonic life, at the time when AT_2 expression is highest in the vasculature.[176] Similar growth inhibition has been described in vascular smooth muscle

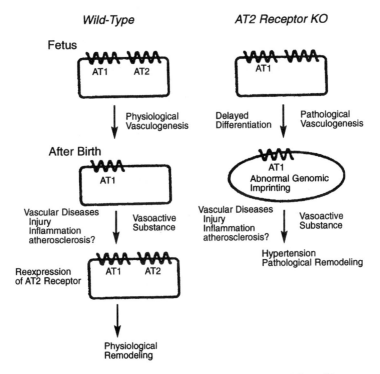

Figure 5. Effect of AT_2 receptor in vasculogenesis and vascular remodeling. AT_2 receptor is expressed abundantly and widely in the fetal vasculature and contributes to physiological vascular development. Disruption of AT_2 receptor gene results in an increase in basal blood pressure as well as increased vasoconstriction in response to angiotensin II. Upregulation of the AT_2 receptor in diseased vessels is induced by injury and inflammation. AT_2 receptor disruption results in increased neointimal formation. KO indicates knockout. (From Horiuchi M, Akishita M, Dzau VJ: Recent progress in angiotensin II type 2 receptor research in the cardiovascular system. Hypertension 33:613–621, 1999, with permission.)

cells,[180] cardiomyocytes,[181] and endothelial cells.[182] AT$_2$ receptors also may play a role in vascular remodeling and differentiaton.[177]

The expression of AT$_2$ in uninduced metanephric mesenchyme suggests that AT$_2$ receptors may play a role in mediating the apoptotic fate of these cells. Developmental abnormalities of the kidney and ureter in AT$_2$ knockout mice have been attributed to an inhibition of apoptosis of undifferentiated mesenchymal cells surrounding the urinary tract.[183] Studies in which smooth muscle cells were transfected with AT$_2$ demonstrated that apoptosis induced by serum withdrawal was enhanced[180]; in contrast, AT$_1$ receptor activation prevented apoptosis under these conditions.[184] AT$_2$ receptor activation activates a caspase cascade that evenuates in apoptosis.[185] AT$_2$ receptors also may mediate vasodilatory responses, since mice lacking the AT$_2$ gene have higher blood pressures than wild-type littermates.[186,187] Therefore, AT$_1$ and AT$_2$ receptors may be mutually antagonistic, with AT$_1$ promoting vasoconstriction, growth, and tissue remodeling and AT$_2$ mediating vasodilitation and growth inhibition.

AT$_2$ Signaling

As mentioned previously, AT$_2$ receptors are also seven-transmembrane G-protein–coupled receptors; to date, the predominant G-protein subtype to which they have been shown to be coupled is the pertussis toxin-sensitive Gα_i.[188–190] In addition, a major mechanism of AT$_2$-mediated cellular responses appears to be activation of protein tyrosine phosphatases that inactivate MAP kinases.[191–193] The serine/threonine phosphatase 2A (PP2A) also has been reported to be activated by AT$_2$ receptor activation.[190,194,195] AT$_2$ receptor activation increases production of nitric oxide in kidney[196,197] and microvessels.[198] Furthermore, in the afferent arteriole, activation of the AT$_2$ receptor may cause endothelium-dependent vasodilatation via a cytochrome P-450 pathway, possibly mediated by EETs.[199]

■ *Conclusion*

Angiotensin II plays a central role in physiologic and pathophysiologic regulation of a broad range of vascular and nonvascular tissues. Our knowledge of the array of signaling events and cellular effects of angiotensin II has expanded greatly in the past decade. We will learn even more in the coming years about its role in hypertrophic and hyperplastic growth and the interaction of angiotensin II receptor subtypes in the mediation of the peptide's biologic effects.

Acknowledgments

This work was supported by funds from the Veterans Administration and National Institutes of Health Grant DK51265.

References

1. Murphy TJ, Alexander RW, Griendling KK, et al: Isolation of a cDNA encoding the vascular type-1 angiotensin II receptor. Nature 351:233–236, 1991.
2. Sasaki K, Yamano Y, Bardhan S, et al: Cloning and expression of a cDNA encoding a bovine adrenal angiotensin II type-1 receptor. Nature 351: 230–233, 1991.
3. Kambayashi Y, Bardhan S, Takahashi K, et al: Molecular cloning of a novel angiotensin II receptor isoform involved in phosphotyrosine phosphatase inhibition. J Biol Chem 268:24543–24546, 1993.
4. Mukoyama M, Nakajima M, Horiuchi M, et al: Expression cloning of type 2 angiotensin II receptor reveals a unique class of seven-transmembrane receptors. J Biol Chem 268:24539–24542, 1993.

5. Gether U, Kobilka BK: G protein-coupled receptors: II. Mechanism of agonist activation. J Biol Chem 273:17979–17982, 1998.

6. Pitcher JA, Freedman NJ, Lefkowitz RJ: G protein-coupled receptor kinases. Annu Rev Biochem 67:653–692, 1998.

7. Dolphin AC: L-type calcium channel modulation. Adv Second Messenger Phosphoprotein Res 33:153–177, 1999.

8. Hughes AD: Molecular and cellular mechanisms of action of angiotensin II (AT1) receptors in vascular smooth muscle. J Hum Hypertens 12:275–281, 1998.

9. van Bilsen M: Signal transduction revisited: Recent developments in angiotensin II signaling in the cardiovascular system. Cardiovasc Res 36:310–322, 1997.

10. Macrez N, Morel JL, Kalkbrenner F, et al: A betagamma dimer derived from G13 transduces the angiotensin AT1 receptor signal to stimulation of Ca2+ channels in rat portal vein myocytes. J Biol Chem 272:23180–23185, 1997.

11. Sayeski PP, Ali MS, Semeniuk DJ, et al: Angiotensin II signal transduction pathways. Regul Pept 78:19–29, 1998.

12. Ohyama K, Yamano Y, Chaki S, et al: Domains for G-protein coupling in angiotensin II receptor type I:studies by site-directed mutagenesis. Biochem Biophys Res Commun 189:677–683, 1992.

13. Conchon S, Barrault MB, Miserey S, et al: The C-terminal third intracellular loop of the rat AT1A angiotensin receptor plays a key role in G protein coupling specificity and transduction of the mitogenic signal. J Biol Chem 272:25566–25572, 1997.

14. Wang C, Jayadev S, Escobedo JA: Identification of a domain in the angiotensin II type 1 receptor determining Gq coupling by the use of receptor chimeras. J Biol Chem 270:16677–16682, 1995.

15. Sano T, Ohyama K, Yamano Y, et al: A domain for G protein coupling in carboxyl-terminal tail of rat angiotensin II receptor type 1A. J Biol Chem 272:23631–23636, 1997.

16. Oppermann M, Freedman NJ, Alexander RW, Lefkowitz RK: Phosphorylation of the type 1A angiotensin II receptor by G protein-coupled receptor kinases and protein kinase C. J Biol Chem 271:13266–13272, 1996.

17. Thomas WG, Baker KM, Booz GW, Thekkumkara TJ: Evidence against a role for protein kinase C in the regulation of the angiotensin II (AT1A) receptor. Eur J Pharmacol 295:119–122, 1996.

18. Sasamura H, Dzau VJ, Pratt RE: Desensitization of angiotensin receptor function. Kidney Int 46:1499–1501, 1994.

19. Tang H, Guo DF, Porter JP, et al: Role of cytoplasmic tail of the type 1A angiotensin II receptor in agonist- and phorbol ester-induced desensitization. Circ Res 82:523–531, 1998.

20. Tang H, Shirai H, Inagami T: Inhibition of protein kinase C prevents rapid desensitization of type 1B angiotensin II receptor. Circ Res 77:239–248, 1995.

21. Balla T, Varnai P, Tian Y, Smith RD: Signaling events activated by angiotensin II receptors: What goes before and after the calcium signals. Endocr Res 24:335–344, 1998.

22. Horowitz A, Menice CB, Laporte R, Morgan KG: Mechanisms of smooth muscle contraction. Physiol Rev 76: 967–1003, 1996.

23. Kureishi Y, Kobayashi S, Amano M, et al: Rho-associated kinase directly induces smooth muscle contraction through myosin light chain phosphorylation. J Biol Chem 272:12257–12260, 1997.

24. Ashida T, Schaeffer J, Goldman WF, et al: Role of sarcoplasmic reticulum in arterial contraction: comparison of ryanodines's effect in a conduit and a muscular artery. Circ Res 62:854–863, 1988.

25. Garcha RS, Hughes AD: Inhibition of norepinephrine and caffeine-induced activation by ryanodine and thapsigargin in rat mesenteric arteries. J Cardiovasc Pharmacol 25:840–846, 1995.

26. Ardaillou R, Chansel D, Chatziantoniou C, Dussaule JC: Mesangial AT1 receptors: expression, signaling, and regulation. J Am Soc Nephrol, 10:S40–S46, 1999.

27. Murasawa S, Mori Y, Nozawa Y, et al: Role of calcium-sensitive tyrosine kinase Pyk2/CAKbeta/RAFTK in angiotensin II induced Ras/ERK signaling. Hypertension 32:668–675, 1998.

28. Hughes AD, Bolton TB: Action of angiotensin II, 5-hydroxytryptamine and adenosine triphosphate on ionic currents in single ear artery cells of the rabbit. Br J Pharmacol 116:2148–2154, 1995.

29. Clement-Chomienne O, Walsh MP, Cole WC: Angiotensin II activation of protein kinase C decreases delayed rectifier K+ current in rabbit vascular myocytes. J Physiol (Lond) 495:689–700, 1996.

30. Kubo M, Quayle JM, Standen NB: Angiotensin II inhibition of ATP-sensitive K+ currents in rat arterial smooth muscle cells through protein kinase C. J Physiol (Lond) 503:489–496, 1997.

31. Miyoshi Y, Nakaya Y: Angiotensin II blocks ATP-sensitive K+ channels in porcine coronary artery smooth muscle cells. Biochem Biophys Res Commun 181:700–706, 1991.

32. Minami K, Hirata Y, Tokumura A, et al: Protein kinase C-independent inhibition of the Ca(2+)-activated K+ channel by angiotensin II and endothelin-1. Biochem Pharmacol 49:1051–1056, 1995.

33. Ling BN, Seal EE, Eaton DC: Regulation of mesangial cell ion channels by insulin and angiotensin II. Possible role in diabetic glomerular hyperfiltration. J Clin Invest 92:2141–2151, 1993.

34. White CR, Elton TS, Shoemaker RL, Brock TA: Calcium-sensitive chloride channels in vascular smooth muscle cells. Proc Soc Exp Biol Med 208:255–262, 1995.

35. Carmines PK: Segment-specific effect of chloride channel blockade on rat renal arteriolar contractile responses to angiotensin II. Am J Hypertens 8:90–94, 1995.

36. Mellor H, Parker PJ: The extended protein kinase C superfamily. Biochem J 332:281–292, 1998.

37. Newton AC: Protein kinase C: Structure, function, and regulation. J Biol Chem 270:28495–28498, 1995.

38. Freeman EJ, Tallant EA: Vascular smooth-muscle cells contain AT1 angiotensin receptors coupled to phospholipase D activation. Biochem J 304:543–548, 1994.

39. Shinoda J, Kozawa O, Suzuki A, et al: Mechanism of angiotensin II-induced arachidonic acid metabolite release in aortic smooth muscle cells: Involvement of phospholipase D. Eur J Endocrinol 136:207–212, 1997.

40. Ushio-Fukai M, Alexander RW, Akers M, et al: Angiotensin II receptor coupling to phospholipase D is mediated by the betagamma subunits of heterotrimeric G proteins in vascular smooth muscle cells. Mol Pharmacol 55:142–149, 1999.

41. Duff JL, Marrero MB, Paxton WG, et al: Angiotensin II signal transduction and the mitogen-activated protein kinase pathway. Card Res 30:511–517, 1995.

42. Bouron A, Soldatov NM, Reuter H: The beta 1-subunit is essential for modulation by protein kinase C of an human and a non-human L-type Ca2+ channel. FEBS Lett 377:159–162, 1995.

43. Maturana AD, Casal AJ, Demaurex N, et al: Angiotensin II negatively modulates L-type calcium channels through a pertussis toxin-sensitive G protein in adrenal glomerulosa cells. J Biol Chem 274:19943–19948, 1999.

44. Weerackody RP, Chatterjee PK, Mistry SK, et al: Selective antagonism of the AT1 receptor inhibits the effect of angiotensin II on DNA and protein synthesis of rat proximal tubular cells. Exp Nephrol 5:253–262, 1997.

45. Okuda M, Kawahara Y, Yokoyama M: Angiotensin II type 1 receptor-mediated activation of Ras in cultured rat vascular smooth muscle cells. Am J Physiol 271:H595–H601, 1996.

46. Cogan MG: Angiotensin II: A powerful controller of sodium transport in the early proximal tubule. Hypertension 15:451–458, 1990.

47. Schuster VL, Kokko JP, Jacobson HR: Angiotensin II directly stimulates sodium transport in rabbit proximal convoluted tubules. J Clin Invest 73:507–515, 1984.

48. Liu F-Y CM: Angiotensin II stimulates early proximal bicarbonate reabsorption in the rat by decreasing cyclic adenosin monophosphate. J Clin Invest 84:83–91, 1989.

49. Liu FY, Cogan MG: Angiotensin II: A potent regulator of acidification in the rat early proximal convoluted tubule. J Clin Invest 80:272–275, 1987.

50. Douglas J, Romero M: Signaling mechanisms coupled to the angiotensin receptor of proximal tubule epithelium. Kidney Int 38:S-43–S-47, 1990.

51. Lamprecht G, Weinman AJ, Yun CH: The role of NHERF and E3KARP in the cAMP-mediated inhibition of NHE3. J Biol Chem 273:29972–29978, 1998.

52. Aperia A, Holtback U, Syren ML, et al: Activation/deactivation of renal Na+,K(+)-ATPase: a final common pathway for regulation of natriuresis. FASEB J 8:436–439, 1994.

53. Bharatula M, Hussain T, Lokhandwala MF: Angiotensin II AT1 receptor/signaling mechanisms in the biphasic effect of the peptide on proximal tubular Na+,K+-ATPase. Clin Exp Hypertens 20:465–480, 1998.

54. Ruiz OS, Qiu YY, Wang LJ, Arruda JA: Regulation of the renal Na-HCO3 cotransporter: IV. Mechanisms of the stimulatory effect of angiotensin II. J A S N 6: 1202–1208, 1995.

55. Burns KD, Inagami T, Harris RC: Cloning of a rabbit kidney cortex AT1 angiotensin II receptor that is present in proximal tubule epithelium. Am J Physiol 264:F645–F654, 1993.

56. Becker BN, Cheng HF, Burns KD, Harris RC: Polarized rabbit type 1 angiotensin II receptors manifest differential rates of endocytosis and recycling. Am J Physiol 269:C1048–C1056, 1995.

57. Baum M, Quigley R, Quan A: Effect of luminal angiotensin II on rabbit proximal convoluted tubule bicarbonate absorption. Am J Physiol 273:F595–F600, 1997.

58. Smith RD, Baukal AJ, Dent P, Catt KJ: Raf-1 kinase activation by angiotensin II in adrenal glomerulosa cells: roles of Gi, phosphatidylinositol 3-kinase, and Ca2+ influx. Endocrinology 140:1385–1391, 1999.

59. Karim Z, Defontaine N, Paillard M, Poggioli J: Protein kinase C isoforms in rat kidney proximal tubule: acute effect of angiotensin II. Am J Physiol 269:C134–C140, 1995.

60. Wang T, Chang Y: Time-and dose-dependent effects of protein kinase C on proximal bicarbonate transport. J Membrane Biol 117:131–139, 1990.

61. Liu F-Y, Cogan MG: Role of protein kinase C in proximal bicarbonate absorption and angiotensin signaling. Am J Physiol 258:F927–F933, 1989.

62. Harris P, et al: Dose-dependent stimulation and inhibition of proximal tubular sodium reabsorption by angiotensin II in the rat kidney. Pflugers Arch 367:295–297, 1977.

63. Chatsudthipong V, Chan YL: Inhibitory effect of angiotensin II on renal tubular transport. Am J Physiol 260:F340–F346, 1991.

64. Madhun ZT, Goldthwait DA, McKay D, et al: An epoxygenase metabolite of arachidonic acid mediates angiotensin II-induced rises in cytosolic calcium in rabbit proximal tubule epithelial cells. J Clin Invest 88:456–461, 1991.

65. Darnell JE Jr: Studies of IFN-induced transcriptional activation uncover the Jak-Stat pathway. J Interferon Cytokine Res 18:549–554, 1998.

66. Hollenberg MD: Tyrosine kinase-mediated signal transduction pathways and the actions of polypeptide growth factors and G-protein-coupled agonists in smooth muscle. Mol Cell Biochem 149–150: 77–85, 1995.

67. Toma C, Jensen PE, Prieto D, et al: Effects of tyrosine kinase inhibitors on the contractility of rat mesenteric resistance arteries. Br J Pharmacol 114:1266–1272, 1995.

68. Di Salvo J, Nelson SR, Kaplan N: Protein tyrosine phosphorylation in smooth muscle: a potential coupling mechanism between receptor activation and intracellular calcium. Proc Soc Exp Biol Med 214:285–301, 1997.

69. Malloy LG, Sauro MD: Tyrosine kinase inhibition suppresses angiotensin contraction in hypertensive and normotensive small resistance arteries. Life Sci 58:PL317–PL324, 1996.

70. Griendling KK, Ushio-Fukai M, Lassegue B, Alexander RW: Angiotensin II signaling in vascular smooth muscle. New concepts. Hypertension 29:366–373, 1997.

71. Linseman DA, Benjamin CW, Jones DA: Convergence of angiotensin II and platelet-derived growth factor receptor signaling cascades in vascular smooth muscle cells. J Biol Chem 270:12563–12568, 1995.

72. Polte TR, Naftilan AJ, Hanks SK: Focal adhesion kinase is abundant in developing blood vessels and elevation of its phosphotyrosine content in vascular smooth muscle cells is a rapid response to angiotensin II. J Cell Biochem 55:106–119, 1994.

73. Kondo S, Becker BN, Homma T, et al: Involvement of calcium and protein kinase C in the signal transduction pathway of p125FAK and paxillin tyrosine phosphorylation by cyclical stretch/relaxation in cultured rat mesangial cells. JASN 7:1680A 1996.

74. Leduc I, Meloche S: Angiotensin II stimulates tyrosine phosphorylation of the focal adhesion-associated protein paxillin in aortic smooth muscle cells. J Biol Chem 270:4401–4404, 1995.

75. Li X, Earp HS: Paxillin is tyrosine-phosphorylated by and preferentially associates with the calcium-dependent tyrosine kinase in rat liver epithelial cells. J Biol Chem 272:14341–14348, 1997.

76. Marrero MB, Schieffer B, Paxton WG, et al: Direct stimulation of Jak/STAT pathway by the angiotensin II AT1 receptor. Nature 375:247–250, 1995.

77. Marrero MB, Paxton WG, Duff JL, et al: Angiotensin II stimulates tyrosine phosphorylation of phospholipase C-gamma 1 in vascular smooth muscle cells. J Biol Chem 269:10935–10939, 1994.

78. Marrero MB, Schieffer B, Ma H, et al: ANG II-induced tyrosine phosphorylation stimulates phospholipase C-gamma 1 and Cl-channels in mesangial cells. Am J Physiol 270:C1834– C1842, 1996.

79. Ali MS, Schieffer B, Delafontaine P, et al: Angiotensin II stimulates tyrosine phosphorylation and activation of insulin receptor substrate 1 and protein-tyrosine phosphatase 1D in vascular smooth muscle cells. J Biol Chem 272:12373–12379, 1997.

80. Duff JL, Marrero MB, Paxton WG, et al: Angiotensin II induces 3CH134, a protein-tyrosine phosphatase, in vascular smooth muscle cells. J Biol Chem 268:26037–26040, 1993.

81. Marrero MB, Venema VJ, Ju H, et al: Regulation of angiotensin II-induced JAK2 tyrosine phosphorylation: roles of SHP-1 and SHP-2. Am J Physiol 275:C1216–C1223, 1998.

82. Venema RC, Venema VJ, Eaton DC, Marrero MB: Angiotensin II-induced tyrosine phosphorylation of signal transducers and activators of transcription 1 is regulated by Janus-activated kinase 2 and Fyn kinases and mitogen-activated protein kinase phosphatase 1. J Biol Chem 273:30795–30800, 1998.

83. Eguchi S, Iwasaki H, Inagami T, et al: Involvement of PYK2 in angiotensin II signaling of vascular smooth muscle cells. Hypertension 33:201–206, 1999.

84. Murasawa S, Mori Y, Nozawa Y, et al: Role of calcium-sensitive tyrosine kinase Pyk2/CAKbeta/RAFTK in angiotensin II induced Ras/ERK signaling. Hypertension 32:668–675, 1998.

85. Yu H, Li X, Marchetto GS, et al:Activation of a novel calcium-dependent protein-tyrosine kinase. Correlation with c-Jun N-terminal kinase but not mitogen-activated protein kinase activation. J Biol Chem 271:29993–29998, 1996.

86. Lev S, Moreno H, Martinez R, et al: Protein tyrosine kinase PYK2 involved in Ca(2+)-induced regulation of ion channel and MAP kinase functions. Nature 376:737–745, 1995.

87. Brinson AE, Harding T, Diliberto PA, et al: Regulation of a calcium-dependent tyrosine kinase in vascular smooth muscle cells by angiotensin II and platelet-derived growth factor. Dependence on calcium and the actin cytoskeleton. J Biol Chem 273:1711–1718, 1998.

88. Schieffer B, Bernstein KE, Marrero MB: The role of tyrosine phosphorylation in angiotensin II mediated intracellular signaling and cell growth. J Mol Medicine 74:85–91, 1996.

89. Ishida M, Marrero MB, Schieffer B, et al: Angiotensin II activates pp60c-src in vascular smooth muscle cells. Circ Res 77:1053–1059, 1995.

90. Ishida M, Ishida T, Thomas SM, Berk BC: Activation of extracellular signal-regulated kinases (ERK1/2) by angiotensin II is dependent on c-Src in vascular smooth muscle cells. Circ Res 82:7–12, 1998.

91. Eguchi S, Numaguchi K, Iwasaki H, et al: Calcium-dependent epidermal growth factor receptor transactivation mediates the angiotensin II-induced mitogen-activated protein kinase activation in vascular smooth muscle cells. J Biol Chem 273:8890–8896, 1998.

92. Venema RC, Ju H, Venema VJ, et al: Angiotensin II-induced association of phospholipase Cgamma1 with the G-protein-coupled AT1 receptor. J Biol Chem 273:7703–7708, 1998.

93. Sadoshima J, Izumo S: The heterotrimeric G q protein-coupled angiotensin II receptor activates p21 ras via the tyrosine kinase-Shc-Grb2-Sos pathway in cardiac myocytes. EMBO J 15:775–787, 1996.

94. Schieffer B, Paxton WG, Chai Q, et al: Angiotensin II controls p21ras activity via pp60c-src. J Biol Chem 271:10329–10333, 1996.

95. Schieffer B, Drexler H, Ling BN, Marrero MB: G protein-coupled receptors control vascular smooth muscle cell proliferation via pp60c-src and p21ras. Am J Physiol 272:C2019–C2130, 1997.

96. Marrero MB, Schieffer B, Paxton WG, et al: Electroporation of pp60c-src antibodies inhibits the angiotensin II activation of phospholipase C-gamma 1 in rat aortic smooth muscle cells. J Biol Chem 270:15734–15738, 1995.

97. Marrero MB, Schieffer B, Ma H, et al: ANG II-induced tyrosine phosphorylation stimulates phospholipase C-gamma 1 and Cl-channels in mesangial cells. Am J Physiol 270:C1834–C1842, 1996.

98. Schelling JR, Nkemere N, Konieczkowski M, et al: Angiotensin II activates the beta 1 isoform of phospholipase C in vascular smooth muscle cells. Am J Physiol 272:C1558–C1566, 1997.

99. Ushio-Fukai M, Griendling KK, Akers M, et al: Temporal dispersion of activation of phospholipase C-beta1 and -gamma isoforms by angiotensin II in vascular smooth muscle cells. Role of alphaq/11, alpha12, and beta gamma G protein subunits. J Biol Chem 273:19772–19777, 1998.

100. Freeman EJ, Chisolm GM, Tallant EA: Role of calcium and protein kinase C in the activation of phospholipase D by angiotensin II in vascular smooth cells. Arch Biochem Biophys 319:84–92, 1995.

101. Suzuki A, Shinoda J, Oiso Y, Kozawa O: Tyrosine kinase is involved in angiotensin II-stimulated phospholipase D activation in aortic smooth muscle cells: Function of Ca2+ influx. Atherosclerosis 121:119–127, 1996.

102. Zou Y, Komuro I, Yamazaki T, et al: Cell type-specific angiotensin II-evoked signal transduction pathways: critical roles of Gbetagamma subunit, Src family, and Ras in cardiac fibroblasts. Circ Res 82:337–345, 1998.

103. Schieffer B, Paxton WG, Chai Q, et al: Angiotensin II controls p21ras activity via pp60c-src. J Biol Chem 271:10329–10333, 1996.

104. Sadoshima J, Izumo S: The heterotrimeric G q protein-coupled angiotensin II receptor activates p21 ras via the tyrosine kinase-Shc-Grb2-Sos pathway in cardiac myocytes. Embo J 15:775–787, 1996.

105. Sayeski PP, Ali MS, Harp JB, et al: Phosphorylation of p130Cas by angiotensin II is dependent on c-Src, intracellular Ca2+, and protein kinase C [see comments]. Circ Res 82:1279–1288, 1998.

106. Tsuganezawa H, Preisig PA, Alpern RJ: Dominant negative c-Src inhibits angiotensin II induced activation of NHE3 in OKP cells. Kidney Int 54:394–398, 1998.

107. Aringer M, Cheng A, Nelson JW, et al: Janus kinases and their role in growth and disease. Life Sci 64:2173–2186, 1999.

108. Shuai K: The STAT family of proteins in cytokine signaling. Prog Biophys Mol Biol 71:405–422, 1999.

109. Marrero MB, Schieffer B, Li B, et al: Role of Janus kinase/signal transducer and activator of transcription and mitogen-activated protein kinase cascades in angiotensin II- and platelet-derived growth factor-induced vascular smooth muscle cell proliferation. J Biol Chem 272:24684–24690, 1997.

110. McWhinney CD, Hunt RA, Conrad KM, et al: The type I angiotensin II receptor couples to Stat1 and Stat3 activation through Jak2 kinase in neonatal rat cardiac myocytes. J Mol Cell Cardiol 29:2513–2524, 1997.

111. Liang H, Venema VJ, Wang X, et al: Regulation of angiotensin II-induced phosphorylation of STAT3 in vascular smooth muscle cells. J Biol Chem 274:19846–19851, 1999.

112. Bhat GJ, Thekkumkara TJ, Thomas WG, et al: Activation of the STAT pathway by angiotensin II in T3CHO/AT1A cells. Cross-talk between angiotensin II and interleukin-6 nuclear signaling. J Biol Chem, 270:19059–19065, 1995.

113. Ali MS, Sayeski PP, Dirksen LB, et al: Dependence on the motif YIPP for the physical association of Jak2 kinase with the intracellular carboxyl tail of the angiotensin II AT1 receptor. J Biol Chem 272:23382–23388, 1997.

114. Shikata Y, Shikata K, Matsuda M, et al: Signaling transduction pathway of angiotensin II in human mesangial cells: mediation of focal adhesion and GTPase activating proteins. Biochem Biophys Res Commun 257:234-238, 1999.

115. Polte TR, Hanks SK: Complexes of focal adhesion kinase (FAK) and Crk-associated substrate (p130(Cas)) are elevated in cytoskeleton-associated fractions following adhesion and Src transformation. Requirements for Src kinase activity and FAK proline-rich motifs. J Biol Chem 272:5501–5509, 1997.

116. Luttrell LM, Della Rocca GJ, van Biesen T, et al: G betagamma subunits mediate Src-dependent phosphorylation of the epidermal growth factor receptor. A scaffold for G protein-coupled receptor-mediated Ras activation. J Biol Chem 272:4637–4644, 1997.

117. Moriguchi Y, Matsubara H, Mori Y, et al: Angiotensin II-induced transactivation of epidermal growth factor receptor regulates fibronectin and transforming growth factor-beta synthesis via transcriptional and posttranscriptional mechanisms. Circ Res 84:1073–1084, 1999.

118. Balsinde J, Balboa MA, Insel PA, Dennis EA: Regulation and inhibition of phospholipase A2. Annu Rev Pharmacol Toxicol 39:175–189, 1999.

119. Lin LL, Wartmann M, Lin AY, et al: cPLA2 is phosphorylated and activated by MAP kinase. Cell 72:269–278, 1993.

120. Shinoda J, Kozawa O, Suzuki A, et al: Mechanism of angiotensin II-induced arachidonic acid metabolite release in aortic smooth muscle cells: Involvement of phospholipase D. Eur J Endocrin 136:207–212, 1997.

121. Needleman P, Turk J, Jakschik BA, et al: Arachidonic acid metabolism. Annu Rev Biochem 55:69–102, 1986.

122. Schramek H, Coroneos E, Dunn MJ: Interactions of the vasoconstrictor peptides, angiotensin II and endothelin-1, with vasodilatory prostaglandins. Semin Nephrol 15:195–204, 1995.

123. Becker BN, Cheng HF, Harris RC: Apical ANG II-stimulated PLA2 activity and Na+ flux: A potential role for Ca2+-independent PLA2. Am J Physiol 273:F554–F562, 1997.

124. Morduchowicz GA, Sheikh-Hamad D, Dwyer BE, et al: Angiotensin II directly increases rabbit renal brush-border membrane sodium transport: presence of local signal transduction system. J Membrane Biol 122:43–53, 1991.

125. Romero MF, Madhun ZT, Hopfer U, Douglas JG: An epoxygenase metabolite of arachidonic acid 5,6 epoxy-eicosatrienoic acid mediates angiotensin-induced natriuresis in proximal tubular epithelium. Adv Prostaglandin Thromboxane Leukotriene Res 21A:205–208, 1991.

126. Omata K, Abraham NG, Schwartzman ML: Renal cytochrome P-450-arachidonic acid metabolism: localization and hormonal regulation in SHR. Am J Physiol 262:F591–F599, 1992.

127. Muthalif M, Benter IF, Karzoun N, et al: 20-Hydroxyeicosatetraenoic acid mediates calcium/calmodulin-dependent protein kinase II-induced mitogen-activated protein kinase activation in vascular smooth muscle cells. Proc Natl Acad Sci U S A 95:12701–12706, 1998.

128. Wang T, Chan Y: Mechanism of angiotensin II action on proximal tubular transport. J Pharmacol Exp Ther 252:689–695, 1990.

129. Reilly AM, Harris PJ, Williams DA: Biphasic effect of angiotensin II on intracellular sodium concentration in rat proximal tubules. Am J Physiol 269:F374–F380, 1995.

130. Li L, Wang YP, Capparell AW, et al: Effect of luminal angiotensin II on proximal tubule fluid transport: role of apical phospholipase A2. Am J Physiol 266:F202–F209, 1994.

131. Ushio-Fukai M, Alexander RW, Akers M, Griendling KK: p38 Mitogen-activated protein kinase is a critical component of the redox-sensitive signaling pathways activated by angiotensin II. Role in vascular smooth muscle cell hypertrophy. J Biol Chem 273:15022–15029, 1998.

132. Fukui T, Ishizaka N, Rajagopalan S, et al: p22phox mRNA expression and NADPH oxidase activity are increased in aortas from hypertensive rats. Circ Res 80:45–51, 1997.

133. Griendling KK, Rittenhouse SE, Brock TA, et al: Sustained diacylglycerol formation from inositol phospholipids in angiotensin II-stimulated vascular smooth muscle cells. J Biol Chem 261:5901–5906, 1986.

134. Delafontaine P, et al: Potassium depletion selectively inhibits sustained diacylglycerol formation from phospatidylinositol in angiotensin II-stimulated smooth muscles. J Biol Chem 262:14549–14554, 1987.

135. Anderson KM, Peach MJ: Receptor binding and internalization of a unique biologically active angiotensin II-colloidal gold conjugate: morphological analysis of angiotensin II processing in isolated vascular strips. J Vascular Res 31:10–17, 1994.

136. Zhang J, Ferguson SSG, Barak LS, et al: Dynamin and beta-arrestin reveal distinct mechanisms for G protein-coupled receptor internalization. J Biol Chem 271:18302–18305, 1996.
137. Ishizaka N, Griendling KK, Lassegue B, Alexander RW: Angiotensin II type 1 receptor: relationship with caveolae and caveolin after initial agonist stimulation. Hypertension 32:459–466, 1998.
138. Schelling JR, Hanson AS, Marzec R, Linas SL: Cytoskeleton-dependent endocytosis is required for apical type 1 angiotensin II receptor-mediated phospholipase C activation in cultured rat proximal tubule cells. J Clin Invest 90:2472–2480, 1992.
139. Schelling JR, Linas SL: Angiotensin II-dependent proximal tubule sodium transport requires receptor-mediated endocytosis. Am J Physiol 266:C669–C675, 1994.
140. van Kats JP, de Lannoy LM, Jan Danser AH, et al: Angiotensin II type 1 (AT1) receptor-mediated accumulation of angiotensin II in tissues and its intracellular half-life in vivo. Hypertension 30:42–49, 1997.
141. Navar LG, Harrison-Bernard LM, Imig JD, et al: Intrarenal angiotensin II generation and renal effects of AT1 receptor blockade. J Am Soc Nephrol 10:S266–S272, 1999.
142. Zou LX, Imig JD, Hymel A, Navar LG: Renal uptake of circulating angiotensin II in Val5-angiotensin II infused rats is mediated by AT1 receptor. Am J Hypertens 11:570–578, 1998.
143. Zou L-X, Imig JD, Von Thun AM, et al: Receptor-mediated intrarenal angiotensin II augmentation in angiotensin II-infused rats. Hypertension 28:669–677, 1996.
144. Robertson AL, Khairallah PA: Angiotensin II: rapid localization in nuclei of smooth and cardiac muscle. Science 172:52–53, 1971.
145. Re RN, Parab M: Effects of angiotensin II on RNA synthesis in isolated nuclei. Life Sci 34:647–651, 1984.
146. Eggena P, Zhu JH, Clegg K, Barrett JD: Nuclear angiotensin receptors induce transcription of renin and angiotensinogen mRNA. Hypertension 22:496–501, 1993.
147. Eggena P, Zhu JH, Sereevinyayut S, et al: Hepatic angiotensin II nuclear receptors and transcription of growth-related factors. J. Hypertension 14:961–968, 1996.
148. Haller H, Lindschau C, Quass P, et al: Nuclear calcium signaling is initiated by cytosolic calcium surges in vascular smooth muscle cells. Kidney Int 46:1653–1662, 1994.
149. Burnier M, Centeno G, Burki E, Brunner HR: Confocal microscopy to analyze cytosolic and nuclear calcium in cultured vascular cells. Am J Physiol 266:C1118–C1127, 1994.
150. Tang SS, Rogg H, Schumacher R, Dzau VJ: Characterization of nuclear angiotensin-II-binding sites in rat liver and comparison with plasma membrane receptors. Endocrinology 131:374–380, 1992.
151. Lu D, Yang H, Shaw G, Raizada MK: Angiotensin II-induced nuclear targeting of the angiotensin type 1 (AT1) receptor in brain neurons. Endocrinology 139:365–375, 1998.
152. Haller H, Lindschau C, Erdmann B, et al: Effects of intracellular angiotensin II in vascular smooth muscle cells. Circ Res 79:765–772, 1996.
153. Kapas S, Hinson JP, Puddefoot JR, et al: Internalization of the type I angiotensin II receptor (AT1) is required for protein kinase C activation but not for inositol trisphosphate release in the angiotensin II stimulated rat adrenal zona glomerulosa cell. Biochem Biophys Res Commun 204:1292–1298, 1994.
154. Lassegue B, Alexander RW, Clark M, Griendling KK: Angiotensin II-induced phosphatidylcholine hydrolysis in cultured vascular smooth-muscle cells. Regulation and localization. Biochem J 276:19–25, 1991.
155. Rosenberg ME, Hostetter TH: Effect of angiotensin II and norepinephrine on early growth response genes in the rat kidney. Kidney Int 43:601–609, 1993.
156. Neyses L, Nouskas J, Luyken J, et al: Induction of immediate-early genes by angiotensin II and endothelin-1 in adult rat cardiomyocytes. J Hypertens 11:927–934, 1993.
157. Wolf G, Killen PD, Neilson EG: Intracellular signaling of transcription and secretion of type IV collagen after angiotensin II-induced cellular hypertrophy in cultured proximal tubular cells. Cell Regul 2:219–227, 1991.
158. Tamura K, Nyui N, Tamura N, et al: Mechanism of angiotensin II-mediated regulation of fibronectin gene in rat vascular smooth muscle cells. J Biol Chem 273:26487–26496, 1998.
159. Naftilan AJ, Pratt RE, Dzau VJ: Induction of platelet-derived growth factor A-chain and c-myc gene expressions by angiotensin II in cultured rat vascular smooth muscle cells. J Clin Invest 83:1419–1424, 1989.
160. Wang DH, Prewitt RL, Beebe SJ: Regulation of PDGF-A: A possible mechanism for angiotensin II-induced vascular growth. Am J Physiol 269: H356–H364, 1995.
161. Gibbons GH, Pratt RE, Dzau VJ: Vascular smooth muscle cell hypertrophy vs. hyperplasia. Autocrine transforming growth factor-beta 1 expression determines growth response to angiotensin II. J Clin Invest 90:456–461, 1992.
162. Koibuchi Y, Lee WS, Gibbons GH, Pratt RE: Role of transforming growth factor-beta 1 in the cellular growth response to angiotensin II. Hypertension 21:1046–1050, 1993.

163. Kagami S, Border WA, Miller DE, Noble NA: Angiotensin II stimulates extracellular matrix protein synthesis through induction of transforming growth factor-beta expression in rat glomerular mesangial cells. J Clin Invest 93:2431–2437, 1994.

164. Eddy AA: Protein restriction reduces transforming growth factor-beta and interstitial fibrosis in nephrotic syndrome. Am J Physiol 266: F884–F893, 1994.

165. Kai T, Kino H, Sugimura K, et al: Significant role of the increase in renin-angiotensin system in cardiac hypertrophy and renal glomerular sclerosis in double transgenic tsukuba hypertensive mice carrying both human renin and angiotensinogen genes. Clin Exp Hypertension 20:439–449, 1998.

166. Kai T, Kino H, Ishikawa K: Role of the renin-angiotensin system in cardiac hypertrophy and renal glomerular sclerosis in transgenic hypertensive mice carrying both human renin and angiotensinogen genes. Hypertens Res 21:39–46, 1998.

167. Daemen MJ, Lombardi DM, Bosman FT, Schwartz SM: Angiotensin II induces smooth muscle cell proliferation in the normal and injured rat arterial wall. Circ Res 68:450–456, 1991.

168. deBlois D, Viswanathan M, Su JE, et al: Smooth muscle DNA replication in response to angiotensin II is regulated differently in the neointima and media at different times after balloon injury in the rat carotid artery. Role of AT1 receptor expression. Arterioscler Thromb Vasc Biol 16:1130–1137, 1996.

169. Geisterfer AA, Peach MJ, Owens GK: Angiotensin II induces hypertrophy, not hyperplasia, of cultured rat aortic smooth muscle cells. Circ Res 62:749–756, 1988.

170. Wolf G, Eg N: Angiotension II induces cellular hypertrophy in cultured murine proximal tubular cells. Am J Physiol 259:F768–F777, 1990.

171. Harris RC: Regulation of S6 kinase activity in renal proximal tubule. Am J Physiol 263:F127–F134, 1992.

172. Burns KD, Harris RC: Signaling and growth responses of LLC-PK1/Cl4 cells transfected with the rabbit AT1 ANG II receptor. Am J Physiol 268:C925–C935, 1995.

173. Chatterjee PK, Weerackody RP, Mistry SK, et al: Selective antagonism of the AT1 receptor inhibits angiotensin II stimulated DNA and protein synthesis in primary cultures of human proximal tubular cells. Kidney Int 52:699–705, 1997.

174. Wolf G, Stahl RA: Angiotensin II-stimulated hypertrophy of LLC-PK1 cells depends on the induction of the cyclin-dependent kinase inhibitor p27Kip1. Kidney Int 50:2112–2119, 1996.

175. Hannken T, Schroeder R, Stahl RA, Wolf G: Angiotensin II-mediated expression of p27Kip1 and induction of cellular hypertrophy in renal tubular cells depend on the generation of oxygen radicals [see comments]. Kidney Int 54:1923–1933, 1998.

176. Nakajima M, Hutchinson HG, Fujinaga M, et al: The angiotensin II type 2 (AT2) receptor antagonizes the growth effects of the AT1 receptor: gain-of-function study using gene transfer. Proc Natl Acad Sci U S A 92:10663–10667, 1995.

177. Horiuchi M, Akishita M, Dzau VJ: Recent progress in angiotensin II type 2 receptor research in the cardiovascular system. Hypertension 33:613–621, 1999.

178. Aguilera G, Kapur S, Feuillan P, et al: Developmental changes in angiotensin II receptor subtypes and AT1 receptor mRNA in rat kidney. Kidney Int 46:973–979, 1994.

179. Norwood VF, Craig MR, Harris JM, Gomez RA: Differential expression of angiotensin II receptors during early renal morphogenesis. Am J Physiol 272:R662–R668, 1997.

180. Yamada T, Akishita M, Pollman MJ, et al: Angiotensin II type 2 receptor mediates vascular smooth muscle cell apoptosis and antagonizes angiotensin II type 1 receptor action: an in vitro gene transfer study. Life Sci 63:PL289–PL295, 1998.

181. Booz GW, Baker KM: Role of type 1 and type 2 angiotensin receptors in angiotensin II- induced cardiomyocyte hypertrophy. Hypertension 28:635–640, 1996.

182. Stoll M, Steckelings UM, Paul M, et al: The angiotensin AT2-receptor mediates inhibition of cell proliferation in coronary endothelial cells. J Clin Invest 95:651–657, 1995.

183. Nishimura H, Yerkes E, Hohenfellner K, et al: Role of the angiotensin type 2 receptor gene in congenital anomalies of the kidney and urinary tract, CAKUT, of mice and men. Mol Cell 3:1–10, 1999.

184. Pollman MJ, Yamada T, Horiuchi M, Gibbons GH: Vasoactive substances regulate vascular smooth muscle cell apoptosis. Countervailing influences of nitric oxide and angiotensin II. Circ Res 79:748–756, 1996.

185. Dimmeler S, Rippmann V, Weiland U, et al: Angiotensin II induces apoptosis of human endothelial cells. Protective effect of nitric oxide. Circ Res 81:970–976, 1997.

186. Hein L, Barsh GS, Pratt RE, et al: Behavioural and cardiovascular effects of disrupting the angiotensin II type-2 receptor in mice. Nature 377:744–747, 1995.

187. Ichiki T, Labosky PA, Shiota C, et al: Effects on blood pressure and exploratory behaviour of mice lacking angiotensin II type-2 receptor. Nature 377:748–750, 1995.

188. Zhang J, Pratt RE: The AT2 receptor selectively associates with Gialpha2 and Gialpha3 in the rat fetus. J Biol Chem 271:15026–15033, 1996.

189. Hayashida W, Horiuchi M, Dzau VJ: Intracellular third loop domain of angiotensin II type-2 receptor. Role in mediating signal transduction and cellular function. J Biol Chem 271:21985–21992, 1996.

190. Kang J, Richards EM, Posner P, Sumners C: Modulation of the delayed rectifier K+ current in neurons by an angiotensin II type 2 receptor fragment. Am J Physiol 268:C278–C282, 1995.

191. Bottari SP, King IN, Reichlin S, et al: The angiotensin AT2 receptor stimulates protein tyrosine phosphatase activity and mediates inhibition of particulate guanylate cyclase. Biochem Biophys Res Commun 183:206–211, 1992.

192. Tsuzuki S, Matoba T, Eguchi S, Inagami T: Angiotensin II type 2 receptor inhibits cell proliferation and activates tyrosine phosphatase. Hypertension 28:916–918, 1996.

193. Bedecs K, Elbaz N, Sutren M, et al: Angiotensin II type 2 receptors mediate inhibition of mitogen-activated protein kinase cascade and functional activation of SHP-1 tyrosine phosphatase. Biochem J 325:449–454, 1997.

194. Huang XC, Richards EM, Sumners C: Mitogen-activated protein kinases in rat brain neuronal cultures are activated by angiotensin II type 1 receptors and inhibited by angiotensin II type 2 receptors. J Biol Chem 271:15635–15641, 1996.

195. Siragy HM, Carey RM: The subtype-2 (AT2) angiotensin receptor regulates renal cyclic guanosine 3′, 5′-monophosphate and AT1 receptor-mediated prostaglandin E2 production in conscious rats [see comments]. J Clin Invest 97:1978–1982, 1996.

196. Siragy HM, Inagami T, Ichiki T, Carey RM: Sustained hypersensitivity to angiotensin II and its mechanism in mice lacking the subtype-2 (AT2) angiotensin receptor. Proc Natl Acad Sci U S A 96:6506–6510, 1999.

197. Siragy HM, Carey RM: The subtype 2 (AT2) angiotensin receptor mediates renal production of nitric oxide in conscious rats. J Clin Invest 100:264–269, 1997.

198. Seyedi N, Xu X, Nasjletti A, Hintze TH: Coronary kinin generation mediates nitric oxide release after angiotensin receptor stimulation. Hypertension 26:164–170, 1995.

199. Arima S, Endo Y, Yaoita H, et al: Possible role of P-450 metabolite of arachidonic acid in vasodilator mechanism of angiotensin II type 2 receptor in the isolated microperfused rabbit afferent arteriole. J Clin Invest 100:2816–2823, 1997.

CHAPTER 5

Circulating versus Tissue Angiotensin II

JÜRG NUSSBERGER, M.D.

■ From Renin-Angiotensin System to Local Angiotensin II Concentration

In their original description of renin some hundred years ago, Tigerstedt and Bergman characterized a protein that the kidneys released as a classic hormone into the blood stream to be transported to specific target tissues where it caused vasoconstriction, high blood pressure, and eventually cardiac hypertrophy.[1] This concept had to be modified when it became evident that a small angiotensin peptide[2,3] was released by the enzyme renin from the hepatogenic alpha-2-globuline angiotensinogen in blood.[4] Three decades ago, Ganten and colleagues described renin-like activity in the brain and led the way to the concept of tissue renin-angiotensin systems in various organs. These systems produced angiotensins independently of renal renin.[5] In a landmark paper in 1987, Campbell proposed the cross-talk between circulating and vascular tissue components of the renin-angiotensin system.[6] Later, in addition to the established role of the circulating renin-angiotensin system in regulating cardiovascular homeostasis, it became clear that the octapeptide angiotensin II (Ang II) also had trophic properties in vitro[7–10] and in vivo.[11]

The degree to which individual tissue production of Ang is in fact independent of renal renin remains controversial,[12–14] but virtually all investigators agree that local Ang concentrations are the key issue in the physiology of any renin-angiotensin system. Furthermore, several nonrenin enzymes, such as tonin, cathepsin, pepsin, trypsin, and kallikrein, generate Ang peptides from angiotensinogen. Thus, angiotensinogen—but not necessarily renin—is required for the production of Ang I or II. In addition, the conversion of Ang I to Ang II does not depend exclusively on the classic angiotensin-converting enzyme (ACE)[15]; it also may be catalyzed in tissues such as the human heart by chymostatin-sensitive chymase.[16] Messenger RNA for angiotensinogen and/or renin has been found in many organs.[17,18] Because the corresponding proteins often were localized in tissues, the question of uptake from plasma or local protein synthesis had to be answered.[19,20] Sadoshima and colleagues found that cultured rat cardiac myocytes released Ang II when they were stretched.[21] It would not be surprising, therefore, if distinct organs, such as brain, testis, ovary, and placenta, could generate Ang II independently of renal renin.

Obviously, theories about any Ang II-producing system in tissues should be based on reliable measurements of tissue concentrations of angiotensins and careful comparison with plasma concentrations and other components of the system. The past decade supported many of these postulated arguments for cardiovascular generation of Ang II. Local concentrations of Ang II appear to be determined largely by circulating renal renin and possibly tissue uptake of hepatogenic angiotensinogen and the number of specific Ang II receptors.[22-24]

Predictability of Plasma Angiotensin Levels from Plasma Components Alone

In humans treated with an oral renin inhibitor, plasma levels of Ang I and II were precisely predicted from measured plasma renin, angiotensinogen, and drug concentration using Michaelis-Menten kinetics for competitive inhibition[25] (Fig. 1). This predictability would not be expected if any nonrenal tissue source contributed plasma Angs in a nonsynchronized manner. Similar observations were made in human volunteers during ACE inhibition.[26]

Link between Plasma and Tissue Angiotensin II

As soon as tissue concentration of Ang II was reliably measured, a striking linear correlation between plasma and tissue concentrations was observed in various organs of rats[27] (Fig. 2) as well as in cardiac tissue of pigs.[22] Tissue concentrations of Ang II were too high to be explained by blood contamination of the tissue extracts. In addition, the slope of the correlation of tissue to plasma Ang II was quite different in different organs, varying from nearly 1 for heart and abdominal muscle to about 10 for liver and lung and close to 1000 for the adrenal glands (see Fig. 2).

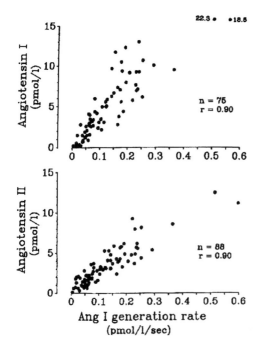

Figure 1. Correlation between actually measured levels of Ang I (upper panel) and Ang II (lower panel) in human plasma and calculated rates of Ang I generation after 600 and 1,200 mg of oral renin inhibitor Ro 42-5892, assuming Michaelis-Menten kinetics for competitive inhibition. For each drug level above the detection limit, the corresponding Ang II level was available; 13 Ang I levels were not obtained. The Ang I generation rate was calculated from plasma components only (renin, renin inhibitor, angiotensinogen concentrations). Tissue contributions out of phase with circulating renin would disturb the correlation. (From Camenzind E, Nussberger J, Juillerat L, et al: Effect of the renin response during renin inhibition: Oral Ro-425892 in normal humans. J Cardiovasc Pharmacol 18:299–307, 1991, with permission.)

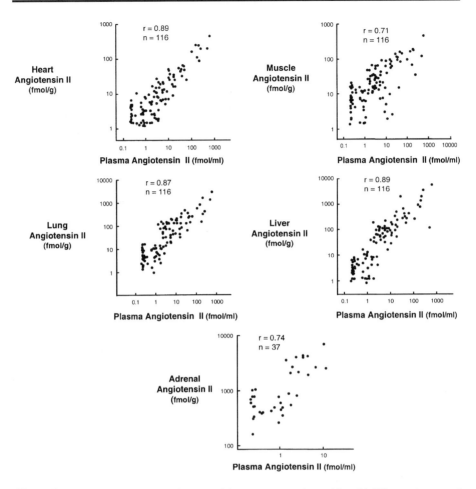

Figure 2. Correlations between plasma and tissue concentrations of Ang II in Wistar rats suggest an influence of circulating renin in both compartments. Different slopes of the correlation in different organs indicate other determinants for local angiotensin II concentrations (e.g., angiotensinogen, converting enzymes, pH).

Parallel Increase in Plasma and Tissue Angiotensin II in Renal Hypertensive Rats and Salt-depleted Rats

The 2-kidney, 1-clip (2K1C) Goldblatt II model of hypertension is characterized by high levels of circulating renin and Ang II. Of interest, these renal hypertensive rats show equally increased tissue levels of Ang II in the heart (Fig. 3) and other organs (Fig. 4). Similarly, salt-depletion in rats raises plasma as well as tissue concentrations of Ang II in the heart (Fig. 5) and other organs (Table 1).

Disappearance of Plasma and Tissue Angiotensin II after Bilateral Nephrectomy

Ang II virtually disappears from plasma after bilateral nephrectomy. In ten anephric patients, Campbell and colleagues[28] found mean circulating Ang II levels of 0.7 fmol/ml. We found similarly low levels in six anephric patients:

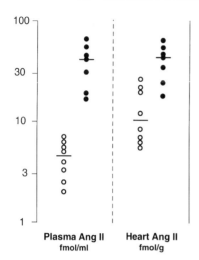

Figure 3.   Parallel increase in plasma and cardiac tissue concentrations of Ang II in renal hypertensive Wistar rats (2K1C, *filled symbols*) compared with sham-operated control rats *(open symbols)*. Circulating renin is high in these hypertensive rats and may raise cardiac tissue concentrations of Ang II. Note the logarithmic scale. Horizontal bar indicates median value.

plasma Ang II levels were below the detection limit of 0.1 fmol/ml in three patients, and the remaining three had mean levels of 0.5 fmol/ml. In rats, plasma Ang II levels fell from the normal value of 4 fmol/ml to < 0.2 fmol/ml within 2 days after binephrectomy when blood was carefully collected in the cold into a protease-inhibitor cocktail containing specific rat renin inhibitor.[29] At the same time, Ang II disappeared in cardiac tissue in 7 of 11 nephrectomized rats, fell to very low levels in three, and remained normal in one rat (Fig. 6; see also Table 1). Ang II levels in adrenal tissue decreased by 81% within 2 days after binephrectomy (Fig. 7). In nephrectomized pigs, Ang II disappeared completely from plasma and cardiac tissue, along with renin.[22] These results emphasize the important role of renal renin in maintaining Ang II concentrations under normal conditions, whereas the small amounts of Ang II in anephric patients with very high levels of circulating angiotensinogen may well be the product of other enzymes (mentioned above) or of newly recruited sources of renin that are of little relevance under more physiologic conditions. Substantially higher levels of circulating Ang II in anephric humans or rats on dialysis treatment were

Table 1.   Angiotensin II Concentrations in Plasma and Tissues of Wistar Rats during Control and Low-salt Conditions and after Bilateral Nephrectomy*

Mean ± SEM	Control (n = 30)	Low salt (n = 9)	Binephrectomy (n = 49)[†]
Plasma (fmol/ml)	4.4 ± 0.4	249 ± 69	0.69 ± 0.09
Heart (fmol/gm)	10.1 ± 1.2	173 ± 39	2.84 ± 0.3
Muscle	30.3 ± 3.5	165 ± 35	9.2 ± 0.9
Liver	69.7 ± 6.9	1176 ± 490	4.1 ± 0.4
Lung	79.5 ± 9.7	891 ± 267	6.4 ± 0.6
Brain	3.2 ± 0.5	9.6 ± 4.9	3.2 ± 0.3
Adrenal glands	3061 ± 159	Not done	572 ± 46

* Concentrations are fmol/ml in plasma and fmol/gm wet weight in tissues. Values are means ± SEM. Data of anephric rats were pooled from several experiments 42–48 hours after nephrectomy.
† n = 11 only for brain and adrenal glands.

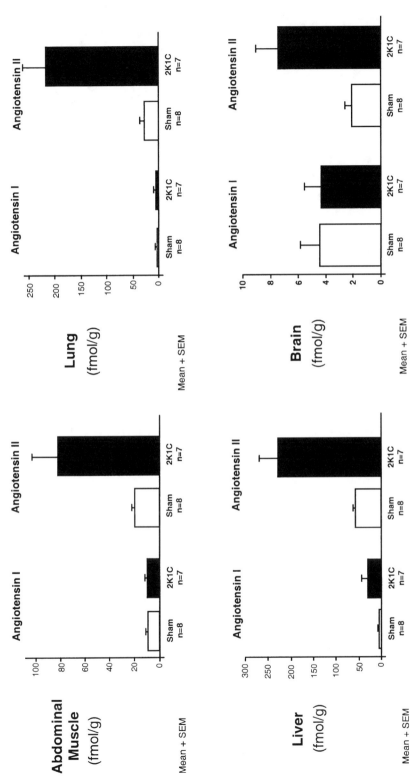

Figure 4. Tissue concentrations of Ang in skeletal muscle, lung, liver, and brain of renal hypertensive rats (2K1C, *filled bars*) and sham-operated control rats (*open bars*). Ang II levels are increased in all organs of the hypertensive rats. Ang I levels are hardly changed and lower than Ang II levels. Bars represent means + SEM (n = 7–8).

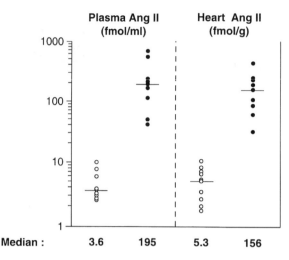

Figure 5. Parallel increase in plasma and cardiac tissue concentrations of Ang II in salt-depleted Wistar rats *(filled symbols)* compared with control rats *(open symbols)*. Circulating renin is high in the salt-depleted rats and may raise Ang II concentrations in cardiac tissue. Note the logarithmic scale. Horizontal bar indicates median value.

reported in several studies.[30–32] These relatively high concentrations of circulating Ang II were seen as evidence of physiologically relevant extrarenal sources of renin. However, different sample handling with less potent enzyme-inhibiting cocktails allows more generation of Ang in vitro, and the specificity of analytic procedures must be questioned when much higher normal values are reported.

■ *Plasma and Tissue Levels of Angiotensin during ACE Inhibition and Angiotensin Receptor Blockade*

Plasma and tissue concentrations of Ang during ACE inhibition and Ang receptor blockade were measured in rats,[33–35] pigs,[24,36] and mice.[11] All ACE inhibitors

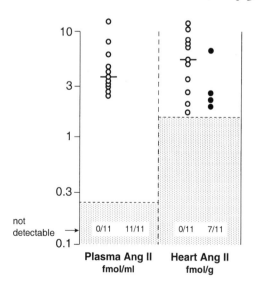

Figure 6. Ang II concentrations in plasma and cardiac tissue of control rats *(open symbols)* and anephric rats *(filled symbols;* 44 hours after binephrectomy). Plasma Ang II was unmeasurably low in all nephrectomized rats; cardiac tissue Ang II was undetectable or very low with one exception (n = 11). Note the logarithmic scale. Horizontal bar indicates median value. The shaded area indicates levels below the detection limit.

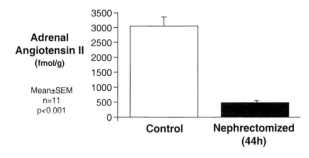

Figure 7. Effect of bilateral nephrectomy on Ang II concentrations in adrenal tissue of Wistar rats. High Ang II levels in control rats are reduced by 81% 2 days after binephrectomy. Renal renin appears essential for adrenal Ang II content, but the half-life of tissue Ang II is longer than the plasma half-life.

decreased Ang II concentrations in plasma and increased Ang I concentrations in plasma and nonrenal tissue. Ang II concentration in cardiac tissue was not consistently decreased. Species or model differences, as well as the use of different ACE inhibitors, may account for discrepant results. Typical results in rats (n = 19) after 2 weeks on a daily oral dose of 14 mg enalapril are shown in Figures 8 and 9.

Ang II type 1 receptor blockade consistently increased circulating levels of Ang I and II as well as tissue levels of Ang I, but tissue levels of Ang II were decreased in mice when insufficient amounts of angiotensinogen were available.[11] This finding supports the concepts that Ang II receptors protect the peptide from metabolism and that receptor blockade exposes both Ang I and Ang II to rapid degradation. Van Kats and colleagues of the Rotterdam group provided evidence that tissues may bind circulating renin and locally liberate Ang I and II, mainly from blood-borne angiotensinogen.[36] Recent measurements of plasma and tissue components of the renin-angiotensin system in mice are compatible with the concept that Ang II concentration in renal tissue is the parameter primarily regulated by the renin-angiotensin system.[11]

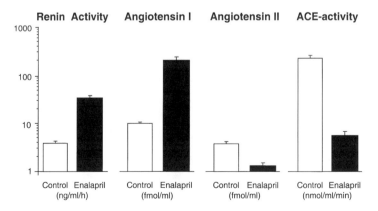

Figure 8. Plasma renin, Ang I, Ang II, and angiotensin-converting enzyme (ACE) activity in Wistar rats after 2 weeks of receiving 14 mg enlapril daily in drinking water *(filled bars)* and under control conditions *(open bars)*. Note the logarithmic scale. With enalapril ACE activity is well suppressed, as are Ang II levels, from already low control levels. Renin activity and Ang I levels are increased with enalapril (n = 19, means + SEM).

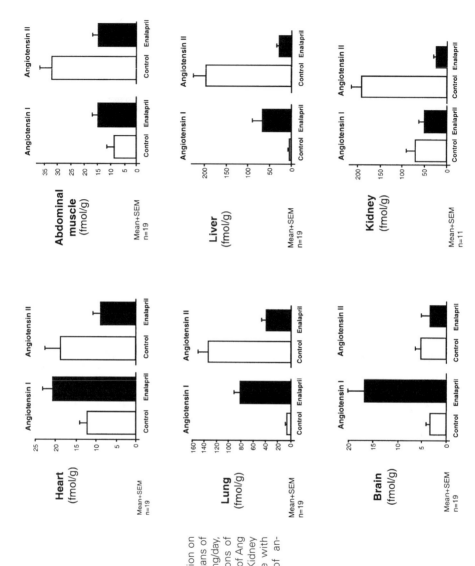

Figure 9. Effect of chronic ACE inhibition on tissue concentrations of Ang in various organs of rats. Two weeks of enalapril ingestion (14 mg/day, *filled bars*) decreased tissue concentrations of Ang II and increased tissue concentrations of Ang I compared with control rats *(open bars)*. Kidney concentrations of Ang I did not increase with enalapril and may reflect exhaustion of angiotensinogen in this high renin state.

■ *Conclusion*

The quest for better understanding of local production and concentration of Ang II has replaced the debate about the existence of multiple independent tissue renin-angiotensin systems. The predictability of circulating Ang levels exclusively from plasma components excludes a major contribution of Ang peptides from renin-angiotensin systems that are out of phase with circulating renin. Plasma and tissue concentrations of Ang II are well correlated but with organ-specific slopes. Ang II disappears from plasma and tissue after binephrectomy. Blockade of the renin-angiotensin system by ACE inhibition or Ang receptor antagonism reveals the importance of uptake of plasma renin and angiotensinogen and local generation of Ang I and II as well as of receptor binding, internalization, and metabolism of Ang II. Renal renin secretion remains an important step in cardiovascular regulation, and Ang II concentration in renal tissue appears to be primarily regulated. The kidneys continue to be linked with circulatory homeostasis, as suggested by Tigerstedt and Bergmann.[1]

References

1. Tigerstedt R, Bergmann PG: Niere und Kreislauf. Skand Arch Physiol 8:223–271, 1898.
2. Munoz JM, Braun-Menendez E, Fasciolo JC, Leloir LF: Hypertensin: The substance causing renal hypertension. Nature 144:980, 1939.
3. Page IH, Helmer OM: A cristalline pressor substance (angiotonin) resulting from the action between renin and renin-activator. J Exp Med 71:29–42, 1940.
4. Skeggs LT, Kahn JR, Lentz KE, Shumway NP: The preparation, purification and amino acid sequence of a polypeptide renin substrate. J Exp Med 106: 439–453, 1957.
5. Ganten D, Merquez-Julio A, Granger P, et al: Renin in dog brain. Am J Physiol 221: 1733–1737, 1971.
6. Campbell DJ: Circulating and tissue angiotensin systems. J Clin Invest 79: 1–6, 1987.
7. Geisterfer AAT, Peach MJ, Owens GK: Angiotensin II induces hypertrophy, not hyperplasia of cultured aortic smooth muscle cells. Circ Res 62:649–656, 1988.
8. Berk BC, Vekhstein V, Gordon HM, Tsuda T: Angiotensin II-stimulated protein synthesis in cultured vascular smooth muscle cells. Hypertension 13:305–314, 1989.
9. Gibbons GH, Pratt RE, Dzau VJ: Angiotensin II is a bifunctional vascular smooth muscle cell growth factor. Hypertension 14: 358, 1989.
10. Baker KM, Aceto JF: Angiotensin II stimulation of protein synthesis and cell growth in chick heart cells. Am J Physiol 259:H610–618, 1990.
11. Mazzolai L, Pedrazzini T, Nicoud F, et al: Increased cardiac angiotensin II levels induce right and left ventricular hypertrophy in normotensive mice. Hypertension 35:985–991, 2000.
12. von Lutterotti N, Catanzaro DF, Sealy JE, Laragh JH: Renin is not synthesized by cardiac and extrarenal vascular tissues: A review of experimental evidence. Circulation 89:458–470, 1994.
13. Dzau VJ, Re RN: Tissue angiotensin system in cardiovascular medicine. A paradigm shift? Circulation 89:493–498, 1994.
14. Dostal DE, Baker KM: The cardiac renin-angiotensin system: Conceptual, or a regulator of cardiac function? Circ Res 85: 643–650, 1999.
15. Yang HYT, Erdös EG, Levin Y: A dipeptidyl carboxypeptidase which converts angiotensin I and inactivates bradykinin. Biochim Biophys Acta 214:374–376, 1970.
16. Urata H, Kinoshita A, Misono KS, et al: Identification of a highly specific chymase as the major angiotensin II-forming enzyme in the human heart. J Biol Chem 265:2348–2357, 1990.
17. Campbell DJ, Habener JF: Angiotensinogen gene is expressed and differentially regulated in multiple tissues of the rat. J Clin Invest 78:31–39, 1986.
18. Dzau VJ, Ellison KE, Brody T, et al: A comparative study of the distributions of renin and angiotensinogen messenger ribonucleic acids in rat and mouse tissues. Endocrinology 120:2334–2338, 1987.
19. Loudon M, Bing RF, Thurston H, Swales JD: Arterial wall uptake of renal renin and blood pressure control. Hypertension 5:629–634, 1983.
20. Danser AHJ, van Kesteren CAM, Bax WA, et al: Prorenin, renin, angiotensinogen and angiotensin converting enzyme in normal and failing hearts: evidence for renin binding. Circulation 96:220–226, 1997.

21. Sadoshima J, Xu Y, Slater HS, Izumo S: Autocrine release of angiotensin II mediates stretch-induced hypertrophy of cardiac myocytes in vitro. Cell 75:977–984, 1993.
22. Danser AHJ, van Kats JP, Admiraal PJJ, et al: Cardiac renin and angiotensins. Uptake from plasma versus in situ synthesis. Hypertension 24:37–48, 1994.
23. de Lannoy LM, Danser AHJ, Bouhuizen AMB, et al: Localization and production of angiotensin II in the isolated perfused rat heart. Hypertension 31:1111–1117, 1998.
24. van Kats JP, Danser AHJ, van Meegen JR, et al: Angiotensin production by the heart: A quantitative study in pigs with the use of radiolabeled angiotensin infusions. Circulation 98:73–81, 1998.
25. Camenzind E, Nussberger J, Juillerat L, et al: Effect of the renin response during renin inhibition: Oral Ro-425892 in normal humans. J Cardiovasc Pharmacol 18:299–307, 1991.
26. Juillerat L, Nussberger J, Ménard J, et al: Determinants of angiotensin II generation during converting enzyme inhibition. Hypertension 16:564–572, 1990.
27. Nussberger J, Nicoud F, Brunner D, et al: Measurement of low angiotensin II concentrations in rat hearts. Hypertension 18:384–385, 1991.
28. Campbell DJ, Kladis A, Skinner SL, Whitworth JA: Characterization of angiotensin peptides in plasma of anephric man. J Hypertens 9:265–274, 1991.
29. Nussberger J, Flückiger JP, Hui KY, et al: Angiotensin I and II disappear completely from circulating blood within 48 hours after binephrectomy: Improved measurement of angiotensins in the rat. J Hypertens 9(Suppl 6): S230–S231, 1991.
30. Mizuno K, Higashimori K, Stone WJ, et al: Re-evaluation of the plasma renin-angiotensin system in anephric patients. Clin Exp Hypertens 12A:1135–1157, 1990.
31. Wilkes BM, Mento PF, Pearl AR, et al: Plasma angiotensins in anephric humans: Evidence for an extrarenal angiotensin system. J Cardiovasc Pharmacol 17:419–423, 1991.
32. Trolliet MR, Phillips MI: The effect of chronic bilateral nephrectomy on plasma and brain angiotensin. J Hypertens 10:29–36, 1992.
33. Campbell DJ, Kladis A, Duncan AM: Effects of converting enzyme inhibitors on angiotensin and bradykinin peptides. Hypertension 23:439–449, 1994.
34. Campbell DJ, Kladis A, Valentijn AJ: Effects of losartan on angiotensin and bradykinin peptides and angiotensin-converting enzyme. J Cardiovasc Pharmacol 26:233–240, 1995.
35. Ruzicka M, Skarda V, Leenen FHH: Effects of ACE inhibitors on circulating versus cardiac angiotensin II in volume overload-induced cardiac hypertrophy in rats. Circulation 92:3568–3573, 1995.
36. van Kats JP, de Lannoy LM, Danser AHJ, et al: Angiotensin II type 1 (AT1) receptor mediated accumulation of angiotensin II in tissues and its intracellular half life in vivo. Hypertension 30:42–49, 1997.

CHAPTER 6

Early Experience with Angiotensin II Receptor Antagonists and Angiotensin-Converting Enzyme Inhibitors

HANS R. BRUNNER, M.D.
HARALAMBOS GAVRAS, M.D.

Interest in the renin-angiotensin-aldosterone system and its relationship to blood pressure homeostasis in hypertensive diseases has increased steadily since the early 1960s when it first became evident that renin secretion is linked closely to sodium metabolism, a factor already known to play a role in the pathogenesis of hypertension. This awareness began with the demonstration that patients with malignant hypertension, unlike those with essential hypertension, have massive oversecretion of aldosterone.[1] It was demonstrated subsequently that angiotensin II exerted a selective stimulating effect on aldosterone secretion in normal volunteers.[2] This finding established the vital connection between the renin-angiotensin system and the control of sodium metabolism via aldosterone and suggested the active involvement of renin excess in severe forms of human hypertension. However, in essential hypertension, by far the most common form of high blood pressure, plasma renin activity usually is within the normal range, and it was generally believed that the renin-angiotensin system was not pathogenetically involved in essential hypertension.[3–5] On the basis of a retrospective analysis of data from hypertensive patients as well as experimental data, we suggested that it may be responsible for vascular complications.[6,7] Moreover, no evidence indicated that the renin system plays a role in normal blood pressure control, and a causal role had not been clearly established in either clinical or experimental renovascular hypertension.

■ Blocking the Renin-Angiotensin System in Experimental Models to Establish Its Pathogenetic Role

Several investigators have actively or passively immunized renal hypertensive rabbits[8,9] or rats[10–12] against angiotensin II. The overall results were inconclusive because some investigators reported blood pressure reduction, whereas others found no effect of the immunization. Already it was apparent that active immunization, i.e. vaccination against angiotensin II, did not induce a hypotensive effect. We chose to administer specific antisera against angiotensin II to two types of animals: one-kidney, one-clip and two-kidney, one-clip hypertensive rats.[13] Antiserum was administered 6 weeks after clipping to one kidney. One-kidney, one-clip hypertensive rats, known to exhibit normal plasma renin activity, showed no reduction in blood pressure. In contrast, in the two-kidney, one-clip hypertensive rats blood pressure was markedly reduced by a specific angiotensin II antiserum. In the same experiment, intravenous administration of saralasin, a novel peptide angiotensin II receptor antagonist, produced the same results: marked blood pressure reduction in the two-kidney, one-clip hypertensive rats but no change in the one-kidney, one-clip hypertensive rats.[13] In a follow-up study, sodium depletion did not alter blood pressure in one-kidney, one-clip hypertensive rats. However, when saralasin was administered to the salt-depleted hypertensive rats, blood pressure fell to almost normal levels.[14] After overnight sodium repletion with saline as drinking fluid, renewed challenge with intravenous infusion of saralasin had no further effect on hypertension.

Given the specificity of the angiotensin II antiserum and the angiotensin receptor antagonist saralasin, these experiments clearly established that angiotensin II can play an active role in causing hypertension in a model characterized by elevated renin levels (i.e., two-kidney, one-clip hypertensive rats). Of equal importance, these experiments demonstrated that, even in a hypertensive model characterized by normal renin levels (i.e., one-kidney, one-clip hypertensive rats), salt depletion with the inherent stimulation of renin secretion can create conditions in which angiotensin II becomes primarily responsible for the hypertensive state.

Two more sets of experiments corroborated the earlier findings. Rats were rendered hypertensive by administration of deoxycorticosterone acetate and salt in the drinking fluid. In this state, characterized by a suppressed plasma renin activity, the infusion of saralasin did not reduce blood pressure but rather increased it slightly, thus exposing the weak agonist effect of saralasin.[15] At the same time, two-kidney, one-clip hypertensive rats were maintained for a longer period of 15 weeks after clipping with no therapy. Although they had responded favorably to the administration of saralasin 6 weeks after clipping, as described previously, hypertension of prolonged duration could be reduced by saralasin only if salt depletion was initiated simultaneously.[16] Thus, with time the two-kidney, one-clip rats behaved similarly to one-kidney, one-clip hypertensive rats.

These experiments further established the important interaction among renin secretion, angiotensin II dependency of hypertension, and sodium metabolism. Hypertension remains exquisitely angiotensin II-dependent as long as pressure-induced natriuresis in the contralateral kidney is intact. With removal of the kidney or impairment of its normal pressure, natriuresis due to prolonged exposure to high blood pressure attenuates the angiotensin II dependency and at the same time exposes the important interaction between sodium handling and angiotensin II.

■ Early Studies in Normotensive and Hypertensive Humans Using Specific Blockade

Early in 1971 we began a first study in which saralasin was given to hypertensive patients. After an initial string of negative results, one patient received a tenfold higher dose than previously approved. This increased dosage resulted in a marked drop in blood pressure. Only after the Food and Drug Administration had approved the use of much higher doses in late 1972 could clinical exploration again proceed. Of the 12 patients included in the original evaluation, 8 exhibited high renin levels. Most of these patients responded to the administration of saralasin with a marked drop in blood pressure, whereas patients with low renin levels showed no change in blood pressure.[17] Of even greater interest, it was demonstrated that coadministration of furosemide markedly enhanced the antihypertensive effect of saralasin, even in previously nonresponding patients, and the infusion of saline with saralasin completely reversed its antihypertensive effect.[18] In one patient who presented with malignant hypertension and marked congestive heart failure bordering on acute pulmonary edema, administration of saralasin immediately reduced dyspnea, and the combined infusion of furosemide and saralasin over a period of 6 days transformed the patient dramatically. This key observation in a single patient soon led to the new concept of treating congestive heart failure with blockade of the renin-angiotensin system.

Shortly afterward, the compound teprotide became available; it blocks the enzyme responsible for the conversion of angiotensin I to angiotensin II.[19] This nonapeptide resulted in a marked reduction in blood pressure in 13 hypertensive patients. In 5 patients who responded suboptimally, salt depletion was induced for 2 days by diuretics; then teprotide was readministered. After sodium depletion, the blood pressure reduction was markedly enhanced; in fact, blood pressure was practically normalized in all patients.[20]

Subsequent studies firmly established the reciprocal relationship between renin dependency and sodium dependency in hypertensive patients[21] and normotensive volunteers.[22] Thus in a short time the concepts developed in hypertensive animals with the use of saralasin were applied successfully to hypertensive patients[17–19,21,23] and normotensive men.[22] This application represents an early example in which specific blockade of a particular vasoactive system established beyond doubt its active involvement in the pathogenesis of hypertension and maintenance of normal blood pressure. With the hindsight of almost 30 years, however, it must be said that we have been quite lucky in using this approach. It proved successful because it triggers relatively little compensatory activation of other vasoactive systems. Subsequent investigations using, for example, alpha-adrenoceptor blockade or vasopressin antagonists have been disappointing because compensation by another vasoactive system, predominantly the renin-angiotensin system, completely covered the effect of a specific blockade.[24,25]

■ *Angiotensin II Receptor Antagonists vs. Angiotensin-Converting Enzyme Inhibitors*

With teprotide a new approach to blockade of the renin-angiotensin system became available. Immediately the specificity of this mechanism was called into question. Indeed, it was well established that the converting enzyme is also responsible for the breakdown of other polypeptide substances, such as bradykinin, and that its blockade can potentiate the effect of bradykinin, a well known vasodilator.[26,27] For this reason, we questioned whether inhibition of the converting enzyme provided the same specificity for the renin system as angiotensin II receptor blockade. To investigate this issue, we administered teprotide to nephrectomized rats and found no effect on blood pressure, even after salt depletion. Administration of teprotide and saralasin, with or without salt depletion, produced no additional effect. Consequently, we concluded that no angiotensin-independent effect of teprotide could be demonstrated.[28] Two years later, the new orally active converting enzyme inhibitor captopril was coadministered to rats rendered hypertensive by infusion of angiotensin II for 9 days. Again, converting enzyme inhibition in purely angiotensin II-induced hypertension had no effect, leading to the conclusion that no angiotensin II-independent effect of a converting enzyme inhibitor could be detected.[29] This finding was important because it clearly demonstrated that converting enzyme inhibition potentiates the vasodilating effect of exogenous bradykinin by almost 100-fold.[30] As a consequence, for all practical purposes, we consider the systemic antihypertensive effect of converting enzyme inhibition to be related almost exclusively to its inhibition of the renin-angiotensin system.

■ *Orally Active Converting Enzyme Inhibitors*

In 1976, an orally active converting enzyme inhibitor became available for clinical use.[31] Until this point, basic concepts had been established using mainly the octapeptide angiotensin II receptor antagonist, saralasin, or, less frequently, the nonapeptide converting enzyme inhibitor, teprotide. There was no fundamental reason to abandon angiotensin II receptor blockade. However, to apply these new concepts to clinical therapy, an orally active nonpeptidic compound capable of blocking the effect of the renin-angiotensin system was badly needed. Captopril was the first such agent. Consequently, most subsequent progress was made with the use of orally active converting enzyme inhibition rather than angiotensin II receptor blockade.

In late 1976 we administered captopril for the first time to normal volunteers challenged with bolus injections of exogenous angiotensin I.[32] It became rapidly apparent that small doses of captopril markedly impaired the pressure response of normal volunteers to exogenous angiotensin I. In fact, 20 mg of captopril administered orally completely abolished the pressor effect of angiotensin I. Thus, the initial administration of captopril to volunteers not only established the potent blocking effect of the pressure response to angiotensin I but also defined a clear dose-response relationship and a relatively short duration of action. The compensatory rise of plasma renin activity in responses to converting enzyme inhibition was also described.

Although the dose-response relationship was defined with this initial observation, for a short time subsequent investigations in hypertensive patients were carried out with substantially higher doses because of the desire to overcome the relatively short duration of action. Quite rapidly it was demonstrated that long-term therapy in patients with essential or renovascular hypertension, using converting enzyme inhibition alone or in combination with a diuretic, could be extremely effective.[33-35]

Other orally active converting enzyme inhibitors followed. Two compounds that later became extremely successful antihypertensive agents were administered for the first time to human volunteers in our research unit: enalapril and lisinopril.[36] Subsequently, many other compounds were also assessed. Drugs with a longer duration of action than captopril became available. Within a rather short period it became evident that blockade of the renin-angiotensin system by converting enzyme inhibition alone or together with diuretic administration is a highly effective treatment of clinical hypertension, thus confirming the concepts developed earlier with angiotensin II antisera and peptide inhibitors.

■ *Renal Effects of Blocking the Renin-Angiotensin System: Unmasking the Key Role of Sodium Chloride*

It was, of course, already known that the kidney plays a key role in blood pressure regulation. Hypertensive patients with impaired renal function due to various causes commonly exhibit severe hypertension that is difficult to control, and in some extreme situations hypertension was treated with bilateral nephrectomy.[37] For these reasons we were eager to use the combination of converting enzyme inhibition and furosemide in hypertensive patients with chronic renal failure, who often are treatment-resistant. Such patients became exquisitely salt-sensitive when the renin system was neutralized by treatment with captopril. Indeed, one of our first patients, whose blood pressure previously could not be normalized with a quadruple combination of antihypertensive drugs, became hypotensive at 90/70 mmHg when an excessive dose of furosemide was added to captopril. For the first time his blood pressure could be reduced and maintained at perfectly normal levels with captopril and adequately titrated furosemide.[38] This finding further underscored the concept that the antihypertensive effect of diuretics—particularly loop diuretics—is often abolished partially or completely by the drug-induced compensatory rise in renin secretion. Simultaneous blockade of the renin-angiotensin system enhances the antihypertensive efficacy of diuretics.

Simultaneously we wished to demonstrate the effect of blockade of the renin-angiotensin system on renal hemodynamics. First, teprotide was administered to dogs that were either salt-depleted or on a normal sodium diet. Redistribution of renal, cardiac, and other regional blood flow was measured with microsphere techniques. Teprotide induced a marked increase in flow in the kidneys and coronary circulation.[39] As soon as captopril became available, it was administered to patients with essential hypertension to quantitate its effect on renal function. Although captopril did not affect glomerular filtration rate, it significantly enhanced renal plasma flow and consequently reduced filtration fraction.[40] This finding confirmed previous observations in normal volunteers[41] and represents a well-recognized pattern of response to blockade of the renin-angiotensin system.

After successful treatment of hypertensive patients with impaired renal function, it was a small step to the use of captopril for treatment of uncontrollable hypertension in patients on maintenance hemodialysis. In view of the close interaction between sodium metabolism and renin secretion and its pathogenetic role in the development of hypertension, it seemed appropriate to try the combination of converting enzyme inhibition with progressive salt subtraction during the hemodialysis session.[42] This approach not only became a highly successful treatment of previously uncontrollable hypertension; it also exposed the difficulty of maintaining an adequate sodium balance in patients on hemodialysis, particularly with the recent trend toward shorter hemodialysis sessions.

■ *Blockade of the Renin-Angiotensin System in Patients with Congestive Heart Failure*

The immediate improvement in hypertensive patients with congestive heart failure after the infusion of saralasin left a lasting impression. When 18 normotensive patients with congestive heart failure received an infusion of saralasin, blood pressure and pulmonary capillary wedge pressure decreased significantly; in addition, left ventricular function curves improved significantly.[43] In a preliminary but carefully documented observation, a hypertensive patient with congestive heart failure markedly improved after infusion of saralasin,[44] providing the first evidence that blockade of the renin-angiotensin system may markedly improve patients with congestive heart failure. It was difficult to get the results published because editors showed little interest in the new mechanism and conceptual aspect of the study and were unimpressed since "the effect was less pronounced than that obtained with sodium nitroprusside." Shortly afterward, teprotide, the peptide-converting enzyme inhibitor, also was administered to patients with congestive heart failure and produced an even better effect.[45] One year later, prolonged treatment of congestive heart failure with the orally active converting enzyme inhibitor captopril proved to be immediately effective in reducing pulmonary pressure and increasing cardiac output.[46] This finding opened the way to a unique and effective treatment of congestive heart failure[47] that years later was demonstrated to alter patient outcome dramatically. Today it is the standard treatment of congestive heart failure.

■ *Nonpeptide AT_1 Receptor Antagonists*

As indicated above, the conceptual exploration of the renin-angiotensin system began with the use of specific antisera against angiotensin II in experimental studies and then expanded to include peptide antagonists of angiotensin II. Receptor blockade was abandoned in favor of converting enzyme inhibition purely for practical reasons (i.e., the availability of an oral compound). It became evident, however, that certain side-effects were linked to converting enzyme inhibition, such as chronic dry cough and angioedema. Furthermore, the use of converting enzyme inhibitors as probes to investigate the pathophysiologic role of the renin-angiotensin system was hampered by the argument that perhaps not all observed effects are due exclusively to blockade of the renin-angiotensin system. Thus an orally active angiotensin II receptor antagonist remained highly desirable.

Losartan was the first such agent.[48] It was particularly exciting when Drs. Timmermans and Lee of DuPont requested that we demonstrate the efficacy of losartan in normal volunteers. In fact, losartan blocked the response to exogenous angiotensin very effectively[49,50]; thus, a new chapter began in therapeutic blockade of the renin-angiotensin system. With the availability of losartan and other agents synthesized by various companies, chronic treatment with specific angiotensin II blockade became possible. This new approach has been rewarded by a high degree of efficacy and a virtual absence of untoward effects. Indeed, for the first time we have an antihypertensive therapeutic principle that has no known class-specific side effects. This fact, together with the therapeutic efficacy of blocking the renin-angiotensin system, closes the circle and brings us back to the question we asked several years ago: Is the renin system necessary?[51]

■ *Is the Renin System Necessary?*

We began with the concept that renin via angiotensin II may have some "vasculotoxic" effect[6,7] that could be blocked. After the initial experiments with antisera and saralasin and clinical experience with saralasin and teprotide, we were extremely impressed by the efficacy and tolerance of the new mode for blocking the renin-angiotensin system. Within a relatively short period orally active substances were available, and their therapeutic efficacy seemed even to exceed our most optimistic expectation with no major untoward effects. Through angiotensin II and stimulation of aldosterone secretion, renin evidently plays an important role in preserving sodium chloride and thus protecting normal body fluid. Angiotensin needed not only to hold back salt excretion by the kidney in case of sodium depletion and hypovolemia but also to maintain normal blood pressure. However, with the availability of excessive amounts of salt, the renin-angiotensin system does not seem to be necessary for maintenance of normal blood pressure, as clearly demonstrated by the excellent tolerance of highly effective converting enzyme inhibitors. Furthermore, in patients with congestive heart failure and rather low blood pressure, converting enzyme inhibitors reduced blood pressure toward net hypotension without deleterious effects. Twenty years later, the new AT_1 receptor antagonists can induce long-term blockade of the system without any known untoward effect. Thus, the question whether the renin-angiotensin system is really necessary under normal living conditions remains as relevant as ever—and the answer "no" becomes more and more acceptable.

Learning to block this enzymatic cascade has been a unique adventure. Even if the system is rather redundant in an industrialized world with excessive availability of salt, it nevertheless plays a key role in the pathogenesis of hypertension and enhances the deleterious effect of ventricular failure. It can be blocked, however, without triggering major compensatory activation of other vasoactive systems—a quality that is rather unique.

References

1. Laragh JH, Ulick S, Januszewicz W, et al: Aldosterone secretion and primary and malignant hypertension. J Clin Invest 39:1091–1106, 1960.
2. Laragh JH, Angers M, Kelly WG, Lieberman S: Hypotensive agents and pressor substances: The effect of epinephrine, norepinephrine, angiotensin II and others in the secretory rate of aldosterone in man. JAMA 174:234–240, 1960.
3. Brown JJ, Davies DL, Lever AF, Robertson JIS: Variations in plasma renin concentration in several physiological and pathological states. Can Med Assoc J 90:201–206, 1964.
4. Veyrat R, De Champlain J, Boucher R, Genest J: Measurement of human arterial renin activity in some physiological and pathological states. Can Med Assoc J 90:215–220, 1964.
5. Helmer OM: Renin activity in blood from patients with hypertension. Can Med Assoc J 90:221, 1964.
6. Brunner HR, Laragh JH, Baer L, et al: Essential hypertension: Renin and aldosterone, heart attack and stroke. N Engl J Med 286:441–449, 1972.
7. Gavras H., Brown JJ, Lever AF, et al: Acute renal failure, tubular necrosis, and myocardial infarction induced in the rabbit by intravenous angiotensin II. Lancet ii:19–22, 1971.
8. Macdonald GJ, Louis WJ, Renzini VE: Renal-clip hypertension in rabbits immunized against angiotensin II. Circ Res 27:197–211, 1970.
9. Eide I, Aars H: Renal hypertension in rabbits immunized with angiotensin II. Scand J Clin Invest 25:119–127., 1970
10. Hedwall PR: Effect of rabbit antibodies against angiotensin-II on the pressor response to angiotensin-II and renal hypertension in the rat. Br J Pharmacol 68:623–629, 1968.
11. Christlieb AR, Biber TU, Hickler RB: Studies on the role of angiotensin in experimental renovascular hypertension: An immunologic approach. J Clin Invest 48:1506–1518, 1969.

12. Bing J, Poulsen K: Effect of anti-angiotensin II on blood pressure and sensitivity to angiotensin and renin: Studies on normal, nephrectomized, ureter-ligated, continuously angiotensin infused, and renal hypertensive rats. Acta Pathol Microbiol Scand 78:6–18, 1970.

13. Brunner HR, Kirshmann JD, Sealey JE, Laragh JH: Hypertension of renal origin: Evidence for two different mechanisms. Science 174:1344–1346, 1971.

14. Gavras H, Brunner HR, Vaughan EDJ, Laragh JH: Angiotensin-sodium interaction in blood pressure maintenance of renal hypertensive and normotensive rats. Science 180:1369–1372, 1973.

15. Gavras H, Brunner HR, Laragh JH, et al: Malignant hypertension resulting from deoxycorticosterone acetate and salt excess: Role of renin and sodium in vascular changes. Circ Res 36:300–309, 1975.

16. Gavras H, Brunner HR, Thurston H, Laragh JH: Reciprocation of renin dependency with sodium volume dependency in renal hypertension. Science 188:1316–1317, 1975.

17. Brunner HR, Gavras H, Laragh JH, Keenan R: Angiotensin II blockade in man by Sar1-ala8-angiotensin II for understanding and treatment of high blood pressure. Lancet ii:1045–1047, 1973.

18. Brunner HR, Gavras H, Laragh JH, Keenan R: Hypertension in man, exposure of the renin and sodium components using angiotensin II blockade. Circ Res 34 (Suppl 1):35–43, 1974.

19. Ondetti MA, Williams NJ, Sabo EF, et al: Angiotensin converting enzyme inhibitors from the venom of *Bothrops jararaca*: Isolation, elucidation of structure and synthesis. Biochemistry 10:4033–4039, 1971.

20. Gavras H, Brunner HR, Laragh JH, J et al: An angiotensin converting enzyme inhibitor to identify and treat vasoconstrictor and volume factors in hypertensive patients. N Engl J Med 291:817–821, 1974.

21. Gavras H, Ribeiro AB, Gavras I, Brunner HR: Reciprocal relation between renin dependency and sodium dependency in essential hypertension. N Engl J Med 295:1278–1283, 1976.

22. Posternak L, Brunner HR, Gavras H, Brunner DB: Angiotensin II blockade in normal man: Interaction of renin and sodium in maintaining blood pressure. Kidney Int 11:197–203, 1977.

23. Streeten DHP, Anderson GH, Freiberg JM, Dalakos TG: Use of an angiotensin II antagonist (saralasin) in the recognition of angiotensinogenic hypertension. N Engl J Med 292:657–662, 1975.

24. Waeber BJ, Nussberger J, Brunner HR: Blood pressure dependency on vasopressin and angiotensin II in prazosin-treated conscious normotensive rats. J Pharmacol Exp Ther 2:442–446, 1983.

25. Burnier M, Biollaz J, Brunner DB, Brunner HR: Blood pressure maintenance in awake dehydrated rats: Role of the renin system, vasopressin and sympathetic activity. Am J Physiol 245:H203–H209, 1983.

26. Green LJ, Camargo ACM, Kreiger EM, et al: Inhibition of the conversion of angiotensin I to angiotensin II and potentiation of bradykinin by small peptides present in *Bothrops jararaca* venom. Circ Res 31(Suppl II):62–71, 1972.

27. Erdös EG: Conversion of angiotensin I to angiotensin II. Am J Med 60:749–759, 1976.

28. Jaeger P, Ferguson RK, Brunner HR, et al: Mechanism of blood pressure reduction by teprotide (SQ 20881) in rats. Kidney Int 13:289–296, 1978.

29. Textor SC, Brunner HR, Gavras H: Converting enzyme inhibition during chronic angiotensin II infusion in rats: Evidence against a non-angiotensin mechanism. Hypertension 3:269–276, 1981.

30. Textor SC, Brunner HR, Gavras H: Evidence for bradykinin potentiation by angiotensin congeners in conscious rats. Am J Physiol 240:H255–H26, 1981.

31. Ondetti MA, Rubin B, Cushman DW: Design of specific inhibitors of angiotensin converting enzyme: New class of orally active antihypertensive agents. Science 196:441–444, 1977.

32. Ferguson RK, Brunner HR, Turini GA, et al: A specific orally active inhibitor of angiotensin converting enzyme in man. Lancet i:775–778, 1977.

33. Gavras H, Brunner HR, Turini GA, et al: Antihypertensive effect of oral angiotensin converting enzyme inhibitor SQ 14225 in man. N Engl J Med 298:991–995, 1978.

34. Brunner HR, Gavras H, Waeber B, et al: Oral angiotensin-converting enzyme inhibitor in long-term treatment of hypertensive patients. Ann Intern Med 90:19–23, 1979.

35. Brunner HR, Gavras H, Waeber B, et al: Clinical use of an orally acting converting enzyme inhibitor: captopril. Hypertension 2:558–565, 1980.

36. Biollaz J, Burnier M, Turini GA, et al: Three new long-acting converting enzyme inhibitors: Relationship between plasma converting enzyme activity and response to angiotensin I. Clin Pharmacol Ther 29:665–670, 1981.

37. Lazarus JM, Hampers CL, Bennett AH, et al: Urgent bilateral nephrectomy for severe hypertension. Ann Intern Med 76:733, 1972

38. Brunner HR, Waeber B, Wauters JP, et al: Inappropriate renin secretion unmasked by captopril (SQ 14,225) in hypertension or chronic renal failure. Lancet ii:704–707, 1978.

39. Gavras H., Liang C, Brunner HR: Redistribution of regional blood flow after inhibition of the angiotensin-converting enzyme. Circ Res 43 (Suppl I):59–63, 1978.

40. Mimran A, Brunner HR, Turini GA, et al: Effect of captopril on renal vascular tone in patients with essential hypertension. Clin Sci 57:421s–423s, 1979.
41. Hollenberg NK, Williams GH, Taub KJ, et al: Renal vascular response to interruption of the renin-angiotensin system in normal man. Kidney Int 12:285–293, 1977.
42. Wauters JP, Waeber B, Brunner HR, et al: Uncontrollable hypertension in patients on hemodialysis: Long-term treatment with captopril and salt subtraction. Clin Nephrol 16:86–92, 1981.
43. Turini GA, Brunner HR, Ferguson RK, et al: Congestive heart failure in normotensive man: Haemodynamics, renin, and angiotensin II blockade. Br Heart J 40:1134–1142, 1978.
44. Gavras H, Flessas A, Ryan TJ, et al: Angiotensin II inhibition: Treatment of congestive heart failure in a high-renin hypertension. JAMA 238:880–882, 1977.
45. Gavras H, Faxon DP, Berkoben J, et al: Angiotensin converting enzyme inhibition in patients with congestive heart failure. Circulation 58:770–775, 1978.
46. Turini GA, Brunner HR, Gribic M, et al: Improvement of chronic congestive heart failure by oral captopril. Lancet 1:1213–1215, 1979.
47. Turini GA, Waeber B, Brunner HR: The renin-angiotensin system in refractory heart failure: Clinical, hemodynamic and hormonal effects of captopril and enalapril. Eur Heart J 4(Suppl A):189–197, 1983.
48. Timmermans PBM, Carini DJ, Chiu AT, et al: Angiotensin II receptor antagonists. Am J Hypertens 3:517–523, 1990.
49. Christen Y, Waeber B, Nussberger J, et al: Oral administration of DuP 753, a specific angiotensin II receptor antagonist, to normal male volunteers: Inhibition of pressor response to exogenous angiotensin I and II. Circulation 83:1333–1342, 1991.
50. Munafo A, Christen Y, Nussberger J, et al: Drug concentration response relationships in normal volunteers after oral administration of losartan (DuP 753, MK 954), an angiotensin II receptor antagonist. Clin Pharmacol Ther 51:513–521, 1992.
51. Brunner HR, Gavras H: Is the renin system necessary? Am J Med 69:739–745, 1980.

CHAPTER 7

Development of Nonpeptidic Angiotensin II Receptor Antagonists

PIETER B.M.W.M. TIMMERMANS, Ph.D.

The renin-angiotensin-aldosterone system (RAAS) has risen from an academically interesting, but obscure, regulatory mechanism to an important hormonal pathway known to play a pivotal role in the regulation of blood pressure and fluid and electrolyte homeostasis.[1] Activation of the RAAS is critically involved in the development and maintenance of hypertension and congestive heart failure. The octapeptide angiotensin II (Ang II) is the primary mediator of the RAAS. Its actions are mediated by specific surface receptors on the various target organs. The most specific and direct way to inhibit the RAAS is by antagonism of the effector hormone Ang II at the level of its target receptors. In theory, Ang II receptor antagonists should be able to inhibit the RAAS completely and selectively, independently of the source of Ang II.

Even before the appearance of Ang I-converting enzyme (ACE) inhibitors, pharmacologic inhibition of the RAAS was achieved in 1971 with saralasin, the first specific peptidic antagonist of Ang II.[2] Although saralasin reduced arterial pressure in hypertensive patients with high circulating plasma renin activity,[3] its therapeutic potential remained limited. Because of its peptidic nature, it has a short plasma half-life, is not orally bioavailable, and still possesses significant Ang II-like agonistic properties. Nonetheless, saralasin showed that the principle of interfering with Ang II at the level of its receptor had therapeutic potential.

Despite considerable efforts, little progress was made in the development of nonpeptidic Ang II receptor antagonists until the publication of two patents granted in 1982 to Furukawa and colleagues at Takeda Chemical Industries.[4,5] They disclosed a series of small-molecule imidazole analogs (see below) that possess Ang II antagonistic properties. Additional studies showed that although their potency was moderate, their oral bioavailability limited, and their duration of action short, they behaved as selective and competitive Ang II receptor antagonists without agonistic properties.[6] These low-molecular-weight imidazole compounds were adopted as leads for further optimization. Structural modification provided important chemical features that led to increasingly more potent and eventually orally active nonpeptidic Ang II receptor antagonists. Such activities culminated into the discovery of losartan,[7] the first clinically useful nonpeptidic Ang II receptor antagonist, followed by eprosartan.[8] Numerous other "sartans" were subsequently created based on modifications of losartan's prototypic chemical structure.[9]

Losartan and nonpeptidic spinacine-derived compounds, such as PD-123,177 and PD-123,319, as well as peptides, such as CGP 42112A, have firmly established the concept of Ang II receptor heterogeneity and have provided critical probes for the isolation and cloning of the two receptors for Ang II characterized in mammals, including humans. According to current nomenclature, losartan represents the prototype antagonist of the Ang II type 1 (AT$_1$) receptor family (further subtypes of rat and mouse AT$_1$ receptors are designated AT$_{1A}$ and AT$_{1B}$) and does not possess significant affinity for the so-called AT$_2$ receptor, for which PD-123,177, PD-123,319 and CGP 42112A exhibit high and selective affinity.[10] Virtually all—if not all—of the known actions of Ang II can be blocked by losartan, emphasizing the major role of the AT$_1$ receptor subtype in mediating the pathologic and physiologic actions of Ang II.[11] It also clearly explains why most of the pharmaceutical effort has been focused on developing nonpeptide AT$_1$ receptor-selective antagonists.

■ Discovery of Losartan and Eprosartan

The origin of the current potent nonpeptide AT$_1$ receptor antagonists, of which losartan is the prototype, can be traced back to the Takeda series of 1-benzylimidazole-5-acetic acid derivatives, such as S-8307 (CV2947) and S-8308 (CV2961) (Fig. 1).[4,5] Losartan[7] and eprosartan[8] were derived from this benzylimidazole series using two different molecular models of putative active conformations of Ang II to align the Takeda derivatives with the C-terminal region of Ang II. The first modeling strategy gave rise to EXP 6155 (see Fig. 1), which showed a 10-fold increase in binding affinity. From this starting point a series of phthalamic acids and related compounds were synthesized with progressively higher affinity for the AT$_1$ receptor. EXP 6803 produced another 10-fold enhancement in binding affinity. All of the compounds, however, were virtually devoid of oral activity, until the amide linker was replaced with a single bond, which resulted in EXP 7711. This biphenyl derivative had only slightly less affinity for the AT$_1$ receptor than EXP 6803 but represented a breakthrough to orally active congeners. To improve the oral activity and duration of action of these biphenyl compounds, a number of acidic groups were systematically evaluated as bioisosteric replacements for the carboxylic acid group. This effort culminated in the identification of the AT$_1$-selective antagonist, losartan, in which a tetrazole moiety substitutes for this carboxylic acid functionality (see Fig. 1).

In many animal species as well as in humans, losartan is metabolized to E3174, the imidazole-5-carboxylic acid, resulting from oxidation of the imidazole 5-hydroxymethyl group. Like losartan, E3174 is a selective AT$_1$ receptor antagonist, but it is appreciably more potent and possesses a much longer duration of action.[12] Like losartan, E3174 has served as a template for the development of many other AT$_1$ receptor antagonists.

A different modeling approach assisted in the synthesis of eprosartan,[8] which is representative of one of the few AT$_1$ receptor antagonists designed independently

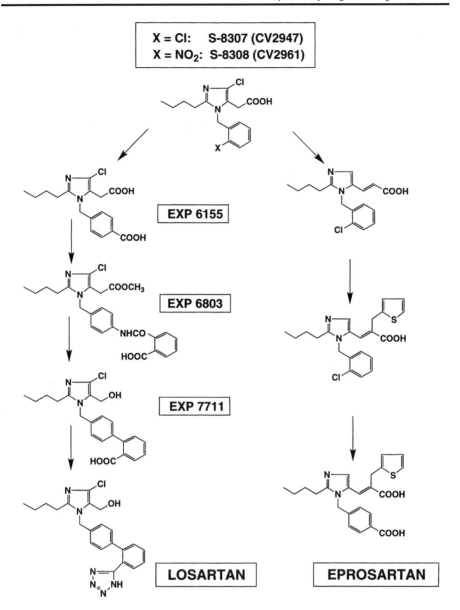

Figure 1. Structural modifications of the initial lead compounds, S-8307 (CV 2947) and S-8308 (CV 2961) that led to the successful discovery of the nonpeptide AT$_1$ receptor antagonists losartan and eprosartan.

of losartan from the Takeda benzylimidazoles. A combination of molecular modeling and knowledge of the structure-activity relationship for Ang II-like peptides resulted in a 15-fold enhancement in binding affinity by chain extension at the imidazole-5-position via a *trans*-5-acrylic acid group followed by addition of an α-benzyl group, which appeared to mimic more closely the Phe[8] side chain in Ang II. Replacement of this α-benzyl group with a 2-thienylmethyl moiety followed by replacement of the 2-chlorobenzyl group with a 4-carboxylbenzyl group to mimic more closely the phenolic moiety of Tyr[4] resulted in eprosartan (see Fig. 1). Eprosartan is a potent, AT_1-selective antagonist.

■ *The Second Wave of Sartans*

Losartan (E3174) is the first but by no means the only potent, selective, orally active and clinically useful nonpeptide AT_1 receptor antagonist. Numerous other antagonists have successfully completed clinical development. Several have been approved and marketed for the treatment of hypertension, and some are approved for congestive heart failure. The number of products within this class will undoubtedly increase. Valsartan (Fig. 2) represents a nonheterocyclic AT_1 receptor selective antagonist in which the imidazole of losartan is replaced with an acylated amino acid. This antagonist is a diacidic compound, like E3174.[13]

A number of additional antagonist designs have replaced the substituted imidazole found in losartan with various five-membered ring heterocycles. The potent AT_1 receptor antagonist irbesartan (see Fig. 2) incorporates an imidazolinone

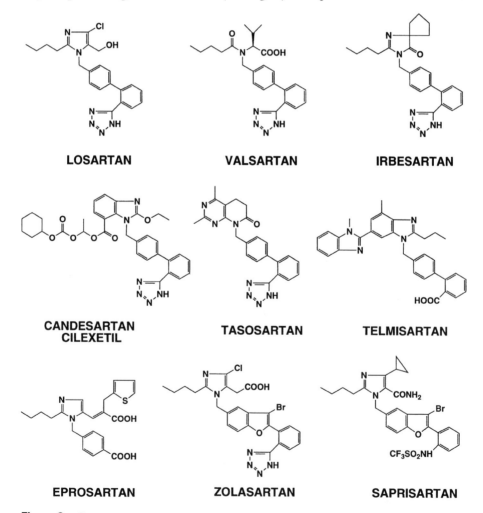

LOSARTAN   **VALSARTAN**   **IRBESARTAN**

CANDESARTAN   **TASOSARTAN**   **TELMISARTAN**
CILEXETIL

EPROSARTAN   **ZOLASARTAN**   **SAPRISARTAN**

Figure 2.   Chemical structures of AT_1 receptor antagonists that have completed clinical development.

ring in which a carbonyl group functions as a hydrogen bond acceptor in place of the hydroxymethyl group of losartan.[14] Potent antagonists have been obtained by joining substituents at the imidazole C_4 and C_5 positions to yield ring-fused imidazoles. The benzimidazole, candesartan cilexetil (see Fig. 2), is an ester carbonate prodrug that is rapidly converted in vivo to the corresponding 7-carboxylic acid candesartan.[15] Potent antagonists also have been obtained by replacing the imidazole of losartan with six-membered ring and fused six-membered ring heterocycles. An example is the AT_1 receptor antagonist tasosartan (see Fig. 2).[16] The enol metabolite, enoltasosartan, is responsible for the long pharmacodynamic action of the drug.[17]

Telmisartan (see Fig. 2) incorporates a carboxylic acid as the biphenyl acidic group. Unlike other series of antagonists, the biphenylcarboxylic acid telmisartan was more potent than its tetrazole analog. Telmisartan is a potent, selective AT_1 receptor antagonist.[18] In zolasartan (see Fig. 2), the "spacer" phenyl ring of E3174 is replaced by a bromobenzofuran. The presence of the 3-bromo substituent is essential for high AT_1 receptor affinity exhibited by this series of compounds. Zolasartan is a potent, selective AT_1 receptor antagonist possessing long-lasting antihypertensive effects in laboratory animals.[19] In saprisartan (see Fig. 2), the imidazolecarboxylic acid of zolasartan is replaced by a neutral imidazole-5-carboxamide to enhance oral bioavailability. This strategy was combined with the replacement of the tetrazole with a triflamide. Saprisartan has high affinity for the AT_1 receptor, and its oral bioavailability in animals and humans exceeds that of zolasartan.[20]

Table 1 lists the affinity of the various AT_1 receptor antagonists discussed so far for the AT_1 receptor as determined by radioligand-binding displacement experiments. The binding affinity is reported as an average value of several published independent measurements using membrane preparations from different tissues. All values are expressed relative to the most potent antagonist (affinity = 1). Candesartan and saprisartan possess the highest affinity for the AT_1 receptor, followed by zolasartan and irbesartan, which have an affinity that is 3- and 5-fold

Table 1. Affinity for AT_1 Receptors, Mode of AT_1 Receptor Antagonism and AT_1 Receptor Off-rate of AT_1 Receptor Antagonists.

AT_1 Receptor Antagonist	AT_1 Receptor Affinity	Mode of AT_1 Receptor Antagonism	AT_1 Receptor Off-Rate
Candesartan cilexetil	280	–	–
(Candesartan)	1	Noncompetitive	Slow
Saprisartan	1	Noncompetitive	N/A
Zolasartan	3	Noncompetitive	Slow
Irbesartan	5	Noncompetitive	Slow
Valsartan	10	Noncompetitive	Slow
Telmisartan	10	Noncompetitive	Slow
Tasosartan	20	Competitive	N/A
(Enoltasosartan)	N/A	N/A	N/A
Losartan	50	Competitive	Fast
(E3174)	10	Noncompetitive	Slow
Eprosartan	100	Competitive	Fast

N/A = not available.

less, respectively. Valsartan, telmisartan, and E3174 (the active metabolite of losartan) show comparable affinities that are 10-fold less than those of candesartan and saprisartan. Losartan's affinity for the AT_1 receptor is approximately 5 times less than that of E3174, whereas the concentration of eprosartan has to be 100-fold higher than that of candesartan to occupy the same number of AT_1 receptors. Finally, the prodrug candesartan cilexetil has a moderate AT_1 receptor binding affinity.

■ Mode of Functional AT_1 Receptor Antagonism

Effects of AT_1 receptor antagonists on the dose/concentration-response curves of Ang II have been characterized as either surmountable or competitive (i.e., the antagonist produces a dose/concentration-dependent, parallel shift to the right of the dose/concentration-response curve of Ang II without a change of the maximally attainable response) or insurmountable or noncompetitive (i.e., the antagonist produces a dose/concentration-dependent, nonparallel shift to the right of the dose/concentration-response curve of Ang II accompanied by a progressive dose/concentration-dependent decrease of the maximally attainable response).[21] Vasopressor responses in vivo and vasoconstrictor effects in vitro to Ang II have been studied to document this distinction. Accordingly, losartan, tasosartan and eprosartan have been classified as competitive AT_1 receptor antagonists, whereas candesartan, saprisartan, zolasartan, irbesartan, valsartan, telmisartan, and E3174 behave as noncompetitive antagonists (see Table 1). True surmountable antagonism presumably requires complete equilibrium among agonist, antagonist, and receptor in the interval between addition of the agonist and development of the response in the tissue, which is usually less than 1 minute.[22] The most common mechanism of insurmountable antagonism is irreversible, covalent binding of the antagonist with the receptor. The receptor number is effectively reduced to the point that the receptor reserve is exhausted and a full agonist response no longer can be obtained. Under certain kinetic conditions, however, antagonists that do not or cannot chemically react with the receptor protein produce insurmountable antagonism.[23] This phenomenon is observed for antagonists that slowly dissociate from the receptor; therefore, the agonist cannot reach equilibrium with the antagonist/receptor complex under the time constraints of the experiment. The more rapid the antagonist can adjust to the presence of the agonist, the more surmountable (competitive) the antagonism becomes. It is likely that slow dissociation kinetics of AT_1 receptor antagonists from the AT_1 receptor underlie insurmountable antagonism. As Table 1 shows, all noncompetitive AT_1 receptor antagonists have a slow off-rate from the AT_1 receptor, whereas all competitive inhibitors dissociate rapidly from the AT_1 receptor protein. In addition, in radioligand-binding displacement assays in which much more time is allowed to approach equilibrium than feasible in functional studies, all AT_1 receptor antagonists show (close to) competitive antagonism of Ang II binding. This subject is discussed in more detail further in chapter 9.

The mode of AT_1 receptor antagonism (competitive vs. noncompetitive) most probably does not play a role in defining the antihypertensive effect of the antagonists because the antagonist has ample time (hours) to reach equilibrium. It is unlikely, therefore, that noncompetitive AT_1 receptor antagonists are more efficacious antihypertensive agents than competitive antagonists. The extensive

Table 2. Characteristics of AT$_1$ Receptor Antagonists in Clinical Practice in the Treatment of Patients with Mild to Moderate Hypertension

Drug (Active Metabolite)	Bioavail-ability (%)	Food Effect	Active Metabolite	Plasma Half-life (h)	% Protein Binding	Dosage (mg)
Losartan (EXP 3174)	33	Minimal	Yes	2 (6–9)	98.7 (99.8)	50–100/day
Valsartan	25	40–50%*	No	6	95.0	80–320/day
Candesartan cilexetil (Candesartan)	42	No	Yes	3.5–4 (3–11)	99.5	4–32/day
Tasosartan† (Enoltasosartan)	N/A	No	Yes	3–7 (36–72)	N/A	50–100/day
Irbesartan	70	No	No	11–15	> 90(?)	150–300/day
Eprosartan	N/A	N/A	No	N/A	97.0	200–400 twice daily
Telmisartan	N/A	N/A	No	~24	N/A	40–120/day
Zolasartan†	20	N/A	No	N/A	N/A	N/A
Saprisartan†	N/A	N/A	N/A	N/A	N/A	N/A

N/A = not available.
* ↓, decrease by
† Clinical development discontinued or marketing application withdrawn
Modified from Brunner HR: The new angiotensin II receptor antagonist, irbesartan. Pharmacokinetic and pharmacodynamic considerations. Hypertension 10:311S–317S, 1997.

preclinical experience with AT$_1$ receptor antagonists clearly documents similar antihypertensive/hypotensive efficacies.[11] However, the slow off-rate from the AT$_1$ receptor exhibited by several antagonists may extend the time of occupancy of the receptor protein and lengthen the duration of the antagonism. Table 2 summarizes the major characteristics of currently available AT$_1$ receptor antagonists. Of interest, eprosartan, which is dosed twice daily, is the only antagonist that is competitive and dissociates rapidly from the AT$_1$ receptor and does not produce an active (noncompetitive) metabolite.

■ Additional AT$_1$ Receptor Antagonists in Advanced Clinical Development

As the database on the clinical efficacy, safety, and tolerability of losartan and subsequent AT$_1$-selective receptor antagonists continues to expand, an increasing number of compounds with potent AT$_1$ receptor antagonistic properties have reached preclinical status. Some of them have been characterized in human subjects.[24] This chapter highlights the three agents that are most advanced in clinical development: milfasartan, embusartan, and elisartan.

Milfasartan (LR-B/081) (Fig. 3) belongs to a series of novel 4-pyrimidinones, which are potent and selective AT$_1$ receptor antagonists[25] that show noncompetitive antagonism in functional studies.[26] In rat adrenal cortical membranes, the affinity of milfasartan for AT$_1$ receptors is about 10-fold higher than that of losartan.[27] When tested orally, milfasartan was as active as losartan in either inhibiting Ang II-induced pressor responses or lowering blood pressure in conscious renal and spontaneously hypertensive rats, although it had a somewhat shorter duration of action.[26] Milfasartan (10, 40, and 80 mg) has been documented to be a potent, well-tolerated, orally active AT$_1$ receptor antagonist in humans.[28] With

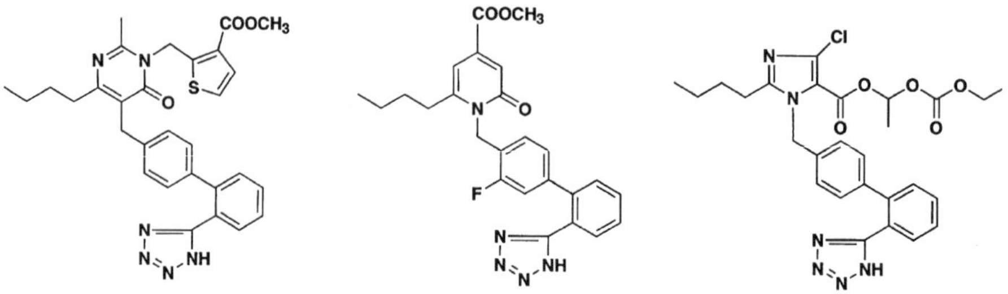

MILFASARTAN (LR-B/081)   EMBUSARTAN (BAY 10-6734)   ELISARTAN (HN-65021)

Figure 3.   Chemical structures of some additional AT_1 receptor antagonists in advanced clinical development.

the highest dose the antagonism remained significant for 24 hours. No active metabolites have been shown to be responsible for its inhibitory effects in humans.[28]

Embusartan (BAY 10-6734) (see Fig. 3) is another newly developed, orally active AT_1 receptor antagonist that has been shown to be efficacious in various animal models of hypertension.[29] In embusartan the imidazole of losartan has been replaced by a six-membered ring, i.e., a dihydropyridinone. In vivo hydrolysis of the ester creates the corresponding carboxylic acid (BAY 10-6735), the predominant therapeutically active moiety of embusartan. Embusartan and its metabolite (BAY 10-6735) have comparable AT_1 receptor-binding affinities, which are superior to that of losartan.[30] Functionally, embusartan behaves as a competitive antagonist, whereas BAY 10-6735 exhibits a noncompetitive mode of antagonism.[31] Embusartan (20, 40, 80, 200, and 300 mg) administered orally to healthy male volunteers dose-dependently induced rightward shifts of the Ang II pressor response curves.[32] All treatments were well tolerated. Single oral doses of 300–400 mg seem to provide a 24-hour antagonistic activity. Circulating concentrations of BAY 10-6735 rose rapidly, reaching levels that were about 10-fold higher than those of the parent compound. The pharmacodynamic and pharmacokinetic half-lives of BAY 10-6735 were nearly identical.[32]

Like losartan, E3174 has served as a starting point for the design of many novel AT_1 receptor antagonists. The limited oral bioavailability of E3174[33] has been addressed through the prodrug approach. One such prodrug is elisartan (HN-65021) (see Fig. 3), which is a prodrug ester of E3174. When given orally to rats and dogs at doses of 0.5 and 1 mg/kg, elisartan antagonized the pressor response produced by Ang II.[34] Elisartan (5, 10, and 100 mg) administered orally to healthy male volunteers was well tolerated and dose-dependently inhibited the Ang II-induced vasoconstriction in the forearm vasculature.[35] Its potency was similar to that of losartan.[35]

■ Development Activities in Japan

Probably a limited number of AT_1 receptor antagonists (the first four to market?) will be adopted to the formularies in Japan, because it is assumed that subsequent agents in the same class will offer no additional benefit (Arakawa, personal communication). Currently, losartan and candesartan have obtained

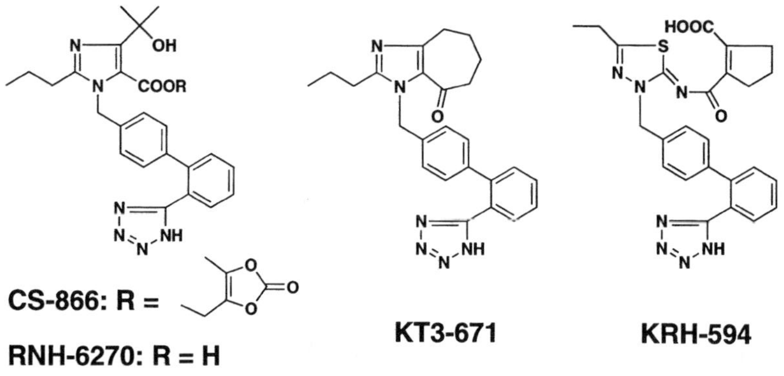

CS-866: R =

RNH-6270: R = H

KT3-671

KRH-594

Figure 4. Chemical structures of some newer AT_1 receptor antagonists in clinical development in Japan.

marketing approval in Japan, and valsartan may be the third to be approved. Because of regulatory and economic pressures in Japan, it is hard to predict which other antagonist(s) will reach approval status. Among the newer agents in clinical development in Japan the most advanced are CS-866, KT3-671, and KRH-594.

CS-866 (olmesartan; Fig. 4) is a prodrug and is hydrolyzed to the active acid RNH-6270. RNH-6270 inhibits the binding of ^{125}I-Ang II to the AT_1 receptors in bovine adrenal cortical membranes at an approximately 10-fold lower concentration than losartan and has negligible affinity for the AT_2 receptor in the same tissue.[36] RNH-6270 showed potent, noncompetitive antagonism against Ang II-induced contractions of the guinea pig aorta. Oral CS-866 produced pronounced and long-lasting inhibition of the pressor effects of Ang II in conscious rats.[36] CS-866 administered orally to salt-restricted hypertensive patients lowered blood pressure and increased plasma renin activity and Ang II concentrations. A single oral dose of 10–20 mg of CS-866 resulted in nearly maximal effect.[37]

KT3-671 (see Fig. 4) contains a seven-membered ring fused to the imidazole (2-propyl-8-oxo-cycloheptimidazole). This newly synthesized agent is a potent, AT_1 receptor subtype selective, competitive antagonist.[38] Its affinity for the AT_1 receptor in rat liver membranes is about 7-fold higher than that of losartan, and it produced parallel rightward shifts of the concentration-contractile response curve to Ang II in isolated rabbit aorta (KT3-671 pA_2 = 10.04; losartan pA_2 = 8.32). KT3-671 produced sustained, long-lasting blood pressure and Ang II pressor inhibitory effects after oral administration to rats and dogs.[38–40]

KRH-594 (see Fig. 4) is an acyliminothiadiazoline; no hepatically produced, active metabolites have been observed. In radioligand displacement experiments, KRH-594 exhibited selective affinity for AT_1 receptors and was found to be as potent as E3174.[41] In functional studies, KRH-594 behaved as a highly active noncompetitive antagonist. Upon oral administration, KRH-594 (1–10 mg/kg) produced sustained antihypertensive effects in spontaneously hypertensive rats and in renal hypertensive rats and dogs.[42]

■ *Selective AT_2 Receptor Antagonists*

The first nonpeptidic compounds that showed selective affinity for the AT_2 receptor were a series of spinacine-derived tetrahydroimidazopyridines, including

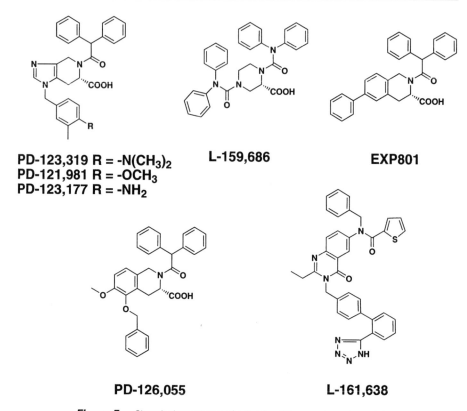

PD-123,319 R = -N(CH₃)₂
PD-121,981 R = -OCH₃
PD-123,177 R = -NH₂

L-159,686

EXP801

PD-126,055

L-161,638

Figure 5. Chemical structures of selective AT_2 receptor antagonists.

PD-123,177, PD-121,981, and PD-123,319 (Fig. 5). Their affinity for the AT_2 receptor (IC_{50} = approximately 100 nM) is about 5000-times higher than their affinity for the AT_1 receptor.[43] These derivatives have been important tools in defining Ang II receptor heterogeneity in tissues and organs from various species, including humans, and in characterizing the AT receptor subtype(s) involved in the multiple actions of Ang II.

Subsequently, potent AT_2 receptor-selective diacylpiperazines, such as L-159,686 (AT_2: IC_{50} = 1.5 nM; AT_1: IC_{50} > 100 nM) (see Fig. 5), were reported. The oral bioavailability and plasma half-life in rats of L-159,686 are 50% and > 6 hours, respectively.[44] Tetrahydroisoquinolines with pronounced AT_2 receptor-binding selectivity have been disclosed, including PD-126,055[45] and EXP801[46] (see Fig. 5). In addition, substituted quinazolinones have yielded potent AT_2 receptor-selective ligands; an example is L-161,638 (AT_2: IC_{50} = 0.06 nM; AT_1: IC_{50} = 200 nM)[47] (see Fig. 5).

Studies involving selective AT_2 receptor antagonists have been confined to the preclinical setting. The extensive pharmacologic analysis performed to date indicates that most, if not all, of the known pathologic and physiologic effects of Ang II are mediated by the AT_1 receptor.[11] However, blockade of AT_1 receptors also causes inhibition of the negative feedback mechanism of Ang II on renin production and release, leading to elevated circulating Ang II concentrations in the plasma with a resultant stimulation of AT_2 receptors. Accumulating evidence indicates that the AT_2 receptor acts as an antagonistic receptor against the AT_1 receptor; that is, AT_2 receptors mediate antigrowth, antihypertrophic, and proapoptotic effects.[48] The added benefits of AT_2 receptor stimulation to the overall clinical effectiveness of AT_1 receptor antagonism remain speculative but intriguing.

■ *Balanced (AT₁/AT₂) Angiotension II Receptor Antagonists*

The exquisite selectivity of losartan and its analogs for the AT_1 receptor as well as the absence of conclusive data about the role of the AT_2 receptor led to early efforts to design compounds possessing equal affinity for AT_1 and AT_2 receptors ("balanced" antagonists).

The hybrid molecule L-162,132 (AT_1: IC_{50} = 15 nM; AT_2: IC_{50} = 180nM) (Fig. 6), which combines structural parts of the AT_1-selective compound losartan and the AT_2-selective ligand L-159,686 (see above), binds moderately to both receptors.[49] However, the most successful approach to balanced AT_1/AT_2 antagonists has been to modify AT_1-selective compounds to enhance their AT_2 affinity. Excellent AT_1/AT_2 balance and potency have been achieved in several heterocyclic series. In most of these molecules, AT_2 affinity and AT_1/AT_2 balance were obtained more readily when an acylsulfonamide group was used as an isosteric replacement for the tetrazole ring. The imidazopyridine antagonist L-163,017 (AT_1: IC_{50} = 0.24 nM; AT_2: IC_{50} = 0.29 nM) (Fig. 7), balanced against AT_1 and AT_2 receptors in rat adrenal tissue, also has balanced affinities for AT_1 and AT_2 receptors in several human tissues, including aorta, kidney, and adrenal gland.[50] L-163,017 exhibited a long duration of action after oral administration to conscious rats and dogs. Its oral bioavailability amounted to 45% in rats and 34% in dogs. Equivalence of AT_1 and AT_2 receptor binding was maintained for longer than 6 hours after oral administration to rats and dogs, as determined by a radioligand displacement assay of plasma samples. The imidazole XR510 (see Fig. 7) showed potent and balanced antagonist activities (AT_1: IC_{50} = 0.26 nM; AT_2: IC_{50} = 0.28 nM) as well as a pronounced oral antihypertensive activity in renal hypertensive rats (ED_{30} = 0.27 mg/kg) with a duration of action longer than 24 hours.[51] The oral bioavailibility of XR510 was 100% in rats and 25% in dogs. The quinazolinone L-163,579 (AT_1: IC_{50} = 0.57 nM; AT_2: IC_{50} = 0.39 nM) and the triazolinone L-163,958 (AT_1: IC_{50} = 0.20 nM; AT_2: IC_{50} = 0.12 nM) (see Fig. 7) are additional examples of potent balanced AT_1/AT_2 receptor antagonists.[52,53] The excellent in vivo properties of all of these agents make them useful tools for in vivo pharmacologic studies.

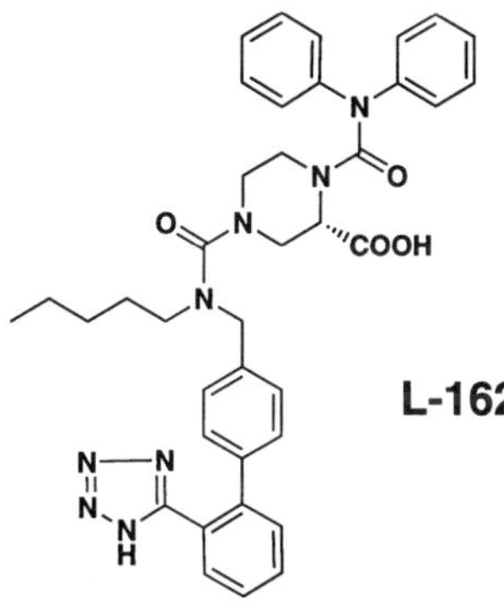

Figure 6.   Chemical structure of the hybrid molecule L-162,132 combining structural elements of the AT_1 receptor selective antagonist losartan and the AT_2 receptor selective antagonist IL-159,686.

L-162,132

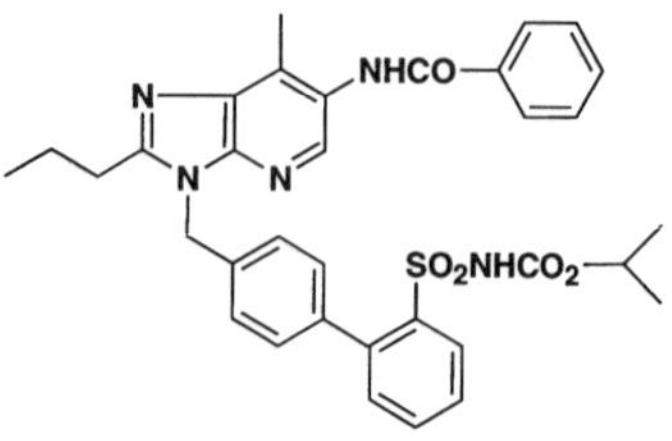

Figure 7. Chemical structures of antagonists with equal affinity for AT_1 and AT_2 receptors ("balanced" antagonists).

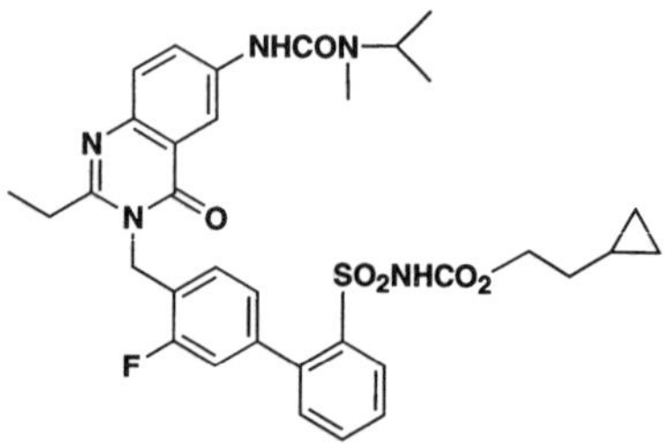

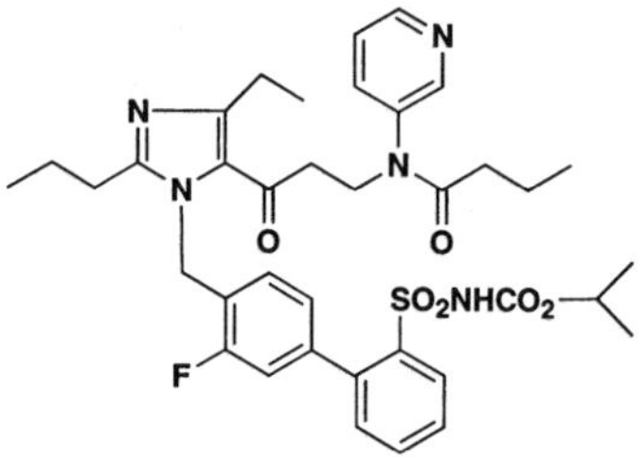

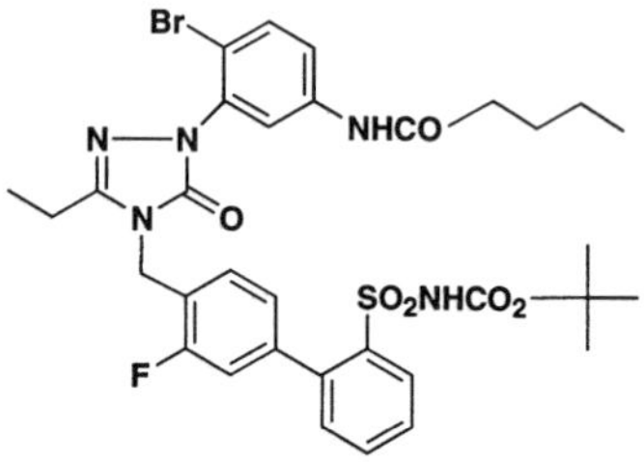

The initial concern over a potential safety liability of AT_1-selective antagonists in the light of unoccupied AT_2 receptors during increased concentrations of circulating Ang II eventually proved unwarranted. In addition, no evidence indicates that additional AT_2 receptor blockade provides increased antihypertensive efficacy over AT_1 receptor blockade alone. Therefore, none of the balanced AT_1/AT_2 receptor antagonists discussed above have reached the stage of clinical development.

■ Conclusion

An appreciation of the full scope of the pathologic and physiologic effects of Ang II (endocrine, paracrine, and autocrine) has been made possible by the discovery and design of specific, potent, long-acting, and orally active nonpeptidic AT_1 receptor antagonists. For the first time, agents have become available to dissect more specifically and to block more completely the actions of Ang II, without the limitations of the earlier peptidic Ang II receptor antagonists and the nonspecificity of the ACE inhibitors. They offer more complete blockade of the RAAS by also antagonizing the actions of Ang II produced by non-ACE dependent pathways. Virtually all of the well-known actions of Ang II are inhibited by AT_1 receptor antagonists, emphasizing the pivotal role of this distinct receptor subtype in mediating an activated RAAS. The extensive preclinical experience with AT_1 receptor antagonists suggests that they produce comparable inhibition of the RAAS to that obtained by ACE and renin inhibitors.[11] In numerous models of experimental and genetic hypertension, AT_1 receptor antagonists are effective antihypertensive agents with similar efficacy to that of ACE and renin inhibitors. This new class of agents also markedly reduces or prevents cardiovascular hypertrophy and remodeling. In animal models of renal disease, AT_1 receptor antagonists significantly decrease protenuria, protect against diabetic glomerulopathy, and increase survival in stroke-prone SH rats. In several models of heart failure, AT_1 receptor antagonists have shown beneficial effects in lowering intracardial pressures, preventing or blunting hypertrophy remodeling, and fibrosis of the heart, and increasing survival after myocardial infarction.

AT_1 receptor antagonists represent the newest addition to the armamentarium of cardiovascular drugs for the treatment of hypertension and congestive heart failure. Their clinical pharmacology is discussed in chapters 18–25. Reviews of the therapeutic usage of AT_1 receptor antagonists have focused on losartan.[24,54] The quality of the therapeutic effect and the excellent tolerability of this class of drugs are expected to enhance patient compliance compared with other commonly used antihypertensives. The place of AT_1 receptor antagonists in therapy ultimately depends in large part on health economic factors and the availability of positive end-point data from several large trials that currently are ongoing. AT_1 receptor antagonists represent a new milestone in the development of cardiovascular therapeutics and add another dimension to the arcenal of drugs manipulating the RAAS.

Acknowledgment

The author wishes to thank Hallie Widlow and Alicia Williams for conducting the literature searches, providing the artwork, and preparing the manuscript.

References

1. Sealy JE, Laragh JH: The renin-angiotensin-aldosterone system for normal regulation of blood Pressure and sodium and potassium homeostasis. In Laragh JH, Brenner B (eds): Hypertension: Pathophysiology, Diagnosis and Management. New York, Raven Press, 1995, pp 1763–1796.
2. Pals DT, Masucci FD, Sipos F, Denning GS: A specific competitive antagonist of the vascular action of angiotensin II. Cir Res 29:664–672, 1971.
3. Brunner HR, Gavras H, Laragh JH, Keenan R: Angiotensin II blockade in man by sar[1]-ala[8]-angiotensin II for understanding and treatment of high blood pressure. Lancet 2:1045–1048, 1973.
4. Furukawa Y, Kishimoto S, Nishikawa K: Hypotensive imidazole derivatives. U.S. Patent 4,340,598. Issued to Takeda Chemical Industries, Ltd, Osaka, Japan, 1982.
5. Furukawa Y, Kishimoto S, Nishikawa K: Hypotensive imidazole-5-acetice acid derivatives. U.S. Patent 4,355,040. Issued to Takeda Chemical Industries, Ltd, Osaka, Japan, 1982.
6. Chiu AT, Carini DJ, Johnson AL, et al: Nonpeptide angiotensin II receptor antagonists. II. Pharmacology of S-8308. Eur J Pharmacol 157:13–21, 1988.
7. Duncia JV, Chiu AT, Carini DJ, et al: The discovery of potent nonpeptide angiotensin II receptor antagonists: A new class of potent antihypertensives. J Med Chem 33:1312–1329, 1990.
8. Weinstock J, Keenan RM, Samanen J, et al: 1-(Carboxybenzyl)imidazole-5-acrylic acids: Potent and selective angiotensin II receptor antagonists. J Med Chem 34:1514–1517, 1991.
9. Wexler RR, Greenlee WJ, Irvin JD, et al: Nonpeptide angiotensin II receptor antagonists: The next generation in antihypertensive therapy. J Med Chem 39:625–656, 1996.
10. de Gasparo M, Husain A, Alexander W, et al: Proposed update of angiotensin receptor nomenclature. Hypertension 25:924–927, 1995.
11. Timmermans PBMWM, Wong PC, Chiu AT, et al: Angiotensin II receptors and angiotensin II receptor antagonists. Pharmacol Rev 45:205–251, 1993.
12. Wong PC, Price WA, Chiu AT, et al: Nonpeptide angiotensin II receptor antagonists XI. Pharmacology of EXP3174: An active metabolite of DuP 753, and orally active antihypertensive agent. J Pharmacol Exp Ther 255:211–217, 1990.
13. Criscione L, de Gasparo M, Buhlmayer P, et al: Pharmacological profile of valsartan: A potent, orally active, nonpeptide antagonist of the angiotensin II AT_1-receptor subtype. Br J Pharmacol 110:761–771, 1993.

14. Cazaubon C, Gougat J, Bousquet F, et al: Pharmacological characterization of SR47436: A new nonpeptide AT_1 subtype angiotensin II receptor antagonist. J Pharmacol Exp Ther 265:826–834, 1993.

15. Shibouta Y, Inada Y, Ojima M, et al: Pharmacological profile of the highly potent and long-acting angiotensin II receptor antagonist, CV-11974, and its prodrug TCV-116. J Pharmacol Exp Ther 266:114–120, 1993.

16. Ellingboe JW, Antane M, Nguyen TT, et al: Pyrido[2,3-d]pyrimidine angiotensin II antagonists. J Med Chem 37:542–550, 1994.

17. Lacourciere Y, Pool JL, Svetkey L, et al: A randomized, double-blind, placebo-controlled, parallel-group, multicenter trial of four doses of tasosartan in patients with essential hypertension. Am J Hypertens 11:454–461, 1998.

18. Wienen W, Hanel N, van Meel JCA, et al: Pharmacological characterization of the novel nonpeptide angiotensin II receptor antagonist, BIBR 277. Br J Pharmacol 110:245–252, 1993.

19. Hilditch A, Hunt AAE, Gardner CJ et al: Cardiovascular effects of GR117289, a novel angiotensin AT_1 receptor antagonist. Br J Pharmacol 111:137–144, 1994.

20. Judd DB, Dowle MD, Middlemiss D, et al: Bromobenzofuran-based non-peptide antagonists of angiotensin II: GR138950, a potent antihypertensive agent with high oral bioavailability. J Med Chem 37:3108–3120, 1994.

21. Gaddum JH, Hameed KA, Hathaway DE, Stephens FF: Quantitative studies of antagonists for 5-hydroxytryptamine. Quart J Exp Physiol 40:49–74, 1955.

22. Rang HP: The kinetics of action of acetylcholine antagonists in smooth muscle. Proc R Soc Lond B Biol Sci 164:488–510, 1996.

23. Kenakin TP: The classification of drugs and drug receptors in isolated tissues. Pharmacol Rev 36:165–222, 1984.

24. Csajka C, Buclin T, Brunner HR, Biollaz J: Pharmacokinetic-pharmacodynamic profile of angiotensin II receptor antagonists. Clin Pharmacokinet 32:1–29, 1997.

25. Salimbeni A, Cavenotti R, Paleari F, et al: N-3-Substituted pyrimidinones as potent, orally active, AT_1 selective angiotensin II receptor antagonists. J Med Chem 38:4806–4820, 1995.

26. Cirillo R, Renzetti AR, Cucchi P, et al: Pharmacology of LR-B/081, a new highly potent, selective and orally active, nonpeptide angiotensin II AT_1 receptor antagonist. Br J Pharmacol 114:1117–1124, 1995.

27. Renzetti AR, Criscuoli M, Salimbeni A, Subissi A: Molecular pharmacology of LR-B/081, a new nonpeptide angiotensin AT_1 receptor antagonist. Eur J Pharmacol 290:151–156, 1995.

28. Noël B, Del Re G, Capone P, et al: Clinical and hormonal effects of the new angiotensin II receptor antagonist LRB081. J Cardiovasc Pharmacol 28:252–258, 1996.

29. Stasch J-P, Knorr A, Hirth-Dietrich C, Krämer T: Long-term blockade of the angiotensin II receptor in renin transgenic rats, salt-loaded Dahl rats, and stroke-prone spontaneously hypertensive rats. Arzneim-Forsch/Drug Res 47:1016–1023, 1997.

30. Iouzalen L, Stepien O, Marche P: Effects of BAY 10-6734 (embusartan), a new angiotensin II type I receptor antagonist, on vascular smooth muscle growth. J Pharmacol Exp Ther 289:181–187, 1999.

31. Knorr A, Stasch J-P, Beuck M, et al: Pharmacology of BAY 10-6734, an AT_1-selective angiotensin II receptor antagonist. Naunyn-Schmiedebergs Arch Pharmacol 353:R69, 1996.

32. Breithaupt-Grögler K, Malerczyk C, Belz GG, et al: Pharmacodynamic and pharmacokinetic properties of an angiotensin II receptor antagonist—Characterization by use of Schild regression technique in man. Intern J Clin Pharmacol Ther 35:434–441, 1997.

33. Sweet CS, Nelson EB: How well have animal studies with losartan predicted responses in humans? J Hypertens 11(3):S63–S67, 1993.

34. Stimmeder D, Stroissnig H, Kuhberger E, et al: HN-65021, a new nonpeptide, highly potent, orally active angiotensin II receptor antagonist in vivo. Can J Physiol Pharmacol 72(Suppl 1):122, 1994.

35. Cockcroft JR, Chowienczyk PJ, Brett SE, et al: The effect of HN-65021 on responses to angiotensin II in human forearm vasculature. Br J Clin Pharmacol 40:591–593, 1995.

36. Mizuno M, Sada T, Ikeda M, et al.: Pharmacology of CS-866, a novel nonpeptide angiotensin II receptor antagonist. Eur J Pharmacol 285:181–188, 1995.

37. Püchler K, Nussberger J, Laeis P, et al: Blood pressure and endocrine effects of single doses of CS-866, a novel angiotensin II antagonist, in salt-restricted hypertensive patients. J Hypertens 15:1809–1812, 1997.

38. Mochizuki S, Sato T, Furuta K, et al: Pharmacological properties of KT3-671, a novel nonpeptide angiotensin II receptor antagonist. J Cardiovasc Pharmacol 25:22–29, 1995.

39. Takata Y, Tajima S, Mochizuki S, et al: Antihypertensive activity and pharmacokinetics of KD3-671, a nonpeptide AT_1-receptor antagonist, in renal hypertensive dogs. J Cardiovasc Pharmacol 32:834–844, 1998.

40. Kawashima K, Amano H, Fujimoto K, et al: Effect of repeated administration of KT3-671, a nonpeptide AT_1 receptor antagonist, on diurnal variation in blood pressure, heart rate, and locomotor activity in stroke-prone spontaneously hypertensive rats as determined by radiotelemetry. J Cardiovasc Pharmacol 27:411–416, 1996.

41. Tamura K, Okuhira M, Amano H, et al: Pharmacologic profiles of KRH-594, a novel nonpeptide angiotensin II receptor antagonist. J Cardiovasc Pharmacol 30:607–615, 1997.

42. Inada Y, Murakami M, Kaido K, Nakao K: Effects of the new angiotensin II receptor type 1 receptor antagonist KRH-594 on several types of experimental hypertension. Arzneim-Forsch/Drug Res 49:13–21, 1999.

43. Blankley CJ, Hodges JC, Klutchko SR, et al: Synthesis and structure-activity relationships of a novel series of non-peptide angiotensin II receptor binding inhibitors specific for the AT_2 subtype. J Med Chem 34:3248–3260, 1991.

44. Wu MT, Ikeler TJ, Ashton WT, et al: Synthesis and structure-activity relationships of a novel series of non-peptide AT_2-selective angiotensin II receptor antagonists. Bioorg Med Chem Lett 3:2023–2028, 1993.

45. Klutchko S, Hamby JM, Hodges JC: Tetrahydroisoquinoline derivatives with AT_2-specific angiotensin II receptor binding inhibitory activity. Bioorg Med Chem Lett 4:57–62, 1994.

46. Van Atten MK, Ensinger SL, Chiu AT, et al: A novel series of selective, non-peptide inhibitors of angiotensin II binding to the AT_2 site. J Med Chem 36:3985–3992, 1993.

47. Glinka TW, de Laszlo SE, Tran J, et al: L-161,638, a potent selective quinazolinone angiotensin II binding inhibitor. Bioorg Med Chem Lett 4: 1479–1484, 1994.

48. Horiuchi M, Akishita M, Dzau VJ: Recent progress in angiotensin type 2 receptor research in the cardiovascular system. Hypertension 33:613–621, 1999.

49. Wu MT, Ikeler TJ, Greenlee WJ: A novel pipezazine angiotensin II antagonist with balanced affinity for angiotensin AT_1 and AT_2 receptor subtypes. Bioorg Med Chem Lett 4:17–22, 1994.

50. Chang RSL, Lotti VJ, Chen TB, et al: In vitro pharmacology of L-163,017: A nonpeptide angiotensin II receptor antagonist with balanced affinity for AT_1 and AT_2 receptors. Eur J Pharmacol 294:429–437, 1995.

51. Wong PC, Quan ML, Hajj-Ali AF, et al: Pharmacology of XR510, a potent orally-active nonpeptide angiotensin II AT_1 receptor antagonist with high affinity for the AT_2 receptor subtype. J Cardiovasc Pharmacol 26:354–362, 1995.

52. Glinka TW, de Laszlo SE, Siegl PKS, et al: Development of balanced angiotensin II antagonists equipotent towards human AT_1 and AT_2 receptor subtypes. Bioorg Med Chem Lett 4:2337–2342, 1994.

53. Ashton WT, Chang LL, Flanagan KL, et al: Optimization of high-affinity AT_1/AT_2-balanced triazolinone angiotensin II antagonists. 208th American Chemical Society National Meeting, Washington, DC, August 21–26, 1994.

54. MacFadyen RJ, Reid JL: Angiotensin receptor antagonists as treatment for hypertension. J Hypertens 12: 1333–1338, 1994.

55. Brunner HR: The new angiotensin II receptor antagonist, irbesartan. Pharmacokinetic and pharmacrodynamic considerations. Hypertension 10: 311S–317S, 1997.

CHAPTER 8

Distinction Between Surmountable and Insurmountable Angiotensin II AT_1 Receptor Antagonists

GEORGES VAUQUELIN, Ph.D.

FREDERIK FIERENS, M.Sc.

PATRICK VANDERHEYDEN, Ph.D.

Angiotensin II (Ang II), the effector peptide of the renin-angiotensin system, produces a variety of biologic actions, including vascular smooth muscle contraction and growth of smooth muscle cells and cardiac myocytes.[1] These actions are mediated by Ang II type I (AT_1) receptors. AT_1 receptors play a major role in the regulation of cardiovascular homeostasis; there has been much interest in developing nonpeptide antagonists for the clinical treatment of hypertension and congestive heart failure.[2]

A fair number of synthetic antagonists have been described during the past decade. Traditionally they are tested for their ability to antagonize Ang II-induced contraction of rabbit aortic rings or strips, a system with small receptor reserve.[3,4] The tissue is preequilibrated with the antagonist for a period ranging between 10 minutes and 2 hours. Then increasing concentrations of Ang II are added to generate a dose-response curve. Based on differences in their ability to depress the maximal response to Ang II in such experiments, the antagonists are commonly divided into two categories:

1. Antagonists that produce only parallel rightward shifts of the dose-response curve without depressing the maximal response are classified as surmountable or competitive antagonists. Losartan is a typical example.[5]

2. Antagonists that also depress the maximal response to Ang II are classified as insurmountable, nonsurmountable, or noncompetitive antagonists. Most of the investigated antagonists fall into this category. The degree by which they depress the maximal response, however, is extremely variable, ranging from a partial decline for irbesartan, valsartan, and EXP3174 (the active metabolite of losartan) to an almost complete effect for antagonists such as GR117289, KRH-594, and candesartan.[5–12]

AT_1 receptors are members of the G protein-coupled receptor superfamily. In primary cultures of vascular smooth muscle cells, they have been shown to stimulate the phosphoinositide signaling system. The resulting elevation of the intracellular free calcium concentration triggers constriction and ultimately cell growth.[13] The initial AT_1 receptor-evoked responses also can be conveniently measured in other primary cell cultures and in cell lines that have been transfected permanently or transiently with the genes coding for the AT_1 receptors from different species. Insurmountable antagonism also has been observed in measuring the inositol triphosphate production in primary cultures of rabbit aortic smooth muscle cells[14,15] and in Chinese hamster ovary cells, which were stably transfected with the gene coding for the AT_1 receptor from rats[16] and humans (i.e., CHO-hAT_1 cells).[17–19]

Several theories have been advanced over the past 10 years to explain the molecular action mechanism of insurmountable AT_1 receptor antagonists and, in particular, the frequently incomplete character of their effect. These theories include the presence of allosteric binding sites on the receptor[20]; slowly interconverting receptor conformations[21–23]; slow dissociation of the antagonist-receptor complex[14,24–29]; slow removal of the antagonist from tissue compartments, cells, or matrix surrounding the receptor[7,15]; coexistence of different receptor subpopulations[30]; and the ability of the antagonist to modulate the amount of internalized receptors.[6]

■ Competitive Nature of Insurmountable Antagonists

To facilitate understanding of the molecular basis of insurmountable antagonism, it is necessary to distinguish the terms "competitive" and "noncompetitive" from the terms "surmountable" and "insurmountable." "Competitive" and "noncompetitive" refer to the ability of two ligands to affect each other's binding to the receptor; these properties, therefore, can be revealed only in experiments in which neither ligand has the unfair advantage of being in contact with the receptor before the other. In other words, only coincubation experiments determine whether two receptor ligands are competitive. When coincubation agonist dose-response experiments are carried out, competitive antagonists do not affect the maximal response, whereas noncompetitive antagonists decrease the maximal response (Fig. 1). The same applies to saturation binding experiments: competitive ligands do not affect the maximal binding of the radioligand, whereas noncompetitive ligands decrease the maximal binding.

In aortic strip contraction studies, the AT_1 receptor antagonists are given to the tissue first. Hence, they are in contact with the receptor before Ang II. Under these experimental conditions, a depression of the maximal response discloses only that Ang II was unable to overcome or surmount the antagonistic action. These antagonists are denoted as "insurmountable." Of interest, both competitive and noncompetitive antagonists may produce insurmountable inhibition (see Fig. 1). Noncompetitive antagonists, for example, act at an allosteric site of the receptor or interfere directly with a cellular process that is necessary for the generation of the response. It is also clear that the action of competitive but irreversible antagonists cannot be overcome during the ensuing exposure of the receptors to an agonist. The same situation applies to competitive antagonists with a reversible but long-lasting action.[31] The ensuing exposure of the receptors to

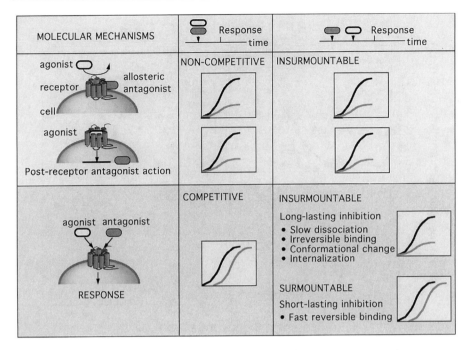

Figure 1. Different modes of antagonism and their consequence on agonist dose-response curves in antagonist coincubation and antagonist preincubation experiments. AT₁ receptor antagonists are competitive (*shaded area below*). In preincubation experiments, they may act surmountably when the inhibition is transient or insurmountably when the inhibition is long-lasting.

the agonist may be too short for their action to be fully overcome. The resulting hemiequilibrium is reflected by the decreased maximal response to the agonist.[32,33] These considerations clearly establish that the terms "insurmountable" and "noncompetitive" should not be used as synonyms.

Even after their preexposure to the receptor, certain antagonists produce full rightward shifts of the agonist dose-response curve. Such antagonists inhibit the response in a competitive fashion, and their antagonistic action is so swiftly reversible that it has been completely overcome or surmounted by the subsequently added agonist at the moment that its response is measured.[32] Because such antagonists are more than simply competitive, it is more appropriate to denote them as "surmountable" (see Fig. 1).

To find out whether an insurmountable antagonist is competitive, it is essential to expose the receptors to the antagonist and the agonist simultaneously. These experimental conditions are difficult to achieve in rabbit aortic strip contraction studies because it implies the absence of a preincubation step with the antagonist and, above all, the addition of a single dose of Ang II per tissue preparation instead of the usual consecutive cumulative dosing. This procedure is adopted only occasionally for contraction studies,[6] but it is routine for radioligand binding experiments as well as for functional experiments on isolated cells. In such test systems, provided that both the agonist and antagonist are added simultaneously to the receptor preparation, AT₁ receptor antagonists produce parallel rightward shifts of the Ang II without decreasing its maximal effect.

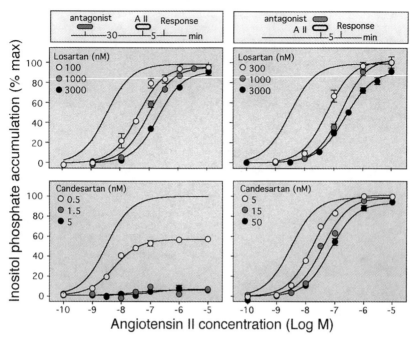

Figure 2. Effect of losartan (*top*) and candesartan (*bottom*) on the angiotensin II-mediated production of inositol triphosphate in CHO-hAT$_1$ cells under preincubation (*left*) and coincubation (*right*) conditions. The control dose-response curve (without symbols) was obtained in the absence of antagonist. Adapted from Vanderheyden P, Fierens FLP, De Backer J-P, et al: Distinction between surmountable and insurmountable selective AT$_1$ receptor antagonists by use of CHO-K1 cells expressing human angiotensin II AT$_1$ receptors. Brit J Pharmacol 126:1057–1065, 1999 and Fierens F, Vanderheyden P, De Backer J-P, Vauquelin G: Insurmountable angiotensin II AT$_1$ receptor antagonists: The role of tight antagonist binding. Eur J Pharmacol 372:199–206, 1999.

Criscione et al. noticed in 1993[8] that valsartan, an insurmountable antagonist in aortic ring contraction studies, inhibited Ang II-induced release of aldosterone in bovine adrenal glomerulosa cells without affecting the maximal response. Even more direct evidence was provided by experiments on CHO-hAT$_1$ cells (Fig. 2). When the Ang II-mediated production of inositol triphosphate was measured, it was found that candesartan, EXP3174 and irbesartan produced parallel rightward shifts of the dose-response curve without affecting the maximal response under coincubation conditions. The same antagonists, however, depressed the maximal response when they were preexposed to the cells.[19] A similar picture also was observed for antagonists such as candesartan, SRL1080277, sarile, and UR-7280 in radioligand-binding studies involving pre- and coincubation experiments.[28,34,35] This finding clearly establishes that nonpeptide AT$_1$ receptor antagonists inhibit the Ang II-mediated response in a competitive fashion.

Contraction studies also revealed that surmountable antagonists can counteract the ability of insurmountable antagonists to depress the maximal response to Ang II.[6,7,12,22,24,27,34] In the same line, insurmountable antagonists no longer depress the maximal Ang II-mediated production of inositol triphosphate in rabbit aortic smooth muscle cells and in CHO-hAT$_1$ cells when losartan is also present during the preincubation step.[14,17] These findings strongly suggest that surmountable and insurmountable antagonists are competitive with each other. Even more direct evidence for the competitive interaction among AT$_1$ receptor antagonists has been provided by a number of radioligand-binding studies in which, under coincubation conditions, the unlabelled antagonists failed to decrease the maximal binding of radiolabelled antagonists.[5,8,14]

■ Long-Lasting Binding of Insurmountable Antagonists

Insurmountable AT$_1$ receptor antagonists inhibit the response to Ang II in a competitive fashion, but when they are preexposed to the receptors, their antagonistic action may be so slowly reversible that it cannot be overcome during the short exposure of the receptors to the Ang II. Wash-out experiments, in which antagonist-pretreated cells or tissues are left in a fresh medium for various periods before the Ang II-mediated response is measured fully agree with this interpretation. For example, Ang II-mediated contraction recovers very slowly in rabbit aortic strips and rat portal vein pretreated with insurmountable antagonists such as candesartan.[29,36] Similarly, Ang II-mediated production of inositol triphosphate recovers quite slowly in candesartan-pretreated CHO-hAT$_1$ cells.[17] The fact that Ang II-mediated responses recover in cells or tissues after pretreatment with insurmountable antagonists indicates that their binding is reversible. Finally, as expected for surmountable antagonists, the recovery of the angiotensin-mediated response is almost instantaneous in losartan-treated cells.

A number of theories have proposed that the antagonist does not need to remain bound to the receptor to produce a long-lasting effect.[21,23,37] In the two-state model,[23,37] the receptor is able to adopt an active and an inactive conformation, and it is assumed that insurmountable antagonists display higher affinity for the inactive conformation. Accordingly, the binding of an insurmountable antagonist creates a new equilibrium with fewer receptors in the active conformation and (because it also is assumed that the interconversion between the two receptor conformations is slower than the ligand binding) reduces the ability of subsequently added agonists to induce a response. In the somewhat related coupling model of de Chaffoy de Courcelles et al.,[21] the crucial conformational change occurs at the cytoplasmic side of the receptor and affects the coupling of a transducing factor involved in generation of the cellular response.

To find out whether such theories apply to insurmountable AT$_1$ receptor antagonists, we compared the binding of [^{3}H]candesartan with its antagonistic action on the Ang II-mediated production of inositol triphosphate in intact CHO-hAT$_1$ cells.[18] When plated in 24 well plates, these cells allow radioligand binding and functional experiments to be carried out under the same conditions. [^{3}H]Candesartan bound with high specificity and affinity (equilibrium dissociation constant [K$_D$] of about 0.06 nM) to the human AT$_1$ receptor, and when the radioligand-containing medium was replaced by a fresh medium, the binding of [^{3}H]candesartan decreased very slowly. Half-maximal decrease was estimated to occur after 8 hours (Fig. 3). This long-lasting binding of candesartan to the AT$_1$ receptor coincided with the slow recovery of the Ang II-mediated production of inostol triphosphate in the wash-out experiments (see Fig. 3). A close match between the binding of candesartan and its antagonistic action also was found in association experiments in which cells were exposed to the antagonist

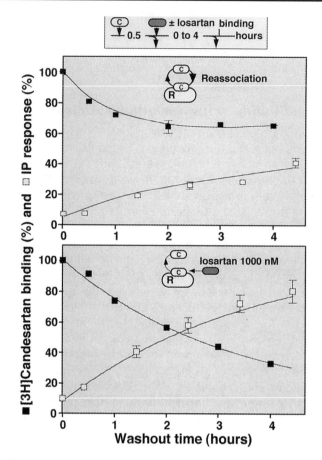

Figure 3.   Time course of [³H]candesartan dissociation and the antagonistic effect of candesartan in CHO-hAT₁ cells. Binding (*filled squares*): [³H]candesartan-pretreated cells were washed and further incubated with fresh medium without (*top*) or with 1 µM losartan (*bottom*). Remaining binding was measured after the indicated periods of time (*abscissa*). Antagonistic effect (*open squares*): candesartan-pretreated cells were washed and further incubated with fresh medium without (*top*) or with 1 µM losartan (*bottom*) and angiotensin II-mediated production of inositol phosphates was measured after the indicated periods. Adapted from Vanderheyden P, Fierens FLP, De Backer J-P, et al: Distinction between surmountable and insurmountable selective AT₁ receptor antagonists by use of CHO-K1 cells expressing human angiotensin II AT₁ receptors. Brit J Pharmacol 126:1057–1065, 1999 and Fierens FLP, Vanderheyden PML, De Backer J-P, Vauquelin G: Binding of the antagonist [³H]candesartan to angiotensin II AT₁ receptor-transfected Chinese hamster ovary cells. Eur J Pharmacol 367:413–422, 1999.

for increasing periods.[18] Taken together, these findings demonstrate that the antagonism by candesartan is directly linked to its occupancy of the AT₁ receptors.

■ Rebinding of Insurmountable Antagonists

The dissociation of antagonists usually is initiated by replacing the medium in functional studies (i.e., wash-out experiments) as opposed to adding an excess of unlabelled ligand to the membranes in radioligand-binding studies. Albeit subtle, this difference may have far-reaching consequences.[38] Indeed, when the medium is simply replaced, dissociated antagonist molecules begin to accumulate in the fresh medium and may bind to the receptor again, especially when they have high affinity for the receptor. This phenomenon, known as "reassociation"[18] or "rebinding"[38] effectively is prevented when another ligand is competitive and present in large excess.

In the wash-out experiments on CHO-hAT₁ cells (see above), rebinding of candesartan to its receptors clearly contributed to its long-lasting receptor occupancy and antagonistic action, as evidenced by (1) the accelerated dissociation of [³H]candesartan from intact CHO-hAT₁ cells in the presence of unlabelled ligands and (2) the accelerated recovery of the Ang II-mediated production of inostol triphosphate when losartan was included in the wash-out medium (see Fig. 3). Without rebinding, the antagonistic action of candesartan and its receptor occupancy declined with a half-life of about 2 hours instead of the 6–8 hours in the simple wash-out experiments (see Fig. 3). A similar losartan-mediated acceleration also has been observed for EXP3174 (half-life of about 30 minutes instead of 90 minutes).

The dissociation of [³H]candesartan from its receptors in CHO-hAT₁ cell membranes is appreciably faster (half-life of 20 minutes) than its dissociation from its receptors in the intact cells (half-life of 2 hours) [unpublished observations]. The reasons for this discrepancy are presently unknown, but it may indicate that an intact cell system is required for the long-lasting binding of insurmountable antagonists to the AT₁ receptor. Findings with candesartan indicate that factors such as rebinding and cellular integrity may contribute to the often dramatic differences between the kinetic properties of insurmountable antagonists in different studies. Additional factors, such as the slow removal of certain AT₁ receptor antagonists from tissue compartments, cells or matrix surrounding the receptor,[7,15] also may intervene. Direct comparisons between the binding properties of AT₁ receptor agonists in cell membrane preparations and their antagonistic action in intact cells or tissues are therefore dubious.

■ Loose and Tight Binding States of the Antagonist-AT₁ Receptor Complex

An intriguing property of many insurmountable AT₁ receptor antagonists is that their effect is often only partial. Indeed, when dose-response curves of Ang II in aortic strip contraction studies are examined, it appears that such antagonists depress the maximal response to a limited degree. When the concentration of these antagonists is further increased, the dose-response curve shifts to the right, but the maximal stimulation by Ang II does not decrease further. This phenomenon is represented even more explicitly by experimental data in the form of inhibition curves.[19] For each inhibition curve, the receptors are preexposed with a wide range of antagonist concentrations (abscissa) and the response is plotted (ordinate) for a single concentration of Ang II (Fig. 4). When the Ang II concentration is sufficiently high, the inhibition curves become biphasic. The most potent component corresponds to insurmountable inhibition (independent of the Ang II concentration) and the least potent component to surmountable inhibition (dependent on the Ang II concentration).[19] The presence of a distinct plateau between the two components is helpful in determining the maximal extent of insurmountable inhibition by an antagonist.

Analysis of the effects of antagonists on the Ang II-mediated production of inositol triphosphate in CHO-hAT₁ cells reveal that this response can be inhibited

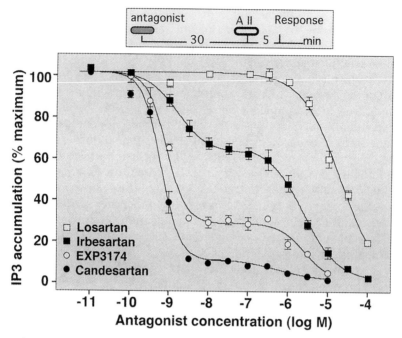

Figure 4.   Inhibition curve of candesartan, EXP3174, irbesartan, and losartan. CHO-hAT$_1$ cells were preincubated for 30 minutes with increasing concentrations of the antagonists (abscissa) and then for 5 minutes with an elevated concentration (10 µM) of angiotensin II to measure its maximal response (production of inositol phosphates). Adapted from Fierens F, Vanderheyden P, De Backer J-P, Vauquelin G: Insurmountable angiotensin II AT$_1$ receptor antagonists: The role of tight antagonist binding. Eur J Pharmacol 372:199–206, 1999.

insurmountably by up to 95% with candesartan, 70% with EXP3174, 30% with irbesartan, and by less than the level of detection for losartan (see Fig. 4).[19] Because these percentages are not affected by the preincubation time (between 10 and 120 minutes), a model can be proposed in which:

1. Antagonist-AT$_1$ receptor complexes may adopt two distinct states: a fast-reversible/surmountable (L.R) state and a tight-binding/insurmountable state (L.R*).

2. Both states reach an early equilibrium.

3. The proportion of receptors residing in each state depends on the nature of the bound antagonist.

Different avenues must be explored to understand the molecular significance of the fast-reversible and tight-binding states of the antagonist-AT$_1$ receptor complexes. Among the many theoretical possibilities, the distinction between the two states may reside at the level of the receptor conformation, its association with other proteins, or even its subcellular localization.

When stimulated by agonists, AT$_1$ receptors are particularly prone to internalize into the cell as part of their recycling process. Several authors have proposed the possibility that antagonists may control or even mimick this process.[6,39,40] It has been established that Ang II binds first to AT$_1$ receptors at the cell surface and that the agonist-receptor complexes are rapidly internalized via coated pits into endosomes. The agonist is then targeted to the lysosomal pathway, whereas the receptors are continuously recycled to the plasma membrane.[41,42] Of interest, binding of Ang II to the AT$_1$ receptor is known to be highly sensitive to acidic pH. This property is commonly exploited in binding studies of intact cells to discriminate between the membrane-associated and internalized forms of the agonist; i.e., brief exposure of the cells to an acidic buffer removes the radio-labelled agonist from the cell surface, and the internalized agonist accounts for the residual, acid-resistant binding.[42]

Because the binding of radio-labelled AT$_1$ receptor antagonists to intact cell systems was also more or less acid-resistant, it has been concluded that antagonist-AT$_1$ receptor complexes may internalize and account for this resistant binding.[39,40] Similarly, recent radioligand-binding experiments in intact CHO-hAT$_1$ cells also indicate that part of the [^{3}H]angiotensin II binding and the totality of [^{3}H]candesartan binding is acid-resistant [manuscript in preparation]. It is, therefore, tempting to postulate that L.R represents a membrane-associated state of the receptor and that L.R* has undergone internalization in the cell. Yet a number of other experiments do not support this model. First, whereas the acid-resistant binding of [^{3}H]angiotensin II to intact CHO-hAT$_1$ cells was rapidly and effectively prevented by a hypertonic concentration of sucrose (known to prevent receptor endocytosis via coated pit formation[43]), this effect was not observed for [^{3}H]candesartan [manuscript in preparation]. In addition, the subcellular distribution of AT$_1$ receptors in human embryonal kidney 293 cells (visualized by fluorescence labelling) was not affected by the AT$_1$-specific antagonist PD 134756. In fact, the Ang II-mediated internalization of these receptors was completely blocked by this antagonist.[42]

It is likely that the tight antagonist binding state of the AT$_1$ receptor is unrelated to its internalization. Whereas differences in acid-sensitivity may be an excellent criterion to distinguish membrane-bound from internalized Ang II, antagonist-receptor complexes are likely to remain at the cell surface and show much less sensitivity to a mild acid exposure.

Alternatively, several authors have proposed that antagonist-AT$_1$ receptor complexes adopt different conformations.[23,44,45] However, because none of the antagonists affects the basal inositol triphosphate levels in CHO-hAT$_1$ cells, it is likely that both L.R or L.R* represent an "inactive"conformation. With this restriction in mind, the equilibrium and possible interconversions between such receptor conformations may be represented by a model similar to the one presented by Leff[46] (Fig. 5).

In examining the chemical structure of AT$_1$ receptor antagonists, it is especially noteworthy that candesartan and EXP3174 contain two negatively charged groups (a carboxyl group and an tetrazole moiety) compared with one such group (tetrazole) for their much less potent precursor molecules, candesartan, cilexetil, and losartan (Fig. 6).[5,10] In fact, many other AT$_1$ receptor antagonists with a pronounced insurmountable character are also diacidic molecules, including valsartan, GR 117289, BMS-180560, CI-996, LR-B/057, UR-7280, KRH-594, and the 6-carboxylate derivative of 5H-pyrazolo[1,5-b][1,2,4]triazole.[7,8,12,14,15,28,47,48] However, the mere presence of two acidic groups is not sufficient for AT$_1$ receptor antagonists to be insurmountable. Experiments with candesartan analogs[10] have stressed the necessity for correct positioning of the carboxyl group. Based on these data, it is reasonable to speculate that the tight-binding component for

$$L+R \underset{K_1}{\overset{K_1}{\rightleftharpoons}} L.R$$

$$K_4 \updownarrow \qquad \updownarrow K_2$$

$$L+R^* \underset{K_3}{\overset{}{\rightleftharpoons}} L.R^*$$

Figure 5.   Equilibrium and possible interconversions between receptor conformations.

antagonists such as candesartan and EXP3174 may be related to the formation of a L.R* complex in which the two negatively charged groups of the antagonist form electrostatic bonds with basic amino acid residues of the receptor (see Fig. 6). The fast-reversible binding component of these antagonists may then be explained by the formation of L.R complexes with only one single electrostatic bond between the antagonist and the receptor (see Fig. 6). Such a model also accounts for the fact that molecules that bear only one negatively charged group, such as candesartan, cilexetil, and losartan, cannot display insurmountable antagonism (see Fig. 6). Obviously, the present model should not overlook the importance of additional interactions (such as π bonding and hydrophobic interactions) between antagonists and receptors.[49,50] For example, it has been reported that the nature of the alkyl substituents on analog of UR-7280, a diacidic antagonist, may determine whether they are surmountable or insurmountable.[28]

Site-directed studies involving the systematic mutagenesis of basic amino acids (Arg, Lys, and His in its protonated state) of the AT_1 receptor into neutral

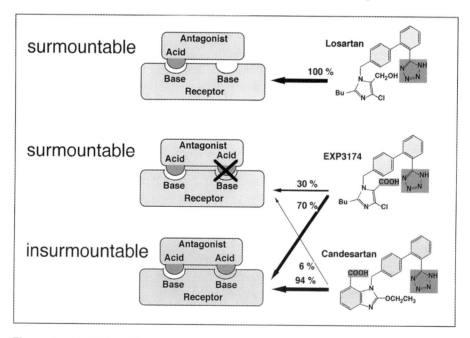

Figure 6.   Model describing the fast-reversible/surmountable and tight-binding/insurmountable binding components for losartan, EXP3174, and candesartan. Fast-reversible binding occurs when one negatively charged group of the antagonist forms an electrostatic bond with basic amino acids of the receptor. Both negatively charged groups of the antagonist are involved in tight-binding.

amino acids suggest that the carboxyl end of Ang II and the tetrazole group of antagonists such as losartan may occupy the same space within the receptor pocket.[50] A basic amino acid of the receptor that matches with the carboxyl group of insurmountable antagonists such as candesartan may be discovered by the same experimental approach. Such amino acid is expected to be crucial for the manifestation of a tight antagonist binding.

Finally, the possibility that tight antagonist binding to AT_1 receptors also involves the interaction of the receptors with other proteins, or even their ability to form dimers, cannot be excluded. It is well known that 7-TM receptors may adopt a tight agonist binding conformation when coupled to G proteins.[51,52] Even G protein-dependent antagonist binding to μ opioid receptors recently has been reported.[53] Therefore, one cannot exclude the possibility that L.R and L.R* are differently associated with certain other proteins from the membrane or cellular matrix or even that they freely diffuse in the cytosol. The faster dissociation of [³H]candesartan from its receptors in cell membranes compared with intact cells is compatible with this hypothesis. Alternatively, it recently has been reported that AT_1 and several other 7-TM receptors may exist as monomers and dimers and that these forms may have distinct functional properties.[54–56] At present, little is known about the impact of such macromolecular interactions on the antagonist-binding properties of receptors, but this issue merits further exploration.

■ Conclusion

Cell lines that have been transfected with the gene encoding for wild type and mutant AT_1 receptors have proved particularly useful for investigating phenomena such as receptor desensitization and internalization. Until recently only limited attention was given to their utilization in pharmacologic studies. However, compared with contraction studies in rabbit aortic strips, such cell lines offer major advantages for the investigation of AT_1 receptor antagonists. Their pharmacologic properties can be investigated by radioligand binding and at the functional level on the same intact cell system under a flexible range of experimental conditions. The receptor population is homogeneous and the untransfected parent cells may serve as useful controls for the detection and exclusion of receptor-unrelated phenomena.

Comparison of radioligand binding and Ang II-mediated production of inositol triphosphate in CHO-hAT₁ cells led to the following major findings (Fig. 7):

1. It was established that insurmountable AT_1 receptor antagonists inhibit the Ang II-mediated response in a competitive fashion. To act insurmountably, they need to bind to the receptor before exposing the cells to Ang II (see Fig. 2).

2. It appears that the antagonist-receptor complexes are able to adopt a fast-reversible and a tight-binding state and that the ratio between the two states depends on the nature of the antagonist (see Figs. 4 and 6). The resulting longevity of part of the antagonist-receptor complexes accounts for the insurmountable inhibition in functional studies (Fig. 7).

At present, the precise nature of the fast-reversible and tight-binding states of the AT_1 receptor is still elusive, but for antagonists such as candesartan and EXP3174, it may be related to the number of electrostatic interactions between the antagonist and the receptor.

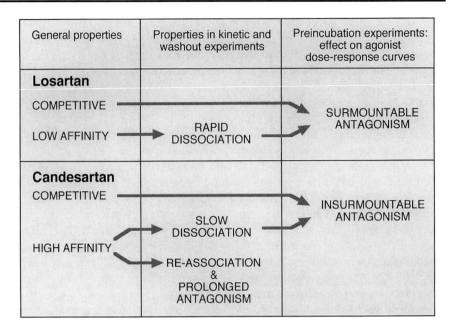

General properties	Properties in kinetic and washout experiments	Preincubation experiments: effect on agonist dose-response curves
Losartan		
COMPETITIVE		
LOW AFFINITY	RAPID DISSOCIATION	SURMOUNTABLE ANTAGONISM
Candesartan		
COMPETITIVE		
HIGH AFFINITY	SLOW DISSOCIATION	INSURMOUNTABLE ANTAGONISM
	RE-ASSOCIATION & PROLONGED ANTAGONISM	

Figure 7. Link between general properties of losartan and candesartan and their behavior under different experimental conditions.

Acknowledgments

We are grateful to Astra-Hässle for material and financial support. We also are obliged to the Queen Elisabeth Foundation of Belgium and the Onderzoeksraad of the Vrije Universiteit Brussel for their kind support. This text presents results of the Belgian program for Interuniversity Poles of Attraction initiated by the Belgian State, Prime Minister's Office, Science Policy Programming. Scientific responsibility is assumed by the authors.

References

1. Timmermans PBMWM, Benfield P, Chiu AT, et al: Angiotensin II receptors and functional correlates. Am J Hypertens 5:221S–235S, 1992.
2. Vallotton MB: The renin-angiotensin system. Trends Pharmacol Sci 8:69–74, 1987.
3. Robertson MJ: Angiotensin antagonists. In Leff P (ed): Receptor-based Drug Design. New York, Marcel Dekker, 1998, pp 207–223.
4. Zhang JC, Van Meel A, Pfaffendorf M, Van Zwieten P: Different types of angiotensin II receptor antagonism induced by BIBS 222 in the rat portal vein and rabbit aorta: The influence of receptor reserve. J Pharmacol Exp Ther 269:509–514, 1993.
5. Mochizuki S, Sato T, Furata K, et al: Pharmacological properties of KT3-671, a novel nonpeptide angiotensin II receptor antagonist. J Cardiovasc Pharmacol 25:22–29, 1995.
6. Liu YJ, Shankley NP, Welsh NJ, Black JW: Evidence that the apparent complexity of receptor antagonism by angiotensin II analogues is due to a reversible and synoptic action. Br J Pharmacol 106:233–241, 1992.
7. Robertson MJ, Barnes JC, Drew GM, et al: Pharmacological profile of GR 117289 in vitro: A novel, potent and specific non-peptide angiotensin AT_1 receptor antagonist. Br J Pharmacol 107:1173–1180, 1992.
8. Criscione L, de Gasparo M, Bühlmayer P, Whitebread S, et al: Pharmacological profile of valsartan: A potent, orally active, nonpeptide antagonist of the angiotensin II AT_1 receptor subtype. Br J Pharmacol 110:761–771, 1993.
9. Cazaubon C, Gougat J, Bousquet F, et al: Pharmacological characterization of SR 47436, a new nonpeptide AT_1 subtype angiotensin II receptor antagonist. J Pharmacol Exp Ther 265:826–834, 1993.

10. Noda M, Shibouta Y, Inada Y, et al: Inhibition of rabbit aortic angiotensin II (AII) receptor by CV-11974, a new neuropeptide AII antagonist. Biochem Pharmacol 46:311–318, 1993.
11. Wong PC, Duncia JV, Santella JP III, et al: EXP597, a nonpeptide angiotensin II receptor antagonist with high affinities for the angiotensin AT_1 and AT_2 receptor subtypes. Eur J Pharmacol 260:261–264, 1994.
12. Tamura K, Okuhira M, Mikoshiba I, Hashimoto K: In vitro pharmacological properties of KRH-594, a novel angiotensin II type 1 receptor antagonist. Biol Pharmacol Bull 20:850–855, 1997.
13. Vincentini LM, Villereal ML: Inositol phosphates turnover, cytosolic Ca^{2+} and pH: Putative signals for the control of cell growth. Life Sci 38:2269–2276, 1986.
14. Dickinson KE, Cohen RB, Skwish S, et al: BMS-180560, an insurmountable inhibitor of angiotensin II-stimulated responses: Comparison with losartan and EXP3174. Br J Pharmacol 113:179–189, 1994.
15. Panek RL, Lu GH, Overhisser RW, et al: Functional studies but not receptor binding can distinguish surmountable from insurmountable AT_1 antagonism. J Pharm Exp Ther 273:753–761, 1995.
16. Perlman S, Schambye HT, Rivero RA, et al: Non-peptide angiotensin agonist. Functional and molecular interaction with the AT_1 receptor. J Biol Chem 270:1493–1496, 1995.
17. Vanderheyden P, Fierens FLP, De Backer J-P, et al: Distinction between surmountable and insurmountable selective AT_1 receptor antagonists by use of CHO-K1 cells expressing human angiotensin II AT_1 receptors. Brit J Pharmacol 126:1057–1065, 1999.
18. Fierens FLP, Vanderheyden PML, De Backer J-P, Vauquelin G: Binding of the antagonist [³H]candesartan to angiotensin II AT_1 receptor-transfected Chinese hamster ovary cells. Eur J Pharmacol 367:413–422, 1999.
19. Fierens F, Vanderheyden P, De Backer J-P, Vauquelin G: Insurmountable angiotensin II AT_1 receptor antagonists: The role of tight antagonist binding. Eur J Pharmacol 372:199–206, 1999.
20. Wienen W, Mauz ABM, Van Meel JCA, Entzeroth M: Different types of receptor interaction of peptide and nonpeptide angiotensin II antagonists revealed by receptor binding and functional studies. Mol Pharmacol 41:1081–1089, 1992.
21. de Chaffoy de Courcelles D, Leysen JE, et al: The serotonin-S2 receptor: A receptor, transducer coupling model to explain insurmountable antagonist effects. Drug Develop Res 8:173–178, 1986.
22. Wong PC, Timmermans PBMWM: Nonpeptide angiotensin II receptor antagonists: Insurmountable angiotensin II antagonism of EXP3892 is reversed by the surmountable antagonist DuP753. J Pharmacol Exp Ther 258:49–57, 1991.
23. Robertson MJ, Dougall IG, Harper D, et al: Agonist-antagonist interactions at angiotensin receptors: Application of a two-state receptor model. Trends Pharmacol Sci 15:364–369, 1994.
24. Wienen W, Hauel N, Van Meel JCA, et al: Pharmacological characterization of the novel nonpeptide angiotensin II receptor antagonist, BIBR 277. Br J Pharmacol 110:245–252, 1993.
25. Olins GM, Chen ST, McMahon EG, et al: Elucidation of the insurmountable nature of an angiotensin receptor antagonist, SC-54629. Mol Pharmacol 47:115–120, 1994.
26. Aiyar N, Baker E, Vickery-Clark L, et al: Pharmacology of a potent long-acting imidazole-5-acrylic acid angiotensin AT_1 receptor antagonist. Eur J Pharmacol 283:63–72, 1995.
27. Cirillo R, Renzetti AR, Cucchi P, et al: Pharmacology of LR-B/081, a new highly potent, selective and orally active, nonpeptide angiotensin II AT_1 receptor antagonist. Br J Pharmacol 114:1117–1124, 1995.
28. De Arriba AF, Gomez-Casajus LA, Cavalcanti F, et al: In vitro pharmacological characterization of a new selective angiotensin AT_1 receptor antagonist, UR-7280. Eur J Pharmacol 318:341–347, 1996.
29. Ojima M, Inada Y, Shibouta Y, et al: Candesartan (CV-11974) dissociates slowly from the angiotensin AT_1 receptor. Eur J Pharmacol 319:137–146, 1997.
30. Zhang J, Pfaffendorf M, Zhang JS, Van Zwieten P: A non-competitive type of angiotensin receptor antagonism by losartan in renal artery preparations. Eur J Pharmacol 252:337–340, 1993.
31. Rang HP: The kinetic action of acetylcholine antagonists in smooth muscle. Proc R Soc Lond 164:488–510, 1965.
32. Rang HP, Dale MM: Mechanisms of drug action. In Rang HP, Dale MM (eds): Pharmacology. New York, Churchill Livingstone, 1987, pp 3–34.
33. Kenakin TP: Drug antagonism. In Kenakin TP (ed): Pharmacological Analysis of Drug-Receptor Interaction. New York, Raven Press, 1987, pp 205–244.
34. Pendleton RG, Gessner G, Horner E: Studies on inhibition of angiotensin II receptors in rabbit adrenal and aorta. J Pharmacol Exp Ther 248:637–643, 1989.
35. Hara M, Kiyama R, Nakajima S, et al: Kinetic studies on the interaction of nonlabeled antagonists with the angiotensin II receptor. Eur J Pharmacol 289:267–273, 1995.
36. Morsing P, Adler G, Brandt-Eliasson U, et al: Mechanistic differences of various AT_1-receptor blockers in isolated vessels of different origin. Hypertension 33:1406–1413, 1999.

37. Gero A: Desensitization, two-state receptors and pharmacological parameters. J Theoret Biol 103:137–161, 1983.

38. Limbird LE (ed): Cell Surface Receptors: A Short Course on Theory and Methods, 2nd ed. Boston, Kluwer, 1996, pp 61–122.

39. Crozat A, Penhoat A, Saez JM: Processing of angiotensin II (A-II) and (sar1,Ala8)A-II by cultured bovine adrenocortical cells. Endocrinol 118:2312–2318, 1986.

40. Conchon S, Monnot C, Teutsch B, et al: Internalization of the rat AT_{1a} and AT_{1b} receptors: Pharmacological and functional requirements. FEBS Lett 349:365–370, 1994.

41. Anderson KM, Murahashi T, Dorstal DE, Peach MJ: Morphological and biochemical analysis of angiotensin II internalization in cultured rat aortic smooth muscle cells. Am J Physiol 264:C179–C188, 1993.

42. Hein L, Meinel L, Pratt RE, et al: Intracellular trafficking of angiotensin II and its AT_1 and AT_2 receptors: Evidence for selective sorting of receptor and ligand. Mol Endocrinol 11:1266–1277, 1997.

43. Renzetti A, Criscuoli M, Salimbeni A, Subissi A: Molecular pharmacology of LR-B/081, a new non-peptide angiotensin AT_1 receptor antagonist. Eur J Pharmacol 290:151–156, 1995.

44. Balforth AJ, Lee AL, Warburton P, et al: The conformational change responsible for AT_1 receptor activation is dependent upon two juxtaposed asparagine residues on transmembrane helices III and VII. J Biol Chem 272:4245–4251, 1997.

45. Leff P: The two-state model of receptor activation. Trends Pharmacol Sci 16:89–97, 1995.

46. Okazaki T, Suga A, Watanabe T, et al: Studies on nonpeptide angiotensin II receptor antagonists. II: Synthesis and biological evaluation of 5H-pyrazolo[1,5-b][1,2,4]triazole derivatives with a C-linked oxygen functional group at the 6-position. Chem Pharm Bull Tokyo 46:287–293, 1998.

47. Yu SS, Lefkowitz RJ, Hausdorff WP: β-Adrenergic receptor sequestration: A potential mechanism of receptor resensitization. J Biol Chem 268:337–341, 1993.

48. Renzetti A, Cucci P, Guelfi M, et al: Pharmacology of LR-B/057, a novel orally active AT_1 receptor antagonist. J Cardiovasc Pharmacol 25:354–360, 1995.

49. Reitz DB, Garland DJ, Norton MB, et al: N1-sterically hindered 2H-imidazole-2-one angiotensin II receptor antagonists: The conversion of surmountable antagonists into insurmountable antagonists. Biorg Med Chem Lett 3:1055–1060, 1993.

50. Noda K, Saad Y, Kinoshita A, et al: Tetrazole and carboxylate groups of angiotensin receptor antagonists bind to the same subsite by different mechanisms. J Biol Chem 270:2284–2289, 1995.

51. De Lean A, Stadel JM, Lefkowitz RJ: A ternary complex model explains the agonist-specific properties of the adenylate cyclase-coupled β adrenergic receptor. J Biol Chem 255:7108–7117, 1980.

52. Severne Y, IJzerman A, Nerme V, et al: Shallow agonist competition binding curves for β-adrenergic receptors: The role for tight agonist binding. Mol Pharmacol 31:69–73, 1986.

53. Brown GP, Pasternak GW: ^{3}H-Naloxone benzoylhydrazone binding in MOR-1-transfected Chinese hamster ovary cells; evidence for G-protein dependent antagonist binding. J Pharmacol Exp Ther 286:376–381, 1998.

54. Monnot C, Bihoreau C, Conchon S, et al: Polar residues in the transmembrane domains of the type 1 angiotensin II receptor are required for binding and coupling: Reconstitution of the binding site by co-expression of two deficient mutants. J Biol Chem 271:1507–1513, 1996.

55. Cvejic S, Devi LA: Dimerization of the δ opioid receptor. J Biol Chem 272:26959–26964, 1997.

56. Gürdal H, Bond RA, Johnson MD, et al: An efficacy-dependent effect of cardiac overexpression of $β_2$-adrenoceptor on ligand affinity in transgenic mice. Mol Pharmacol 52:187–194, 1997.

CHAPTER 9

Does the Renin-Angiotensin System Exert an Important Stimulatory Influence on the Sympathetic Nervous System?

MURRAY ESLER, M.D., Ph.D.
HANS PETER BRUNNER-LA ROCCA, M.D.

Interaction between the renin-angiotensin system and the sympathetic nervous system traditionally has been regarded as bidirectional. The contribution of the renal sympathetic nerves to renal renin release, one component of this synergy, is explicit and well documented.[1] The juxtaglomerular apparatus receives a rich postganglionic sympathetic innervation, and even with stimuli such as restriction of dietary sodium intake, for which the mechanisms stimulating renal renin release might be expected to exclude an influence of the renal sympathetic outflow, the sympathoneural element is important. In humans, a low salt diet markedly and preferentially stimulates the renal sympathetic nerves[2] so that the homeostatic adjustment to sodium depletion includes neural renin release.

The other component of this presumed angiotensin-sympathetic nervous synergy—facilitation of the sympathetic nervous system by angiotensin—also has a long research pedigree, dating back to the seminal observations of Dickinson[3] and Bickerton and Buckley,[4] who observed that angiotensin injected into the dog carotid or vertebral artery activated the sympathetic nervous system. Angiotensin receptors and other components in the renin-angiotensin cascade are widely distributed in the brain,[5] giving support to the idea that angiotensin generated in the brain is an important regulator of sympathetic outflow. Over time, the stimulatory influence of angiotensin on the sympathetic nervous system was understood to extend beyond the central control of sympathetic outflow and to involve almost all elements of the neuraxis, including facilitation of ganglionic transmission, presynaptic augmentation of norepinephrine release from sympathetic nerves, inhibition of neuronal norepinephrine reuptake, sensitization of adrenoceptors, enhancement of adrenoceptor signal transduction, and stimulation of catecholamine release by the adrenal medulla.[6]

In our opinion the notion that angiotensin augments the sympathetic nervous system in such an all-encompassing fashion has been badly overstated and is quite out of keeping with the generally rather trifling antiadrenergic effects that accompany blockade of the renin-angiotensin system by angiotensin-converting enzyme (ACE) inhibitors and angiotensin receptor blockers in humans. There is a striking mismatch between the common absence of significant direct antiadrenergic effects when the renin angiotensin system is blocked in humans[7-13] and the prominent sympathoneural stimulation produced by angiotensin in laboratory experiments.[14-18] This mismatch has arisen in part from flaws in experimental design, which are discussed below. In addition, other processes appear to have been at work, tending to maximize the importance of any possible antiadrenergic activities of ACE inhibitors and angiotensin receptor blockers. Pharmaceutical industry marketing strategies have no doubt helped to perpetuate the misconception that these drug classes rank on an equal footing with beta-adrenergic blockers and centrally acting sympathetic suppressants as antiadrenergic agents, at a time when inhibition of the sympathetic nervous system in heart failure in particular is seen as highly beneficial.[19]

■ Angiotensin Augmentation of the Sympathetic Nervous System: Confounding Influences and Sources of Experimental Artifact

Following the first suggestions 30 years ago that angiotensin stimulated the sympathetic nervous system, there has been so little concordance of subsequent research findings[6] that an appraisal of methodology and potential sources of artifact is needed.

Administration of Angiotensin versus Angiotensin Blockade

Evidence supporting a stimulatory influence of angiotensin on the sympathetic nervous system has been drawn more commonly from studies involving the administration of angiotensin than from studies involving its blockade. In laboratory experiments the doses and concentrations of angiotensin used have often been so extraordinarily high,[14,16,20,21] sometimes even in micromolar concentrations,[17] as to have doubtful relevance to mammalian biology. The difficulty of judging the appropriateness of an administered dose applies particularly in the case of central nervous system administration of angiotensin. The focal injection of perhaps 100 pmoles[18] may be justified as physiologically relevant in that it is many times less than the dose needed to produce a systemic response when administered intravenously, but the interstitial angiotensin concentration achieved by this "small" dose might still be markedly supraphysiologic. In general, the results obtained through blockade of the renin-angiotensin system, assessing a sympathetic influence by the measured subtraction of sympathetic activity achieved,[7,9,10,12,13] are more trustworthy than the results from experiments in which angiotensin is administered, more often than not in inappropriately high doses.

Use of Blood Pressure "Normalizing" Procedures

The assessment of the influence of angiotensin on sympathetic activity is complicated by the change in blood pressure that commonly results from angiotensin administration or blockade, such that reflex sympathetic stimulation or inhibition is a confounder. Typically blood pressure is restored (appropriately raised or lowered pharmacologically) to what it was before the intervention in order to estimate what the angiotensin effect would be in the absence of blood pressure change and reflex sympathetic adjustment.[22,23] Clearly there is some justification to this widely used approach, but errors may result from rapid resetting of the arterial baroreflex, a well-documented phenomenon.[24] This resetting produces a surprisingly rapid change in the set point of the baroreflex, so that the "restored" blood pressure is not registered as the starting blood pressure. For example, with intravenous infusion of angiotensin in sufficient dose in humans, blood pressure rises and sympathetic nerve-firing rates reflexly fall. With restoration of pressure to the starting level by a vasodilator, nerve-firing rate may be elevated above baseline, but this elevation does not necessarily represent sympathetic stimulation by the administered angiotensin, as is often assumed. This response is to be expected from rapid upward resetting of the arterial baroreflex during the period of pressure elevation produced by the infused angiotensin.[24] Similarly, experiments involving compensatory upward adjustment of blood pressure by a pharmacologic pressor agent during angiotensin blockade can lead to an equivalent misinterpretation of the direct effect of angiotensin on the sympathetic nervous system.

Special Characteristics of Studies in Humans

In general, small or no antiadrenergic effects are observed with blockade of the renin-angiotensin system by ACE inhibitors and angiotensin receptor blockers in humans.[7-13] Such results are strikingly discordant with those obtained in many laboratory experiments.[14-18] This discordance is not due, as has been claimed, to the insensitivity of available methods for the clinical study of sympathetic nervous function. Contemporary methods for measuring sympathetic nerve firing by microneurography[25] and rates of norepinephrine release from sympathetic nerves by isotope dilution[26] are sophisticated and sensitive; they are not inferior to the methodology available in the experimental animal laboratory.

The difference in results derives from other aspects of design, such as the absence of anesthesia in the clinical studies (individual anesthetic agents profoundly modify sympathetic activity[27]); the avoidance in humans, on the grounds of safety and ethics, of studies involving peripheral administration of angiotensin in supraphysiologic doses and central nervous system administration in any dose; and a preference for study designs involving renin-angiotensin blockade rather than angiotensin administration.[7-11,13]

Influence of Diseases Such as Cardiac Failure

The case for a facilitatory influence of angiotensin on the sympathetic nervous system is perhaps stronger in experimental and human cardiac failure than in any other context, based on apparent reduction of sympathetic tone during renin-angiotensin system inhibition.[28-30] On closer appraisal, however, explanations other than a direct effect of angiotensin are more likely.

One source of error has been the misinterpretation of changing plasma norepinephrine values during heart failure therapy. The plasma concentration of norepinephrine, widely used as a measure of overall sympathetic activity, falls during the course of treatment of cardiac failure with ACE inhibitors. This fall has been taken to signify sympathetic inhibition. Plasma norepinephrine concentrations, however, are determined both by rates of transmitter release from sympathetic nerves, and by rates of removal of norepinephrine from plasma after its release.[26] Norepinephrine plasma clearance is influenced by cardiac output and regional blood flows and is subnormal in patients with cardiac failure.[26,31,32] During treatment of heart failure, improvement in cardiac output and restoration of regional blood flows toward normal increase the plasma clearance of norepinephrine, lowering its plasma concentration, so that a fall in plasma norepinephrine concentration cannot be equated with a reduction in sympathetic nervous system activity.

Sympathetic nervous activity, in fact, can fall during treatment of heart failure, but this appears not to be due specifically to renin-angiotensin inhibition. Sympathetic tone in the failing human heart is approximately three times higher in minimally treated patients with New York Heart Association class III and IV failure than in optimally treated patients with the same severity of heart failure,[32,33] independent of which antifailure drugs are used. The basis of the reduction in sympathetic nervous activity during heart failure therapy is not entirely clear but seems to involve removal of reflex sympathetic drive by lowering of elevated right-sided intracardiac pressures; acute pharmacologic reduction of pulmonary wedge pressure in patients with heart failure by any means lowers cardiac sympathetic tone.[34,35]

■ *Does Angiotensin Exert Significant Effects at Any Particular Site in the Sympathetic Neuraxis?*

The conclusions from experiments designed to assess whether angiotensin in the central nervous system exerts a controlling influence on sympathetic nervous system activity depend very much on the experimental conditions: whether angiotensin or an angiotensin blocker is administered, whether the experimental animal is conscious or anesthetized, whether the animal has been preconditioned by sodium depletion, and whether heart failure is present.

Central Nervous System Administration of Angiotensin or Its Antagonists

In general, the administration of angiotensin intracerebroventricularly or into brain regions such as the rostral ventrolateral medulla is more likely to show effects on sympathetic activity than the central administration of ACE inhibitors or angiotensin receptor blockers. Often the doses of angiotensin used, such as 100 pmoles microinjected into the rat rostral ventrolateral medulla,[18] have been so large as to call into question the validity of the experiment.

In anesthetized animals the common[14,18,36] response to central angiotensin administration is sympathetic excitation, which is neutralized by the central administration of an angiotensin receptor blocker. In contrast, when de novo administration of an angiotensin blocker is used, sympathetic activity typically does not change.[15,36] The sympathetic excitation produced by central administration of angiotensin is observed more consistently and is of larger magnitude in sodium-depleted animals.[37,38]

In studies conducted on conscious animals, although angiotensin-induced sympathetic excitation may be seen,[15,39] the direct effect of administration of angiotensin into the central nervous system often differs; sometimes *sympathetic inhibition* is noted rather than sympathetic activation.[40,41] In elegant studies in conscious sheep, May and McAllen observed that subpressor doses of angiotensin II administered into the lateral ventricle caused renal sympathetic inhibition, which was blocked by losartan.[40,41] The findings of Gaudet and colleagues in conscious rabbits were similar; losartan administered into the fourth ventricle raised renal sympathetic nerve firing.[42] The basis for this difference between findings in anesthetized and awake animals is unclear, but it certainly would be unjustified to conclude that within the central nervous system angiotensin sympathoexcitation is the norm.

An inhibitory influence of angiotensin within the central nervous system is also evident with some sympathetic reflexes, again studied in awake animals. Angiotensin appears to mediate the inhibition of the renal sympathetic outflow produced by infusion of hypertonic saline into the lateral ventricle of sheep[41] and to exert an inhibitory influence over the renal sympathetic activation seen with hypoxia in rabbits.[43,44]

Presynaptic Facilitation of Norepinephrine Release From Sympathetic Nerves

Receptors on sympathetic neurons have the capacity to modulate the amount of transmitter released per neural discharge. This phenomenon is best documented with presynaptic neural α_2-adrenoceptors, which, when stimulated by released norepinephrine or α_2-adrenergic agonists such as clonidine, reduce quantal exocytic norepinephrine release. The available evidence suggests that angiotensin also can act presynaptically in this fashion to reduce norepinephrine release from sympathetic nerves; this is perhaps the best demonstrated effect of angiotensin on the sympathetic neuraxis.

Presynaptic modulation of release of norepinephrine by angiotensin has been studied by measuring the rate of transmitter released during electrically induced sympathetic nerve discharge in experimental animal preparations. The electrical discharge of sympathetic nerves typically has been achieved in pithed rats with stimulation via the spinal canal[45] or in isolated animal preparations by stimulation of the cut sympathetic nerves of supply[46] or field stimulation of the tissue.[47] A neuromodulatory influence of angiotensin can be sought by measurement of rates of release of transmitter, either of endogenous norepinephrine or after loading of neuronal stores with 3H-norepinephrine, at predetermined levels of nerve firing in the presence of angiotensin and angiotensin receptor blockers.

Angiotensin facilitation of norepinephrine release was evident in early studies,[16,20,21] but angiotensin concentrations typically used to achieve this effect (300–1000 pM) were clearly too high to be biologically relevant. More recent studies, using angiotensin concentrations of 10–30 pM,[46–49] have confirmed a rather small but significant neuromodulatory effect, abolished by angiotensin receptor blockers. Angiotensin receptor blockers typically have no presynaptic effects on baseline norepinephrine release.[20,46,50]

In humans, the infusion of low doses of angiotensin into the brachial artery results, very much for the animal experiments, in a small increase in norepinephrine release.[51]

Influences on Adrenal Medullary Secretion of Catecholamines

Although angiotensin receptors exist in the adrenal medulla,[6] earlier claims for an important role for the renin-angiotensin system in regulating adrenal catecholamine secretion have not been supported by recent studies in humans. In humans the plasma concentration of adrenaline is not changed by infusion of low doses of angiotensin or renin-angiotensin system inhibition.[7,10,11] A report that antagonism of the renin-angiotensin system, with captopril reduced adrenaline secretion during insulin-induced hypoglycemia[52] was not supported by a later study, in which angiotensin receptor blockade was without effect.[10]

■ Angiotensin Effects on the Human Sympathetic Nervous System

The findings from studies in healthy humans and patient populations are often out of step with the findings from studies in experimental animals, but because they are potentially of greater validity and relevance to human disease and therapies, they deserve special mention. This mismatching of clinical and experimental findings is not due to insensitivity of available methods for studying sympathetic nervous function in humans; it derives instead from other aspects of experimental design. Not least among these are the avoidance in humans, on the grounds of safety and ethics, of studies involving peripheral administration of angiotensin in supraphysiologic doses and of central nervous system administration of angiotensin in any dose and a preference in clinical research for study designs involving renin-angiotensin blockade rather than angiotensin administration.

Healthy Humans

Contemporary methods for measuring human sympathetic nerve firing by microneurography[25] and by measurement of rates of norepinephrine release from sympathetic nerves by isotope dilution[26] can be used to quantify sympathetic nervous activity at rest[7,9,11-13] or during reflex responses, such as those driven by the arterial baroreflex.[9] Presynaptic neuromodulatory influences of angiotensin can be studied clinically by measuring norepinephrine spillover into the venous effluent of the forearm during infusion of low doses of angiotensin into the brachial artery.[51]

In healthy humans low-dose angiotensin infusion or blockade of the renin-angiotensin system by ACE inhibition or angiotensin receptor antagonists produces minimal or no reduction in plasma norepinephrine concentration, whole body norepinephrine spillover to plasma, or sympathetic outflow to the skeletal muscle vasculature as measured by microneurography.[7,10,11,30] Preconditioning by dietary sodium restriction does not modify these findings.[11]

These negative effects contrast with evidence from several sources documenting a presynaptic neuromodulatory influence of angiotensin. In one study,[51] when angiotensin was infused into the brachial artery in low dose, a small increase in facilitated norepinephrine release was seen. A 15% increase in norepinephrine spillover from the forearm occurred at an estimated achieved plasma angiotensin concentration of 25 pM.[51] Presynaptic facilitation of norepinephrine release by angiotensin also has been demonstrated in human heart[47] and kidney cortex[49] preparations studied in vitro with electrical field stimulation and bath concentrations of angiotensin as low as 10 pM. On balance, any augmentation of sympathetic nervous activity by the renin-angiotensin system in healthy humans is minimal, although some presynaptic facilitation of norepinephrine release is demonstrable.

Heart Failure

In patients with heart failure low-dose angiotensin infusion does not increase sympathetic activity; the total body norepinephrine spillover rate remains unchanged.[12] ACE inhibition with enalapril has been reported to lower muscle sympathetic nerve activity as measured by microneurography[30] but to leave total body norepinephrine spillover unchanged.[12] The case for a direct facilitatory influence of angiotensin on the sympathetic nervous system in heart failure is thus not strong. The widely held view to the contrary seems to be a misconception based on two sources of error.

The first of these sources is misinterpretation of the significance of changing plasma norepinephrine values under therapy. The plasma concentration of norepinephrine typically falls during the course of treatment of cardiac failure with ACE inhibitors, but this fall is due in part to hemodynamic improvement increasing regional blood flow and the plasma clearance of norepinephrine. The second basis for misconception is that sympathetic nervous activity may, in fact, fall during treatment of heart failure, but due to hemodynamic improvement and reduction of right-sided intracardiac pressures removing the reflex basis for sympathetic nervous stimulation[34,35] rather than a specific effect of renin-angiotensin system inhibition.

Angiotensin blockade has been demonstrated to increase the gain of the arterial baroreflex in clinical heart failure[30] and in animal models of heart failure,[53] in part through facilitation of the central integration of the reflex.[28] This increase does not necessarily represent a direct effect, since unloading of the low-pressure baroreceptors by any heart failure therapies achieving volume depletion would be expected to increase interactively the gain of the arterial baroreflex.[54]

Hypertension

In essential hypertension there is no evidence of augmentation of sympathetic activity by the renin-angiotensin system. Reflex sympathetically mediated hemodynamic responses to a variety of stimuli in hypertensive patients were not modified by ACE inhibition.[8] Grassi and colleagues reported that in patients with essential hypertension ACE inhibition with lisinopril had no effect on plasma norepinephrine concentration or sympathetic outflow to the skeletal muscle vasculature at rest and did not change the gain of the arterial baroreflex for either heart rate or muscle sympathetic nervous activity.[9] It is possible that at high interstitial concentrations of angiotensin achieved by release of renin in the kidneys, particularly in renovascular hypertension, local enhancement of renal sympathetic neurotransmission might occur, but this effect has not yet been demonstrated.

Renal Failure

In patients with chronic renal failure sympathetic nervous system activity is increased.[55] The mechanism is not entirely clear, but the stimulus for sympathetic activation seems to come from the diseased kidneys, perhaps via renal afferent nerves,[56] and disappears with nephrectomy.[55] ACE inhibition with enalapril recently has been shown to reduce strikingly the muscle sympathetic nerve-firing rate in patients with renal failure.[57] How this sympathetic inhibition occurs is uncertain, whether from a direct action of the drug antagonizing the renin-angiotensin system or, less specifically, from a more general clinical improvement under therapy.

■ Conclusion

There is a longstanding viewpoint that the renin-angiotensin system exerts an important regulatory influence over the sympathetic nervous system. Review of the published evidence discloses that such an effect is much more likely to be evident in experimental studies in which angiotensin is administered peripherally or within the central nervous system, often in inappropriately high doses, than when the renin-angiotensin system is blocked pharmacologically by ACE inhibitors or angiotensin receptor antagonists. In healthy humans, there is minimal evidence of sympathetic nervous augmentation by administration of angiotensin, other than a rather small but well-documented facilitatory effect of locally administered angiotensin acting presynaptically on sympathetic neurons, and little evidence of reduction in sympathetic tone with inhibition of the renin-angiotensin system. Substantial sympathetic inhibition recently has been described with ACE inhibition in patients with renal failure; whether this represents a direct effect or a general response to treatment is uncertain. Sympathetic inhibition during ACE inhibitor treatment of patients with heart failure is largely a consequence of hemodynamic improvement, which removes the reflex drive for sympathetic stimulation, rather than a direct effect of renin-angiotensin system inhibition. The direct antiadrenergic effect of drugs blocking the renin-angiotensin system does not rank in potency with that achieved by beta-adrenergic blockers or centrally acting sympathetic nervous suppressants.

References

1. Keeton TK, Campbell WB: The pharmacologic alteration of renin release. Pharmacol Rev 32:81–227, 1980.
2. Friberg P, Meredith I, Jennings G, et al: Evidence of increased renal noradrenaline spillover rate during sodium restriction in man. Hypertension 16:121–130, 1990.
3. Dickinson CJ: Neurogenic Hypertension. Oxford, Blackwell Scientific Publications, 1965.
4. Bickerton RK, Buckley JP: Evidence for a central mechanism in angiotensin induced hypertension. Proc Soc Exp Biol Med 106:832–846, 1961.
5. Ganten D, Lang RE, Lehmann E, Unger T: Brain angiotensin: On the way to becoming a well-studied neuropeptide system. Biochem Pharmacol 33:3523–3528, 1984.
6. Reid IA: Interactions between ANG II, sympathetic nervous system, and baroreceptor reflexes in regulation of blood pressure. Am J Physiol 262:E763–E778, 1992.
7. Rongen GA, Brooks SC, Ando S-I, et al: Angiotensin AT1 receptor blockade abolishes the reflex sympatho-excitatory response to adenosine. J Clin Invest 101:769–776, 1998.
8. Ajayi AA, Reid JL: Renin-angiotensin modulation of sympathetic reflex function in essential hypertension and in the elderly. Int J Clin Pharm Res 8:327–333, 1988.
9. Grassi G, Turri C, Dell'Oro R, et al: Effect of chronic angiotensin converting enzyme inhibition on sympathetic nerve traffic and baroreflex control of the circulation in essential hypertension. J Hypertens 16:1789–1796, 1998.
10. Worck RH, Ibsen H, Frandsen E, Dige-Petersen H: AT1 receptor blockade and the sympatho-adrenal response to insulin-induced hypoglycemia in humans. Am J Physiol 272:E415–E421, 1997.
11. Lang CC, Stein M, He HB, Wood AJJ: Angiotensin converting enzyme inhibition and sympathetic activity in healthy subjects. Clin Pharmacol Ther 59:668–674, 1996.

12. Goldsmith SR, Hasking GJ, Miller E: Angiotensin II and sympathetic activity in patients with congestive heart failure. J Am Coll Cardiol21:1107–1113, 1993.

13. Noll G, Wenzell RR, de Marchi S, Shaw S, Luscher TF: Differential effects of captopril and nitrates on muscle sympathetic activity in volunteers. Circulation 95;2286–2292, 1997.

14. Weekley LB: Angiotensin-II acts centrally to alter renal sympathetic nerve activity and the intrarenal renin-angiotensin system. Cardiovasc Res 25:353–363, 1991.

15. Dorward PK, Rudd CD: Influence of brain renin-angiotensin system on renal sympathetic and cardiac baroreflexes in conscious rabbits. Am J Physiol 260:H770–H778, 1991.

16. Li CG, Majewski H, Rand MJ: Facilitation of noradrenaline release from sympathetic nerves in rat anococcygeus muscle by activation of prejunctional beta-adrenoceptors and angiotensin receptors. Br J Pharmacol 95:385–392, 1988.

17. Cox SL, Ben A, Story DF, Ziogas J: Evidence for the involvement of different receptor subtypes in the pre- and postjunctional actions of angiotensin II at rat sympathetic neuroeffector sites. Br J Pharmacol114:1057–1063, 1995.

18. Averill DB et al: Losartan, nonpeptide angiotensin II-type 1 (AT1) receptor antagonist, attenuates pressor and sympathoexcitatory responses evoked by angiotensin II and L-glutamate in rostral ventrolateral medulla. Brain Res 665:245–252, 1994.

19. Packer M, Bristow MR, Colucci WS, Fowler MB, Gilbert EM, Shusterman NH: The effect of carvedilol on morbidity and mortality in patients with chronic heart failure: US Carvedilol Heart Failure Study Group. N Engl J Med 334:1349–1355, 1996.

20. Mian MA, Majewski H, Rand MJ: Facilitation of noradrenaline release by isoprenaline in rat isolated atria does not involve angiotensin II formation. Clin Exp Pharmacol Physiol 16:905–911, 1989.

21. Garcia-Sevilla JA, Dubocovich ML, Langer SZ: Interaction between presynaptic facilitatory angiotensin II receptors and inhibitory mucarinic cholinoceptors on 3H-noradrenaline release in the rabbit heart. Naunyn Schmiedebergs Arch Pharmacol 330:9–15, 1985.

22. Niederberger M, Aubert J-F, Nussberger J, Brunner HR, Waeber B: Sympathetic nerve activity in conscious renal hypertensive rats treated with an angiotensin converting enzyme inhibitor or an angiotensin II antagonist. J Hypertens 13:439–445, 1995.

23. Xu L, Brooks VL: ANG II chronically supports renal and lumbar sympathetic activity in sodium-deprived conscious rats. Am J Physiol 271:H2591–H2598, 1996.

24. Korner PI. Central nervous control of autonomic cardiovascular function. In Berne RM, Sperelakis N, Geiger SR (eds). Handbook of Physiology. The Cardiovascular System: The Heart vol 1, sect 2. American Physiological Society, Bethesda, 1979, pp 691–739.

25. Wallin BG, Esler M, Dorward P, Eisenhofer G, Ferrier C, Westerman R, Jennings G: Simultaneous measurements of cardiac norepinephrine spillover and sympathetic outflow to skeletal muscle in humans. J Physiol 453:45–56, 1992.

26. Esler M, Jennings G, Lambert G, Meredith I, Horne M, Eisenhofer G: Overflow of catecholamine neurotransmitters to the circulation: Source, fate and functions. Physiol Rev 70:963–985, 1990.

27. Best JD, Taborsky GJ Jr, Flatness DE, Halter JB: Effect of pentobarbital anesthesia on plasma norepinephrine kinetics in dogs. Endocrinology 115:853–857, 1984.

28. Ma R, Zucker IH, Wang W: Central gain of the cardiac sympathetic afferent reflex in dogs with heart failure. Am J Physiol 272:H2664–H2671, 1997.

29. Noshiro T, Way D, McGrath BP: Angiotensin converting enzyme inhibition improves baroreflex-induced noradrenaline spillover responses in rabbits with heart failure. J Auton Nerv Syst 66: 87–93, 1997.

30. Dibner-Dunlap ME, Smith ML, Kinugawa T, Thames MD: Enalaprilat augments arterial and cardiopulmonary baroreflex control of sympathetic nerve activity in patients with heart failure. J Am Coll Cardiol 27:358–364, 1996.

31. Davis D, Baily R, Zelis GJ: Abnormalities in systemic norepinephrine kinetics in human congestive heart failure.Am J Physiol254:H760–H766, 1988.

32. Hasking G, Esler M, Jennings G, Burton D, Johns J, Korner P: Norepinephrine spillover to plasma in congestive heart failure: evidence of increased overall and cardiorenal sympathetic nervous activity. Circulation 73:615–621, 1986.

33. Kaye DM, Lefkovits J, Jennings GL, Bergin P, Broughton A, Esler MD: Adverse consequences of high sympathetic nervous activity in the failing human heart. J Am Coll Cardiol 26:1257–1263, 1995.

34. Newton GE, Parker JD: Cardiac sympathetic response to acute vasodilatation: Normal ventricular function versus congestive cardiac failure. Circulation 94:3161–3167, 1996.

35. Kaye DM, Jennings GL, Dart AM, Esler MD: Differential effect of acute baroreceptor unloading on cardiac and systemic sympathetic tone in congestive heart failure. J Am Coll Cardiol 31:583–587, 1998.

36. Hirooka Y, Potts PD, Dampney RA: Role of angiotensin II receptor subtypes in mediating the sympathoexcitatory effects of exogenous and endogenous angiotensin peptides in the rostral ventrolateral medulla of the rabbit. Brain Res 772:107–114, 1997.

37. DiBona GF, Jones SY, Sawin LL: Effect of endogenous angiotensin II on renal nerve activity and its arterial baroreflex regulation. Am J Physiol 271:R361–R367, 1996.
38. DiBona GF, Jones SY, Sawin LL: Effect of endogenous angiotensin II on renal nerve activity and its cardiac baroreflex regulation. J Am Soc Nephrol 9:1983–1989, 1998.
39. Head GA: Role of AT1 receptors in the central control of sympathetic vasomotor function. Clin Exp Pharmacol Physiol 3(Suppl):S93–S98, 1996.
40. May CN, McAllen RM: Baroreceptor-independent renal nerve inhibition by intracerebroventricular angiotensin II in conscious sheep. Am J Physiol 273:R560–R567, 1997.
41. May CN, McAllen RM: Brain angiotensinergic pathways mediate renal nerve inhibition by central hypertonic NaCl. Am J Physiol 272:R593–R600, 1997.
42. Gaudet EA, Godwin SJ, Head GA: Role of central catecholaminergic pathways in the actions of endogenous ANG II on sympathetic reflexes. Am J Physiol 275:R1174–R1184, 1998.
43. Gaudet EA, Godwin SJ, Lukoshkova E, Head GA: Effect of central endogenous angiotensin II on sympathetic activation induced by hypoxia. Clin Exp Hypertens 19:913–923, 1997.
44. Bendle RD, Malpas SC, Head GA: Role of endogenous angiotensin II on sympathetic reflexes in conscious rabbits. Am J Physiol 272:R1816–R1825, 1997.
45. Ohlstein EH, et al: Inhibition of sympathetic outflow by the angiotensin II receptor, eprosartan, but not by losartan, valsartan or irbesartan: Relationship to differences in prejunctional angiotensin II receptor blockade. Pharmacology 55:244–251, 1997.
46. Schwieler JH, Kahan T, Nussberger J, Hjemdahl P: Influence of the renin-angiotensin system on sympathetic neurotransmission in canine skeletal muscle in vivo. Naunyn Schmiedebergs Arch Pharmacol 343:166–172, 1991.
47. Rump LC, Schwertfeger E, Schaible U, et al: Beta 2-adrenergic receptor and angiotensin II receptor modulation of sympathetic neurotransmission in human atria. Circ Res 74:434–440, 1994.
48. Foucart S, Patrick SK, Oster L, de Champlain J: Effects of chronic treatment with losartan and enalaprilat on [3H]-norepinephrine release from isolated atria of Wistar-Kyoto and spontaneously hypertensive rats. Am J Hypertens 9:61–69, 1996.
49. Rump LC, Bohmann C, Schaible U, et al: Beta-adrenergic, angiotensin II, and bradykinin receptors enhance neurotransmission in human kidney. Hypertension 26:445–451, 1995.
50. Yasuda G, Shionoiri H, Kubo T, Misu Y: Presynaptic angiotensin II receptors and captopril-induced adrenergic transmission failure probably not via converting enzyme inhibition in guinea-pig pulmonary arteries. J Hypertens 5(Suppl):S39–S45, 1987.
51. Clemson B, Gaul L, Gubin SS, et al: Prejunctional angiotensin II receptors. Facilitation of norepinephrine release in the human forearm. J Clin Invest 93:684–691, 1994.
52. Madsen BK, Holmer P, Ibsen H, Christiansen NJ: The influence of captopril on the epinephrine response to insulin-induced hypoglycemia in humans. The interaction between the renin-angiotensin system and the sympathetic nervous system. Am J Hypertens 5:361–365, 1992.
53. Nishiro T, Way D, McGrath BP: Angiotensin converting enzyme inhibition improves baroreflex-induced noradrenaline spillover responses in rabbits with heart failure. J Auton Nerv Syst 66:87–93, 1997.
54. Korner PI: Integrative neural cardiovascular control. Physiol Rev 51:312–367, 1971.
55. Converse RJ Jr, Jacobsen TN, Toto RD, et al: Sympathetic overactivity in patients with chronic renal failure. N Engl J Med 329:998–1008, 1992.
56. Campese V, Kogosov E: Renal afferent denervation prevents hypertension in rats with chronic renal failure. Hypertension 25:878–882, 1995.
57. Ligtenberg G, Blankestijn PJ, Oey PL, et al: Reduction of sympathetic hyperactivity by enalapril in patients with chronic renal failure. N Engl J Med 340:1321–1328, 1999.

CHAPTER 10

Angiotensin and the Central Nervous System

ANDREW M. ALLEN, Ph.D.
MICHAEL J. MCKINLEY, Ph.D., D.Sc.
JOOHYUNG H. LEE, B.Sc. (Hons.)
FREDERICK A. O. MENDELSOHN, M.D., Ph.D., FRACP

Angiotensin (Ang) affects the central nervous system (CNS) at several different sites to cause an array of different physiologic effects, including cardiovascular, neuroendocrine, and behavioral responses. Consistent with the diversity of its physiologic actions is the variety of paths it uses to reach its target receptors in the brain. Angiotensin that influences brain function may come from the bloodstream (in which case only neurons that are located in regions lacking the blood-brain barrier are influenced directly), or it may be synaptically released subsequent to its generation in the brain by glia and possibly neurons. In this analysis, therefore, a distinction is made between the effects of blood-borne Ang II acting on the circumventricular organs of the brain (which are devoid of a blood-brain barrier) and the effects of Ang that may be released as a neurotransmitter or neuromodulator from neurons within the CNS, although the neural pathways subserving these two aspects of central Ang action may not be completely independent.

This review of the neural mechanisms that mediate the various physiologic responses involving an action of Ang on the CNS also considers the localization of the various components of the renin-Ang system that may or may not exist within various compartments of the brain. Examples include angiotensinogen, angiotensin-converting enzyme (ACE), renin and other processing enzymes, and Ang receptors.

■ Angiotensinogen and Processing Enzymes

The existence of an endogenous source of brain Ang is a long-established concept.[1-5] Ang II-like immunoreactivity occurs in a discrete pattern throughout the nervous system[6,7] but is associated predominantly with regions involved in fluid and electrolyte homeostasis, cardiovascular control, and neuroendocrine regulation. The high correlation between the distributions of Ang II-like immunoreactive nerve terminals and Ang II (AT_1 and AT_2) receptors suggests that Ang II may act via direct release across synapses.[7-9] However, it also has been suggested that Ang II may act by volume transmission through the extracellular space. This suggestion is substantiated by the high concentrations of angiotensinogen in the cerebrospinal fluid.[10]

How neuronal Ang is formed is a perplexing question. Although all components of the renin-Ang system occur in the brain, correlating their distributions has proved extremely difficult.

1. Angiotensinogen is synthesized predominantly by astrocytes,[11] but recent evidence also indicates that some neurons may express angiotensinogen mRNA.[12] Although immunohistochemical studies indicate the presence of angiotensinogen in neurons, this finding has been questioned.[13,14]

2. Renin mRNA occurs in brain but in extremely low concentrations.[15] Consequently, it has not proved possible to localize accurately the distribution of renin in the brain.

3. ACE occurs in a widespread pattern in the nervous system with a partial overlap in distribution with that of Ang II-like immunoreactivity in neuronal cell bodies.[16] It is likely that ACE in other regions is processing neuropeptides other than angiotensin I.[17]

4. Receptors for Ang occur in a characteristic pattern throughout the nervous system at sites both accessible to systemically derived Ang II (the circumventricular organs [CVOs]) and sites behind the blood-brain barrier.[18]

Thus there are several possible mechanisms by which neuronal Ang II might be formed.

1. It is possible that all components are present within neurons but that the very low levels, particularly of angiotensinogen and renin, make their detection difficult. In this case, extracellular angiotensinogen derived from astrocytes may play another role.

2. Alternatively, astrocytic angiotensinogen is secreted and taken up into select neurons, either intact or in a metabolized form. Further processing and trafficking may then occur. Because ACE is generally considered to be an ectoenzyme, it is possible that Ang II is formed extracellularly and then sequestered into the neuron.

3. It is possible that some neurons, with processes in the CVOs, sequester systemic Ang II, which then may be used as a central neurotransmitter. However, this theory does not explain the existence of neurons behind the blood-brain barrier that possess Ang II-like immunoreactivity, such as those in the parvocellular division of the hypothalamic paraventricular nucleus[7] or the rostral ventrolateral medulla.[19]

4. Neuronal Ang II may not be produced by a classical renin-angiotensin system at all; angiotensinogen, or another substrate, may be metabolized by other enzymes. Many enzymes capable of performing this task occur in the brain.

■ Angiotensin Receptors

Ang II elicits its biologic actions by binding to specific membrane-bound receptors on target cells to activate multiple intracellular transduction pathways. Using selective receptor ligands, two major Ang II receptor subtypes—AT_1 and

AT_2—were identified[20] and subsequently cloned.[20–24] Physiologic and pharmacologic studies with the receptor subtype-selective blockers have revealed that the known biologic actions of Ang II are mediated by AT_1 receptors.[20] By contrast, although AT_2 receptors have been reported to show biologic activities in cultured cell lines in vitro, including cellular antiproliferation and apoptosis,[25,26] their physiologic role in vivo is still being elucidated.[27]

The AT_1 receptor gene (cDNA) encodes a 359-amino acid protein with a structure typical of seven transmembrane G-protein-coupled receptors.[21,22] Stimulation of AT_1 receptors by Ang II activates phospholipase C_β, resulting in increased intracellular calcium and inositol 1,4,5-triphosphate (IP3) concentrations.[21,22] Ang II also activates the mitogen-activated protein (MAP)-kinases, such as extracellular regulated kinases (ERK 1/2), via Src and Ras (small G-proteins belonging to the Ras family of G-proteins) as well as JAK/STAT pathways.[28]

The two highly homologous subtypes of AT_1 receptors in rodents are termed AT_{1A} and AT_{1B}.[29] These AT_1 receptor isoforms share 94% identity in amino acid sequence, but only 60% identical nucleotide sequence in the 5' and 3' untranslated regions. In rats, the AT_{1A} gene is localized on chromosome 17 and the AT_{1B} gene on chromosome 2.[30,31] AT_{1A} receptors are expressed predominantly in the vascular smooth muscle, liver, lung, and kidney, whereas the AT_{1B} receptors occur mainly in the adrenal gland and anterior pituitary.[21,22] Humans have only one AT_1 receptor gene, which is located on chromosome 3.[32]

The AT_2 receptor gene, initially cloned from rat fetus and rat pheochromocytoma cells, encodes a 363-amino acid protein, which has only 32–34% amino acid identity with the AT_{1A} receptor protein.[23,24] Although the AT_2 receptor is also a seven transmembrane G-protein-coupled receptor, its mode of signal transduction is uncertain. AT_2 receptor activation results in growth inhibition and promotion of apoptosis associated with inhibition of MAP kinases, such as ERK 1/2, probably via activation of phosphotyrosine phosphatases.[28] The AT_2 receptor gene is located on chromosome X.[23,24,33] Northern blot analysis shows that AT_2 receptors are expressed predominantly in the adrenal medulla, myometrium, and myocardium in adults and in the fetal mesenchyme.[23,24,34]

In addition to AT_1 and AT_2 receptors, other receptors for Ang peptides have been proposed, but none has yet been cloned or definitively identified. Examples include receptors for Ang III, Ang [1-7], and Ang [3-8].[35] Of interest, recent data suggest that the active ligand at AT_1 receptors may in fact be Ang III.[36,37]

Distribution of Ang AT_1 and AT_2 Receptors in the Brain

The distribution of Ang AT_1 and AT_2 receptors in the central nervous system has been mapped in detail using in vitro autoradiography, with displacement of the radioligand, ^{125}I-[Sar^1, Ile^8] Ang II, by subtype specific antagonists[38–41]; in situ hybridization histochemistry with riboprobes directed against specific sequences of the AT_{1A}, AT_{1B}, and AT_2 receptor mRNA[9,42–44]; and immunohistochemistry.[45] These studies have been performed in a number of species, including humans.[46–48] Detailed maps of the distributions of these receptors are included in several recent comprehensive reviews.[9,49,50] A brief summary of the main sites of high receptor densities is included below and in Figure 1.

Most circumventricular organs, including the subfornical organ, vascular organ of the lamina terminalis (OVLT), median eminence, anterior pituitary,

AT$_1$ RECEPTORS

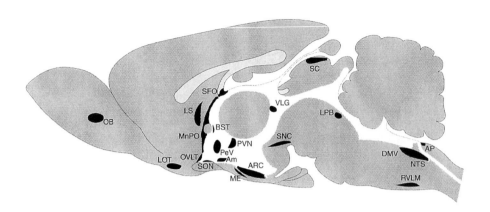

AT$_2$ RECEPTORS

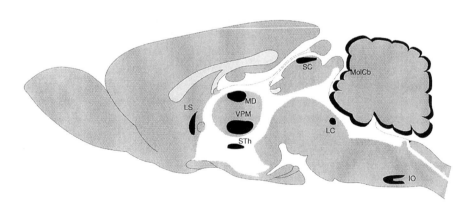

Figure 1. Diagram of the main sites of angiotensin AT$_1$ and AT$_2$ receptors in mammalian brains, summarizing the major sites of Ang II receptors that have been observed in human, rat, rabbit, and monkey brains (see references 8, 9, 18, 40, 41, 43, and 45–50). These receptor locations are projected onto a midsagittal diagram of a rat brain, although some sites (e.g., the supraoptic nucleus) do not exhibit Ang receptors in rats. Am = amygdala, ARC = arcuate nucleus, AP = area postrema, BST = bed nucleus of the stria terminalis, DMV = dorsal motor nucleus of the vagus, IO = inferior olive, LC = locus ceruleus, LPB = lateral parabrachial nucleus, LOT = nucleus of the lateral olfactory tract, LS = lateral septum, MD = medial dorsal thalamic nucleus, ME = median eminence, MnPO = median preoptic nucleus, Mol Cb = molecular layer of the cerebellum, NTS = nucleus tractus solitarii, OB = olfactory bulb, OVLT = organum vasculosum of the lamina terminalis, PeV = periventricular nucleus, PVN = hypothalamic paraventricular nucleus, RVLM = rostral ventrolateral medulla, SC = superior colliculus, SFO = subfornical organ, SNC = substantia nigra pars compactus, SON = supraoptic nucleus, STh = subthalamic nucleus, VLG = ventrolateral geniculate nucleus, VPM = ventroposterior thalamic nucleus medial part. (Modified from Swanson LW: Brain Maps: Structure of the Rat Brain. Amsterdam, Elsevier Science, 1992.)

and the area postrema of the hindbrain, contain high densities of AT_1 receptors.[9,42] These regions are exposed to blood-borne Ang II and are the sites where systemic Ang II may act to alter drinking and salt appetite, blood pressure, and pituitary hormone release. In the forebrain, AT_1 receptors also occur at many regions within the blood-brain barrier, such as the median preoptic nucleus; hypothalamic paraventricular nucleus; anteroventral preoptic, suprachiasmatic, and periventricular nuclei; and discrete regions of the lateral and dorsomedial hypothalamus.[9,42]

In the hindbrain, a striking distribution of AT_1 receptors is observed in regions involved in regulation of autonomic activity and cardiovascular reflexes—for example, the lateral parabrachial nucleus, nucleus of the solitary tract, dorsal motor nucleus of vagus, intermediate reticular nucleus, and rostral and caudal ventrolateral medulla.[9,42] In the sympathetic preganglionic neurons of the spinal cord, a high density of AT_1 receptors is also found. Thus, AT1 receptors occur in the brainstem nuclei involved in the baroreceptor reflex regulation of heart rate, sympathetic vasomotor activity, and blood pressure.[49]

Overall, the distribution of the AT_1 receptor is highly conserved across all studied species and is associated with regions of the brain known to be involved in fluid and electrolyte balance, control of neuroendocrine function, and central regulation of autonomic activity.[49] In contrast, the AT_2 receptor distribution is highly variable between species, and the only constant site of expression in the adult brain is in the molecular layer of the cerebellar cortex.[50] Despite a wide distribution in the rat, the AT_2 receptor occurs in a limited number of sites in other species.[44,46,47] Little is known about the function of the AT_2 receptor in the brain, although the AT_2 receptor knockout mouse has some behavioral deficits indicative of altered brain function.[51,52]

■ Actions of Circulating Ang II on the Brain

Blood-borne Ang II exerts a number of actions on the brain, despite its lack of passage across the blood-brain barrier. Included among the centrally mediated responses stimulated by circulating Ang II are water drinking and salt hunger, vasopressin (AVP) and adrenocorticotropic hormone (ACTH) secretion, and a centrally mediated increase in arterial pressure.

Pressor Responses

The proposal that the pressor response to systemic Ang II, which primarily involves constriction of vascular smooth muscle, also involves an action on the brain came from the work of Bickerton and Buckley.[53] Initially these observations were dismissed because supraphysiologic doses of Ang were used; however, it later was shown that much lower doses were required when Ang was infused into the circulation supplying the brain.[54-56] The central pressor response to systemic Ang II involves direct sympatho-excitation, AVP release, and inhibition of baroreceptor activity.[55,57-59,60-63]

Recent experiments, using specific AT_1 receptor antagonists or ACE inhibitors, have shown that under many physiologic and pathologic conditions systemic Ang II supports blood pressure by activation of sympathetic efferent pathways and inhibition of baroreceptor reflex gain.[64-68] Systemic Ang II can affect either sympathetic vasomotor nerve activity or baroreceptor reflex gain through several sites, including the subfornical organ and area postrema centrally and at the sympathetic ganglia and sympathetic nerve terminals peripherally.[69–73] The relative importance of these sites has not been determined.

Thirst

Following the early demonstrations by Fitzsimons and colleagues that water drinking was a response to stimulation of the renin-Ang system[74] or to systemically administered Ang II,[75] the question arose in regard to its site of action in the brain. How could a circulating peptide like Ang II, which is unable to cross the blood-brain barrier, induce water drinking? The studies of Simpson and colleagues showed that the subfornical organ, a circumventricular organ lacking the blood-brain barrier, was the cerebral site at which Ang induced drinking in rats and dogs.[76] In addition, another circumventricular organ, the organum vasculosum of the lamina terminalis (OVLT), which also lacks a blood-brain barrier, may play a role in Ang-induced drinking in dogs.[77] Neurons in both of these regions are rich in AT_1 receptors[41] and are activated (as shown by *c-fos* expression) by intravenous Ang II.[78] Central administration of AT_1 receptor antagonists (but not AT_2 receptor antagonists) blocks drinking induced by blood-borne or intracerebroventricularly administered Ang II[79–82] as well as Ang-induced activation of neurons, as shown electrophysiologically[83,84] by calcium imaging[85] or *c-fos* expression[86] in the subfornical organ and OVLT. Although the neural pathways subserving Ang-induced thirst are not well understood, a pathway via the median preoptic nucleus is probably involved.[87]

Demonstration of a central dipsogenic action of Ang II in humans is lacking at present. Intravenously infused Ang II at doses producing moderate physiologic blood levels did not significantly increase thirst scores in human volunteers.[89] However, the increase in arterial pressure that accompanies systemic infusion of Ang II may activate baroreceptors, providing a strong inhibitory influence on water drinking. Such an inhibitory effect has been demonstrated in rats[90] but would not be expected to result from increased endogenously generated Ang II under physiologic conditions of hypovolemia or sodium depletion, when blood pressure does not rise. Evidence suggestive of a central dipsogenic effect of circulating Ang II in humans is the intense thirst observed in patients with chronic renal failure who undergo intermittent renal hemodialysis.[90,91] Such patients have elevated plasma levels of renin and Ang II, and their intense thirst is extinguished by treatment with ACE inhibitors.[91]

An interesting, and seemingly paradoxical, dipsogenic effect of ACE inhibitors (such as captopril and enalapril) has been observed in rats.[92–94] The likely explanation of this effect is that, although certain doses of ACE inhibitors can block conversion of Ang I to Ang II, they are insufficient to block the extremely high concentrations of ACE in the subfornical organ.[94,95] Thus, the resulting high circulating Ang I levels are converted locally in the subfornical organ and OVLT to Ang II with resultant stimulation of AT_1 receptors in these circumventricular organs.[95] Subsequent water drinking can be blocked by systemic administration of an AT_1 receptor antagonist.[95]

Vasopressin Secretion

Systemic infusion of Ang II also can result in AVP secretion if the dose is high enough in conscious rats and dogs[96] or if the concomitant pressor response to the infused Ang II is counteracted.[97] The site of action of blood-borne Ang II that results in AVP secretion appears to be the subfornical organ; however, the OVLT also may play a role. There are direct projections from the subfornical organ to the sites of the AVP-secreting neurons in the supraoptic and paraventricular nuclei,[98,99] and ablation of the subfornical organ prevents AVP secretion in response to systemically administered Ang II.[100] Neurons in the subfornical organ that project to the supraoptic and paraventricular nuclei are stimulated by systemic Ang II, suggesting a direct neural pathway from Ang receptors in the subfornical organ to the vasopressin-secreting neurons of the hypothalamus.[101] Another pathway via the median preoptic nucleus from the subfornical organ also may be involved.[102] However, functional neuroanatomic studies of *c-fos* expression in the subfornical organ show that many neurons in the rostral and outer parts of the subfornical organ, with efferent projections to the supraoptic nucleus, are activated by intravenous infusion of Ang II in conscious rats.[103] Fewer such neurons in the median preoptic nucleus and OVLT are activated by systemic Ang II.[103] It seems likely that the predominant neural pathway in the rat that mediates circulating Ang-induced vasopressin secretion is a direct pathway from the AT_1 receptor-rich neurons in the outer parts of the subfornical organ to the magnocellular neurons of the supraoptic and paraventricular nuclei. In addition, a role for the OVLT in Ang-mediated vasopressin secretion is possible because ablation of this site blocks vasopressin secretion in response to intravenous infusion of Ang II in dogs.[77]

Adrenocorticotropic Hormone Secretion

Increased circulating levels of adrenocorticotropic hormone (ACTH) and corticosteroids may be stimulated by systemic infusion of Ang II in dogs and rats.[96,97,105,106] This increased steroid secretion is more pronounced if the infusion is made directly into the carotid artery.[97] Because secretion of corticotropin-releasing hormone in the pituitary portal blood is observed, an action of Ang II on the brain is likely to be responsible. The circumventricular organs have been suggested as the sites at which Ang II exerts this response,[106] but which of the circumventricular organs mediates this response is still unresolved. The median eminence seems a likely site of action in view of the high levels of Ang receptors there and evidence that the subfornical organ is not the site of action of Ang II for this response.[106] Ablation of the OVLT does not prevent circulating Ang-induced ACTH secretion, although it does abolish the associated vasopressin release,[77] indicating, firstly, that the OVLT is not involved in the ACTH response and, secondly, that this response is not explained by Ang-stimulated vasopressin acting as a corticotropin-releasing factor.

Sodium Intake

Although considerable attention initially focused on the possibility that centrally generated Ang had a role in the hunger for salt exhibited by a number of species,[107] recent evidence suggests that circulating Ang II acting on circumventricular organs plays a significant role in the initiation of sodium appetite in salt-deficient animals. In rats, systemic infusion of Ang II increases sodium intake,[108] and high doses of ACE inhibitors block salt appetite during sodium depletion.[109–111]

In sodium-deficient sheep, systemic infusion of captopril reduces sodium intake, which can be restored by intravenous infusion of Ang II designed to reinstate the circulating levels of Ang II.[112] This effect has been subsequently observed in rats. Although the high dose of captopril needed to inhibit salt appetite blocked the conversion of peripherally administered Ang I, it did not block conversion of intracerebroventricularly injected Ang I.[111,113] This result is consistent with the idea that circulating Ang II acting on the circumventricular organs generates a hunger for salt. Lesions in the subfornical organ and also the OVLT block salt appetite caused by diuretic-induced sodium loss,[114] and microinjection of Ang II into the region of the OVLT stimulates salt intake in rats.[115] It seems likely that salt appetite may depend on blood-borne Ang II acting at AT_1 receptors in both the subfornical organ and OVLT.

■ Actions of Centrally Generated Ang

In addition to an action of blood-borne Ang II on circumventricular organs to stimulate water drinking, AVP secretion, sodium hunger, ACTH release, and centrally mediated pressor response, considerable evidence indicates that Ang generated within the brain may influence central neural pathways and regulate a number of functions.

Pressor Responses

Depending on the cerebral site stimulated, the pressor response to Ang II in the brain involves changes in autonomic efferent activity, inhibition of baroreceptor reflex function, and stimulation of vasopressin release. This section concentrates on the first two effects. Vasopressin release is discussed below.

Sympathetic Nerve Activity

Intracerebroventricular (ICV) administration of Ang II results in increases in blood pressure due to a combination of increased vasopressin release and sympathetic nerve activity.[116,117] However, direct recordings in the rat suggest that the changes in sympathetic nerve activity are not the primary cause of increased blood pressure in response to ICV Ang II.[118] In addition, renal sympathetic nerve activity appears to be inhibited by central Ang, independent of changes in blood pressure and baroreceptor reflex alterations.[119]

Microinjections of Ang II into distinct brain nuclei induce sympathetically mediated increases in blood pressure. Ang excites neurons in the hypothalamic paraventricular nucleus with identified projections to the spinal cord.[120] Activation of these neurons may explain the increase in blood pressure produced by direct microinjection of Ang II into the paraventricular nucleus.[121] Microinjection of Ang II into the nucleus of the solitary tract produces depressor (low dose) and pressor responses.[122,123] The pressor response involves activation of sympathetic efferent pathways. The rostral ventrolateral medulla contains a population of sympathetic premotor neurons whose tonic activity is essential for the maintenance of sympathetic vasomotor tone and normal resting blood pressure.[124] Microinjection of Ang II into the rostral ventrolateral medulla causes a sympathetically mediated pressor response.[125–127] Similarly, intrathecal injections of Ang II induce a sympathetically mediated increase in blood pressure, presumably by activation of sympathetic preganglionic neurons in the intermediolateral cell column.[128]

The precise site in the brain at which ICV-administered Ang II inhibits renal sympathetic nerve activity is not known; however, stimulation of the hypothalamic paraventricular nucleus (PVN) can produce an inhibition of the renal nerve activity.[129] Microinjections of Ang II into the caudal ventrolateral medulla inhibit sympathetic vasomotor activity and produce a decrease in blood pressure.[130] The physiologic role of Ang II at this site is not clear.

Vagal Efferent Nerve Activity

Microinjections of Ang II into the dorsal motor nucleus of the vagus induce a decrease in blood pressure and heart rate, which is proposed to be due to inhibition of cardiac vagal motor neurons.[131]

Modulation of Baroreceptor Reflex Function

Microinjections of Ang II into the nucleus of the solitary tract inhibit baroreceptor reflex control of sympathetic nerve activity and heart rate.[132,133] Although the mechanism is not yet elucidated, it is proposed that this action of Ang II plays an important role during the developmental switch from postnatal to adult blood pressures.[134]

In addition, a direct effect of Ang II on baroreceptor afferents has been proposed but not proved. Ang AT_1 receptors are located on the presynaptic terminals of vagal afferent neurons in the nucleus tractus solitarius, and at least some of these are associated with baroreceptor afferent neurons.[135,136] Ang II has been shown, in an in vitro slice preparation, to alter the release of substance P via a presynaptic mechanism.[137] The physiologic role of this action is not clear.

Thirst Mechanisms

Probably the most spectacular manifestation that Ang may act within the brain as a neurotransmitter in neural circuits subserving thirst is the rapid and copious water drinking that occurs within seconds of an injection of the octapeptide into the hypothalamic/preoptic region of the brain or the cerebral ventricles of many species.[138]

A likely site of action of Ang as a neurotransmitter is the median preoptic nucleus in the anterior wall of the third ventricle. This nucleus is rich in both AT_1 receptors and Ang-containing nerve terminalis.[7,41] Direct injection of Ang II into the median preoptic nucleus rapidly stimulates water drinking,[139] and studies of *c-fos* expression in the brain of rats administered Ang II either centrally or systemically show that neurons are activated predominantly in the median preoptic nucleus by centrally administered Ang II, whereas neurons in the subfornical organ and OVLT are the main targets of circulating Ang.[140] Ablation of the median preoptic nucleus[87] but not of the subfornical organ[141] abolishes drinking induced by centrally injected Ang II. Administration directly into the brain of peptide antagonists, such as saralasin and sarthran, or nonpeptide AT_1 receptor antagonists, such as losartan, effectively blocks some types of drinking responses.[142–145] This finding may be evidence of a neurotransmitter function of Ang II, although it is possible that the inhibition occurred because of pharmacologic blockade of circulating Ang II at central sites such as the subfornical organ or OVLT. Recent studies using central injections of antisense oligonucleotides complementary to parts of angiotensinogen mRNA, designed to suppress centrally generated Ang, show inhibition of isoproterenol-induced drinking (a blood-borne Ang II-dependent thirst) as well as drinking caused by ICV injection of renin.[146] These results support the idea that centrally generated Ang may be used within the neural pathways, subserving drinking stimulated initially by the action of blood-borne Ang on the circumventricular organs.

Vasopressin Secretion

ICV injection of Ang II also is a potent stimulator of vasopressin secretion.[147] It is unlikely that this effect results from direct action on the AVP-containing neurons of the supraoptic and paraventricular nuclei of the hypothalamus because in rats these nuclei lack Ang receptors.[9,41] Neuronal inputs to the supraoptic and paraventricular nuclei from the caudal ventrolateral medulla, nucleus of the solitary tract, and the lamina terminalis[148] come from regions rich in Ang receptors and Ang-containing terminalis. Thus, they may be sites at which Ang acts as a neurotransmitter to influence vasopressin release.[149] Indeed, injection of an Ang antagonist into the caudal ventrolateral medulla suppresses hemorrhage-induced AVP secretion, and electrophysiologic evidence supports the idea that an angiotensinergic synapse in the median preoptic nucleus is involved with vasopressin release.[102]

Adrenocorticotropic Hormone Secretion

In addition to stimulation of the hypothalamo-pituitary-adrenal (HPA) axis by Ang II from the circulation, there is also evidence of a central angiotensinergic influence on corticotropin-releasing hormone and ACTH secretion. Infusions of Ang II into the lateral or third cerebral ventricle increase plasma concentrations of corticosteroids or ACTH in a number of species.[106,150,151] This effect of Ang II is most likely due to an action behind the blood-brain barrier because blockade of Ang II receptors in the circumventricular organs (but not other brain regions) by means of systemically administered saralasin does not inhibit the the increase in ACTH release that occurs in response to ICV infusion of Ang II.[106] A possible site of action of Ang II to influence the HPA axis is the corticotropin-releasing hormone-containing parvocellular neurons of the paraventricular nucleus. These neurons are rich in AT_1 receptors, as shown by in vitro autoradiographic studies and in situ hybridization, which reveals the presence of mRNA encoding the AT_1 receptor.[152] ICV injection of Ang II increases the corticotropin-releasing hormone mRNA in conscious rats.[151,152] Several stressors, as well as glucocorticoid treatment, increase levels of AT_1 mRNA in the paraventricular nucleus, whereas adrenalectomy reduces these levels.[153] However, the physiologic role of AT_1 receptors in the parvocellular paraventricular nucleus in stress-induced activation is unclear at present; stressor-induced changes in AT_1 receptor expression in the paraventricular nucleus do not reflect the effects of particular stressors on ACTH secretion.[153] In addition, centrally administered losartan does not affect basal or stress-induced plasma levels of ACTH or corticosterone,[154] although plasma catecholamine secretion and CRH mRNA increases in response to immobilization-stress were reduced.

Sodium Appetite

Centrally administered renin or Ang II can cause a long-lasting stimulation of salt intake in species as diverse as rats, pigeons, sheep, and pigs,[155] suggesting that angiotensinergic mechanisms within the brain participate in regulating sodium appetite. In contrast to the water drinking that is quickly initiated after central injection of Ang II, the increased sodium intake may occur only after several hours and may persist for days. Interpretation of this Ang-induced sodium hunger is difficult because of its long latency and long-lasting effect. In addition, part of it (but not all) may be secondary to sodium depletion resulting from a natriuretic response that also occurs in response to centrally administered Ang II.[156] Central administration of AT_2 and AT_1 antagonists reduces sodium intake in response to ICV Ang II.[143] Regions of the brain that have been implicated in central Ang-induced sodium appetite include the ventral lamina terminalis and amygdala.[115,157]

Natriuresis

Contrasting with the sodium-retaining effect that results when circulating Ang increases aldosterone secretion is the natriuretic effect that occurs in response to ICV administration of Ang II in a number of species.[156,158] The rapid natriuresis after ICV injection of Ang II may come about because blood pressure increases (causing a pressure natriuresis), renal sympathetic nerve activity is suppressed,[119] plasma levels of renin fall,[159] vasopressin secretion increases,[147,160] or a natriuretic agent is released into the circulation. One of these factors, alone or in combination with one or more of the others, may be the link between brain and kidney that mediates this response. Ablation of the Ang receptor-rich region of the AV3V region of the brain abolishes the natriuretic response to ICV Ang II in sheep (Pennington and McKinley, unpublished observations), suggesting that the median preoptic nucleus and/or OVLT may be sites of such central Ang action. Relatively few data (see below) are available about the effects of centrally administered Ang antagonists on renal sodium excretion during various physiologic conditions of high sodium loss. The natriuretic responses to ICV infusion of hypertonic saline or Ang II are blocked by centrally administered losartan in sheep and rats,[160–163] suggesting the possibility of a central angiotensinergic AT_1 involvement in osmotically stimulated natriuresis. The exact physiologic role of central angiotensinergic pathways in regulating renal sodium excretion, however, awaits further study.

Renin Secretion

Circulating Ang II exerts a powerful inhibitory influence on renin secretion by the kidney. Evidence also suggests that a central angiotensinergic influence may inhibit renal renin secretion. In several species ICV infusion of Ang II reduces renin secretion by the kidney and plasma renin levels fall.[159,161,164,165] Although this effect may be secondary to baroreceptor activation due to the pressor response caused by ICV Ang II, ICV infusion still reduces plasma renin levels in sodium-depleted sheep, in which no pressor response occurs.[161] This finding suggests that either a nervous or humoral pathway from the brain to the kidney is involved. Prior treatment with losartan blocks this response. In fact, central losartan treatment further increases plasma renin levels in sodium-depleted sheep,[161] indicating AT_1 receptor involvement. Central administration of Ang II also causes reduced renal sympathetic nerve activity,[119] which may contribute to the reduction in plasma renin levels.

Osmoregulation

ICV administration of hypertonic saline stimulates a number of responses, including water drinking, vasopressin secretion, natriuresis, reduced renin secretion, reduced renal sympathetic nerve activity and a pressor response, all of which are similar to the responses when Ang II is infused into the cerebral ventricles.[147,158-165] Recent studies in rats and sheep show that central administration of the AT_1 receptor antagonist losartan blocks all of these responses to ICV infusion of hypertonic saline.[145,160,161-163,166] This finding may indicate that a brain angiotensinergic influence is common to virtually all central osmoregulatory mechanisms.

Thermoregulation

Indications that central angiotensinergic mechanisms participate in thermoregulation came initially from observations that centrally administered Ang II produced a reduction in body temperature in monkeys and rabbits.[167,168] This effect is due to increased heat radiation from the skin and decreased metabolic heat production.[168,169] The effects of ICV Ang II on thermoregulation in rats can be blocked by losartan,[170] indicating an AT_1 receptor-mediated response. We recently observed that centrally administered losartan caused a greater increase in core temperature of rats exposed to a hot environment (39°C) for 60 minutes.[171] This finding is consistent with a physiologic role for central angiotensinergic mechanisms in thermoregulation in rats. The cerebral location of this thermoregulatory action of Ang in the brain has not been precisely identified, although thermoregulatory responses were obtained in response to microinjections of Ang II into several cerebral regions, including preoptic, hypothalamic, thalamic, and midbrain sites.[172]

Memory

Considerable evidence links brain Ang with a role in cognition. Behavioral studies have reported that exogenous administration of renin or Ang II, acting through AT_1 receptors, disrupts learning and memory in passive avoidance, operant, and retention behavior paradigms.[173-176] In line with this behavioral observation, Ang II inhibits depolarization-induced release of acetylcholine from rat entorhinal and human temporal cortex.[177,178] Thus, Ang II may inhibit cognitive performance by inhibiting cholinergic function. Of interest, ACE inhibitors improve the cognitive performance of mice and rats.[179]

Some evidence also suggests a positive role for Ang II in memory and learning via modulation of dopaminergic neurons.[180-182] Baranowska et al.[183] noted that high doses of Ang II (1–2 µg), administered intracerebroventricularly, facilitated acquisition in the conditioned avoidance tests, whereas low doses (0.5 µg) were disruptive. Because the improvements in cognitive performance were not blocked by Ang II receptor antagonists, it was concluded that the facilitatory effect of Ang II was not mediated via a known Ang II receptor. Later studies have indicated that a C-terminal fragment of Ang II may be responsible for facilitatory effects.[180,184]

A specific binding site for Ang II [3–8] (Ang IV) is distributed widely in the brain and has been termed the AT_4 receptor.[185] It is present in high density in structures important for cognition, including the neocortex, septum, hippocampus, thalamus, and cerebellum.[185-187] Ang IV and related peptides potentiate cognitive processes in associative and spatial tasks,[184,186–189] whereas specific antagonism of the AT_4 receptor impairs learning in spatial tasks.[189] These findings suggest that Ang IV acting via the AT_4 receptor may be responsible for the cognitive improvements seen with administration of Ang II. We have shown that the decapeptide LVV-hemorphin 7 is a potent and specific ligand for the AT_4 receptor and may represent its endogenous ligand.[190]

■ Conclusion

Angiotensin II and III coexert a wide range of actions in the brain, following either delivery from the circulation to AT_1 receptors in the circumventricular organs or generation within the brain to access AT_1 receptors at sites within the blood-brain barrier. Many of these actions concern central pressor, autonomic, and renal effects, which in concert with neuroendocrine and behavioral actions help to maintain blood pressure and body fluid and electrolyte homeostasis. Central angiotensinergic pathways are involved in many of these actions as well as the cerebral response to hyperosmolality. In addition, angiotensin has actions in other areas, including thermoregulation, modulation of catecholaminergic and cholinergic neurotransmission, and effects on cognition. In contrast to these AT_1 receptor-mediated effects, the role of angiotensin acting at brain AT_2 receptors is poorly understood. Abundant AT_4 receptors in the brain may mediate cognitive actions of exogenous Ang IV, but their endogenous ligand may be peptides, such as LVV-hemorphan-7, that are unrelated to angiotensin. Although much has been learned about angiotensin receptors and actions in the brain, details of the biochemical and cellular pathways of its formation in the brain remain unclear.

Acknowledgments

The work of the authors is supported by an Institute Block Grant (No 983001) from the National Health and Medical Research Council of Australia. We thank Helen Mansour and Michelle Giles for help with the manuscript and figure.

References

1. Phillips MI: Functions of angiotensin in the central nervous system. Ann Rev Physiol 49: 413–435, 1987.
2. Fischer-Ferraro C, Nahmod VE, Goldstein DJ, Finkelman S: Angiotensin and renin in rat and dog brain. J Exp Med 133:353–361, 1971.
3. Ganten D, Minnich JL, Granger P, et al: Angiotensin-forming enzyme in the brain tissue. Science 173:64–65, 1971.
4. Hirose S, Yokosawa H, Inagami T: Immunochemical identification of renin in rat brain and distinction from acid proteases. Nature 274:392–393, 1978.
5. Campbell DJ: Angiotensin peptides in the brain. Adv Exp Med Biol 377:349–355, 1995.
6. Fuxe K, Ganten D, Hokfelt T, Bolme P: Immunohistochemical evidence for the existence of angiotensin II-containing nerve terminals in the brain and spinal cord of the rat. Neurosci Lett 2:229–234, 1976.
7. Lind RW, Swanson LW, Ganten D: Organization of angiotensin II immunoreactive cells and fibres in the rat central nervous system. Neuroendocrinology 40:2–24, 1985.
8. Allen AM, Paxinos G, Song KF, Mendelsohn FAO: Localization of angiotensin receptor binding sites in the rat brain. In Bjorkland A, Hokfelt T, Kuhar MJ (eds): Handbook of Chemical Neuroanatomy: Neuropeptide Receptors in the CNS, vol. 11. Amsterdam, Elsevier, 1992, pp 1–35.
9. Lenkei Z, Palkovits M, Corvol P, Llorens-Cortes C: Expression of angiotensin type-1 (AT_1) and type-2 (AT_2) receptor mRNAs in the adult rat brain: A functional anatomical review. Front Neuroendocrinol 18:383–439, 1997.
10. Hilgenfeld U: Angiotensinogen in rat cerebrospinal fluid. Clin Exp Hypertens 6:1815–1824, 1984.
11. Stornetta RL, Hawelu-Johnson CL, Guyenet PG, Lynch KR: Astrocytes synthesize angiotensinogen in brain. Science 242:1444–1446, 1988.

12. Yang G, Gray TS, Sigmund CD, Cassell MD: The angiotensinogen gene is expressed in both astrocytes and neurons in murine central nervous system. Brain Res 817:123–131, 1999.

13. Sernia C, Zeng T, Kerr D, Wyse B: Novel perspectives on pituitary and brain angiotensinogen. Front Neuroendocrinol 18:174–208, 1997.

14. Campbell DJ, Sernia C, Thomas WJ, Oldfield BJ: Immunochemical localization of angiotensinogen in rat brain: Dependence of neuronal immunoreactivity on method of tissue processing. J. Neuroendocrinol 3:653–660, 1991.

15. Dzau VJ, Ingelfinger J, Pratt RE, Ellison KE: Identification of renin and angiotensinogen messenger RNA sequences in mouse and rat brains. Hypertension 8:544–548, 1986.

16. Chai SY, Mendelsohn FAO, Paxinos G: Angiotensin converting enzyme in rat brain visualized by quantitative in vitro autoradiography. Neuroscience 20:615–627, 1987.

17. Erdos EG, Skidgel RA: The unusual substrate specificity and the distribution of human angiotensin I converting enzyme. Hypertension 8(Suppl I):I-34–I-37, 1986.

18. Allen AM, Moeller I, Jenkins TA, et al: Angiotensin receptors in the nervous system. Brain Res Bull 47:17–28, 1998.

19. Covenas R, Fuxe K, Cintra A, et al: Evidence for the existence of angiotensin II like immunoreactivity in subpopulations of tyrosine hydroxylase immunoreactive neurons in the A1 and C1 area of the ventral medulla of the male rat. Neurosci Lett 114:160–166, 1990.

20. Timmermans PBMW, Wong PC, Chiu AT, et al: Angiotensin II receptors and angiotensin II receptor antagonists. Pharmacol Rev 45:205–251, 1993.

21. Murphy TJ, Alexander RW, Griendling KK, et al: Isolation of a cDNA encoding the vascular type-1 angiotensin II receptor. Nature 351:233–236, 1991.

22. Sasaki K, Yamano Y, Bardhan S, et al: Cloning and expression of a complementary DNA encoding a bovine adrenal angiotensin II type-1 receptor. Nature 351:230–233, 1991.

23. Kambayashi Y, Bardhan S, Takahashi K, et al: Molecular cloning of a novel angiotensin II receptor isoform involved in phosphotyrosine phosphatase inhibition. J Biol Chem 268:24543–24546, 1993.

24. Mukoyama M, Nakajima M, Horiuchi M, et al: Expression cloning of type 2 angiotensin II receptor reveals a unique class of seven-transmembrane receptors. J Biol Chem 268:24539–24542, 1993.

25. Stoll M, Steckelings UM, Paul M, et al: The angiotensin AT_2-receptor mediates inhibition of cell proliferation in coronary endothelial cells. J Clin Invest 95:651–657, 1995.

26. Yamada T, Horiuchi M, Dzau VJ: Angiotensin II type 2 receptor mediates programmed cell death. Proc Natl Acad Sci USA 93:156–160, 1996.

27. Horiuchi M, Akishita M, Dzau VJ: Recent progress in angiotensin II type 2 receptor research in the cardiovascular system. Hypertension 33:613–621, 1999.

28. Schmitz U, Berk BC: Angiotensin II signal transduction: Stimulation of multiple mitogen-activated protein kinase pathways. Trends Endocrinol Metab 8:261–266, 1997.

29. Iwai N, Inagami T: Identification of two subtypes in the rat type I angiotensin II receptor. FEBS Lett 298:257–260, 1992.

30. Szpirer C, Riviere M, Szpirer J, et al: Chromosomal assignment of human and rat hypertension candidate genes: Type 1 angiotensin II receptor genes and the SA gene. J Hypertens 11:919–925, 1993.

31. Lewis JL, Serikawa T, Warnock DG: Chromosomal localization of angiotensin II type 1 receptor isoforms in the rat. Biochem Biophys Res Commun 194:677–682, 1993.

32. Curnow KM, Pascoe L, White PC: Genetic analysis of the human type-1 angiotensin II receptor. Mol Endocrinol 6:1113–1118, 1992.

33. Lazard D, Briend-Sutren MM, Villageois P, et al: Molecular characterization and chromosomal localization of a human angiotensin II AT_2 receptor gene highly expressed in fetal tissues. Receptors-Channels 2:271–280, 1994.

34. Wharton J, Morgan K, Rutherford RA, et al: Differential distribution of angiotensin AT_2 receptors in the normal and failing human heart. J Pharmacol Exp Ther 284:323–336, 1998.

35. Moeller IM, Allen AM, Chai SY, et al: Bioactive angiotensin peptides. J Human Hypertens 12:289–293, 1998.

36. Harding JW, Felix D: The effects of aminopeptidase inhibitors amastatin and bestatin on angiotensin-evoked neuronal activity in rat brain. Brain Res 424:299–304, 1987.

37. Zini S, Fournie-Zaluski MC, Chauvel E, et al: Identification of metabolic pathways of brain angiotensin II and III using specific aminopeptidase inhibitors: Predominant role of angiotensin III in the control of vasopressin release. Proc Natl Acad Sci 93:11968–11973, 1996.

38. Rowe BP, Grove KL, Saylor DL, Speth RC: Angiotensin II receptor subtypes in the rat brain. Eur J Pharmacol 186:339–342, 1990.

39. Wamsley JK, Herblin WF, Hunt M: Evidence for the presence of angiotensin II type receptors in brain. Brain Res Bull 25:397–400, 1990.

40. Song K, Allen AM, Paxinos G, Mendelsohn FAO: Angiotensin II receptor subtypes in rat brain. Clin Exp Pharmacol Physiol 18:93–96, 1991.
41. Song K, Allen AM, Paxinos G, Mendelsohn FAO: Mapping of angiotensin II receptor subtype heterogeneity in rat brain. J Comp Neurol 316:467–484, 1992.
42. Bunnemann B, Iwai N, Metzger R, et al: The distribution of angiotensin II AT_1 receptor subtype mRNA in the rat brain. Neurosci Lett 142:155–158, 1992.
43. Lenkei Z, Corvol P, Llorens-Cortes C: The angiotensin receptor subtype AT_{1A} predominates in rat forebrain areas involved in blood pressure, body fluid homeostasis and neuroendocrine control. Mol Brain Res 30:53–60, 1995.
44. Lenkei Z, Palkovits M, Corvol P, Llorens-Cortes C: Distribution of angiotensin II type-2 receptor (AT_2) mRNA expression in the adult rat brain. J Comp Neurol 373:322–339, 1996.
45. Giles ME, Fernley RT, Nakamura Y, et al: Characterization of a specific antibody to the rat AT_1 receptor. J Histochem Cytochem 47:507–515, 1999.
46. Aldred GP, Chai SY, Song K, et al: Distribution of angiotensin II receptor subtypes in the rabbit brain. Regul Pept 44:119–130, 1993.
47. MacGregor DP, Murone C, Song K, et al: Angiotensin II receptor subtypes in the human central nervous system. Brain Res 675:231–240, 1995.
48. Barnes JM, Steward U, Barber PC, Barnes NM: Identification and characterization of angiotensin II receptor subtypes in human brain. Eur J Pharmacol 231:251–258, 1993.
49. Allen AM, Oldfield BJ, Giles ME, et al Localization of angiotensin receptors in the nervous system. In Quirion R, Bjorklund A, Hokfelt T (eds): Handbook of Chemical Neuroanatomy. Amsterdam, Elsevier, 1999.
50. Allen AM, MacGregor DP, McKinley MJ, Mendelsohn FAO: Angiotensin II receptors in the human brain. Reg Pept 79:1–7, 1999.
51. Hein L, Barch GS, Pratt RE, et al: Behavioural and cardiovascular effects of disrupting the angiotensin II type-2 receptor gene in mice. Nature 377:744–747, 1995.
52. Ichiki T, Labosky PA, Shiota C, et al: Effects on blood pressure and exploratory behaviour of mice lacking angiotensin II type-2 receptor. Nature 377:748–750, 1995.
53. Bickerton RK, Buckley JP: Evidence of a central mechanism in angiotensin-induced hypertension. Proc Soc Exper Biol Med 106:834–836, 1961.
54. Dickinson CJ, Lawrence JR: A slowly developing pressor response to small concentrations of angiotensin: Its bearing on the pathogenesis of chronic renal hypertension. Lancet i:1354–1356, 1963.
55. Scroop GC, Lowe RD: Efferent pathways of the cardiovascular response to vertebral artery infusions of angiotensin in the dog. Clin Sci 37:605–619, 1969.
56. Ferrario CM, Dickinson CJ, McCubbin JW: Central vasomotor stimulation by angiotensin. Clin Sci 39:239–243, 1970.
57. Ferrario CM, Gildenberg PL, McCubbin JW: Cardiovascular effects of angiotensin mediated by the central nervous system. Circ Res 30:257–262, 1972.
58. Fukiyama K: Central action of angiotensin and hypertension increased vasomotor outflow by angiotensin. Jpn Circ J 36:599–603, 1972.
59. Bonjour JP, Malvin RL: Stimulation of ADH release by the renin-angiotensin system. Am J Physiol 218:1555–1559, 1970.
60. Lumbers ER, McClosky DI, Potter EK: Inhibition by angiotensin II of baroreceptor-evoked activity in cardiac vagal efferent nerves in the dog. J Physiol 294:69–80, 1979.
61. Guo GB, Abboud FM: Angiotensin II attenuates baroreflex control of heart rate and sympathetic activity. Am J Physiol 246:H80–H89, 1984.
62. Stein RD, Stephenson RB, Weaver LC: Central actions of angiotensin II oppose baroreceptor-induced sympathoinhibition. Am J Physiol 246:R13–R19, 1984.
63. Keil LC, Summy-Long J, Severs WB: Release of vasopressin by angiotensin II. Endocrinology 96:1063–1068, 1975.
64. Brooks VL: Interactions between angiotensin II and the sympathetic nervous system in the long-term control of arterial pressure. Clin Exp Pharmacol Physiol 24:83–90, 1997.
65. DiBona GF, Jones SY, Brooks VL: Ang II receptor blockade and arterial baroreflex regulation of renal nerve activity in cardiac failure. Am J Physiol 269: R1189–R1196, 1995.
66. Dibner-Dunlap ME, Smith ML, Kinugawa T, Thames MD: Enalaprilat augments arterial and cardiopulmonary baroreflex control of sympathetic nerve activity in patients with heart failure. Am Coll Cardiol 27: 358–364, 1996.
67. Xu L, Brooks VL: Ang II chronically supports renal and lumbar sympathetic activity in sodium-deprived, conscious rats. Hypertension 271:H2591, 1996.
68. Heesch CM, Crandall ME, Turbek JA: Converting enzyme inhibitors cause pressure-independent resetting of baroreflex control of sympathetic outflow. Am J Physiol 270: R728–R737, 1996.
69. Mangiapane ML, Simpson JB: Subfornical organ lesions reduce the pressor effects of systemic angiotensin. Neuroendocrinology 31:380–384, 1980.

70. Gildenberg PL, Ferrario CM, McCubbin JW: Two sites of cardiovascular actions of angiotensin II in the brain of the dog. Clin Sci 44:417–422, 1973.
71. Lewis GP, Reit E: The action of angiotensin and bradykinin on the superior cervical ganglion of the cat. J Physiol 179 538–553, 1965.
72. Zimmerman BG: Effect of acute sympathectomy on responses to angiotensin and norepinephrine. Circ Res 11:780–787, 1962.
73. Hughes J, Roth RH: Evidence that angiotensin enhances transmitter release during sympathetic nerve stimulation. Br J Pharmacol 41:239–255, 1971.
74. Fitzsimons JT: The role of a renal thirst factor in drinking induced by extracellular stimuli. J Physiol (Lond) 201:349–368, 1969.
75. Fitzsimons JT, Simons B: The effect on drinking in the rat of intravenous infusion of angiotensin, given alone or in combination with other stimuli of thirst. J Physiol 203:45–57, 1969.
76. Simpson JB, Epstein AN, Cammardo JS: Localization of receptors for the dipsogenic action of angiotensin II in the subfornical organ of rat. J Comp Physiol Psychol 92:581–608, 1978.
77. Thrasher TN: Circumventricular organs, thirst, and vasopressin secretion. In Schrier RW (ed): Vasopressin. New York, Raven Press, 1985, pp 311–318.
78. McKinley MJ, Badoer E, Oldfield BJ: Intravenous angiotensin II induces Fos-immunoreactivity in circumventricular organs of the lamina terminalis. Brain Res 294:295–300, 1992.
79. Fregly MJ, Rowland NE: Effect of a nonpeptide angiotensin II receptor antagonist (DUP-753) on angiotensin related water intake. Brain Res Bull 27:97–100, 1991.
80. Beresford MJ, Fitzsimons JT: Intracerebroventricular angiotensin II induced thirst and sodium appetite in rat are blocked by the AT_1 receptor antagonist, losartan (DUP 753), but not by the AT_2 antagonist CGP 42112B. Exp Physiol 77, 1992.
81. Dourish CT, Duggan JA, Bank RJA: Drinking induced by subcutaneous injection of angiotensin II in the rat is blocked by the selective AT_1 receptor antagonist DUP 753 but not by the selective AT_2 receptor antagonist WL 19. Eur J Pharmacol 211:113–116, 1992.
82. McKinley MJ, McAllen RM, Pennington GL, et al: Physiological actions of angiotensin II mediated by AT_1 and AT_2 receptors in the brain. Clin Exp Pharmacol Physiol Suppl 3:S99–S104, 1996.
83. Schmid HA, Rauch M, Koch J: Effect of calcitonin on the activity of Ang II-responsive neurons in the rat subfornical organ. Am J Physiol 274:R1646–R1652, 1998.
84. Ferguson AV, Bains JS: Electrophysiology of the circumventricular organs. Front Neuroendocrinol 17:440–475, 1996.
85. Gebke E, Mulller AR, Jurzak M, Gerstberger R: Angiotensin II-induced calcium signalling in neurons and astrocytes of rat circumventricular organs. Neuroscience 85:509–520, 1998.
86. McKinley MJ, Oldfield BJ: Distribution of Fos in rat brain resulting from endogenously-generated angiotensin II. Kidney Int 46:1567–1569, 1994.
87. Cunningham JT, Beltz TG, Johnson RF, Johnson AK: The effects of ibotenate lesions of the median preoptic nucleus on experimentally induced and circadian drinking behaviours in rats. Brain Res 580:325–330, 1992.
88. Phillips PA, Rolls BJ, Ledingham JG: Angiotensin II-induced thirst and vasopressin release in man. Clin Sci 68:669–674, 1995.
89. Robinson MM, Evered MD: Pressor action of intravenous angiotensin II reduces drinking in rats. Am J Physiol 252:R754–R759, 1987.
90. Rogers PW, Kurzman NA: Renal failure, uncontrollable thirst and hyper-reninaemia. Cessation of thirst with bilateral nephrectomy. JAMA 225:1236–1238, 1973.
91. Yamamoto T, Shimuzu M, Morioka M: Role of angiotensin II in the pathogenesis of hyperdipsia in chronic renal failure. JAMA 25:604–608, 1986.
92. Lehr D, Goldman HW, Casner P: Renin-angiotensin role in thirst: Paradoxical enhancement of drinking by angiotensin converting enzyme inhibitor. Science 182:1031–1034, 1973.
93. Schiffrin EL: Mechanism of captopril-induced drinking. Am J Physiol 242:R136–R140, 1982.
94. Thunhorst RL, Fitts DA, Simpson JB: Angiotensin converting enzyme in subfornical organ mediates captopril-induced drinking. Behav Neurosci 103:1302–1310, 1989.
95. McKinley MJ, Colvill LM, Giles ME, Oldfield BJ: Distribution of Fos-immunoreactivity in rat brain following a dipsogenic dose of captopril and effects of angiotensin receptor blockade. Brain Res 747:43–51, 1997.
96. Ramsay DJ, Keil LC, Sharpe MC, Shinsaki J: Angiotensin II infusion increases vasopressin, ACTH and 11-hydroxycorticosteroid secretion. Am J Physiol 234:R66–R71, 1978.
97. Reid IA: Actions of angiotensin II on the brain: Mechanisms and physiologic role. Am J Physiol 246:F533–F543, 1984.
98. Miselis RR: The efferent projections of the subfornical organ of the rat: A circumventricular organ with a neural network subserving water balance. Brain Res 230:1–23, 1981.
99. Lind RW, van Hoesen GW, Johnson AK: An HRP study of the connections of the subfornical organ of the rat. J Comp Neurol 210:265–277, 1982.

100. Mangiapane ML, Thrasher TN, Keil LC, et al: Role for the subfornical organ in vasopressin release. Brain Res Bull 1984;13:43–47.
101. Gutman MB, Ciriello J, Mogenson GJ: Effects of plasma angiotensin II and hypernatremia on subfornical organ neurons. Am J Physiol 254:R746–R754, 1988.
102. Tanaka J, Saito H, Kaba H: Subfornical organ and hypothalamic paraventricular nucleus connections with median preoptic nucleus neurons: An electrophysiological study in the rat. Exp Brain Res 68:579–585, 1987.
103. Oldfield B, Hards DK, McKinley MJ: Projections from the subfornical organ to the supraoptic nucleus in the rat: Ultrastructural identification of an interposed synapse in the median preoptic nucleus using a combination of neural tracers. Brain Res 558:13–19, 1991.
104. Oldfield BJ, Badoer E, Hards DK, McKinley MJ: Fos production in retrogradely labelled neurons of the lamina terminalis following intravenous infusion of either hypertonic saline or angiotensin II. Neuroscience 60:255–262, 1994.
105. Reid IA, Brooks VL, Rudolph CD, Keil LC: Analysis of the action of angiotensin on the central nervous system of conscious dogs. Am J Physiol 243:R82–R91, 1982.
106. Ganong WF, Murakami K: The role of angiotensin II in the regulation of ACTH release. Ann N Y Acad Sci 512:176–186, 1987.
107. Buggy J, Fisher AE: Evidence for a dual central role for angiotensin in water and sodium intake. Nature 250:733–735, 1974.
108. Findlay ALR, Epstein AN: Increased sodium intake is somehow induced in rats by intravenous angiotensin II. Horm Behav 14:86-92, 1980.
109. Moe KE, Weiss ML, Epstein AN: Sodium appetite during captopril blockade of endogenous angiotensin II formation. Am J Physiol 247:R356–R365, 1984.
110. Weisinger RS, Denton DA, Di Nicolantonio R, McKinley MJ: The effect of captopril or enalaprilic on the Na appetite of Na-deplete rats. Clin Exp Pharmacol Physiol 15:55–65, 1988.
111. Thunhorst RL, Fitts DA: Peripheral angiotensin causes salt appetite in rats. Am J Physiol 2267:R171–R177, 1994.
112. Weisinger RS, Denton DA, Di Nicolantonio R, et al: Role of angiotensin in sodium appetite of sodium-deplete sheep. Am J Physiol 253:R482–R488, 1987.
113. Weisinger RS, Blair-West JR, Burns P, et al: The role of angiotensin II in ingestive behaviour: a brief review of angiotensin II thirst and Na appetite. Reg Pept 661:73–81, 1996.
114. Weisinger RS, Denton DA, Hards DK, McKinley MJ: Subfornical organ lesion decreases sodium appetite in the sodium-depleted rat. Brain Res 526:23–30, 1990.
115. Fitts DA, Mason DB: Preoptic angiotensin and salt appetite. Behav Neurosci 28:89–98, 1990.
116. Falcon JE, Phillips MI, Hoffman WE, Brody MJ: Effects of intraventricular angiotensin II mediated by the sympathetic nervous system. Am J Physiol 235:H392–H397, 1978.
117. Severs WB, Daniels-Severs A: Effects of angiotensin on the central nervous system. Pharmacol Rev 25:415–463, 1973.
118. Unger T, Becker H, Petty M, et al: Differential effects of central angiotensin II and substance P on sympathetic nerve activity in conscious rats. Circ Res 156:563–575, 1985.
119. May CN, McAllen RM: Baroreceptor-independent renal nerve inhibition by icv angiotensin II in conscious sheep. Am J Physiol 273:R560–R567, 1997.
120. Bains JS, Ferguson AV: Paraventricular nucleus neurons projecting to the spinal cord receive excitatory input from the subfornical organ. Am J Physiol 268: R625–R633, 1995.
121. Bains JS, Potyok A, Ferguson AV: Angiotensin II actions in paraventricular nucleus: Functional evidence for a neurotransmitter role in efferents originating in subfornical organ. Brain Res 599:223–229, 1992.
122. Casto R, Philips MI:Cardiovascular actions of microinjections of angiotensin II on the brain stem of rats. Am J Physiol 246: R811–R816, 1984.
123. Rettig R, Healy DP, Printz MP: Cardiovascular effects of microinjections of angiotensin II into the nucleus tractus solitarii. Brain Res 364: 233–240, 1986.
124. Dampney RAL: Functional organisation of central pathways regulating the cardiovascular system. Physiol Rev 74:323–364, 1994.
125. Allen AM, Dampney RAL, Mendelsohn FAO: Angiotensin receptor binding and pressor effects in the cat subretrofacial nucleus. Am J Physiol 255:H1011–H1017, 1988.
126. Andreatta SH, Averill DB, Santos RAS, Ferrario CM: The ventrolateral medulla: A new site of action of the renin-angiotensin system. Hypertension 11(Suppl I): I-163–I-166, 1988.
127. Sasaki S, Dampney RAL: Tonic cardiovascular effects of angiotensin II in the ventrolateral medulla. Hypertension 15:274–283, 1990.
128. Lewis DI, Coote JH: Angiotensin II in the spinal cord of the rat and its sympatho-excitatory effects. Brain Res 614:1–9, 1993.
129. Gardner J, Coote JH: Cluster analysis of the effects on renal and adrenal nerve activity of stimulation of the paraventricular nucleus in the rabbit. J Physiol 497:17, 1996.

130. Allen AM, Mendelsohn FAO, Gieroba ZJ, Blessing WW: Vasopressin release following microinjection of angiotensin II into the caudal ventrolateral medulla in the anaesthetized rabbit. J Neuroendocrinol 2:867–874, 1990.

131. Diz DI, Barnes KL, Ferrario CM: Hypotensive actions of microinjections of angiotensin II into the dorsal motor nucleus of the vagus. J Hypertens 2(Suppl 3):53–56, 1984.

132. Casto R, Phillips MI: Angiotensin II attenuates baroreflexes at nucleus tractus solitarius of rats. Am J Physiol 250:R193–R198, 1986.

133. Campagnole-Santos MJ, Diz DI, Ferrario CM: Baroreceptor reflex modulation by angiotensin II at the nucleus tractus solitarii. Hypertension 11(Suppl I):I-167–I-171, 1988.

134. Kasparov S, Butcher JW, Paton JFR: Angiotensin II receptors within the nucleus of the solitary tract mediate the developmental attenuation of the baroreceptor vagal reflex in pre-weaned rats. J Auton Nerv Syst 74:160–168, 1998.

135. Lewis SJ, Allen AM, Verberne AJM,et al: Angiotensin II receptor binding in the rat nucleus tractus solitarii is reduced after unilateral nodose ganglionectomy or vagotomy. Eur J Pharmacol 125:305–307, 1986.

136. Diz DI, Barnes KL, Ferrario CM: Contribution of the vagus nerve to angiotensin II binding sites in the canine medulla. Brain Res Bull 17:497–506, 1986.

137. Qu L, McQueeney AJ, Barnes KL: Presynaptic or postsynaptic location of receptors for angiotensin II and substance P in the medial solitary tract nucleus. J Neurophysiol 75:2220–2228, 1996.

138. Fitzsimons JT: Angiotensin stimulation of the central nervous system. Rev Physiol Biochem Pharmacol 87:117–167, 1980.

139. O'Neill TP, Brody MJ: Role for the median preoptic nucleus in centrally evoked pressor responses. Am J Physiol 252:R1165–R1172, 1987.

140. McKinley MJ, Badoer E, Vivas L, Oldfield BJ: Comparison of C-fos expression in the lamina terminalis of conscious rats after intravenous or intracerebroventricular angiotensin. Brain Res Bull 37:131–137, 1995.

141. Buggy J, Fisher AE: Anteroventral third ventricle site of action of angiotensin induced thirst. Pharmacol Biochem Behav 4:651–660, 1976.

142. Fregly MJ, Rowland NE: Effect of DuP 753, a non-peptide angiotensin II receptor antagonist, on the drinking responses to acutely administered dipsogenic agents in rats. Proc Soc Exp Biol Med 199:158–164, 1992.

143. Rowland NE, Rozelle A, Riley PJ, Fregly MJ: Effect of non-peptide angiotensin receptor antagonists on water and salt intake in rats. Brain Res Bull 29:389–393, 1992.

144. Blair-West JR, Denton DA, McKinley MJ, Weisinger RS: Thirst and brain angiotensin in cattle. Am J Physiol 262:R204–R210, 1992.

145. Mathai M, Evered MD, McKinley MJ: Intracerebroventricular losartan inhibits post-prandial drinking in sheep. Am J Physiol 272:R1055–R1059, 1997.

146. Sinnayah P, Kachab E, Haralambidis J, et al: Effects of angiotensinogen antisense oligonucleotides on fluid intake in response to different dipsogenic stimuli in the rat. Brain Res 50:43–50, 1997.

147. Andersson B, Eriksson L, Fernandez O, et al: Centrally mediated effects of sodium and angiotensin II on arterial pressure and fluid balance. Acta Physiol Scand 85:398–407, 1972.

148. Wilkin LD, Mitchell LD, Ganten D, Johnson AK: The supraoptic nucleus: Afferents from areas involved in control of body fluid homeostasis. Neuroscience 28:573–583, 1989.

149. Bealer S, Phillips MI, Johnson AK, Schmid PG: Anteroventral third ventricle lesions reduce antidiuretic responses to angiotensin II. Am J Physiol 236:E610–E615, 1979.

150. Scholkens BA, Jung W, Rasher W, et al: Intracerebroventricular angiotensin II increases arterial blood pressure in Rhesus Monkeys by stimulation of pituitary hormones and the sympathetic nervous system. Experientia 38:469–473, 1982.

151. Sumitomo T, Suda T, Nakano Y, et al: Angiotensin II increases the corticotropin releasing factor messenger ribonucleic acid level in the rat hypothalamus. Endocrinology 128:2248–2252, 1991.

152. Aguilera G, Young WS, Kiss A, Bathia A: Direct regulation of hypothalmic corticotropin releasing hormone neurons by angiotensin II. Neuroendocrinology 61:437, 1995.

153. Aguilera G, Kiss A, Luo X: Increased expression of type-1 angiotensin II receptors in the hypothalamic paraventricular nucleus following stress and glucocorticoid administration. J Neuroendocrinol 7:775–783, 1995.

154. Jezova D, Ochedalski T, Kiss A, Aguilera G: Brain angiotensin II modulates sympathoadrenal and hypothalamic pituitary adrenocortical activation during stress. J Neuroendocrinol 10:67–72, 1998.

155. Fitzsimons JT: Angiotensin, thirst and sodium appetite. Physiol Rev 78:583–682, 1998.

156. Coghlan JP, Considine PJ, Denton DA, et al: Sodium appetite in sheep induced by cerebral ventricular infusion of angiotensin: Comparison with sodium deficiency. Science 214:195–197, 1980.

157. Galaverna O, Deluca LA, Schulkin J, et al: Deficits in NaCl ingestion after damage to the central nucleus of the amygdala in the rat. Brain Res Bull 28:89–98, 1992.

158. Unger T, Horst PJ, Bauer M, et al: Natriuretic action of central angiotensin II in conscious rats. Brain Res 486:33–38, 1999.

159. Eriksson L, Fyhrquist F: Plasma renin activity following central infusions of and altered CSF sodium concentration in the conscious goat. Acta Physiol Scand 48:209–216, 1976.

160. Mathai ML, Evered MD, McKinley MJ: Central losartan blocks natriuretic, vasopressin and pressor responses to central hypertonic NaCl in sheep. Am J Physiol 275:R548–R554, 1998.

161. McKinley MJ, Evered M, Mathai M, Coghlan JP: Effects of central losartan on plasma renin and centrally mediated natriuresis. Kidney Int 46:1479–1482, 1994.

162. Rohmeiss P, Beyer C, Nagy E, et al: Sodium chloride injections in the brain induce natriuresis and blood pressure responses sensitive to AT_1 receptors. Am J Physiol 269:F282–F288, 1995.

163. Rohmeiss P, Beyer C, Hocher B, et al: Osmotically induced natriuresis and blood pressure involves angiotensin AT_1 receptors in the subfornical organ. J Hypertens 13:1399–1404, 1995.

164. Malayan SA, Keil LC, Ramsay DJ, Reid IA: Mechanism of suppression of plasma renin activity by centrally administred angiotensin II. Endocrinology 104:672–675, 1979.

165. Weekly LB: Renal renin secretion and norepinephrine secretion rate in response to centrally administered angiotensin II: Role of medial basal forebrain. Clin Exp Hypertens 14:923–945, 1992.

166. McKinley MJ, Mathai ML: Centrally administered losartan inhibits the reduction in plasma renin concentration caused by intracerebroventricular hypertonic saline in Na-depleted sheep. Reg Pept 66:37–40, 1996.

167. Sharpe LG, Swanson LW: Drinking induced by injections of angiotensin into forebrain and midbrain sites of the monkey. J Physiol (Lond.) 239:595–622, 1974.

168. Lin MT: Effects of angiotensin II on metabolic, respiratory and vasomotor activities as well as body temperature in the rabbit. J Neur Transmiss 49:197–204, 1980.

169. Shido O, Nagasaka T: Effects of intraventricular angiotensin II on heat balance at various ambient termperatures in rats. Jpn J Physiol 35:163–167, 1985.

170. Fregly MJ, Rowland NE: Effect of losartan potassium and deoxycorticosterone acetate on tail skin temperature response to acute amdinistration of angiotensin II. Pharmacol Biochem Behav 43:229–233, 1992.

171. Mathai ML, Huebschle T, McKinley MJ, Mendelsohn FAO: Central angiotensin AT_1 receptor blockade impairs <u>66</u>, 37 thermoregulation and thirst following heat stress in rats. Soc Neurosci 24:121, 1998.

172. Sharpe LG, Garnett JE, Olsen NS: Thermoregulatory changes to cholinomimetics and angiotensin II, but not to the monoamines microinjected into the brain stem of the rabbit. Neuropharmacology 18:117–125, 1979.

173. Melo JC, Graeff FG: Effect of intracerebroventricular bradykinin and related peptides on rabbit operant behaviour. J Pharmacol Exp Ther 193:1–10, 1975.

174. Morgan TM, Routtenberg A: Angiotensin injected into the neostriatum after learning disrupts retention performance. Science 196:87–89, 1977.

175. Koller M, Krause HP, Hoffmeister F, Ganten D: Endogenous brain angiotensin II disrupts passive avoidance behaviour in rats. Neurosci Lett 14:71–75, 1979.

176. DeNoble VJ, DeNoble KF, Spencer KR, et al: Non-peptide angiotensin II receptor antagonist and angiotensin-converting enzyme inhibitor: Effect on a renin-induced deficit of a passive avoidance response in rats. Brain Res 561:230–235, 1991.

177. Barnes JM, Barnes NM, Costall B, et al: Angiotensin II inhibits cortical cholinergic function: Implications for cognition. J Cardiovasc Pharmacol 16:234–238, 1990.

178. Barnes JM, Barnes NM, Costall B, et al: Angiotensin II inhibits acetylcholine release from human temporal cortex: Implications for cognition. Brain Res 507:341–343, 1990.

179. Costall B, Coughlan J, Horovitz ZP, et al: The effects of ACE inhibitors captopril and SQ29852 in rodent tests of cognition. Pharmacol Biochem Behav 33:573–580, 1989.

180. Braszko JJ, Wisniewski K: Effective angiotensin II and saralasin on motor activity in the passive avoidance behaviour of rats. Peptides 9:475–479, 1988.

181. Wiasienko J, Braszko JJ, Koziolkiewicz W, et al: Psychotropic activity of angiotensin II and its fragments: Val-Tyr-Ile-NH2 and Val-Tyr-Ile-His-NH2. Biomed Biochim Acta 48:707–713, 1989.

182. Georgiev VP, Yonkov DI, Kambourova TS: Interactions between angiotensin II and baclofen in shuttle-box and passive avoidance performance. Neuropeptides 12:155–158, 1988.

183. Baranowska D, Braszko JJ, Wisniewski K: Effect of angiotensin II and vasopressin on acquisition and extinction of conditioned avoidance in rats. Psychopharmacology 81:247–251, 1983.

184. Braszko JJ, Wiasienko J, Koziolliewicz W, et al: The 3-7 fragment of angiotensin II is probably responsible for its psychoactive properties. Brain Res 542:49–54, 1991.

185. Miller-Wing AV, Hanesworth JM, Sardinia MF, et al: Central angiotensin IV receptor: Distribution and specificity in guinea pig brain. J Pharmacol Exp Ther 266:1718–1726, 1993.

186. Wright JW, Miller-Wing AV, Shaffer MJ, Harding JW: Angiotensin II (3-8) (Ang IV) hippocampal binding: Potential role in the facilitation of memory. Brain Res Bull 32:497–502, 1993.
187. Moeller I, Paxinos G, Mendelsohn FAO, et al: Distribution of AT_4 receptors in the Macaca fasicularis brain. Brain Res 712:307–324, 1996.
188. Pederson ES, Harding JW, Wright JW: Attenuation of scopolamine-induced spatial learning impairments by an angiotensin IV analog. Reg Pept 74:97-103, 1998.
189. Wright JW, Stubley L, Pederson ES, et al: Contributions of the brain angiotensin IV-AT_4 receptor subtype system to spatial learning. J Neurosci 19: 3952–3961, 1999.
190. Moeller I, Lew RA, Mendelsohn FAO, et al: The globin fragment LVV-Hemorphan-7 is an endogenous ligand for the AT_4 receptor in the brain. J Neurochem 68:2530–2537, 1997.

CHAPTER 11

Interaction of AT_1 Receptor Antagonists and Other Vasoactive Factors

AHMED G. ADAM, M.D., Ph.D.
AREEF ISHANI, M.D.
RAHUL KOUSHIK, M.D.
LEOPOLDO RAIJ, M.D.

The efficacy of angiotensin-converting enzyme (ACE) inhibitors in some cardiovascular and renal diseases has encouraged the development of other drugs to inhibit the renin-angiotensin system (RAS). The newest of these are the specific antagonists of angiotensin II (Ang II) receptors[1]; in the near future, vasopeptidase inhibitors—molecules that concomitantly inhibit both ACE and neutral endopeptidase (NEP)—should become available.

The current Ang II receptor antagonists interfere only with actions of Ang II mediated by type 1 (AT_1) receptors. The result is disinhibition of renin release and increased formation of all angiotensin peptides.[1,2] There is growing interest in the physiologic roles of these peptides,[1–8] the actions of which are unaffected by AT_1 antagonists and hence may have important pathophysiologic implications in hypertension and target organ damage.[1,3,4]

This chapter reviews the major actions of angiotensin and Ang II receptor blockers (mainly AT_1 blockers) and their interactions with other vasoactive factors, including nitric oxide (NO), endothelin (ET), and bradykinin (BK) (Fig. 1). We explore these interactions in regard to vascular endothelial function and tone as well as other renal and systemic organ interactions.

■ What Are the Vasoactive Factors?

The discovery of ACE inhibitors and, more recently, AT_1 blockers, paves the way for more knowledge about the interactions among the RAS, vascular biology, and organ damage in general as well as interactions with other factors affecting the vascular system—in particular, vasoactive factors. There appears to be a link between (1) end-organ damage and (2) hypertension, endothelial function, the NO–Ang II axis, and other vasoactive factors. Antihypertensive agents that can restore endothelial function in addition to exerting an antihypertensive effect may

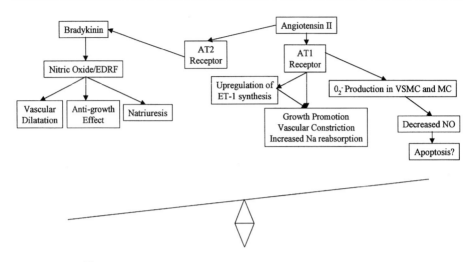

Figure 1. Angiotensin II interactions with other vasoactive factors.

be better in preventing or at least slowing end-organ damage.

Numerous molecules are implicated in the integrity, physiology, and pathophysiology of the vascular system, including Ang II, NO, ET, BK, endothelium-derived contracting factor (EDCF), aldosterone, atrial natriuretic peptide, arginine-vasopressin, prostaglandins (PGs), and thromboxane. We stress the notion, however, that the absolute concentration of these molecules does not condition their biologic effect. Instead, the balance among them is what matters in relationship to cardiovascular and renal physiology and pathophysiology. Their proper or improper presence, either in time or place, and their relative bioavailability make each of these molecules either injurious or protective of the target organs.[5–7]

■ Interactions with Nitric Oxide

NO—previously known as endothelium-derived relaxing factor—is synthesized by a family of enzymes known as nitric oxide synthases (NOSs).[8,9] This family consists of two main groups:[10–12]

1. Constitutive NOS (cNOS) includes two isoforms: the brain isoform (bNOS or NOS I), which is present in the brain and peripheral neural tissue, and the endothelial (vascular) isoform (eNOS or NOS III). Both are calcium- and calmodulin-dependent. Neurohumoral substances, such as acetylcholine, substance P, BK, and adenosine diphosphate (ADP), can activate the endothelial constitutive isoforms. Mechanical stimuli or physical forces (e.g., shear stress) and cyclic strain also can activate eNOSs as well as upregulate their synthesis. These two physical forces, under physiologic conditions such as exercise, upregulate eNOSs and contribute to vasodilation and increased blood flow to the organs in need.[8,9,11,13]

2. The inducible NOS isoform (iNOS or NOS II) can be induced in macrophages, neutrophils, Kupffer cells, hepatocytes, and renal mesangial and tubular cells by different factors, including tumor necrosis factor (TNF), PGs, other cytokines, and bacterial products. It is not normally expressed constitutively, and it is calcium-independent. It is implicated mainly in conditions of inflammation,

immunologic injury, sepsis, and shock.

The localization of these different NOS isoforms in different organs, including the heart, vessels, and kidneys, affects not only the role of NO in these organs but also its interaction with the RAS and other vasoactive factors.[12,14,15] Once released, NO is rapidly inactivated either by superoxide anions (O_2^-) or by binding to hemoglobin.[15] Under normal conditions NO has a short half-life of around 7 seconds. Under pathologic conditions increased levels of O_2^- may dramatically shorten the bioactivity of NO and/or transform it into a toxic metabolite.[10,16]

The actions of NO can be inhibited by NOS inhibitors, whereas the actions of Ang II can be inhibited by AT$_1$ receptor antagonists, which block its binding to receptors that enable it to exert its action, as well as by ACE inhibitors, which inhibit the conversion of Ang I to Ang II.[17,18]

General Principles of the Interactions of Nitric Oxide with Angiotensin II and AT Blockers

The loss of NO and, more importantly, the imbalance among Ang II, NO, and superoxide anion production, may contribute to the development and/or maintenance of both hypertension and abnormal vascular remodeling,[19–21] as seen in atherosclerosis and after myocardial injury.[20,21]

Renin is the key rate-limiting enzyme, secreted predominantly by the juxtaglomerular cells in the kidney, that converts angiotensinogen to angiotensin I. It is both stimulated and inhibited by NO in a complex, variable fashion. Renin production stimulated by NO is counteracted by Ang II. Other investigators have shown that under certain conditions NO inhibits renin secretion.[22–25]

The endothelium is a site of the final step in the synthesis of both Ang II and NO; hence, it is also a major site for their interactions. The endothelial cells contain ACE, which converts Ang I to Ang II. NO downregulates the synthesis of ACE in the endothelium and thus can affect Ang II production.[26]

The two main G-protein–coupled transmembrane[27] subtypes of AT receptors, designated AT$_1$ and AT$_2$,[17,28] are discussed in detail in chapter 3. The AT$_1$ subtype mediates the vasoconstrictor effect of Ang II and also the Ang II-induced growth in cardiovascular and renal tissue.[1] NO can downregulate AT$_1$ receptors in vascular tissue[29] and the adrenal gland[30] and thus mitigate the actions of Ang II. On the other hand, the actions of AT$_2$ receptors are less understood. These receptors are expressed in greater abundance in fetal tissues; their expression declines after birth. However, AT$_2$ receptors may be upregulated in adult animals in response to injury. They have been associated with the synthesis and/or release of both PGs and NO.[31–33]

Endothelial Dysfunction

The endothelial response to hypertension is to organize a complex local milieu that includes upregulation of NO and inhibition of the effects of Ang II. Through this endothelial function end-organs may be spared from the effects of hypertension.[10,16,34–36] Impairment of endothelium-dependent relaxation mediated by NO occurs in people with essential hypertension.[37,38] At times it even precedes hypertension, as observed in some normotensive blacks[39] and normotensive offspring of hypertensive parents.[40]

The endothelium and vascular smooth muscle cells produce superoxide anion in response to various stimuli, including oxidized lipoproteins, hyperglycemia,[41] ischemia,[42] and Ang II. Ang II activates nicotinamide adeninine dinucleotide (NAD) and reduced NAD phosphate oxidase in vascular smooth muscle[43] and mesangial cells,[44,45] leading to the synthesis of O_2^-. The O_2^- diffuses extracellularly and inactivates NO, whereas intracellularly, through activation of mitogen-activated protein (MAP) kinase, O_2^- drives responses related to cell growth.[14,46,47] On the other hand, NO was reported to quench superoxide radicals.[10,48,49] Besides NO and superoxide anions, many other endothelium-derived factors have been identified, including ET-1, thromboxane, and EDGF.

Mounting evidence suggests that the effects of NO are modulated by concomitant changes in the synthesis or release of other vasoactive agents, including ET-1 and Ang II.[12,16,50] The interaction between NO and ET-1 appears to be more important under pathologic than under physiologic conditions,[51,52] because ET-1 synthesis is upregulated by Ang II, and downregulated by NO.[53,54]

Vascular Tone

NO and Ang II have numerous effects on the regulation of vascular tone; these effects vary by organ system. This section concentrates on the systemic and renovascular effects of NO and Ang II.

Ang II is a potent constrictor of systemic vasculature, whereas NO contributes to the maintenance of resting vascular tone and to the tonic maintenance of normal blood pressure. Numerous studies have demonstrated that chronic administration of an NOS inhibitor leads to a dose-dependent, progressive increase in blood pressure.[51,55,56] Acute rescue with Ang II receptor antagonists in the chronic NOS inhibitor model have yielded inconclusive results. Some studies have demonstrated large reductions in blood pressure with AT_1 receptor antagonists,[57] whereas others have demonstrated little effect of Ang II receptor antagonists on blood pressure.[58] These conflicting results lead to the possibility that other vasoactive substances have a role in the maintenance of hypertension. In fact, acute inhibition of both the RAS and alpha-adrenergic receptors leads to almost complete reversal of chronic hypertension induced by ^{N}G-nitro-L-arginine methyl ester (L-NAME).[59] Chronic administration of an Ang II receptor antagonist in L-NAME–induced hypertension reverses the hypertension and prevents renal injury and cardiac hypertrophy.[60,61] Taken together, these studies suggest that Ang II may play a causative role in the initiation of hypertension linked to NO deficiency and a permissive role once hypertension has been established.

Other models have been used to corroborate the above findings. Angiotensinogen-knockout mice show a threefold increase in NO activity in the macula densa as well as chronic hypotension. Similarly AT_{1A}-knockout mice also exhibit chronic hypotension, renin overproduction, and an increase in NO activity (although to a lesser degree than angiotensinogen-knockout mice).[62] This finding also demonstrates the permissive effect of Ang II on hypertension.

The role of Ang II in hypertension and increased blood pressure can occur without an increase in renal concentrations of Ang II.[63] Most studies[64–66] demonstrate that inhibitors of NOS reduce renal secretion of renin. However, other in vitro observations[67,68] and experiments in isolated perfused kidneys[69] suggest that NO may stimulate the synthesis and/or secretion of renin. Along with a variable effect on renal secretion of renin, NOS inhibition also appears to have a varying effect on plasma renin activity (PRA). PRA has been reported to increase,[60] decrease,[61] or remain unchanged.[70] Taken as a whole, these studies suggest a balance between Ang II and NO. An increase or decrease in the concentration of either molecule is equivalent to a functional increase or decrease in the other. The sum effect of this balance contributes to changes in vascular tone.

A similar interaction occurs between Ang II and NO in the renal vasculature. Inhibition of NO decreases renal blood flow and glomerular filtration rate (GFR) but increases filtration fraction.[71] Micropuncture studies demonstrate that NOS inhibition causes afferent, but not efferent, arteriolar vasoconstriction[72] and a decrease in single-nephron GFR.[73] The renal effects of NOS inhibitors are similar to those produced by intrarenal infusion of Ang II. Specifically, Ang II infusion results in renal vasoconstriction with a decrease in GFR and an increased filtration fraction.[74,75] Prior blockade of Ang II with losartan eliminates the afferent arteriolar vasoconstriction and decrease in GFR caused by NOS inhibition.[76] Alternatively, losartan by itself has been shown to increase renal plasma flow and GFR in spontaneously hypertensive rats (SHRs). This effect is reduced by pretreatment with L-NAME.[77] These results demonstrate that NO buffers the constrictor action of Ang II in the renal vasculature.

Growth Promotion and End-organ Damage

In addition to its effect on vascular tone, Ang II is a potent inducer of growth (hypertrophy and/or hyperplasia).[78-80] In vivo studies demonstrate that Ang II induces cell hypertrophy in many preparations, including mesangial cells,[81] proximal tubules,[82] cardiomyocytes, and fibroblasts.[83] These stimulatory effects are reduced by AT$_1$ receptor blockade[84] and by NO,[14] again suggesting a counterregulatory function between NO and Ang II. In fact, NO is an endogenous inhibitor of hypertrophy and hyperplasia of mesangial cells[14] and growth of vascular smooth muscle cells.[53] Thus, the in vivo effect of Ang II is to promote growth, which can be retarded by administration of an AT$_1$ receptor blocker and/or NO.

The effect of Ang II on growth has been demonstrated not only in vitro, but also in numerous in vivo models. Continuous Ang II infusion in rats enhanced vascular smooth muscle cell proliferation in normal and injured arterial walls.[85] This proliferation can be blunted by the administration of an Ang II receptor blocker after injury.[86] The proliferative effect of Ang II also has been demonstrated with other models. Rats with the ACE gene transfected into the carotid artery show a local increase in ACE activity. The local increase in Ang II concentrations results in medial layer hypertrophy and an increase in wall-lumen ratio of the transfected carotid artery. These changes occur without a change in systemic blood pressure.[87] Such results confirm the role of Ang II in modulating growth. Hence rats respond similarly to administration of Ang II and inhibition of NO synthesis.

Hypertensive Dahl salt-sensitive rats on 4% salt diets have four times less NO activity in the renal medulla than SHRs, despite similar levels of hypertension.[34] Associated with this decrease in NO activity are increases in proteinuria, tubulointerstitial injury, glomerular sclerosis, and left ventricular mass. These effects can be normalized with addition of an AT$_1$ receptor blocker or an ACE inhibitor.[87a] Moreover, long-term blockade of NOS with L-NAME in rats causes systemic arterial hypertension associated with microvascular structural changes, including medial thickening, perivascular fibrosis, and myocardial hypertrophy. Such changes are prevented by concomitant administration of an AT_1 receptor blocker.[16,88] These studies once again demonstrate the contrasting effect of NO and Ang II.

Sodium Balance and Excretion

The RAS is a paracrine as well as an endocrine system. Current evidence suggests that the entire RAS exists in the kidney and numerous other tissues.[27,89,90] The presence of the RAS in the kidney—in addition to its systemic distribution—may play a crucial role in renal handling of sodium and water.[5,25,91–94] Ang II regulates blood pressure by controlling sodium reabsorption in the proximal tubule, altering GFR and renal blood flow, and modifying the production and release of aldosterone in the adrenal gland.[5,25,27,91–95]

Most of the effects of Ang II in the kidney, however, are not seen in sodium-repleted people. Ang II appears to work not only at the basolateral membrane of the proximal convoluted tubule (PCT), but also at the luminal membrane brush border, where the AT_1 receptor increases sodium transport.[27,96] Stimulation of AT_1 receptors causes an increase in tubular sodium, water, and bicarbonate reabsorption and a decrease in glomerular/medullary blood flow. In addition, AT_1 receptor stimulation in the glomerulus increases GFR.[97] In the juxtaglomerular apparatus, AT_1 receptor stimulation leads to a decrease in renin formation and renin release by a short feedback-loop mechanism.[96]

Ang II stimulation of the AT_1 receptor reduces the filtration coefficient by directly affecting the contractility of the mesangial cells. On the other hand, because of its greater constricting effect on efferent than afferent renal arterioles, Ang II leads to a higher filtration fraction. Via AT_1 receptors, Ang II enhances the sensitivity of the vascular elements of the nephron that mediate tubuloglomerular feedback.[27,98]

It also has been reported that intrarenal blockade of Ang II receptors, under conditions in which decreases in arterial pressure are minimal, causes substantial increases in renal blood flow and GFR as well as several-fold increases in total and fractional sodium excretion in normotensive as well hypertensive rats. This substantial increase in sodium excretion may be caused not only by hemodynamic effects but also by the effects of blocking intraluminal Ang II receptors.[99–101] Cervenka et al. have shown similar effects by administration of candesartan into the renal artery of the nonclipped kidney in the two-kidney, one-clipped (2K1C) rat model. Significant increases in GFR, renal blood flow, sodium excretion, and fractional sodium excretion suggest synergistic actions on tubular transport and vascular smooth muscle cells.[99,102]

These effects vary in humans according to which AT_1 receptor blocker is used. In one study, the use of losartan (50 mg once daily) in patients with essential hypertension did not cause renal vasodilation effect, whereas irbesartan (100 mg once daily) and candesartan (8 mg once daily) produced an increase in renal plasma flow, no change in GFR, and a decrease in filtration fraction. In hypertensive patients with renal impairment, candesartan (8 mg once daily for 5 days) produced a renal dilatory effect and a decrease in filtration fraction similar to that observed with enalapril or losartan. This finding may predict a favorable effect on the evolution of renal function in patients with chronic renal failure.[103] Candesartan has the combined effect of increasing sodium excretion and reducing Ang II-dependent vascular tone.[27,104]

It also was found that during dietary sodium restriction the PCT angiotensin protein, its mRNA, and renin are increased, suggesting local regulation of RAS activity in the kidney. In addition, expression of AT_2 receptors was increased in the glomeruli and interstitial cells.[1,27,105,106]

Ang II increases the release of aldosterone. On the other hand, AT_1 receptor blockers reduce the secretion of aldosterone by the adrenal cortex, an effect that undoubtedly contributes to their antihypertensive action.[107] This inhibition is not complete; some secretion of aldosterone persists. Residual aldosterone secretion may explain why severe hyperkalemia has not been reported in clinical trials of AT_1 receptor blockers. However, such results should not be interpreted to mean that treatment with AT_1 receptor blockers involves no risk of hyperkalemia.[1]

AT_2 receptors have been shown to increase renal production of NO, which can affect renal hemodynamics. AT_2 receptors also affect renal hemodynamics by dilating the afferent arteriole.[27,108,109]

NO may participate in salt excretion, either directly (by decreasing tubular sodium reabsorption) or indirectly (through modulation of the renal medullary blood flow).[45,73–75,110,111]

Salt-sensitive hypertension may be linked to a decrease in renal production of NO, inappropriate activation of the RAS, or both. However, a causal relationship between salt sensitivity and NO deficiency has not been clearly identified.[112,113] Haykawa and Raij[34,87b,114] have shown impaired NOS activity in salt-sensitive experimental models of hypertension; however, the decrease in NOS activity occurs after the development of hypertension—not before.

In hypertensive humans, independent of the effects of salt on blood pressure, salt sensitivity may be a marker for the susceptibility to develop endothelial dysfunction as well as cardiovascular and renal vascular injury.[10,112,113,116] Of interest, both aging and diabetes are characterized by increased prevalence of hypertension, salt sensitivity, and decreased endothelium-dependent relaxation mediated by NO.[117,118]

Moreover, differences in end-organ susceptibility to hypertensive injury may be linked to a genetic, familial, environmental, or acquired inability to upregulate eNOS in response to hypertension. The absolute risk of developing end-organ damage at the same level of blood pressure varies substantially in different parts of the world.[119]

■ *Interactions with Endothelin*

The identification of ET-1 by Yanagisawa et al. in 1988[120] added an important player to the arena of potential causes of arterial hypertension and related cardiovascular and target-organ disease. Over the years, it has been increasingly appreciated that any newly discovered agent cannot be investigated singularly but should be assessed in the context of all other known mechanisms.[121] The RAS and the endothelin system entail the most potent vasopressor mechanism identified to date.[122–124] They have been investigated extensively in relation to arterial hypertension and related cardiovascular disease.[121]

ET-1, which consists of 21 amino acids,[120] is considered the most potent endogenous vasoconstrictor peptide and an obvious candidate for contributing to the development of hypertension and cardiovascular disease. Since ET-1 was identified in 1988,[125] a steadily increasing body of impressive data supports its likely role in the regulation of vascular tone and in the pathophysiology of several conditions associated with vasoconstriction, including hypertension, Raynaud's disease, renal failure, and congestive heart failure.[126] In addition to its direct vasoconstrictor properties, ET exerts long-term effects on vascular smooth muscle cell proliferation and phenotype.[127]

ET is synthesized as a large preprohormone (big ET-1), which is cleaved to pro-ET and then undergoes further modification by one of several endothelin-converting enzymes (ECEs) to yield mature ET. Three isoforms have been cloned and sequenced: ET-1, ET-2, and ET-3. ET-1, the predominant isoform synthesized in human vasculature, is the most potent. ET-2 is not found in human plasma but is present in the kidney and intestine, where it has vasoconstrictor properties similar to ET-1. ET-3 has minimal vasoconstrictor properties; its major source is unclear. Endothelins are rapidly cleared from the circulation by the lung, liver, and kidneys.[125]

ET can bind to two receptors: ET_A, which is found in vascular smooth muscle cells and mediates vasoconstriction, and ET_B, which is found predominately in endothelial cells and mediates vasodilation through the release of NO and prostacyclin.[125,128,129] In one study of healthy subjects, selective antagonism of ET_A caused vasodilation associated with an increase in NO generation. Inhibition of NO synthesis or antagonism of ET_B receptors attenuated this response.[130,131]

The effects of ET are potentially relevant in several pathologic conditions, even more so than under normal circumstances. These conditions occur when endothelial damage, hypertension, and hyperaldosteronism coexist; examples include congestive heart failure, malignant and severe hypertension, and endotoxemia.[121]

Potential Sites of Interactions

Several potential sites of interactions between the RAS and ET system, spanning from the molecular level to in vivo hormonal and hemodynamic regulation, can be speculated. Ang II affects the synthesis of ET-1, which in turn can influence the RAS. An important site of interactions is at the level of ET-1 biosynthesis. Although the predominant ET biosynthetic pathway involves the specific cleavage of big ET-1 by ECE-1, it is possible that big ETs also are cleaved by human chymase, an enzyme responsible for conversion of Ang I to Ang II in the myocardium.[132,133] It was shown that rat chymase cleaves big-ETs at the Try^{31}-Gly^{32} bond,[134] leading to novel 1-31 endothelin isopeptides [ETs (1-31)]. These ETs (1-31) were shown in vitro to exert a less potent and more slowly developing but longer-lasting contraction than ETs (1-21) in porcine coronary artery and rat aorta. The vasoconstrictive effect of ETs (1-31) also was found to be inhibited by either the ET_A antagonist BQ-485 or the ET_B antagonist BQ-788. This finding suggests that ET (1-31) isopeptides may act in a different manner from endothelins, possibly through different receptors.[135]

Effects of Angiotensin II on the Endothelin System

The identification of consensus sequences for *jun* in the regulatory region of the preproendothelin-1 (ppET-1) and ECE-1 genes raised the possibility of its transcriptional regulation by Ang II through AT_1 receptors via protein kinase C (PKC)-mediated mechanisms. This was confirmed by the finding that stimulation with Ang II of cultured vascular smooth muscle cells[136-138] and endothelial cells[139,140] induced expression of the ppET-1 gene and synthesis of ET-1.[138,139,141,142] However, the possibility of complex cross-talk between several other signaling pathways that can be activated by a number of humoral factors, such as insulin, catecholamines, components of the clotting / fibrinolysis cascade, and cytokines, also should be considered.[121]

It also was found that Ang II mediates the elevated plasma concentration of ET in congestive heart failure.[143] If this process occurs in humans, part of the beneficial actions of ACE inhibitors in patients with congestive heart failure may be diminished release of ET.

Effects of Endothelin on the Renin-Angiotensin System

Endogenously produced ET-1 was found to contribute to the hypertrophic response of cardiomyocytes to Ang II and ET-3 and thereby to cardiac hypertrophy.[141] Furthermore, ET-1 exerts multifaceted effects on the RAS, such as dose-dependent inhibition of renin synthesis and stimulation of aldosterone secretion. The finding of abundant specific ET-1 receptors in the adrenocortical zona glomerulosa suggests a direct secretagogue effect of ET-1.[144,145]

Studies of the in vivo interactions between ETs and the RAS have given conflicting results. Some suggest the participation of ET-1 in the pressor and cellular effects of exogenously administered Ang II, whereas others (in transgenic TGR [Ren2m]27 and 2K1C rats) do not.[121]

Besides its potent hemodynamic effects, the intravenous infusion of ET-1 in animals and humans deeply affects the RAS. Renin secretion from juxtaglomerular cells generally was decreased by ET-1 both in vitro and in vivo. ET-1 exerts its inhibitory effect on renin through both direct and indirect mechanisms, including increases in aldosterone, plasma volume, calcium, NO, protaglandin I_2, and cyclic adenosine monophosphate as well as possible effects through phospholipase C and PKC.[146-149]

Despite its inhibitory effect on renin, ET-1 markedly stimulates aldosterone secretion in both animals and humans. This finding suggests a direct effect on the adrenal cortex.[144] The ET_B receptor subtype mediates the direct secretagogue effect of ET-1 on aldosterone in animals,[150-152] but both ET_A and ET_B receptors are involved in the transcriptional regulation of the aldosterone synthase gene in humans.[153,154] ET-1 was found to be equipotent to Ang II,[155] the most important physiologic secretagogue of aldosterone.

Pretreatment with bosentan (a mixed ET_A-ET_B antagonist) blunted the increase in blood pressure as well as the decrease in cardiac output and arterial conductance evoked by an infusion of Ang II in Wistar-Kyoto (WKY) rats and SHRs, although the effects are more pronounced in SHRs.[156] This blunting effect was more evident at lower (2–10 ng/kg/min) than higher (> 30 ng/kg/min) doses of Ang II, thereby suggesting the possibility of an ET-1 component only in the initial pressor effect of Ang II.[121]

ET-1 may play a role not only in the hemodynamic effects of Ang II but also in the mechanisms of related cardiovascular damage. This theory is supported by the finding that bosentan entirely prevented the development of hypertension, the reduction in renal blood flow, and the marked increase in albuminuria and heart weight induced by 10-day infusion of Ang II (200 ng/kg/min).[157] Also bosentan was found to have an additive hypotensive effect to that of losartan (an AT_1 receptor blocker) in both the Page canine model (kidney wrapping) of hypertension and rats with renin-dependent hypertension.[158,159]

Endothelin in Hypertension

Animal studies suggest that ET plays a role in certain models of hypertension.[160-162] In addition, ET-1 may mediate the cardiovascular and renal effects of Ang II, as discussed later.[157]

On the other hand, plasma ET levels are usually normal in hypertensive patients.[160,163] However, sensitivity to ET may be increased in patients with essential hypertension.[120] Other studies showed an increase in the circulating levels of ET in patients with symptomatic heart failure, suggesting that it may contribute to the progression of left ventricular dysfunction.[126,164,165]

An increased ET-1 mRNA content has been found in the kidney of male HanRen2/Edinburg rats, derived from crossing the homozygote transgenic TGR (mREN-2)27 with Edinburgh Sprague-Dawley rats. HanRen2/Edinburg rats also show a 73.5% incidence of the malignant phase of hypertension.[166] Nonetheless, bosentan was found to have no effect on blood pressure.[167]

The ET-1 dependency of hypertension differs according to the different models of hypertension. It is most pronounced in 1K1C Goldblatt rats and rats with deoxycorticosterone acetate (DOCA)- and salt-induced hypertension; it is least pronounced in transgenic Ren2 and HanRen2/Edinburg rats. The Ang II infusion and chronic L-NAME–induced models of hypertension are in the middle of the spectrum. This finding may suggest a more reciprocal effect of Ang II and NO on ET-1.[121,168-171]

The reasons that ET-1 may take part in hypertension induced by exogenously administered Ang II but not in models with an enhanced endogenous production of Ang II are still unclear. They may depend on the different tissue levels attained by Ang II and/or the different gradient between the blood stream, endothelium, and vascular smooth muscle cells of the blood vessels (tunica media) in the two types of models. In fact, it is well documented that in heterozygote TGR(mREN-2)27 rats, a high tissue expression of Ang II is accompanied by a low plasma level of Ang II, whereas in models of exogenous administration, Ang II concentrations are likely to be higher in plasma and lower in tissues.[121]

In contrast with the controversial data about the involvement of ET-1 in renin-dependent forms of hypertension, data about the role of ET-1 in mineralocorticoid-dependent forms of hypertension are fairly concordant.[160] Increased levels of immunoreactive ET-1 were found in the plasma and arterial wall of rats with DOCA-salt–induced hypertension.[172-174] In the same model Day et al.[175] showed enhanced expression of the ppET-1 gene in the vessel wall. In addition, treatment with bosentan was effective in preventing vascular hypertrophy. This finding may support the contention of a direct involvement of ET-1 in target-organ damage in this model of low-renin hypertension.[121,176]

The contention that ET-1 plays a role in salt-dependent hypertension is supported by the work of Haykawa and Raij,[115] who showed upregulation of ET in

Dahl salt-sensitive rats, and by Barton et al.,[177] who reported that the ET$_A$-specific antagonist LU135252 partially prevented the development of hypertension and the structural and functional alterations caused by chronic salt administration in DS rats. In addition, a role for ET-1 in cardiovascular damage of salt-sensitive hypertension is suggested by data in humans.[178]

The applicability of these findings to hypertension in humans is uncertain, but an increasing number of studies suggest that ET antagonists will be useful clinically.[179] Regardless of the initial ET-1 dependency of hypertension, the pathogenic role of the ET system is deemed to become more important as endothelial and target-organ damage supervenes.[121]

In contrast, ET-1 transgenic mice develop glomerulosclerosis, interstitial fibrosis, and renal cysts—but not hypertension. This finding may suggest a new blood pressure-independent animal model of ET-induced renal pathology. In another transgenic model elevation of ET-2 expression did not induce hypertension but led to changes at the end-organ level. Normotension is thought to be due to compensatory mechanisms, such as increased NO formation.[180,181]

Endothelin Mediation of the Actions of Angiotensin II

Considerable evidence indicates that ET-1 may mediate the cardiovascular and renal effects of Ang II.[157] In 1997, several studies suggested that ET-1 may play an important role in the structural changes induced by Ang II infusion. Two weeks of Ang II infusion (200 ng/kg min) increased media thickness, the media-lumen ratio, and the cross-sectional area of mesenteric and cerebral arterioles and nearly doubled the content of ET-1 in mesenteric tissue. The underlying mechanism most likely involves the ET$_A$ receptor, because the ET$_A$-specific antagonist LU135252 prevented development of medial hypertrophy and increased peptide content in both types of vessels.[161] A similar dose of Ang II infusion led to enhanced vascular ECE activity and renal ET-1 content in WKY rats[182]; in addition, LU135252 lowered the Ang II-induced increase in blood pressure and improved endothelium-dependent relaxation.[183]

Effects of Endothelin Blockers on the Renin-Angiotensin System

As discussed above, ET-1 antagonism may offer an additional weapon for therapeutic interventions aimed at preventing progression of cardiovascular damage. Long-term treatment with ET antagonists greatly improved the survival of rats with chronic heart failure and also prevented ventricular remodeling. ET antagonists also ameliorate the increase in left ventricular mass and cavity enlargement[184] as well as the increase in collagen density.[185]

Administration of the ET$_A$-selective antagonist PD 155080 abolished the rise in blood pressure induced by Ang II infusion, as did the AT$_1$ receptor blocker, losartan.[186] In another study an ET receptor antagonist prevented the increase in systemic blood pressure and the reduction in renal blood flow induced by Ang II infusion.[157]

A recent randomized trial included 293 patients with essential hypertension who were treated with bosentan, enalapril, or placebo.[187] Bosentan and enalapril produced equivalent reductions in blood pressure. The fall in blood pressure with bosentan was achieved without reflex activation of the sympathetic nervous system or the RAS.

Therapeutic Implications of Combined Blockade of the Renin-Angiotensin and Endothelin Systems

The interactions between the RAS and ET systems at multiple levels in the pathogenesis and pathophysiology of hypertension and related cardiovascular and other end-organ damage suggest the potential usefulness of a therapeutic strategy targeted at both systems.[121]

Hypertension

The potential synergistic effects of combined inhibition on mean arterial pressure (MAP) have been investigated in SHRs. Inhibition of the ET-1 system by maximally effective doses of either Ro 61-1790 (ET_A-selective receptor antagonist) or phosphoramidon (a mixed NEP24.11/ECE inhibitor) similarly decreased MAP by about –30 mmHg. The effect of the two agents was equipotent to maximal ACE inhibition. Of greater interest, the combination of phosphoramidon and cilazapril or phosphoramidon and Ro 61-1790 enhanced the maximal decrease in MAP by 100% (–60 mmHg) and thus almost normalized blood pressure in SHRs.[121]

Congestive Heart Failure

Chronic administration of an ET receptor antagonist in experimental congestive heart failure improves left ventricular function, prevents remodeling, and leads to an approximate doubling of survival.[184]

Synergism between blocking of the two systems also was found in patients with class III New York Heart Association (NYHA) congestive heart failure, who were hemodynamically stable on ACE inhibitors and diuretics. The addition of the mixed ET_A/ET_B receptor antagonist bosentan elicited a clear-cut decrease in systemic and pulmonary vascular resistance along with an increase in cardiac index.[188] Furthermore, the use of ACE inhibitors and ET receptor antagonists in patients with congestive heart failure already receiving an ACE inhibitor increased forearm blood flow by 30–50% as a result of decreased vascular resistance.[189]

Experimental research has begun to unravel the interactions between the RAS and ET system. Pilot clinical trials gave promising results.[179] But whether they are clinically relevant in humans and have therapeutic implications is still unanswered.

■ *Interactions with Bradykinin*

BK is liberated from its substrate, kininogen, by the action of kallikrein.[190] It causes vasodilatation through NO synthase and increased synthesis of vasodilatory prostaglandins.[191,192] The effects of BK and other kinins are mediated through their binding of specific receptors. Both receptors for BK have been cloned. The BK_1 receptor is expressed mainly under pathologic conditions and is thought to mediate inflammation. Whereas the BK_1 receptor is responsible for inflammation, the BK_2 receptors are responsible for most of the cardiovascular and renal effects of kinins.[193,194] BK stimulation of the BK_2 receptor in the vasculature has been shown to stimulate production of NO.[53] In addition, intravenous and intraarterial administration of BK produces a dose-dependent dilatation of arterial and venous vessels.[195] These vascular effects are attenuated by the inhibition of NO synthesis or by antagonism of the BK_2 receptor.[195] Stimulation of the BK receptor has been shown to cause vasodilatation and NO production, whereas chronic blockade of BK_2 receptors with icatibant increases blood pressure in rats, provided that administration of the antagonist is combined with nonpressor doses of Ang II.[196]

New insights into the role of the bradykinin system can be obtained from recent studies using a mouse strain with a targeted disruption of the BK_2 receptor gene. Mice lacking a functional BK_2 receptor have higher blood pressure and heavier hearts than wild-type mice. They also have an exaggerated pressor response to Ang II and chronic salt supplementation.[197] Chronic administration of an AT_1 receptor blocker reduced blood pressure in mice without a functional BK_2 receptor to levels similar to those of wild-type mice. In addition, administration of a BK_2 receptor antagonist or L-NAME increased the blood pressure of wild-type mice to the level in the mice with a functional BK_2 receptor.[197] Taken together, these results suggest that BK plays an important protective role in the vascular endothelium that is mediated through the BK_2 receptor and stimulation of NO.

In addition to the clear link between BK and NO, there also appears to be an interaction between Ang II and BK through the AT_2 receptor. The AT_2 receptor is abundant in fetal tissue; in adults it has been described in the adrenal gland, brain, uterine myometrium, and atretic ovarian follicles.[198] However, after vascular injury the AT_2 receptor is reexpressed, constituting 10% of all Ang II receptor mRNA.[199] Several studies have demonstrated an antigrowth role of the AT_2 receptor in the cardiovascular system. In myopathic hamsters, stimulation of the AT_2 receptor inhibits the progression of interstitial fibrosis in myopathic lesions.[200] AT_2 receptor stimulation also prevents Ang II-induced growth of cultured neonatal rat myocytes.[201]

The protective effect of the AT_2 receptor probably is mediated through stimulation of NO and BK. AT_2 receptor-mediated activation of the kinin/NO system has been demonstrated in numerous models.[202] Binding of Ang II to the AT_2 receptor increased the release of BK and, subsequently, aortic cyclic guanosine monophosphate (cGMP), a marker or NO production.[203] Liu et al.[204] reported that in rats with heart failure administration of an Ang II receptor blocker improved left ventricular remodeling and cardiac function. This benefit was abolished by concomitant administration of an AT_2 receptor blocker. The benefit observed with the Ang II receptor blocker also was partially blocked by concomitant administration of a BK antagonist. Finally, concentrations of both BK and cGMP in normal mice were shown to increase in response to Ang II infusion; this increase was not demonstrated in mice lacking the AT_2 receptor.[205] These studies suggest that the effect of AT_2 stimulation is suppression of growth and that this effect is mediated through stimulation of both BK and NO.

■ *Interactions with Other Vasoactive Factors*

Ang II and AT receptor blockers also interact with other vasoactive factors, including aldosterone, atrial natriuretic peptide, EDCFs (e.g., thromboxane 2, prostaglandin H_2), arginine-vasopressin, and others. The discussion of these interactions is beyond the scope of this chapter.

■ *Conclusions*

- Vascular biology and hemodynamics constitute milestones in understanding the pathophysiologic mechanism of hypertension and target-organ damage.
- The functional balance of bioavailability among vasoactive factors, both constrictive and relaxing, rather than their absolute concentrations conditions the response to different stimuli.
- These vasoactive factors, including angiotensin II, nitric oxide, endothelin, prostaglandins, and bradykinin, have an enormous network of interactions among themselves and in relation to vascular integrity that govern their cumulative effects and determine whether they are protective or injurious to the body.
- These interactions are not constant; they differ according to circumstances and different pathologic conditions.
- Angiotensin receptor type 1 blockers have proved their efficacy as antihypertensives and, to a certain extent, as target-organ protective agents.
- Endothelin antagonists have emerged as possible synergistic agents in the treatment of hypertension and end-organ disease, at least in experiments. More clinical trials are needed to verify their actual benefits in humans.
- The role of angiotensin receptors type 2 and their stimulation and inhibition and the role of the nitric oxide-arginine pathway and its substrates and inhibitors as possible agents in the clinical treatment of hypertension and target-organ damage remain to be established.
- At present it is not known whether vasopeptidase inhibitors—molecules that concomitantly inhibit both angiotensin-converting enzyme and neutral endopeptidase—will add a new and/or different dimension to the treatment of hypertension and cardiovascular diseases.

Acknowledgments

This study was supported with research funds from the Department of Veterans Affairs. We thank Ms. Barb Devereaux for secretarial support.

References

1. Goodfriend T, Elliott M, Catt K: Angiotensin receptors and their antagonists. N Engl J Med 334:1649–1654, 1999.
2. Goldberg M, Bradstreet T, McWilliams E: Biochemical effects of losartan, a nonpeptide angiotensin II receptor antagonist, on the renin-angiotensin-aldosterone system in hypertensive patients. Hypertension 25:37–46, 1995.
3. Jaiswal N, Tallant E, Jaiswal R, et al: Differential regulation of prostaglandin synthesis by angiotensin peptides in porcine aortic smooth muscle cell: Subtypes of angiotensin receptors involved. J Pharmacol Exp Ther 265:644–673, 1993.
4. Wright J, Krebs L, Stobb J, Harding J: The angiotensin IV system functional implications. Front Neuroendocrinol 16:23–52, 1995.
5. Gabbai F: Introduction. Semin Nephrol 19:213–214, 1999.
6. Klahr S: Can L-arginine manipulation reduce renal disease. Semin Nephrol 19:304–309, 1999.
7. Klahr S, Morrissey J: Comparative study of ACE inhibitors and AII receptor antagonists in interstitial scarring. Kidney Int 52(Suppl 63):S111–S114, 1997.
8. Nathan C, Xie Q: Nitric oxide syntheses, roles, tolls and controls. Cell 78:915–918, 1994.
9. Pollock S, Forstermann U, Mitchell J: Purification and characterization of particulate endothelium-derived relaxing factor synthase from cultured and native bovine aortic endothelial cells. Proc Natl Acad Sci USA 88:10480–10484, 1991.
10. Bataineh A, Raij L: Angiotensin II, nitric oxide, and endorgan damage in hypertension. Kidney Int 54(Suppl 68):S14–S19, 1998.

11. Lamas S, Marsden P, Lie G: Endothelial nitric oxide synthase: Molecular cloning and characterization of a distinct constitiutive enzyme isoform. Proc Natl Acad Sci USA 89:6348–6453, 1992.
12. Raij L, Hayakawa H, Jaimes E: Cardiorenal injury and nitric oxide synthase activity in hypertension. J Hypertens 16(Suppl 8):S69–S73, 1998.
13. Vanhoutte P, Rubany G, Miller V, Houston D: Modulation of vascular smooth muscle contraction by the endothelium. Annu Rev Physiol 48:307–320, 1986.
14. Raij L, Baylis C: Glomerular actions of nitric oxide. Kidney Int 48:20–32, 1995.
15. Moncada S, Palmer R, Higgs E: Nitric oxide: Physiology, pathophysiology, and pharmacology. Pharmacol Rev 43:109–142, 1991.
16. Ishani A, Raij L: Hypertension, nitric oxide, and endorgan damage. Curr Opin Nephrol Hypertens 9:237–241, 1999.
17. Timmermans P, Wong P, Chiu A: Angiotensin II receptors and angiotensin II receptor antagonists. Pharmacol Rev 45:205–251, 1993.
18. Griendling K, Lassegue B, Alexander R: Angiotensin receptors and their therapeutic implications.:Annu Rev Pharmacol Toxicol 36:281–306, 1996.
19. Cayette A, Palcino J, Hortens K, Cohen R: Chronic inhibition of nitric oxide production accelerates neointima formation and impairs endothelial function in hypercholesterolemic rabbits. Arterioscler Thromb 14:753–759, 1994.
20. Hokimoto S, Yasue H, Fujimoto K: Expression of angiotensin-converting enzyme in remaining viable myocytes of human ventricles after myocardial infarction. Circulation 94:1513, 1996.
21. Potter D, Sobey C, Tompkins P, et al: Evidence that macrophages in atherosclerotic lesions contain angiotensin II. Circulation 98:800–807, 1998.
22. Gardes J, Poux J, Gonzalez M: Decreased renin release and constant kallikrein secretion after injection of L-NAME in isolated perfused rat kidney. Life Sci 50:987–993, 1992.
23. Kurtz A, Kaissling B, Busse R, Baier W: Endothelial cells modulate renin secretion from isolated mouse juxtaglomerular cells. J Clin Invest 88:1147–1154, 1991.
24. Sigmon D, Carretero O, Belierwaltes W: Endothelium-derived relaxing factor regulates renin release in-vivo. Am J Physiol 263:F256–261, 1992.
25. He X, Greenberg S, Schnermann J, Brigss J: Role of nitric oxide in regulation of macula densa mediated renin secretion. FASEB J 7:1267A, 1993.
26. Higashi Y, Oshima T, Ng O: Intravenous administration of L-arginine inhibits angiotensin converting enzyme in humans. J Clin Endocrinol Metab 80:198–202, 1995.
27. Zitnay C, Siragy H: Action of angiotensin receptor subtypes on the renal tubules and vasculature: Implications for volume homeostasis and atherosclerosis: Miner Electrolyte Metab 24:362–370, 1998.
28. Denton K, Fennessy P, Alcorn D, Anderson W: Morphometric analysis of the actions of angiotensin II on renal arterioles and glomeruli. Am J Physiol 262(3 Pt 2):F367–F372, 1992.
29. Ichiki T, Usui M, Kato M: Downregulation of angiotensin II type I receptor gene transcription by nitric oxide. Hypertension 31(Pt 2):342–348, 1998.
30. Usui M, Ichiki T, Katoh M: Regulation of angiotensin II receptor expression by nitric oxide in rat adrenal gland. Hypertension 32:527–533, 1998.
31. Tsutsumi K, Saavedra J: Characterization and development of angiotensin receptor subtypes (AT1 and AT2) in rat brain. Am J Physiol 261:R209–R216, 1991.
32. Grady E, Sechi L, Griffin C: Expression of AT2 receptors in the developing rat fetus. J Clin Invest 88:921–933, 1991.
33. Stoll M, Steckelings M, Paul M: The angiotensin AT2 receptor mediates inhibition of cell proliferation in coronary endothelial cells. J Clin Invest 95:651–657, 1995.
34. Hayakawa H, Raij L: The link among nitric oxide synthase activity, endothelial function, and aortic and ventricular hypertrophy in hypertension. Hypertension 29(Pt 2):235–241, 1997.
35. Hayakawa H, Coffee K, Raij L: Does vascular nitric oxide synthase activity mitigate end-organ injury in hypertension? Am J Hypertens 10:160A, 1997.
36. Awolesi M, Widmann M, Sessa W, Sumpio B: Cyclic strain increases endothelial nitric oxide synthase activity. Surgery 116:439–444, 1994.
37. Panza J, Quyyumi A, Brush J, Epstein S: Abnormal endothelial dependent relaxation in patients with essential hypertension. N Engl J Med 323:22–27, 1990.
38. Panz J, Casino P, Kelcyne C, Quyyumi A: Role of endothelium-derived nitric oxide in the abnormal endothelium dependent vascular relaxation in patients with essential hypertension. Circulation 87:1468–1474, 1993.
39. Cardillo C, Kilcoyne C, Cannon R, Panza J: Racial differences in nitric oxide-mediated vasodilator response to mental stress in forearm circulation. Hypertension 31:1235–1239, 1998.
40. Taddei S, Virdis A, Mattei P: Defective L-arginine nitric oxide pathway in offspring of essential hypertensive patients. Circulation 94:1298–1303, 1996.

41. Maziere C, Avclair M, Rose R: Glucose-enriched medium enhanced cell mediated low density lipoprotein peroxidation. FEBS Lett 363:277–279, 1995.
42. Crawford L, Milliken E, Irani K: Superoxide mediated actin response in post-hypoxic endothelial cells. J Biol Chem 43:26863–26867, 1996.
43. Griendling K, Minieri C, Ollerenshaw J, Alexander R: Angiotensin II stimulates NAD and NADPH oxidase activity in cultured vascular smooth muscle cells. Cir Res 74:1141–1148, 1994.
44. Galceran J, Jaimes E, Raij L: Pathogenetic role of angiotensin II in glomerular injury: Is superoxide O_2^- the missing link? J Am Soc Nephrol 7:1631A, 1996.
45. Jaimes E, Galceran J, Raij L: Angiotensin II induces superoxide anion production by mesangial cells. Kidney Int 54:775–784, 1998.
46. Rajagopalan S, kurz S, Munzel T: Angiotensin II mediated hypertension in the rat increases vascular superoxide production via membrane NADH/NADPH oxidase activation. J Clin Invest 97:1916–1923, 1996.
47. Gryglewski R, Palmer R, Moncada S: Superoxide anion involved in the breakdown of endothelium-derived vascular relaxing factor. Nature 320:454–456, 1986.
48. Schnackenberg C, Wilkins F, Granger J: Role of nitric oxide in modulating the vasoconstrictor actions of angiotensin II in preglomerular and postglomerular vessels in dogs. Hypertension 26(6 Pt 2):1024–1029, 1995.
49. Lefer A: Vasculoprotective actions of nitric oxide. In Weissman B (ed): Biochemical, Pharmacological and Clinical Aspects of Nitric Oxide. New York, Plenum Press, 1995, pp 167–173.
50. King A, Brenner B, Anderson S: Endothelin: A potent renal and systemic vasoconstrictor peptide. Am J Physiol 256:1051–1058, 1989.
51. Baylis C, Mitruka B, Deng A: Chronic blockade of nitric oxide synthesis in the rat produces systemic hypertension and glomerular damage. J Clin Invest 90:278–281, 1992.
52. Peiro C, Redondo J, Rodriguez-Martinez M: Influence of endothelium on cultured vascular smooth muscle cell proliferation. Hypertension 25:748–751, 1995.
53. Garg V, Hassid A: Nitric oxide-generating vasodilators and 8-bromo-cyclic guanosine monophosphate inhibit mitogenesis and proliferaton of cultured rat vascular smooth muscle cells. J Clin Invest 83:1774–1777, 1989.
54. Rudic R, Shesely E, Maeda N, et al: Direct evidence for the importance of endothelium-derived nitric oxide in vascular remodeling. J Clin Invest 101:731–736, 1998.
55. Navarro J, Sanchez A, Siz J, et al: Hormonal, renal and metabolic alteration during hypertension induced by chronic inhibition of NO in rats. Am J Physiol 267:R1516–R1521, 1994.
56. Tolins J, Raij L, et al: Role of endothelium derived relaxing factor in regulation of vascular tone and remodeling. Update on humoral regulation of vascular tone. Hypertension 17(6 Pt 2):909–916, 1991.
57. Zanchi A, Schaad N, Osterheld M, et al: Effects of chronic NO synthase inhibition in rats on renin-angiotensin system and sympatheic nervous system. Am J Physiol 268:H2267–H2273, 1995.
58. Bank N, Aynedjian H, Khan G: Mechanism of vasoconstriction induced by chronic inhibition of nitric oxide in rats. Hypertension 24:322–328, 1994.
59. Qui C, Engles K, Baylis C: AII and alpha 1 adrenergic tone in chronic nitric oxide blockade induced hyertension: Am J Physol 266:R1470–R1476, 1994.
60. Ribeiro M, Antunes E, deNucci G, et al: Chronic inhibition of nitric oxide synthesis: A new model of arterial hypertension. Hypertension 20:298–303, 1992.
61. Pollock D, Polakowsky J, Divish B, Opgenorth T: Angiotensin blockade reverses hypertension during long-term nitric-oxide synthase inhibition. Hypertension 21:660–666, 1993.
62. Kihara M, Umemura S, Sumida Y, et al: Genetic deficiency of angiotensinogen produces an impaired urine concentrating ability in mice. Kidney Int 53:548–555, 1998.
63. Marjan A, Verhagen G, Braam B, et al: Losartan-sensitive renal damage caused by chronic NOS inhibition does not involve increased renal angiotensin II concentrations. Kidney Int 56:222–231, 1999.
64. Persson P, Baumann J, Ehmke H, et al: Endothelium-derived NO stimulates pressure-dependent renin release in conscious dogs. Am J Physiol 264:F943–F947, 1993.
65. Vidal M, Romero J, Vanhoutte P: Endothelium-derived relaxing factor inhibits renin release. Eur J Pharmacol 149:401–402, 1988.
66. Wagner C, Jensen B, Kramer B, Kurtz A: Control of the renal renin system by local factors. Kidney Int 54(Suppl 67):S78–S83, 1998.
67. Kramer B, Tritthaler, Ackermann M, et al: Endothelium-mediated regulation of renin secretion. Kidney Int 46:1577–1579, 1994.
68. Gardes J, Gonzalez M, Alhenc-Gelas F, Menard J: Influence of sodium diet on L-NAME effects on renin release and renal vasoconstriction. Am J Physiol 267:F798–F804, 1994.

69. Bosse H, Bohm R, Resch S, Backmann S: Parallel regulation of constitutive NO synthase and renin at JGA of rat kidney under various stimuli. Am J Physiol 269:F793–F805, 1995.

70. Jover B, Herizi A, Ventre F, et al: Sodium and angiotensin in hypertension induced by long-term nitric oxide synthase inhibition. Hypertension 21:944–948, 1993.

71. Baylis C, Hartoon P, Engles K: Endothelial derived relaxing factor controls renal hemodynamics in the normal rat kidney. J Am Soc Nephrol 1:875–881, 1990.

72. Ito S, Armina S, Ren Y, et al: Endothelium-derived relaxing factor/nitric oxide modulates angiotensin II action in the isolated microperfused rabbit afferent but not efferent arteriole. J Clin Invest 91:2012–2019, 1993.

73. DeNicola L, Blantz R, Gabbai F: Nitric oxide and AII. Glomerular and tubular interaction in the rat. J Clin Invest 89:1248–1256, 1992.

74. Lohmeier T, Cowley A: Hypertensive and renal effects of chronic low level intrarenal angiotensin infusion in the dog. Circ Res 44:154–160, 1979.

75. Rosivall L, Naval G: Effects on renal hemodynamics of intraarterial infusion of angiotensin I and II. Am J Physiol 254:F181–F187, 1983.

76. Ohishi K, Carmines P, Inscho E, Navar L: EDRF-AII interactions in rat juxtamedullary afferent and efferent arterioles. Am J Physiol 263:F900–F906, 1992.

77. Munoz-Garcia R, Maeso R, Rodrigo E, et al: Acute renal excretory actions of losartan in spontaneously hypertensive rats: Role of AT2 receptors, prostaglandins, kinins and nitric oxide. J Hypertens 13:1779–1784, 1995.

78. Geisterfer A, Peach M, Owens G: Angiotensin II induces hypertrophy, not hyperplasia, of cultured rat aortic smooth muscle cells. Circ Res 62:749–756, 1988.

79. Itoh H, Mukoyama M, Pratt R, et al: Multiple autocrine growth factors modulate vascular smooth muscle cell growth response to angiotensin II. J Clin Invest 91:2268–2274, 1993.

80. Gibbons G, Pratt R, Dzau V: Vascular smooth muscle cell hypertrophy vs. hyperplasia: Autocrine transforming growth factor-B1 expression determines growth response to angiotensin II. J Clin Invest 90:456–461, 1992.

81. Chansel D, Czekalski S, Pham P, Ardaillou R: Characterization of angiotensin II receptor subtypes in human glomeruli and mesangial cells. Am J Physiol 262:F432–F441, 1992.

82. Wolf G: Regulation of renal tubular cell growth: Effects of angiotensin II. Exp Nephrol 2:107–114, 1994.

83. Sadoshima J, Izumo S: Molecular characterization of angiotensin II-induced hypertrophy of cardiac myocytes and hyperplasia of cardiac fibroblasts: Critical role of AT1 receptor subtype. Circ Res 73:412–423, 1993.

84. Ardaillou R: Angiotensin II receptors. J Am Soc Nephrol 10:S30–S39, 1999.

85. Daemen M, Lombardi D, Bosman F, Schwartz S: Angiotensin II induces smooth muscle cell proliferation in the normal and injured rat arterial wall. Circ Res 68:450–456, 1991.

86. Kawamura M, Terashita Z, Okuda H, et al: TCV-116, a novel angiotensin II receptor antagonist, prevents intimal thickening and impairment of vascular function after carotid injury in rats. J Pharmacol Exp Ther 266:1664–1669, 1993.

87. Gibbons GH: Cardioprotective mechanisms of ACE inhibition: The angiotensin II–nitric oxide balance: Drugs 54(Suppl 5):1–11, 1997.

87a. Raij L, Johnston B, Coffee K: Does functional upregulation of angiotensin II mediate end-organ injury in salt sensitive hypertension? Presented at the Ninth European Meeting on Hypertension, Milan, June 11–15, 1999 [abstract].

87b. Hayakawa H, Coffee K, Raij L: Endothelial dysfunction and cardiorenal injury in experimental salt-sensitive hypertension. Effects of antihypertensive therapy. Circulation 96:2407–2413, 1997.

88. Amal J, Amrani A, Chatellier G, ete al: Cardiac weight in hypertension induced by nitric oxide synthase blockade. Hypertension 22:380–387, 1993.

89. Ohkubo H, Nakayayama K, Tanaka T, Nakamshi S: Tissue distribution of rat angiotensinogen mRNA and structural analysis of its heterogeneity. J Biol Chem 262:319–323, 1986.

90. Navar L, Inscho E, Majid S, et al: Paracrine regulation of the renal microcirculation. Physiol Rev 76:425–436, 1996.

91. Llinas M, Gonzalez J, Salazar F: Interactions between angiotensin and nitric oxide in the renal response to volume expansion. Am J Physiol 269:R504–510, 1995.

92. Hollemberg N, Williams G: The renal response to converting enzyme inhibition and the treatment of sodium sensitive hypertension. Clin Exp Hypertens 91:531–541, 1987.

93. Goligorsky M, Noiri E: Duality of nitric oxide in acute renal failure. Semin Nephrol 19:263–271, 1999.

94. Braam B, Koomans H: Renal response to antagonism of the renin-angiotensin system. Curr Opin Nephrol Hypertens 5:89–96, 1996.

95. Johnston C, Fabris B, Jandeleit K: Intrarenal renin-angiotensin system in renal physiology and pathophysiology. Kidney Int 44(Suppl 42):S59–S63, 1993.

96. Lorenz J, Weihprecht H, He X, et al: Effects of adenosine and angiotensin on macula densa-stimulated renin secretion. Am J Physiol 265:F187–F194, 1993.

97. Xie M, Liu F, Wong P, Timmerman P, Cogan M: Proximal nephron and renal effects of DuPt53, a nonpeptide angiotensin II receptor antagonist. Kidney Int 38:473–479, 1990.

98. Lo M, Liu K, Lantelme P, Sassard J: Subtype 2 of angiotensin II receptors controls pressure natriuresis in rats. J Clin Invest 95:1394–1397, 1995.

99. Navar L, Harrison-Bernard L, Imig J, et al: Intrarenal angiotensin II generation and renal effects of AT1 receptor blockade. J Am Soc Nephrol 10(Suppl 10):S266–S272, 1999.

100. Cervenka L, Wang C, Mitchell K, Navar L: Proximal tubular angiotensin II levels and renal functional responses to AT1 receptor blockade in nonclipped kidneys of Goldblatt hypertensive rats. Hypertension 33:102–107, 1999.

101. Cervenka L, Wang C, Navar L: Effects of acute AT1 receptor blockade by candesartan on arterial pressure and renal function in rats. Am J Physiol 274:F940–F945, 1998.

102. Cervenka L, Navar L: Renal responses of the nonclipped kidney of 2 kidney, 1 clip Goldblatt hypertensive rats to AT1 receptor blockade with candesartan. J Am Soc Nephrol 10(Suppl 11):S197–S201, 1999.

103. Mimarn A, Ribstein J: Angiotensin receptor blockers: Pharmacology and clinical significance: J Am Soc Nephol 10(Suppl 12):S273–S277, 1999.

104. Navar L: The kidney in blood pressure regulation and development of hypertension. Med Clin North Am 81:1165–1198, 1997.

105. Ozono R, Wang Z, Moore A, et al: Expression of the subtype 2 angiotensin (AT2) receptor protein in rat kidney. Hypertension 30:1238–1246, 1997.

106. Burnier M, Rutschmann B, Nussberger J: Salt-dependent renal effects of an angiotensin II antagonist in healthy subjects. Hypertension 22:339–347, 1993.

107. Balla T, Baukal A, Eng S, Catt K: Angiotensin II receptor subtypes and biological responses in the adrenal cortex and medulla. Mol Pharmacol 40:401–406, 1991.

108. Arima S, Eado Y, Yaoita H, et al: Possible role of p450 metabolite of arachidonic acid in vasodilator mechanism of angiotensin type 2 receptors in isolated microperfused rabbit afferent arteriole. J Clin Invest 100:2816–2823, 1997.

109. Ajikobi D, Novak P, Salevsky F, Cupples W: Pharmacologic modulation of spontaneous renal blood flow dynamics. Can J Physiol Pharmcol 74:964–972, 1996.

110. Mattson D, Lu S, Nakanishi K: Effect of chronic renal medullary nitric oxide inhibition on blood pressure. Am J Physiol 266:H1918–H1926, 1994.

111. Gabbai F, Blantz R: Role of nitric oxide in renal hemodynamics. Semin Nephrol 19:242–250, 1999.

112. Luscher T, Dohi Y, Tachdi M: Endothelium dependent regulation of resistance arteries: Alterations with aging and hypertension. J Cardiovasc Pharmacol 19(Suppl 5):S34–S42, 1992.

113. Salazar F, Alberola A, Pinilla J: Salt-induced increase in arterial pressure during nitric oxide synthesis inhibition. Hypertension 22:49–55, 1993.

114. Luscher T, Raij L, Vanhoutte P: Endothelium-dependent vascular responses in normotensive and hypertensive Dahl rats. Hypertension 9:157–163, 1987.

115. Reference deleted.

116. Campese V: Salt sensitivity in hypertension. Renal and cardiovascular implications [clinical conference]. Hypertension 23:531–535, 1994.

117. Overlack A, Rupper M, Kollock R: Age is a major determinant of the divergent blood pressure responses to varying salt intake in essential hypertension. Am J Hypertens 8:829–836, 1995.

118. Miyoshi A, Suzuki H, Fujiwara M: Impairment of endothelial function in salt-sensitive hypertension in humans. Am J Hypertens 10:1083–1090, 1997.

119. VanDenHoogen P, Feskens E, Nagelkerke N, et al: The relation between blood pressure and mortality due to coronary heart disease among men in different parts of the world. N Engl J Med 342:1–8, 2000.

120. Yanagisawa M, Kurihara H, Kimura S: A novel potent vasoconstrictor peptide produced by vascular endothelial cells. Nature 332:411–415, 1988.

121. Rossi G, Sacchetto A, Cesari M, Pessina A: Interactions between endothelin-1 and the renin-angiotensin-aldosterone system. Cardiovasc Res 43:300–307, 1999.

122. Masaki T: Possible role of endothelin in endothelial regulation of vascular tone. Annu Rev Pharmacol Toxicol 35:235–255, 1995.

123. Rubanyl G, Botelho L: Endothelins. FASEB J 5:2713–2720, 1991.

124. Johnston C, Volhard F: Renin-angiotensin system: A dual tissue and hormonal system for cardiovascular control. J Hypertens 10:S13–S26, 1992.

125. Fukuroda T, Fujikawa T, Ozaki S, et al: Clearance of circulating endothelin-1 by ETB receptors in rats. Biochem Biophys Res Commun 199:1461–1465, 1994.

126. Colucci W: Myocardial endothelin. Does it play a role in myocardial failure? [editorial comment]. Circulation 93:1069–1072, 1996.
127. Komuro I, Kurihara H, Sugiyama T, et al: Endothelin stimulates *c-fos* and *c-myc* expression and proliferation of vascular smooth muscle cells. FEBS Lett 238:249–252, 1988.
128. Karne S, Jayawickreme C, Lerner M: Cloning and characterization of an endothelin-3 specific receptor (ETC receptor) from *Xenopus laevis* dermal melanophores. J Biol Chem 268:19126–19133, 1993.
129. Fujise K, Stacy L, Beck P, et al: Differential effects of endothelin receptor activation on cyclic flow variations in rat mesenteric arteries. Circulation 96:3641–3646, 1997.
130. Bialecki R, Fisher C, Murdoch W, et al: Functional comparison of endothelin receptors in human and rat pulmonary artery. Am J Physiol 272(2 Pt 1):L211–L218, 1997.
131. Verhaar M, Strachan F, Newby D, et al: Endothelin-A receptor antagonist-mediated vasodilatation is attenuated by inhibition of nitric oxide synthesis and by endothelin-B receptor blockade. Circulation 97:752–756, 1998.
132. De-Nucci G, Thomas R, D'Orleans-Juste P, et al: Pressor effects of circulating endothelin are limited by its removal in the pulmonary circulation and by the release of prostacyclin and endothelium-derived relaxing factor. Proc Natl Acad Sci USA 85:9797–9800, 1988.
133. Urata H, Kinoshita A, Perez D: Cloning of the gene and cDNA for human heart chymase. J Biol Chem 266:17173–17179, 1991.
134. Nakano A, Kishi F, Minami K: Selective conversion of big endothelins to tracheal smooth muscle-constricting 31 amino acid-length endothelins by chymase from human mast cells. J Immunol 159:1987–1992, 1997.
135. Kishi F, Minami K, Okishima N: Novel 31-amino-acid-length endothelins cause constriction of vascular smooth muscle. Biochem Biophys Res Commun 248:387–390, 1998.
136. Hahn A, Resink T, Scott-Burden T: Stimulation of endothelin mRNA and secretion in rat vascular smooth muscle cells, a novel autocrine function. Cell Regul 1:649–659, 1990.
137. Resink T, Scott-Burden T, Buhler F: Endothelin stimulates phospholipase C in cultured vascular smooth muscle cells. Biochem Biophys Res Commun 157:1360–1368, 1988.
138. Sung C, Arleth A, Storer B, Ohlstein E: Angiotensin type 1 receptors mediate smooth muscle proliferation and endothelin biosynthesis in rat vascular smooth muscle. J Pharmacol Exp Ther 271:429–437, 1994.
139. Imai T, Hirata Y, Emori T: Induction of endothelin-1 gene by angiotensin and vasopressin in endothelial cells. Hypertension 19:753–757, 1992.
140. Chua B, Chua C, Diglio C, Siu B: Regulation of endothelin-1 mRNA by angiotensin II in rat heart endothelial cells. Biochim Biophys Acta 178:201–206, 1993.
141. Ito H, Hirata Y, Adachi S: Endothelin-1 is an autocrine/paracrine factor in the mechanism of angiotensin II-induced hypertrophy in cultured rat cardiomyocytes. J Clin Invest 92:398–403, 1993.
142. Ishiye M, Umemura K, Uematsu T, Nakashima M: Angiotensin AT1 receptor-mediated attenuation of cardiac hypertrophy due to volume load: Involvement of endothelin. Eur J Pharmacol 280:11–17, 1995.
143. Good J, Nihoyannopoulos P, Ghatei M, et al: Elevated plasma endothelin concentrations in heat failure: An effect of angiotensin II? Eur Heart J 15:1634–1640, 1994.
144. Nussdorfer G, Rossi G, Belloni A: The role of endothelins in the paracrine control of the secretion and growth of the adrenal cortex. Int Rev Cytol 171:267–308, 1997.
145. Rossi G, Albertin G, Belloni A: Gene expression, localization, and characterization of endothelin A and B receptors in the human adrenal cortex. J Clin Invest 94:1226–1234, 1994.
146. Beierwaltes W, Carretero O: Nonprostanoid endothelium-derived factors inhibit renin release. Hypertension 19(Suppl 2):1168–1173, 1992.
147. Moe O, Tejedor A, Campbell W, et al: Effects of endothelin on in vitro renin secretion. Am J Physiol 260:E521–E525, 1991.
148. Kramer B, Schricker K, Scholz H: Role of endothelins for renin regulation. Kidney Int 55:S119–S121, 1996.
149. Polonia J, Ferreira-de-Almeida J, Matias A: Renin-angiotensin-aldosterone, sympathetic and endothelin systems in normal and hypertensive pregnancy: Response to postural and volume load stimuli. J Hypertens 11(Suppl 5):S242–S243, 1993.
150. Imai T, Hirata Y, Eguchi S: Concomitant expression of receptor subtype and isopeptide of endothelin by human adrenal gland. Biochem Biophys Res Commun 182:1115–1121, 1992.
151. Cozza E, Chiou S, Gomez-Sanchez C: Endothelin-1 potentiation of angiotensin II stimulation of aldosterone production. Am J Physiol 262:R85–R89, 1992.
152. Gomez-Sanchez C, Cozza E, Foeching M, et al: Endothelin receptors subtypes and stimulation of aldosterone secretion. Hypertension 15:744–747, 1990.
153. Belloni A, Rossi G, Andreis P: Endothelin adrenocortical secretagogue effect is mediated by the B receptor in rats. Hypertension 27:1153–1159, 1996.

154. Rossi G, Alberin G, Neri G: Endothelin-1 stimulates steroid secretion of human adrenocortical cells ex vivo via both ETA and ETB receptor subtypes. J Clin Endocrinol Metab 82:3445–3449, 1997.

155. Rossi G, Albertin G, Bova S: Autocrine-paracrine role of endothelin-1 in the regulation of aldosterone synthase expression and intracellular Ca^{2+} in human adrenocortical carcinoma. Endocrinology 138:4421–4426, 1997.

156. Balakrishnan S, Wang H, Gopalakrishnan V, et al: Effect of an endothelin antagonist on hemodynamic responses to angiotensin II. Hypertension 28:806–809, 1996.

157. Herizi A, Jover B, Bouriquet N, Mimran A: Prevention of the cardiovascular and renal effects of angiotensin II by endothelin blockade. Hypertension 31:10–14, 1998.

158. Massart P, Hodeige D, Van-Mechelen H: Angiotensin II and endothelin-1 receptor antagonists have cumulative hypotensive effects in canine Page hypertension. Circulation 84:2476–2484, 1991.

159. Gardiner S, March J, Kemp P, et al: Hemodynamic effects of losartan and the endothelin antagonist, SB 209670, in conscious, transgenic ((mRen-2)27), hypertensive rats. Br J Pharmacol 116:2237–2244, 1995.

160. Schiffrin E: Endothelin: Potential role in hypertension and vascular hypertrophy. Hypertension 25:1135–1143, 1995.

161. Moreau P, d'Uscio L, Shaw S: Angiotensin II increases tissue endothelin and induces vascular hypertrophy: Reversal by ET(A)-receptor antagonist. Circulation 96:1593–1597, 1997.

162. Donckier J, Massart P, Hodeige D, et al: Additional hypotensive effect of endothelin-1 receptor antagonism in hypertensive dogs under angiotensin-converting enzyme inhibition. Circulation 96:1250–1256, 1997.

163. Nava E, Luscher T: Endothelium-derived vasoactive factors in hypertension: Nitric oxide and endothelin [review]. J Hypertens 13(Suppl):S39–S48, 1995.

164. McMurray J, Ray S, Abdullah I, et al: Plasma endothelin in chronic heart failure. Circulation ;85:1374–1379, 1992.

165. Cody R, Haas G, Binkley P, et al: Plasma endothelin correlates with the extent of pulmonary hypertension in patients with congestive heart failure. Circulation 85:504–509, 1992.

166. Whitworth C, Veniant M, Firth J, et al: Endothelin in the kidney in malignant phase hypertension. Hypertension 26:925–931, 1995.

167. Clozel M, Breu V, Gray G: Pharmacological characterization of bosentan, a new potent orally active nonpeptide endothelin receptor antagonist. J Pharmacol Exp Ther 270:228–235, 1994.

168. Ganten D, Lindpaintner K, Ganten U: Transgenic rats: New animal models in hypertension research. Hypertension 17:843–855, 1991.

169. Cargnelli G, Rossi G, Pessina A: Changes of blood pressure and aortic strip contractile responses to ET-1 to heterozygous female transgenic rats, TGR(mRen2)27. Pharmacol Res 37:207–211, 1998.

170. Gardiner S, Kemp P, March J, Bennett T: Enhanced involvement of endothelin in the hemodynamic sequelae of endotoxemia in conscious, hypertensive, transgenic ((mRen-2)27) rats. Br J Pharmacol 123:1403–1408, 1998.

171. Schricker K, Scholz H, Hamann M: Role of endogenous endothelins in the renin system of normal and two-kidney, one clip rats. Hypertension 25:1025–1029, 1995.

172. Lariviere R, Day R, Schiffrin E: Increased expression of endothelin-1 gene in blood vessels of doxycorticosterone acetate salt hypertensive rats. Hypertension 21:916–920, 1993.

173. Lariviere R, Deng L, Day R: Increased endothelin-1 gene expression in the endothelium of coronary arteries and endocardium in the DOCA-salt hypertensive rat. J Mol Cell Cardiol 27:2123–2131, 1995.

174. Lariviere R, Sventek P, Thibault G, Schiffrin E: Endothelin-1 expression in blood vessels of DOCA-salt hypertensive rats treated with the combined ETA/ETB endothelin receptor antagonist bosentan. Can J Physiol Pharmacol 73:390–398, 1995.

175. Day R, Lariviere R, Schiffrin E: In situ hybridization shows increased endothelin-1 mRNA levels in endothelial cells of blood vessels of deoxycorticosterone acetate-salt hypertensive rats. Am J Hypertens 8:294–300, 1995.

176. Li J, Lariviere R, Schiffrin E: Effect of a nonselective endothelin antagonist on vascular remodeling in deoxycorticosterone acetate salt hypertensive rats. Evidence for a role of endothelin in vascular hypertrophy. Hypertension 24:183–188, 1994.

177. Barton M, d'Uscio L, Shaw S: ET(A) receptor blockade prevents increased tissue endothelin-1, vascular hypertrophy, and endothelial dysfunction in salt sensitive hypertension. Hypertension 31:499–504, 1998.

178. Ferri C, Bellini C, Desideri G: Elevated plasma and urinary endothelin-1 levels in human in salt-sensitive hypertension. Clin Sci (Colch) 93:35–41, 1996.

179. Webb D, Strachan F: Clinical experience with endothelial antagonists [review]. Am J Hypertens 11(4 Pt 3):71S–79S, 1998.

180. Hocher B, Thone-Reineke C, Rohmeiss P, et al: Endothelin-1 transgenic mice develop glomeru-losclerosis, interstitial fibrosis, and renal cysts but not hypertension. JCI 99:1380–1389, 1997.

181. Liefeldt L, Schonfelder G, Bocker W, et al: Transgenic rats expressing the human ET-2 gene: A model for study of endothelin actions in vivo. J Mol Med 77:565–574, 1999.

182. Barton M, Shaw S, d'Uscio L, et al: Angiotensin II increases vascular and renal endothelin-1 and functional endothelin converting enzyme activity in vivo: Role of ETA receptors for endothelin regulation. Biochem Biophys Res Commun 238:861–865, 1997.

183. d'Uscio L, Moreau P, Shaw S: Effects of chronic ET(A) receptor blockade in angiotensin II-induced hypertension. Hypertension 29:435–441, 1997.

184. Sakai S, Miyauchi T, Kobayashi M, et al: Inhibition of myocardial endothelin pathway improves long-term survival in heart failure. Nature 384:353–355, 1996.

185. Mulder P, Richard V, Derumeaux G: Role of endogenous endothelin in chronic heart failure: Effect of long-term treatment with an endothelin antagonist on survival hemodynamics, and cardiac remodeling. Circulation 96:1976–1982, 1997.

186. Rajagopalan S, Laursen J, Borthayre A: Role for endothelin-1 in angiotensin II-mediated hypertension. Hypertension 30:29–34, 1997.

187. Krum H, Viskoper R, Lacourciere Y, et al: The effect of an endothelin receptor antagonist, bosentan on blood pressure in patients with essential hypertension. N Engl J Med 338:784–790, 1998.

188. Kiowski W, Sutsch G, Hunziker P: Evidence for endothelin-1 mediated vasoconstriction in severe chronic heart failure. Lancet 236:732–736, 1995.

189. Love M, Haynes W, Gray G: Vasodilator effects of endothelin-converting enzyme inhibition and endothelin receptor (ETA) blockade in chronic heart failure patients treated with ACE inhibitors. Circulation 94:2131, 1996

190. Regoli D, Barabe J: Pharmacology of bradykinin and related kinins. Pharmacol Rev 32:1–46, 1990.

191. Seyedi N, Xu X, Nasjletti A, Hintze T: Coronary kinin generation mediates nitric oxide release after angiotensin receptor stimulation. Hypertension 26:164–170, 1995.

192. Cachoeiro V, Sakakibara T, Nasjletti A: Kinins, nitric oxide, and the hypotensive effect of captopril and ramiprilat in hypertension. Hypertension 19:138–145, 1992.

193. Tscope C, Gohlke Y, Zhu W, et al: Antihypertensive and cardioprotective effects after angiotensin-converting enzyme inhibition: Role of kinins. J Card Fail 3:133–148, 1997.

194. Rhaleb N, Telemaque S, Roussi N, et al: Structure-activity studies of bradykinin and related peptides: B2-receptor antagonists. Hypertension 17:107–115, 1991.

195. Bonner G: The role of kinins in the antihypertensive and cardioprotective effects of ACE inhibitors: Drugs 54(Suppl 5):23–30, 1997.

196. Madeddu P, Parpaglia PP, Demontis M, et al: Chronic inhibition of bradykinin B2 receptors enhances the slow vasopressor response to angiotensin II. Hypertension 23:646–652, 1993.

197. Madeddu P, Varoni M, Paomba D, et al: Cardiovascular phenotype of a mouse strain with disruption of the bradykinin B2-receptor gene. Circulation 96:3570–3578, 1997.

198. Carey R, Zhi-Qin W, Siragy H: Role of the angiotensin type 2 receptor in the regulation of blood pressure and renal function. Hypertension 35:155–163, 2000.

199. Hutchinson H, Hein L, Fujinaga M, Pratt R: Modulation of vascular development and injury by angiotensin II. Cardiovasc Res 41:689–700, 1998.

200. Ohkubo N, Matsubara H, Nozawa Y, et al: Angiotensin type 2 receptors are re-expressed by cardiac fibroblasts from failing myopathic hamster hearts and inhibit cell growth and fibrillar collage metabolism. Circulation 96:3954–3962, 1997.

201. Booz G, Baker K: Role of type and type 2 angiotensin receptors in angiotensin II-induced cardiomyocyte hypertrophy. Hypertension 28:635–640, 1996.

202. Matsubara H: Pathophysiological role of angiotensin II type 2 receptor in cardiovascular and renal diseases. Circ Res 83:1182–1191, 1998.

203. Gohlke P, Pees C, Unger R: AT2 receptor stimulation increases aortic cyclic GMP in SHRSP by kinin-dependent mechanisms. Hypertension 31:349–355, 1998.

204. Liu Y-H, Yang X-P, Sharov VG, et al: Effects of angiotensin-converting enzyme inhibitors and angiotensin II type 1 receptor antagonists in rats with heart failure: J Clin Invest 99:1926–1935, 1997.

205. Siragy HM, Inagami T, Ichiki T, Carey RM: Sustained hypersensitivity to angiotensin II and its mechanism in mice lacking the subtype (AT2) angiotensin receptor. Proc Natl Acad Sci USA 96:6506–6510, 1999.

CHAPTER 12

Mechanism for Chronic Antihypertensive Effect of Angiotensin II Blockade

MICHAEL W. BRANDS, Ph.D.
JOHN E. HALL, Ph.D.

The renin-angiotensin system has long been recognized as a principal component of the body's systems for regulating circulatory homeostasis. Because angiotensin II (Ang II) has both a powerful vasoconstrictor effect and renal sodium- and volume-retaining actions, pharmacologic inhibition of this hormonal system offers a powerful treatment for high blood pressure and other cardiovascular diseases. The mechanisms underlying the effect of Ang II—or Ang II blockade—on chronic blood pressure control are somewhat confusing, however, mainly because accurate interpretation of measurements of total peripheral resistance and renal sodium excretion is complex and at first glance even counterintuitive. For example, the measurement of sodium balance in a high-renin hypertensive patient documents a central role for the renal actions of Ang II in sustaining high blood pressure, and measurement of increased total peripheral resistance does not prove that the hypertension is caused by Ang II-mediated systemic vasoconstriction. This chapter clarifies these relationships as well as the mechanisms through which changes in circulating Ang II levels influence the control system for chronic blood pressure.

■ Renal Excretion and Long-Term Blood Pressure Control

The Circulation Functions as an "Open" Circuit

A closed circulatory system is characteristic of the phylum Chordata, but it often is helpful to consider the human circulation as an open system when linking renal function to arterial pressure control. In 1909, Starling proposed that circulatory homeostasis is achieved through the interdependence of fluid balance and circulatory stability and that both are maintained through the regulatory function of the kidneys.[1] Cardiac performance is tied directly to the volume and pressure in the circulation. The heart, in turn, communicates via arterial pressure the state of the circulation to the kidneys, which adjust volume excretion as needed to maintain circulatory homeostasis. Using an example of overfilling or high pressure in the circulation, the kidneys can be viewed as pressure-relief valves. By being open to the external environment, the kidneys enable the restoration and maintenance of stable arterial pressure by releasing volume from the circulation. This function becomes even clearer in considering arterial pressure control in patients without kidneys; the closed nature of their circulatory system makes arterial pressure extremely sensitive to changes in sodium intake and blood volume.[2]

The Renal Pressure-Natriuresis Relationship Determines the Set Point for Arterial Pressure Control

Starling's theory suggests that renal fluid excretion is an essential control mechanism that enables maintenance of circulatory homeostasis, but in his scheme the kidneys function mainly to adjust fluid excretion as compensation for changes in cardiac performance. In 1963, however, Borst and Borst-de Geus, drawing extensively from the work of Starling, hypothesized that "blood pressure will be maintained at the exact level required for the maintenance of sodium balance."[3] This hypothesis set in motion the concept that renal sodium excretory function, or the "willingness of the kidneys to excrete sodium," as stated by Borst and Borst-de Geus,[3] is in fact the overriding determinant of mean 'arterial pressure. As demonstrated by Guyton and Coleman[4] and others,[5-11] there is only one arterial pressure at which sodium balance can be maintained. Changes in blood pressure above or below that set point cause sufficient sodium loss or retention, respectively, to correct the change in pressure. Moreover, it was demonstrated that this control system actually has infinite feedback gain; therefore, it is the only mechanism capable of restoring blood pressure completely to control levels.[4,8,10]

Two points, therefore, are fundamental to understanding how renal function determines the set point at which mean arterial pressure is regulated: (1) blood pressure per se has a powerful natriuretic action; and (2) sodium balance must be maintained in the steady state. The natriuretic effect of increased blood pressure commonly is referred to as the pressure-natriuresis relationship.[11] Numerous experiments in humans and animals have shown clearly that an increase in renal perfusion pressure rapidly increases sodium and volume excretion by the kidneys[10-15] (Fig. 1). This control system operates effectively on both sides of the set point; thus, decreases in renal perfusion pressure cause fluid retention by the kidneys.[10,11] Pressure-natriuresis can be modified by neural and humoral inputs (e.g., high levels of Ang II), but it is an intrinsic characteristic of the kidneys and can operate even in the absence of extrarenal control, although neurohumoral control increases its efficiency.[10,11] However, although pressure-natriuresis clearly is demonstrable in an acute setting, its role in chronic blood pressure control is more difficult to understand. At this point it becomes necessary to consider the requirement for sodium balance.

If urinary sodium excretion is continuously lower than sodium intake, progressive volume expansion and circulatory congestion ensue; likewise, continuous sodium excretion in excess of intake leads to circulatory collapse. Maintenance of sodium balance, therefore, is essential for life. But how is it achieved? Changes in sodium intake are sensed by numerous neural and humoral systems, such as the renin-angiotensin system, and changes in their activity help to effect the required change in sodium excretion that restores balance. However, blood pressure also is an important, though often overlooked, controller of sodium

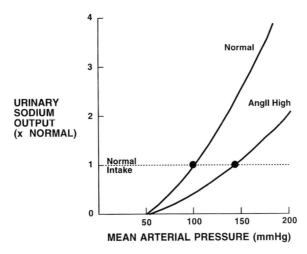

Figure 1.   The pressure-natriuresis relationship under normal conditions and during chronic angiotensin II infusion. In each instance there is only one blood pressure at which sodium balance is maintained. An increase in arterial pressure above this point raises sodium excretion and a decrease in arterial pressure below that point causes sodium retention. To determine the effect of increased angiotensin II, compare the dots on each curve. Angiotensin II imparts an antinatriuretic shift in the pressure-natriuresis relationship so that a higher blood pressure is needed to achieve the same level of sodium excretion.

excretion, and changes in blood pressure also help to restore sodium balance. For example, the increase in arterial pressure that accompanies chronic administration of antinatriuretic hormones is essential for "escape" from sodium retention and restoration of sodium balance.[16–20] The kidneys, therefore, have a set point for the arterial pressure level that allows maintenance of sodium balance; deviations from that level in either direction have a direct effect on sodium excretion that persists until the pressure set point is restored.[10,11]

Extrarenal Vascular Resistance Is Not a Primary Long-term Controller of Arterial Pressure

With chronic hypertension, total peripheral resistance is almost invariably increased, leading many to conclude that the change in resistance is the mediator of the change in pressure. In many cases, however, the increase in resistance may be an autoregulatory response rather than a cause of the increase in arterial pressure.[3–5,7,8] Huang et al.[21] addressed this issue by chronically administering the peripheral vasodilator, minoxidil, to rats with hypertension induced by deoxycorticosterone acetate (DOCA). The treatment significantly decreased total peripheral resistance but did not decrease arterial pressure. How was the same level of hypertension maintained with a lower peripheral vascular resistance? The minoxidil-treated group retained more sodium and had greater cardiac output than the control rats. Thus, the kidneys, which were not markedly vasodilated by minoxidil, compensated for peripheral vasodilation by retaining volume sufficient to maintain the level of hypertension determined by the effects of DOCA on the kidneys.

Most tissues autoregulate their own blood flow in accordance with metabolic needs, and vascular tone is adjusted to maintain the flow appropriate for nutrient delivery and waste removal.[3,4,7,22,23] Because tissue blood flow most often is normal in hypertension and because cardiac output is the sum of blood flow in all tissues, cardiac output essentially is normal in most forms of sustained hypertension—even if volume retention initiated the pressure rise.[3–10,24] In short-term experimental hypertension, such as 7-day aldosterone infusion, total peripheral resistance increases as a result of vasoconstriction to maintain normal tissue blood flow in the face of the elevated blood pressure.[4,24] With long-term hypertension, structural changes in the arterioles and vascular rarefaction gradually become more important for maintaining normal blood flow and increasing total peripheral resistance.[4,24,25] Thus, peripheral vascular resistance in the steady state is a function primarily of vascular adjustments to maintain appropriate tissue blood flow and does not determine the set point for blood pressure control unless renal vascular resistance is altered.[4,10,24] Rather, the set point is determined by the sodium excretory capability of the kidneys. Forcing changes in peripheral vascular tone, as in the minoxidil study,[21] simply causes the kidneys to adjust volume until blood pressure returns to the level needed to maintain sodium balance.[3,4,10,11,24]

How do vasoactive drugs change blood pressure? A drug that causes only systemic vasoconstriction, without affecting the kidneys, initially causes an increase in arterial pressure; however, because there has been no change in renal sodium excretory capability, natriuresis ensues and continues until enough volume has been lost to restore arterial pressure to normal levels[10,11] (Fig. 2). Many vasoactive drugs, however, are known to cause chronic changes in arterial pressure. How are such changes explained in terms of the pressure-natriuresis relationship? Most vasoactive agents affect the renal vasculature as well as blood vessels throughout the body, altering renal excretory capability and enabling the maintenance of a chronic change in arterial pressure. Thus, the effect of drugs or hormones to change systemic vascular resistance may have significant acute effects on arterial pressure, but it is their effect on *renal* vascular resistance and excretory capability that induces a sustained change in pressure.[10,11]

■ Modulation of Pressure-Natriuresis by Angiotensin II

Clearly, changes in arterial and, hence, renal perfusion pressure have direct effects on sodium excretion, and this pressure-natriuresis relationship is a means by which sodium balance is restored. However, healthy adults do not normally experience wide variations in blood pressure throughout the day to regulate sodium excretion because neural and hormonal systems are responsive to changes in blood pressure and capable of regulating sodium excretion. The renin-angiotensin system is perhaps the most powerful of these systems.

Figure 3 shows the pressure-natriuresis relationship as it is evaluated in the chronic steady state.[26] The relationship is determined by measuring arterial pressure after sodium balance has been attained at various levels of sodium intake. Because sodium intake and excretion are equal at that point, arterial pressure is plotted against sodium excretion to facilitate discussion of the pressure-natriuresis relationship. The steepness of the curve in the normal condition indicates that only minimal changes in arterial pressure occur in response to changes in sodium intake over an extremely wide range. If pressure-natriuresis is so important in restoring sodium balance, why does arterial pressure not change to a

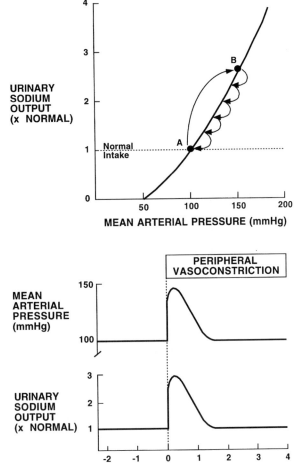

Figure 2. Predicted response to increased total peripheral resistance with no change in renal pressure natriuresis (e.g., no renal vasoconstriction). Arterial pressure increases along the same renal function curve from A to B (because pressure natriuresis was not affected). Arterial pressure increase causes an increase in sodium excretion that persists until enough volume is lost to return arterial pressure to the level that matches renal sodium excretory capability (i.e., the set point for maintenance of sodium balance).

greater extent? The answer is the underlying change in Ang II levels and its consequent action on renal sodium excretory function. Ang II is the most powerful sodium-retaining hormone in the body, and with increases in sodium intake, Ang II levels decrease.[27] Thus, the decrease in the sodium-retaining influence of Ang II increases the sodium excretory capability of the kidneys, and sodium excretion can rise to a level that matches intake with only a minimal increase in renal perfusion pressure. The opposite occurs with decreases in sodium intake. Sodium balance, therefore, is the result of a balance among all of the natriuretic and antinatriuretic forces, including blood pressure, acting on the kidneys.

Angiotensin II Blockade or Angiotensin II Infusion Decreases the Slope of Pressure-Natriuresis

How the renin-angiotensin system and arterial pressure interact to maintain sodium balance is illustrated by the marked change in the slope of the pressure-natriuresis curves in Figure 3 with ACE inhibition or Ang II infusion. If sodium

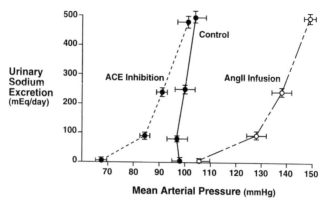

Figure 3. Relationship between mean arterial pressure and sodium excretion after steady state was achieved at four levels of sodium intake (i.e., after sodium balance was achieved). Sodium intakes ranging from approximately 5–500 mEq/day were provided under normal conditions with a functional renin-angiotensin system, after blockade of angiotensin II formation with chronic angiotensin-converting enzyme inhibitor, and after infusing angiotensin II continuously at 5 ng/kg/min to prevent plasma angiotensin II levels from being suppressed on the high-salt diet. Note the sensitivity of blood pressure to sodium intake when angiotensin II levels are prevented from changing (Redrawn from data in Hall JE, Guyton AC, Smith MJ Jr, Coleman TG: Blood pressure and renal function during chronic changes in sodium intake: Role of angiotensin. Am J Physiol 239:F271–F280, 1980.)

intake is decreased and compensatory increases in Ang II are prevented by an ACE inhibitor, arterial pressure decreases markedly. Moreover, this decrease in arterial pressure is the means by which sodium balance is restored.[11] Thus, with a decrease in sodium intake, the kidneys must switch to a more sodium-retaining state so that sodium excretion can be decreased accordingly. Normally, an increase in Ang II accomplishes this goal; however, without Ang II the decrease in sodium excretory capability is achieved through the effect of decreased arterial pressure. Sodium balance, therefore, is maintained at the expense of a decrease in arterial pressure. This process demonstrates that Ang II has a powerful effect on the pressure-natriuresis relationship and also shows that the ability to change circulating Ang II levels in accordance with changes in sodium intake is essential to minimize salt-induced changes in arterial pressure.[11]

Inability to Modulate Angiotensin II Levels Causes Salt-Sensitive Hypertension

An inability to suppress Ang II levels while changing from a low- to high-salt intake causes an increase in arterial pressure. This inability to modulate Ang II formation appropriately also may be important in causing salt-sensitivity of blood pressure in several types of clinical hypertension. For example, patients with low renin levels tend to be salt-sensitive, in part because they are unable to suppress Ang II further as salt intake is raised. The experiment in Figure 3 demonstrated this point by infusing Ang II chronically so that Ang II levels were held constant and were unable to be suppressed with high sodium intake. In patients who have subpopulations of ischemic nephrons, renin secretion is increased by the ischemic nephrons.[28] The other nephrons, however, are overperfused to excrete the urine that would have been excreted by the ischemic nephrons; renin secretion, therefore, is greatly suppressed. Both ischemic nephrons (with increased renin release) and overperfused nephrons (with suppressed renin release) are unable to appropriately modulate renin release and Ang II formation with changes in salt intake. As a result, blood pressure is salt-sensitive. The experimental correlate is the two-kidney, 1-clip Goldblatt model of hypertension, in which the clipped and nonclipped kidneys secrete high and low amounts of renin, respectively. The result may not be marked increases in circulating Ang II levels, but the underperfused nephrons (or kidney) are unable to suppress renin secretion appropriately when sodium intake increases. Thus, at a time when sodium excretory capability needs to increase to help eliminate the increased salt load, Ang II levels do not decrease sufficiently to accomplish this goal; thus, arterial pressure increases as a compensatory mechanism to maintain sodium balance.[11]

Ang II blockade also renders blood pressure salt-sensitive.[26] This fact often is not appreciated, primarily because the focus on salt sensitivity in general is in the hypertensive range of arterial pressure. In Figure 3, however, the slope of the pressure-natriuresis relationship decreases markedly with both infusion and blockade of Ang II, and a decrease in the slope of this curve in essence defines salt sensitivity.[11] A clinical ramification of this relationship is that maintenance of a relatively high salt intake prevents Ang II blockade from decreasing arterial pressure, whereas restricted salt intake greatly enhances the depressor response.

Escape from Sodium Retention in Angiotensin II-Mediated Hypertension: Role of Pressure-Natriuresis

In a patient with chronic, stable hypertension, clinical determination of sodium balance often is interpreted as evidence that the kidneys are not involved in the etiology of the hypertension. Similarly, Ang II infusion can cause marked sodium retention initially, but with continued administration escape occurs and sodium balance soon is restored.[16] This finding often leads to the conclusion that the renal actions of Ang II are involved only in the initiation of the hypertension and that peripheral vasoconstrictor actions maintain the hypertension. Finally, the "slow pressor" action of Ang II, reported during chronic, low-dose infusions, is attributed to peripheral vasoconstrictor actions because increased sodium balance is not measured.[29,30] However, because increased blood pressure has a natriuretic action and sodium balance must be maintained in the steady state, these three examples, in fact, indicate that the kidneys underlie the hypertension in each case.

Considering sodium escape, for example, Ang II obviously cannot cause continued sodium retention if circulatory homeostasis is to be maintained; however, the restoration of sodium balance is *not* due to a decrease in the antinatriuretic actions of Ang II. Rather, the increase in arterial pressure *compensates* for the antinatriuretic action and is essential for the restoration of sodium balance.[11] As shown in Figure 4, if the kidneys are prevented from "seeing" the hypertension during chronic Ang II infusion, sodium retention continues unabated.[16] Thus, the maintenance of sodium balance during Ang II infusion is due to a balance between the antinatriuretic actions of Ang II and the natriuretic effect of increased blood pressure. The same can be said for all chronic hypertension. Thus, the maintenance of sodium balance in any state of

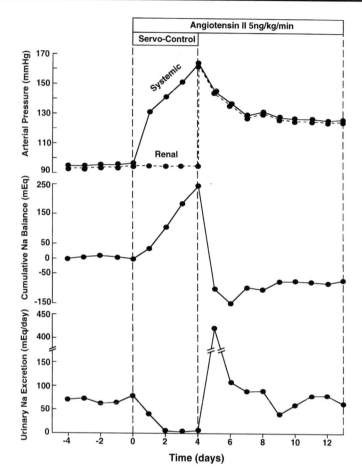

Figure 4. Mean arterial pressure, cumulative sodium balance, and sodium excretion during chronic intravenous infusion of angiotensin II at 5 ng/kg/min with an inflatable occluder on the renal artery to prevent the kidneys from experiencing the hypertension. Renal artery pressure was not decreased below normal but was maintained at control levels by continuous servo-controlled adjustment of the occluder. Sodium escape was prevented until the occluder was released. (Redrawn from data in Hall JE, Granger JP, Hester RL, et al: Mechanisms of escape from sodium retention during angiotensin II hypertension. Am J Physiol 246:F627–F634, 1984.)

chronic hypertension indicates that the kidneys are under an antinatriuretic influence, due, for example, to Ang II, aldosterone, norepinephrine, or a renal artery clip in some models of secondary hypertension; glomerular injury in the hypertension of diabetic nephropathy; or unknown factors in essential hypertension. Therefore, one cannot measure an actual decrease in sodium excretion in steady-state hypertension. Knowing that elevated arterial pressure causes natriuresis in a normal kidney, however, one can conclude that sodium excretory *capability* is decreased.

Thus, the multiple intrarenal actions of Ang II that contribute to its sodium-retaining capability are central to its long-term effect on blood pressure, regardless of whether a change in sodium excretion is measured. The specific intrarenal actions of Ang II are discussed in relation to the mechanisms underlying the hypotensive response to Ang II blockade.

Peripheral Vasoconstrictor Actions of Angiotensin II

Emphasis on the renal basis for chronic blood pressure control does not preclude an important role for the peripheral vasoconstrictor actions of Ang II. The importance of this mechanism in the short-term control of blood pressure, as observed in severe hemorrhage, for example, has been demonstrated clearly. However, vasoconstriction of the veins also serves an important function during chronic increases in Ang II. By reducing the capacitance in the venous system, venoconstriction significantly reduces the amount of renal sodium and volume retention required to raise blood pressure.[24] Thus, although the vasoconstrictor action of Ang II cannot cause hypertension by itself (because it results in natriuresis and volume loss), it appears to work in concert with the intrarenal actions of Ang II to facilitate the rise in blood pressure.

Of interest, the vasoconstrictor action of Ang II also explains, in part, why the role of its renal actions in determining chronic blood pressure sometimes is underestimated. Ang II infusions that produce physiologic increases in plasma levels cause transient sodium retention and subsequent escape as arterial pressure increases.[16] However, supraphysiologic doses in fact cause an initial natriuresis,[31–33] because the vasoconstrictor systems are activated more powerfully and rapidly than normal and raise arterial pressure above the renal set point, thereby promoting natriuresis. This finding might be interpreted as evidence that Ang II has a direct natriuretic action at high doses, but studies have demonstrated that the natriuresis is secondary to the rapid rise in systemic arterial pressure.[16]

At the other end of the spectrum, some studies postulate a "slow pressor" action of Ang II that mediates the hypertension associated with chronic infusion of low doses of Ang II.[29,30] Little or no sodium retention is measured in such studies, although total peripheral resistance is increased in the steady state. However, Ang II increases renal sodium reabsorption through actions on the tubules and efferent arterioles at concentrations as low as 10^{-13} M and 10^{-12} M, respectively,[34,35] which are much lower than concentrations that constrict extrarenal blood vessels. In addition, other investigators have measured transient sodium retention at low-dose infusion rates,[36–38] with escape from this effect as arterial pressure increases. Moreover, peripheral vasoconstriction probably is an autoregulatory response to increased arterial pressure.[3,10,24]

■ *Renal Actions of Angiotensin II Blockade*

Angiotensin II Blockade Increases Renal Sodium Excretory Capability

Chronic administration of either an ACE inhibitor or an Ang II receptor antagonist induces a sustained decrease in mean arterial pressure by decreasing circulating levels of Ang II or blocking its action. Despite interest in the possibility that ACE inhibitors lower arterial pressure by alternative mechanisms, most evidence indicates that decreases in Ang II levels mediate the chronic decrease in arterial pressure. Because Ang II blockade enhances the ability of the kidneys to excrete sodium, sodium balance can be maintained at a lower arterial pressure.

There are two possible mechanisms for increasing sodium excretory capability: an increase in glomerular filtration rate (GFR) or a decrease in tubular sodium reabsorption. Ang II has powerful renal vasoconstrictor actions that affect renal vascular resistance as well as direct effects that increase tubular sodium reabsorption, but considerable evidence indicates that the physiologic effects of Ang II on sodium excretion are exerted mainly through its tubular actions.[27,39] In some pathophysiologic conditions, however, excessive Ang II may reduce GFR by causing glomerular injury, and blockade of Ang II may increase sodium excretory capability by preventing such injury.

Control of GFR by Angiotensin II Blockade

The renin-angiotensin system works cooperatively with other autoregulatory mechanisms, such as tubuloglomerular feedback (TGF) and myogenic activity, to maintain a relatively constant GFR.[27,39] The primary renal vascular site of action of Ang II is the efferent arteriole, where vasoconstriction prevents decreases in GFR in conditions of circulatory depression or sodium depletion.[27,39–43] This action enables the maintenance of normal excretion of metabolic waste products while Ang II acts through multiple mechanisms to increase renal tubular sodium and water reabsorption.

Ang II blockade predictably decreases efferent arteriolar resistance, but in normal kidneys this decrease has a minimal effect on GFR because other autoregulatory mechanisms help to maintain a steady filtration rate.[39] This effect is fortunate because the predicted response would be a decrease in GFR, which tends to cause sodium retention—opposite to the actual response to Ang II blockade.

Ang II blockade may further reduce GFR in underperfused kidneys. The effect of Ang II on the efferent arteriole and GFR appears to be most important when renal perfusion pressure is reduced to low levels, near the limits of autoregulation, or when other disturbances such as sodium depletion are superimposed on low renal perfusion pressure.[27,39] Clinically, the importance of the constrictor effect of Ang II on efferent arterioles becomes especially important in patients with bilateral renal artery stenosis or stenosis of a solitary kidney. In such cases, Ang II blockade may cause severe decreases in GFR.[44,45]

Ang II blockade is protective in overperfused kidneys. Normally, renin-angiotensin system activity is decreased under conditions of increased glomerular pressure, but in diabetes mellitus and certain forms of hypertension associated with glomerulosclerosis and nephron loss, the suppression in activity often is incomplete.[46–51] In such instances, Ang II blockade, by decreasing efferent arteriolar resistance, lowers hydrostatic pressure and wall stress in the overperfused glomerular capillaries, which is of considerable benefit in attenuating the progression of renal injury as well as the hypertension.[46–51] Glomerular injury decreases renal sodium excretory capability, thus shifting the pressure-natriuresis relationship so that a higher arterial pressure becomes necessary to raise renal perfusion pressure sufficiently to maintain sodium balance. However, the further rise in glomerular hydrostatic pressure causes additional glomerular injury, and a vicious cycle is set in motion.[52–55]

Under conditions of nephron overperfusion, therefore, Ang II blockade increases sodium excretory capability, in part by preventing or attenuating further decreases in GFR. This protection of the glomeruli is due partly to the efferent arteriolar dilator effect of Ang II blockade. Clinical and experimental studies indicate that Ang II blockers, in fact, are more effective than other anti-hypertensive agents in preventing glomerular injury, even with similar reductions in systemic arterial pressure.[46–51] Thus, the efferent arteriolar dilator effect of Ang II blockade can be exploited as an additional mechanism for protecting the glomerulus from the injurious effects of chronic increases in nephron perfusion pressure and becomes an important component of the antihypertensive effect of Ang II blockade by preserving renal sodium excretory capability.

Does Angiotensin II Blockade Protect the Glomerulus through Nonhemodynamic Effects?

In addition to its hemodynamic effects, Ang II has been hypothesized to cause glomerular injury through direct actions that promote growth of vascular smooth muscle, increased collagen formation, and production of extracellular matrix by glomerular mesangial cells.[56,57] It follows, therefore, that the glomeruloprotective effect of Ang II blockade may be due to attenuation of direct tissue effects of Ang II. However, most evidence supporting this role for Ang II in modulating glomerular structure comes from in vitro studies, which often use supraphysiologic concentrations (10^{-6} or higher) to demonstrate such effects. In addition, although some in vivo studies have reported greater renoprotective effects of Ang II blockers compared with other antihypertensive drugs, the studies in many cases did not control for differences in hemodynamic effects, especially the decreases in glomerular hydrostatic pressure and wall stress that result from efferent arteriolar dilation.

An observation that is difficult to reconcile with the concept that Ang II directly mediates renal injury through nonhemodynamic mechanisms is the finding that physiologic activation of the renin-angiotensin system by renal artery stenosis or sodium depletion is not associated with vascular, glomerular, or tubulointerstitial injury as long as the kidney is not overperfused or exposed to increased blood pressure.[58,59] For example, the clipped kidney of the two-kidney, one-clip Goldblatt model of hypertension is exposed to high levels of Ang II, but it is protected from increased arterial pressure by the clip on the renal artery and has no visible glomerulosclerosis or interstitial injury.[58] On the other hand, the nonclipped kidney, exposed to lower Ang II concentrations but much higher renal perfusion pressure, has marked glomerular and tubulointerstitial injury.[58] These observations suggest that the hemodynamic effects of Ang II rather than some direct action at the tissue or cellular level are responsible for renal injury. It also is possible that Ang II has direct growth-promoting effects that require increased blood pressure (or glomerular pressure) for expression. In either case, the glomeruloprotective effect of Ang II blockade may be due, in large part, to lowering of glomerular hydrostatic pressure through dilation of the different arteriole and decreased systemic arterial pressure.

Angiotensin II Increases Renal Tubular Sodium Reabsorption

Although Ang II blockade preserves GFR in overperfused kidneys by lowering glomerular hydrostatic pressure, in most physiologic conditions Ang II controls sodium excretion by increasing tubular reabsorption.[27,39] However, inappropriately elevated Ang II levels may shift natriuresis to higher pressures due to cumulative glomerular injury that occurs over years (Fig. 5). Thus Ang II can have

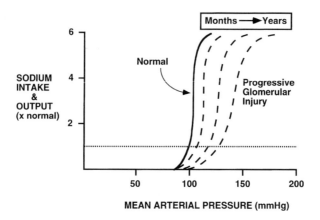

Figure 5. Predicted shift of the renal pressure-natriuresis relationship during prolonged exposure of the glomeruli to increased hydrostatic pressure. With progressive nephron loss under these conditions, as experienced in poorly controlled diabetes, the kidneys have a growing impairment in sodium excretory capability. Thus, sodium balance is maintained at the expense of higher arterial pressure, which contributes further to the glomerular injury process. A gradual decrease in slope may occur, denoting salt-sensitivity, because heterogeneity of nephrons in the damaged kidneys may impair the responsiveness of renin secretion to varying sodium intakes. (Laragh JH, Sealey JE: Renin system understanding for analysis and treatment of hypertensive patients. In Laragh JH, Brenner BM (eds): Hypertension: Pathophysiology, Diagnosis, and Management, 2nd ed. New York, Raven Press, 1995.)

a significant effect on GFR over the long term, but it normally functions to control blood pressure via its effect of increasing renal tubular sodium reabsorption. The rapid and powerful effect of Ang II blockade to enhance renal sodium excretory capability and lower arterial pressure, therefore, occurs mainly through prevention of the effects of Ang II on renal sodium reabsorption.

The sodium-retaining actions of Ang II are mediated, in part, through its effect to stimulate aldosterone secretion.[39] This mechanism is important, and at least some basal amount of aldosterone must be present to prevent unabated renal sodium loss. However, the direct intrarenal actions of Ang II appear to be quantitatively more important than the effects of aldosterone in causing sodium retention.[39] This effect is due to the vascular and tubular actions of Ang II within the kidneys.

Ang II increases reabsorption in part through its vasoconstrictor actions. Ang II-mediated constriction of efferent arterioles not only stabilizes GFR but also reduces renal blood flow and peritubular capillary hydrostatic pressure and increases peritubular colloid osmotic pressure as a result of increased filtration fraction. These changes reduce renal interstitial fluid hydrostatic pressure and raise interstitial fluid colloid osmotic pressure, thereby increasing the driving force for fluid reabsorption across tubular epithelial cells.[60] The decreased interstitial fluid hydrostatic pressure also may reduce the permeability of luminal membrane tight junctions, thereby reducing backleak of sodium actively transported into the intercellular spaces.[60] Although such changes in the Starling forces are well documented in the proximal tubule, evidence also suggests that renal medullary blood flow and tubular reabsorption in more distal nephron segments can be affected similarly.[60,61]

Ang II also stimulates proximal tubular epithelial transport. The proximal tubule was the first site in the nephron at which Ang II was shown to stimulate epithelial transport directly. This effect occurs at low physiologic concentrations of Ang II (10^{-13} to 10^{-10} M), whereas higher concentrations (10^{-9} M or higher) inhibit reabsorption.[34,62] The stimulatory effect of Ang II is mediated by actions on the luminal and basolateral membranes, due at least in part to inhibition of adenyl cyclase and increased phospholipase C activity.[63,64] Ang II stimulates the sodium-hydrogen antiporter on the luminal membrane and increases sodium-potassium-adenosine triphosphatase activity and sodium/bicarbonate cotransport on the basolateral membrane.[63,65,66] These actions greatly increase proximal tubular reabsorption by increasing sodium entry into epithelial cells and sodium extrusion into the interstitial fluid for uptake by the peritubular capillaries.

There is much less information about the effects of angiotensin on segments beyond the proximal tubule, but several lines of evidence suggest that Ang II directly increases reabsorption in most of these segments. Indirect evidence supporting this effect is that Ang II can reduce sodium excretion to virtually zero without decreases in GFR, suggesting a powerful effect at distal nephron sites, where final processing of the urine takes place. Specific binding of Ang II has been demonstrated in the ascending limb of the loop of Henle, the distal convoluted tubule, and the cortical medullary collecting tubules. In addition, autoradiographic studies indicate a high concentration of Ang II receptors in the renal medulla.[67] In vivo microperfusion studies also have demonstrated that Ang II increases bicarbonate reabsorption in the loop of Henle[68] and stimulates sodium/potassium/chloride transport in the medullary thick ascending loop of Henle.[69] Thus, it is likely that Ang II acts at multiple nephron sites in addition to the proximal tubule to increase sodium reabsorption.

Angiotensin II Increases Tubuloglomerular Feedback Sensitivity

Tubuloglomerular feedback (TGF) describes the mechanism whereby increases in sodium chloride delivery to the macula densa generates a signal for constriction of the afferent arteriole.[39] Decreases in delivery have the opposite effect, and GFR is adjusted to return macula densa sodium chloride delivery toward normal. Thus, this feedback mechanism is an important controller of renal sodium chloride excretion. The precise signal sensed by the macula densa is uncertain, but it is closely related to sodium chloride transport by these cells.[70]

Multiple studies have shown that Ang II enhances and Ang II blockade decreases TGF sensitivity.[71] It is unlikely that Ang II mediates its effect on TGF by acting directly on the afferent arteriole, however, because Ang II has essentially no direct constrictor effect on the afferent arteriole at physiologic concentrations. Other vasoconstrictors that have such a direct effect (e.g., norepinephrine) do not increase TGF sensitivity. Considerable evidence, on the other hand, indicates that Ang II may amplify TGF sensitivity by stimulating macula densa transport of sodium chloride. AT1 binding receptors are present on macula densa cells,[72] and recent studies by Bell and Petri-Peterdi indicate that Ang II, in physiologic concentrations, stimulates macula densa basolateral sodium-hydrogen exchange.[73] Whether Ang II stimulates other transporters in macula densa cells, such as the sodium-potassium-chloride cotransporter, remains to be determined, but a stimulatory effect of Ang II on this transporter in the neighboring cells of the thick ascending loop of Henle renders this theory plausible. Thus, if Ang II

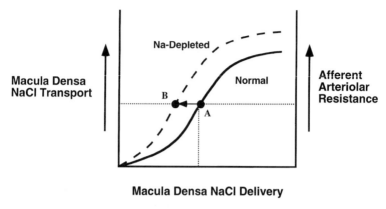

Macula Densa NaCl Delivery

Figure 6.   Postulated relationships between macula densa sodium chloride delivery and transport and afferent arteriolar resistance under normal conditions and when angiotensin II levels are increased on a low-sodium diet. The effect of angiotensin II in increasing TGF sensitivity prevents the decrease in afferent resistance that otherwise would occur at the same rate of delivery.

stimulates sodium-chloride transport by the macula densa cells, as it does in other cells, including the loop of Henle, it also shifts the relationship between distal sodium chloride delivery and macula densa transport, thereby amplifying TGF sensitivity (Fig. 6). For a given rate of sodium chloride delivery, a greater rate of sodium chloride transport by the macula densa cells and a greater degree of afferent arteriolar constriction will occur in the presence of Ang II.

The effect of Ang II on macula densa sodium chloride transport and TGF sensitivity is a key factor underlying the powerful antinatriuretic effect of Ang II, because it permits decreases in distal sodium chloride delivery without compensatory increases in GFR via TGF. Similarly, by attenuating TGF sensitivity, Ang II blockade can increase distal sodium chloride delivery without compensatory constriction of the afferent arteriole and decreases in GFR. Without blocking the effect of Ang II on macula densa cells, all of the other renal actions of Ang II blockade to increase sodium excretory capability would be much less effective because of the powerful counterregulation by TGF. The effect of Ang II blockade to blunt TGF sensitivity, therefore, can be considered an important action underlying increased renal excretory capability and the chronic antihypertensive response.

■ Conclusion

The level at which arterial pressure is maintained in the steady state, whether in a normotensive or hypertensive person, is the pressure necessary to maintain sodium balance. The volume changes that accompany changes in renal sodium handling do not permit homeostasis within the circulatory system. The maintenance of sodium balance, in turn, is determined by a balance among all of the natriuretic and antinatriuretic forces acting on the kidneys. One of the most important antinatriuretic forces is Ang II, which changes in accordance with sodium intake to adjust sodium excretion appropriately. Another important force is arterial pressure, which restores sodium balance when other mechanisms fail—for example when Ang II levels cannot be suppressed in patients on a high-salt diet.

Ang II increases renal tubular sodium reabsorption by stimulating tubular transport at multiple sites and through the effect of efferent arteriolar constriction to change peritubular capillary forces to favor reabsorption. These actions are beneficial when sodium intake is low but deleterious when Ang II levels are not adequately suppressed on a high-salt diet or when arterial pressure increases through other mechanisms. By remaining elevated, Ang II keeps arterial pressure elevated, which may lead to injury throughout the circulatory system. This effect is compounded in the kidneys, because the efferent arteriolar constrictor action causes even higher elevations in glomerular capillary pressure. The increased pressure leads to further glomerular injury, and even greater increases in arterial pressure become necessary to maintain sodium balance. Hence, a vicious cycle, culminating in renal failure, ensues. Because of the influence that Ang II exerts on arterial pressure control and glomerular capillary integrity, Ang II blockade is highly effective in treating hypertension. Moreover, because the influence of Ang II is so powerful, blockade of Ang II when plasma levels are normal or even reduced can be of considerable benefit, particularly when many factors, as in diabetes, conspire to raise glomerular hydrostatic pressure.

Acknowledgments

The authors' research is supported by National Heart Lung and Blood Institute grants HL51971 and HL56259 and by the American Heart Association.

References

1. Starling EH: The Mercer's Company Lectures on the Fluids of the Body. London, Constable 1909.
2. Coleman TG, Bower JD, Langford HG, Guyton AC: Regulation of arterial pressure in the anephric state. Circulation 42:509–514, 1970.
3. Borst JGG, Borst-de Geus A: Hypertension explained by Starling's theory of circulatory homeostasis. Lancet 1:677–682, 1963.
4. Guyton AC, Coleman TG: Quantitative analysis of the pathophysiology of hypertension. Circ Res 24(Suppl I):I-1–I-19, 1969.
5. Ledingham JH, Cohen RD: Changes in the extracellular fluid volume and cardiac output during the development of experimental renal hypertension. Canad Med Ass J 90:292–297, 1964.
6. Guyton AC, Coleman TG, Bower JD, Granger HJ: Circulatory control in hypertension. Circ Res 24(Suppl II):I-1–I-19, 1970.
7. Guyton AC, Granger HJ, Coleman TG: Autoregulation of the total systemic circulation and its relation to control of cardiac output and arterial pressure. Circ Res 28(Suppl I):I-93–I-97, 1971.
8. Coleman TG, Granger HJ, Guyton AC: Whole-body circulatory autoregulation and hypertension. Circ Res 28(Suppl II):II-76–II-87, 1971.
9. Guyton AC, Coleman TG, Granger HJ: Circulation: Overall regulation. Annu Rev Physiol 34:13–46, 1972.
10. Guyton AC, Coleman TG, Cowley AW Jr, et al: Arterial pressure regulation. Am J Med 52:584–594, 1972.
11. Hall JE, Mizelle HL, Hildebrandt DA, Brands MW: Abnormal pressure natriuresis: A cause or consequence of hypertension? Hypertension 15:547–559, 1990.
12. Selkurt EE: Effect of pulse pressure and mean arterial pressure modification on renal hemodynamics and electrolyte and water excretion. Circulation 4:541–549, 1951.
13. Langston JB, Guyton AC, Gillespie WJ: Acute effect of changes in renal arterial pressure and sympathetic blockade on kidney function. Am J Physiol 197:595–601, 1959.
14. Guyton AC: Physiologic regulation of arterial pressure. Am J Cardiol 8:401–407, 1961.
15. Roman RJ: Pressure diuresis mechanisms in the control of renal function and arterial pressure. Fed Proc 45:2878–2884, 1986.
16. Hall JE, Granger JP, Hester RL, et al: Mechanisms of escape from sodium retention during angiotensin II hypertension. Am J Physiol 246:F627–F634, 1984.
17. Hall JE, Granger JP, Smith MJ Jr, Premen AJ: Role of renal hemodynamics and arterial pressure in aldosterone "escape." Hypertension 6(Suppl I):I-1183–I192, 1984.

18. Hall JE, Mizelle HL, Woods LL, Montani J-P: Pressure natriuresis and control of arterial pressure during chronic norepinephrine infusion. J Hypertens 6:723–731, 1988.
19. Woods LL, Mizelle HL, Hall JE: Control of sodium excretion in NE-ACTH hypertension: Role of pressure natriuresis. Am J Physiol 255:R894–R900, 1988.
20. Brands MW, Hall JE: Renal perfusion pressure is an important determinant of sodium and calcium excretion in DOC-salt hypertension. Am J Hypertens 11:1199–1207, 1998.
21. Huang M, Hester RL, Coleman TG, et al: Development of hypertension in animals with reduced total peripheral resistance. Hypertension 20:828–833, 1992.
22. Guyton AC: Circulatory Physiology: Cardiac Output and Its Regulation. Philadelphia, W.B. Saunders, 1963.
23. Guyton AC: Regulation of cardiac output. N Eng J Med 277:805–812, 1967.
24. Guyton AC: Long-term arterial pressure control: An analysis from animal experiments and computer and graphic models. Am J Physiol 259:R865–R877, 1990.
25. Folkow B, Hallback M, Lundgren Y, et al: Importance of adaptive changes in vascular design for establishment of primary hypertension, studied in man and in spontaneously hypertensive rats. Circ Res 32/33(Suppl I):12–38, 1973.
26. Hall JE, Guyton AC, Smith MJ Jr, Coleman TG: Blood pressure and renal function during chronic changes in sodium intake: Role of angiotensin. Am J Physiol 239:F271–F280, 1980.
27. Hall JE: Control of sodium excretion by angiotensin II: Intrarenal mechanisms and blood pressure regulation. Am J Physiol 250:R960–R972, 1986.
28. Laragh JH, Sealey JE: Renin system understanding for analysis and treatment of hypertensive patients. In Laragh JH, Brenner BM (eds): Hypertension: Pathophysiology, Diagnosis, and Management, 2nd ed. New York, Raven Press, 1995.
29. Melaragno MG, Fink GD: Slow pressor effect of angiotensin II in normotensive rats with renal artery stenosis. Clin Exp Pharm Physiol 23:140–144, 1996.
30. Simon G, Cserep G, Limas C: Development of structural vascular changes with subpressor angiotensin II administration in rats. Am J Hypertens 8:67–73, 1995.
31. Olsen ME, Hall JE, Montani J-P, et al: Mechanisms of angiotensin II natriuresis and antinatriuresis. Am J Physiol 249:F299–F307, 1985.
32. Louis WJ, Doyle AE: The effects of varying doses of angiotensin on renal function and blood pressure in man and dogs. Clin Sci 29:489–504, 1965.
33. Navar LG, Langford HG: Effects of angiotensin on the renal circulation. In Page IH, Bumpus FM (eds): Angiotensin. New York, Springer-Verlag, 1974, pp 455–474.
34. Harris PJ, Young JA: Dose-dependent stimulation and inhibition of proximal tubular sodium reabsorption by angiotensin II in the rat kidney. Pflugers Archiv 367:295–297, 1977.
35. Edwards RM: Segmental effects of norepinephrine and angiotensin II on isolated renal microvessels. Am J Physiol 244:F526–F534, 1983.
36. DeClue JW, Guyton AC, Cowley AW Jr, et al: Subpressor angiotensin infusion: Renal sodium handling and salt-induced hypertension in the dog. Circ Res 43:503–512, 1978.
37. Hall JE, Guyton AC, Salgado HC, et al: Renal hemodynamics in acute and chronic angiotensin II hypertension. Am J Physiol 235:F174–F179, 1978.
38. Lohmeier TE, Cowley AW Jr: Hypertensive and renal effects of chronic low level intrarenal angiotensin infusion in the dog. Circ Res 44:154–160, 1979.
39. Hall JE, Guyton AC, Brands MW: Control of sodium excretion and arterial pressure by intrarenal mechanisms and the renin-angiotensin system. In Laragh JH, Brenner BM (eds): Hypertension: Pathophysiology, Diagnosis and Management, 2nd ed. New York, Raven Press, 1995, pp 1451–1475.
40. Hall JE, Guyton AC, Jackson TE, et al: Control of glomerular filtration rate by the renin-angiotensin system. Am J Physiol 233:F355–F372, 1977.
41. Hall JE, Guyton AC, Cowley AW Jr: Dissociation of renal blood flow and filtration rate autoregulation by renin depletion. Am J Physiol 232:F215–F221, 1977.
42. Hall JE, Guyton AC, Smith MJ Jr, Coleman TG: Chronic blockade of angiotensin II formation during sodium deprivation. Am J Physiol 237:F424–F432, 1979.
43. Hall JE, Coleman TG, Guyton AC, et al: Intrarenal role of angiotensin II and [des-asp1]angiotensin II. Am J Physiol 236:F232–F239, 1979.
44. Hricik DE: Captopril-induced renal insufficiency and the role of sodium balance. Ann Intern Med 103:222–223, 1985.
45. Textor SC, Tarazi RC, Novick AC, et al: Regulation of renal haemodynamics and glomerular filtration in patients with reno vascular hypertension during converting enzyme inhibition with captopril. Am J Med 76:29–37, 1984.
46. Anderson S, Rennke HG, Brenner BM: Therapeutic advantage of converting enzyme inhibitors in arresting progressive renal disease associated with systemic hypertension in the rat. J Clin Invest 77:1993–2000, 1986.

47. Perico N, Amuchastegui CS, Malanchini B, et al: Angiotensin-converting enzyme inhibition and calcium channel blockade both normalize early hyperfiltration in experimental diabetes, but only the former prevents late renal structural damage. Exp Nephrol 2:220–228, 1994.

48. Zatz R, Dunn BR, Meyer TW, et al: Prevention of diabetic glomerulopathy by pharmacological amelioration of glomerular capillary hypertension. J Clin Invest 77:1925–1930, 1986.

49. Bohlen L, de Courten M, Weidmann P: Comparative study of the effect of ACE inhibitors and other antihypertensive agents on proteinuria in diabetic patients. Am J Hypertens 7:84S–92S, 1994.

50. Breyer JA: Medical management of nephropathy in type I diabetes mellitus: Current recommendations. J Am Soc Nephrol 6:1523–1529, 1995.

51. Cooper ME: Renal protection and angiotensin converting enzyme inhibition in microalbuminuric type I and type II diabetic patients. J Hypertens 14(Suppl 6):S11–S14, 1996.

52. Ritz E, Fliser D, Nowicki M: Hypertension and vascular disease as complications of diabetes. In Laragh JH, Brenner BM (eds): Hypertension: Pathophysiology, Diagnosis, and Management, 2nd ed. New York, Raven Press, 1995, pp 2321–2334.

53. Hostetter TH: Diabetic nephropathy. In Brenner BM, Recter FC Jr (eds): The Kidney, 4th ed. Philadelphia, W.B. Saunders, 1991, pp 1695–1727.

54. Mogensen CE: Management of the diabetic patient with elevated blood pressure or renal disease. In Laragh JH, Brenner BM (eds): Hypertension: Pathophysiology, Diagnosis, and Management, 2nd ed. New York, Raven Press, 1995, pp 2335–2365.

55. Parving HH, Smidt UM, Hommel E, et al: Effective antihypertensive treatment postpones renal insufficiency in diabetic nephropathy. Am J Kidney Dis 22:188–195, 1993.

56. Matsuaka M, Hymes J, Ichikawa I: Angiotensin in progressive renal diseases: Theory and practice. J Am Soc Nephrol 7:2025–2043, 1996.

57. Ketteler M, Noble NA, Border WA: Transforming growth factor-B and angiotensin: The missing link from glomerular hyperfiltration to glomerulosclerosis? Annu Rev Physiol 57:279–295, 1995.

58. Eng E, Veniants M, Floege J, et al: Renal proliferative and phenotypic changes in rats with two-kidney, one-clip Goldblatt hypertension. Am J Hypertens 7:177–185, 1994.

59. Mauer SM, Steffes MW, Azar S, et al: The effects of Goldblatt hypertension on development of the glomerular lesions of diabetes mellitus in the rat. Diabetes 27:738–744, 1978.

60. Knox FG, Burnett JC Jr, Kohran DE, et al: Escape from the sodium-retaining effects of mineralocorticoids. Kidney Int 17:263–276, 1980.

61. Cowley AW Jr: Long-term control of arterial blood pressure. Physiol Rev 72:231–300, 1992.

62. Schuster VL: Effects of angiotensin on proximal tubular reabsorption. Fed Proc 45:1444–1447, 1986.

63. Liu FY, Cogan MG: Angiotensin II stimulates early proximal bicarbonate absorption in the rat by decreasing cyclic adenosine monophosphate. J Clin Invest 84:83–91, 1989.

64. Schelling JR, Singh H, Marzec R, Linas S: Angiotensin II-dependent proximal tubular sodium transport is mediated by cAMP modulation of phospholipase C. Am J Physiol 267:C1239–C1245, 1994.

65. Garvin JL: Angiotensin stimulates bicarbonate transport and Na^+/K^+ ATPase in rat proximal straight tubules. J Am Soc Nephrol 1:1146–1152, 1991.

66. Geibel J, Giebisch G, Boron WF: Angiotensin II stimulates both Na^+-H^+ exchange and Na^+/HCO_3^- cotransport in the rabbit proximal tubule. Proc Nat Acad Sci 87:7917–7920, 1990.

67. Mendelsohn FAO, Dunbar M, Allen A, et al: Angiotensin II receptors in the kidney. Fed Proc 45:1420–1425, 1986.

68. Capasso G, Unwin R, Ciani F, et al: Bicarbonate transport along the loop of Henle. II: Effects of acid-base, dietary and neurohumoral determinants. J Clin Invest 94:830–838, 1994.

69. Amlal H, LeGoff C, Vernimmen C, et al: Ang II controls Na^+-$K^+(NH_4^+)$-$2Cl^-$ cotransport via 20-HETE and PKC in medullary thick ascending limb. Am J Physiol 274:C1047–C1056, 1998.

70. Schnermann J: Juxtaglomerular cell complex in the regulation of renal salt excretion. Am J Physiol 274:R263–R279, 1998.

71. Navar LG, Inscho EW, Majid DSA, et al: Paracrine regulation of the renal microcirculation. Physiol Rev 76:425–536, 1996.

72. Harrison-Bernard LM, Navar LG, Ho MM, et al: Immunohistochemical localization of Ang II, AT_1 receptor in adult rat kidney using a monoclonal antibody. Am J Physiol 273:F170–F177, 1997.

73. Bell PD, Peti-Peterdi J: Angiotensin II stimulates macula densa basolateral sodium/hydrogen exchange via type 1 angiotensin II receptors. J Am Soc Nephrol 10(Suppl 11):S225–S229, 1999.

CHAPTER 13

Renal Actions of Angiotensin II and AT$_1$ Receptor Blockers

L. GABRIEL NAVAR, Ph.D.
LISA M. HARRISON-BERNARD, Ph.D.
JOHN D. IMIG, Ph.D.
KENNETH D. MITCHELL, Ph.D.

The renin-angiotensin system, in general, and intrarenal angiotensin II (Ang II), in particular, exert a cardinal role in the pathophysiology of many forms of hypertension.[1-3] Inappropriate overactivity of the renin-angiotensin system leads to powerful hypertensinogenic actions mediated, for the most part, by activation of AT$_1$ receptors, which are widely distributed among many different organs and cell types.[4,5] The development of highly selective AT$_1$ receptor antagonists that block these actions offers great promise for the treatment of many forms of hypertension.[6] The ever-increasing use of these therapeutic agents highlights the need to obtain more detailed knowledge about the multiple actions of Ang II and the consequences of both acute and long-term treatment with AT$_1$ receptor blockers.

Although several other angiotensin peptides have biologic effects,[7-10] Ang II is of greatest significance in mediating hypertension.[1,4] Ang II is derived from angiotensinogen, which is formed primarily by the liver and constitutively secreted,[11] but it also is formed in other organs, including the kidney (Fig. 1).[12-15] Circulating angiotensinogen concentrations are high in most species—many times greater than the concentrations of Ang I and Ang II.[16,17] Because substrate is so abundant, the rate of Ang I formation in the circulation is limited primarily by available active renin, which is released by the juxtaglomerular cells of the kidney. Ang II is generated by angiotensin-converting enzyme (ACE) located on endothelial cells in many vascular beds and on membranes of various other cell types.[18] The resultant increases in Ang II exert powerful actions throughout the body. Ang II directly constricts vascular smooth muscle cells, enhances myocardial contractility, stimulates aldosterone release, stimulates release of catecholamines from the adrenal medulla and sympathetic nerve endings, increases sympathetic nervous system activity, stimulates thirst and salt appetite, and regulates sodium transport by epithelial cells in intestine and kidney.[1,19-24] Ang II

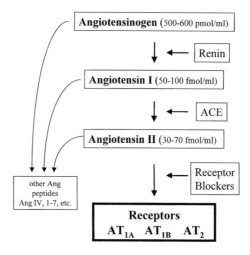

Figure 1. The renin-angiotensin system with representative plasma concentrations from rats. The key steps by which pharmacologic antagonists or blockers interfere with the system are shown.

also exerts significant long-term proliferative effects that can lead to tissue injury when inappropriately activated.[25-29]

Of the two major Ang II receptor subtypes, AT_1 and AT_2 (Fig. 2), AT_1 is the most abundant in adults. The major hypertensinogenic effects are caused by activation of AT_1 receptors. Indeed, several studies have suggested that AT_2 receptors exert counter actions that partially buffer the effects of the AT_1 receptors.[30-32] In rodents, two AT_1 receptor subtypes have been identified—AT_{1A} and AT_{1B}[33-35]—but their actions are thought to be similar. Both are blocked by AT_1 receptor blockers. This chapter focuses on the critical role exerted by intrarenal Ang II in the development and maintenance of hypertension, the unique mechanisms responsible for the regulation of intrarenal Ang II, the cascading effects of Ang II that lead to

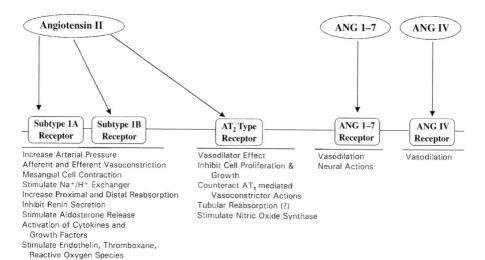

Figure 2. Types of angiotensin receptors and their demonstrated or suggested actions.

sodium retention through both vascular and tubular mechanisms, and the ability of AT_1 receptor antagonists to block these effects.

■ *Intrarenal Angiotensin II Receptors*

The AT_1 and AT_2 subtypes have been characterized pharmacologically[36] and cloned.[37–43] Both AT_{1A} and AT_{1B} subtypes in rodents[33,34] have seven transmembrane domains typical of G protein-coupled receptors. Ang II-mediated signal transduction through the AT_{1A} and AT_{1B} subtypes involves activation of G-proteins of the Gq/G11 family, which subsequently activate phospholipase C and thus result in mobilization of intracellular calcium (Ca^{2+}) and activation of protein kinase C.[35,44–50] Stimulation of the AT_2 receptor has been shown to activate protein-phosphotyrosine phosphatase.[51,52]

Intrarenal Ang II receptors are widely distributed on the luminal and basolateral membranes of several segments of the nephron as well as on the renal microvasculature in both cortex and medulla.[53–60] In vitro autoradiographic studies by Mendelsohn and associates[54,57,61] localized Ang II receptor-binding in afferent and efferent arterioles, glomerular mesangial cells, the inner stripe of the outer medulla, and renal medullary interstitial cells. Radioligand-binding experiments confirmed that most of the angiotensin receptors on the renal vasculature are of the AT_1 type.[5,62] Studies using both polyclonal and monoclonal antibodies to the AT_1 receptor also have identified abundant AT_1 receptors widely distributed throughout the kidney. AT_1 receptor protein has been localized to afferent and efferent arteriolar smooth muscle cells, epithelia of the thick ascending limb of the loop of Henle, proximal tubular brush border, and mesangial cells.[56] Harrison-Bernard et al.[58] extended these findings using a monoclonal antibody that recognized both AT_{1A} and AT_{1B} receptors. They found AT_1 receptors in proximal tubule brush border and basolateral membranes, distal tubules, collecting ducts, glomerular podocytes, and macula densa cells.[58] Extensive luminal localization of AT_1 receptors in both proximal and distal nephron segments was observed (Fig. 3). More recent studies using an AT_{1A}-specific polyclonal antibody[59] and a polyclonal AT_1 receptor antibody[60] have reported a similar distribution. AT_1 and AT_2 receptors also have been found on glomerular epithelial cells; of interest, Ang II caused accumulation of cyclic adenosine monophosphate (cAMP), which was blocked only by the combined use of both AT_1 and AT_2 receptor blockers.[63]

In situ hybridization histochemistry has been used to localize the AT_1 mRNA in various segments of the kidney. AT_1 mRNA has been localized to tubule cells of the outer medulla, proximal tubules, thick ascending limb of the loop of Henle,[64] glomeruli, arterial vasculature, vasa recta,[65] and juxtaglomerular cells.[66] Using the RT-PCR technique in microdissected nephron segments, Terada et al.[67] detected AT_1 transcripts in glomeruli, proximal convoluted and straight tubules, medullary thick ascending limbs, medullary collecting ducts, cortical collecting ducts, vasa recta bundles and arcuate arteries. High levels of AT_1 mRNA also have been shown in proximal tubule primary cultures, freshly isolated proximal tubule segments,[35,55] and immortalized rabbit cortical collecting-duct cells.[68] AT_{1B} mRNA expression also has been demonstrated in proximal tubules and collecting tubules.[69] AT_{1A} and AT_{1B} mRNAs have been demonstrated in the glomerulus and all nephron segments, including the proximal tubule, distal tubule, thick ascending limb, and collecting ducts.[35,60] The AT_{1A} mRNA was the predominant

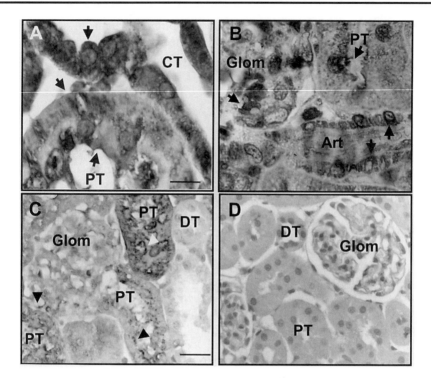

Figure 3.   Immunohistochemical localization of AT_1 receptors *(A, B, arrows)* and angiotensinogen *(C, arrowheads)* in the rat renal cortex. *A*, AT_1 receptors on luminal and basolateral membranes of a proximal tubule (PT) and connecting tubule/collecting duct (CT). *B*, AT_1 receptors located on vascular smooth muscle cells of the afferent arteriole (Art), glomerular (Glom) mesangial cells, and PT. *C*, Predominant PT localization of angiotensinogen. Glomerular capillary endothelia also show angiotensinogen immunostaining. Distal tubules (DT) do not contain angiotensinogen. When primary antibody is omitted, no positive immunostaining is detected *(D)*. Bars are 10 microns for *A* and *B* and 25 microns for *C* and *D*.

subtype (72–94% of total AT_1 mRNA) in all nephron segments, whereas the AT_{1B} (60%) was more abundant than AT_{1A} only in the glomerulus. A similar ratio of AT_{1A} and AT_{1B} expression has been reported for isolated preglomerular resistance vessels of the kidney.[35,70]

In rats the AT_2 receptor is highly expressed in the kidney during fetal life and decreases dramatically in adulthood.[71] The AT_2 receptor protein has been localized to the glomeruli of the adult rat using immunohistochemical staining.[59] AT_2 receptor immunostaining also has been localized in proximal tubules, collecting ducts, and parts of the renal vasculature.[60] The role of AT_2 receptors in regulating renal function remains uncertain, but recent findings indicate that AT_2 activation counteracts AT_1 receptor effects by stimulating formation of bradykinin and nitric oxide, thus increasing renal interstitial fluid concentrations of cyclic guanosine monophosphate (GMP).[30–32,51] Ang II infusions into AT_2 knockout mice caused a greater degree of hypertension and reductions in renal function, which were thought to be due to the lack of increased renal interstitial fluid levels of bradykinin and cyclic GMP available to counteract the direct effects of Ang II.[32]

■ *Intrarenal Angiotensin II*

Intrarenal Ang II is formed primarily as a consequence of the actions of ACE, which is abundantly distributed on tubules and vascular tissue.[18,72–74] Although much of the Ang I is converted to Ang II in the circulation, Ang II formed within the kidney may contribute to a greater extent to the intrarenal Ang II content.[1,75–78] In many organs, it is difficult to delineate the influences of locally generated Ang II versus those of systemically delivered Ang II. In a few tissues, such as the adrenal gland and the kidney, however, the high tissue levels of Ang II provide clear evidence that local concentrations of Ang II are far greater than can be explained solely on the basis of equilibration with circulating concentrations.[16,17,79,80] These findings thus indicate that a major fraction of Ang II in the kidney is formed locally. Because substantial metabolism and degradation of the angiotensin peptides also occur intrarenally, estimates of intrarenal Ang II generation based on differences in arterial and venous concentrations do not reveal the extent of intrarenal formation.[81]

All of the precursors and enzymatic mechanisms needed for Ang II formation are present in the kidney and lead to a complex processing system (Fig. 4). Ang II can be formed intrarenally from Ang I delivered in the circulation as well as from locally generated Ang I. Likewise, Ang I may be derived from the circulation or from locally synthesized angiotensinogen.[3] Both angiotensinogen and angiotensinogen mRNA have been localized in the cells of the proximal tubule.[12–14,82] Angiotensinogen secretion was demonstrated recently in proximal tubule cell cultures treated with dexamethasone and isoproterenol.[83] Renin is secreted by the cells of the juxtaglomerular apparatus into the renal interstitium and thus can act on intrarenal angiotensinogen to generate Ang I. ACE is abundant in the kidney and is located at several sites, including endothelial cells of the renal microvessels and proximal tubule brush border membranes. Recent studies indicate that intrarenal ACE activity is increased in experimental hypertension.[84–87]

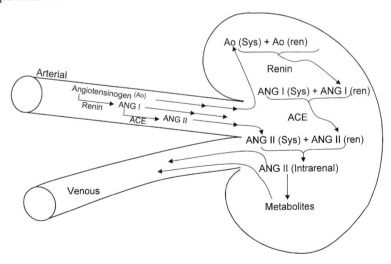

Figure 4.   Intrarenal processing of the renin-angiotensin system. All components of the renin-angiotensin system are present in the kidney. Sys = systemically delivered, ren = synthesized in the kidney.

The abundance of all components of the renin-angiotensin system within the kidney helps to explain why intrarenal tissue levels of Ang II expressed per gram of wet weight are much greater than plasma Ang II concentrations expressed per ml of plasma.[17,84,86] This principle also applies to Ang I content, which is higher than plasma concentrations. In addition, as a result of regional compartmentalization, the medullary Ang II content per gram of tissue is much greater than the cortical Ang II contents.[3,88] Within the cortex, both intratubular fluid and interstitial fluid concentrations are much higher than plasma concentrations. Recent evidence also has indicated that the greater intrarenal Ang II levels are due, in part, to accumulation of intact Ang II, some of which has been internalized via AT$_1$ receptors.[89]

Studies from experimental models of hypertension have contributed to our knowledge of AT$_1$ receptor-mediated internalization of Ang II. Several experimental models of hypertension, including two-kidney, one-clip (2K1C) Goldblatt hypertensive rats, Ang II-induced hypertensive rats, and Ren-2 transgenic rats, have shown that the high intrarenal levels of Ang II can be dissociated not only from circulating Ang II concentrations but also from kidney renin content.[16,84,86,90] Ang II contents in the nonclipped kidney from 2K1C Goldblatt hypertensive rats and in kidneys from Ang II-infused rats and Ren-2 transgenic rats are higher than can be explained on the basis of the circulating Ang II concentrations, even though these kidneys have been shown to be renin-depleted (Fig. 5). The Ang II-infused rats accumulate Ang II gradually over 2 weeks. The increased Ang II is functionally active and contributes to hypertension. Chronic treatment with AT$_1$ receptor blockers prevents the development of hypertension and the associated renal injury in Goldblatt hypertensive rats and Ang II-infused rats.[91,92] The observation that the increases in kidney Ang II contents were decreased by chronic treatment with the AT$_1$ receptor blocker, losartan, suggested that in this hypertensive model the augmentation of intrarenal Ang II depends in part on an AT$_1$ receptor-mediated process, perhaps involving internalization of the receptor peptide complex.[16] These results indicate that the intrarenal levels of Ang II are

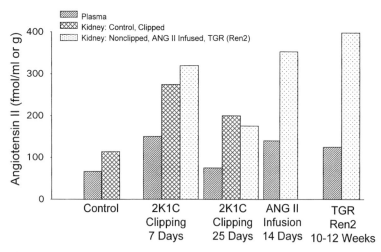

Figure 5. Comparison of kidney Ang II contents of control and hypertensive rats with corresponding plasma concentrations. Intrarenal Ang II contents expressed as fmoles/gm consistently exceed the plasma Ang II concentrations expressed as fmoles/ml.

the consequence not only of the amount delivered to the kidney but also of the amount newly formed by the kidney. They also indicate that part of the total kidney Ang II content is mediated by AT$_1$ receptor-mediated uptake of Ang II.

The finding that much of the Ang II coupled to the AT$_1$ receptor may be internalized via receptor-mediated endocytosis raises the question of how much of the kidney Ang II content in Ang II-infused hypertensive rats is internalized Ang II. Zou et al.[93] determined the relative contributions of exogenously administered and endogenously formed Ang II to the observed enhancement of intrarenal Ang II in Ang II-infused hypertensive rats. When a different form of Ang II (Val^5-Ang II) was infused, up to two-thirds of the kidney Ang II was accumulated from exogenous Ang II. The AT$_1$ receptor antagonist, losartan, prevented the intrarenal Ang II accumulation,[89] supporting the concept that Ang II is actively taken up in renal cells via AT$_1$ receptors and presumably stored in intracellular sites where it is protected from degradation.

Accumulating evidence suggests that the internalization of the AT$_1$ receptor Ang II complex does not occur for the sole purpose of trafficking Ang II to the lysosomes for degradation and recycling of the receptor. Rather, this process may be vital for some of the cellular actions of Ang II. Endocytosis of the Ang II–AT$_1$ receptor complex is important for the full expression of physiologic responses to Ang II.[94,95] In proximal tubule cells, binding of Ang II and endocytosis of the Ang II–AT$_1$ receptor complex is coupled to the activation of signal transduction pathways and sodium transport.[96–99] Studies using cultured proximal tubule cells demonstrated that endocytosis of apical AT$_1$ receptors was coupled to increases in phospholipase C, inhibition of cyclic AMP, increases in intracellular Ca^{2+}, and Ang II-induced sodium flux.[97–99] In a tubule cell line expressing rabbit AT$_1$ receptors (LLC-PK-AT1R), apical membrane AT$_1$ receptor-mediated endocytosis of Ang II stimulates phospholipase A$_2$, which is necessary for sodium flux and recycling of the AT$_1$ receptor.[96,100] Compared with the rapid internalization of the apical membrane AT$_1$ receptor complex, the basolateral membrane internalization of the AT$_1$ receptor is a slow process, not linked to activation of phospholipase A$_2$.[100] Thus, intracellular trafficking of Ang II may be important for directing Ang II to certain cellular locations for full expression of its biologic response.

Although many studies have demonstrated that Ang II is internalized via an AT$_1$ receptor-mediated process,[94,99,101–103] the amount of Ang II in intracellular compartments and its regulation have not been well delineated. A recent study by Imig et al.[104] using flow cytometry combined with radioimmunoassay analysis demonstrated the presence of Ang I, Ang II, ACE activity, and AT$_{1A}$ receptors in renal intermicrovillar clefts, an apically derived membrane fraction, and endosomes, a true intracellular compartment. Although previous studies have shown that the kidney and proximal tubule ratio of Ang I to Ang II is close to one,[3,80,105] the ratio of Ang I to Ang II in the intermicrovillar clefts and endosomes was less than 0.2. These results provide further evidence that Ang II is actively transported to the endosomal compartment. Although the endosomal contents of Ang II were not significantly different in rats fed diets containing different amounts of sodium, the rats fed a low sodium diet exhibited significantly greater AT$_{1A}$ receptor-binding than rats fed a high salt diet. In addition, inhibition of ACE activity by enalapril decreased intermicrovillar cleft and endosomal levels of Ang II. These findings support the concepts that Ang I is converted to Ang II at the proximal tubule brush border membrane; that Ang II is internalized into the cell complexed to the AT_1 receptor; and that intracellular Ang II levels are influenced by ACE activity.[106]

Regional regulation of Ang II levels within the kidney during hypertension is of interest because many studies suggest that Ang II strongly influences renal medullary hemodynamics.[76,107-109] As an example of regional differences, Ang II levels are substantially higher in the renal medulla than in the renal cortex[3,88] (Fig. 6). Both cortical and medullary Ang II contents are much greater than circulatory concentrations. Furthermore, the increase in both cortical and medullary Ang II contents in Ang II-infused rats was substantially greater than the increases in plasma concentrations. These data support the notion that elevated Ang II levels during the development of hypertension contribute significantly to functional alterations in the renal cortex and medulla. The elevated Ang II levels in the medulla may have powerful effects on renal medullary hemodynamics and tubular function. Receptor-binding studies have shown that Ang II receptor density is much greater in the medulla than in the cortex.[54,110-112]

■ Intratubular Concentrations of Angiotensin II

Interest in the generation and actions of intratubular Ang II continues to increase. As already mentioned, angiotensinogen has been localized in proximal tubule cells by immunohistochemistry,[13,113] and angiotensinogen mRNA in the kidney is expressed primarily in proximal tubule cells.[12,14,67,82] The presence of angiotensinogen mRNA in proximal tubule cells and the demonstration of Ang II receptors on the brush border membranes of proximal tubule cells are consistent with physiologic studies demonstrating an action of intratubular Ang II in the control of transport function.[114-118] Recent studies in a rat proximal tubule cell line directly support the hypothesis that Ang II can serve a positive amplification function by directly stimulating angiotensinogen mRNA production via activation of AT_1 receptors.[114] The presence of angiotensinogen in proximal tubule cells (see Fig. 3) provides evidence that at least part of the intrarenally derived Ang II is from intrarenally synthesized angiotensinogen. Much of the intrarenally formed

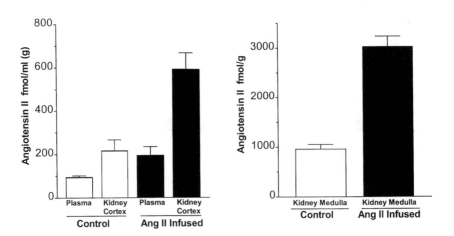

Figure 6. Comparison of plasma, renal cortical and medullary Ang II levels in normotensive and Ang II-infused hypertensive rats.

Ang II may be derived from the proximal tubule stores of angiotensinogen, but the relative contributions of intrarenal angiotensinogen and liver-derived angiotensinogen to the intrarenally formed Ang II remain undetermined.

Micropuncture studies have shown that proximal tubule fluid concentrations of Ang I and Ang II are in the range of 3–10 pmoles/ml—much higher than can be explained on the basis of the plasma concentrations.[119-121] In microperfusion experiments, Braam et al.[120] determined that concentrations of Ang II in fluid collected from perfused tubules were similar to concentrations measured in tubular fluid samples collected from filtering nephrons. These data indicate that Ang II or a precursor is secreted directly into the proximal tubule lumen by the surrounding tubular cells. In subsequent experiments, Ang I and angiotensinogen also were found in high concentrations in proximal tubule fluid, suggesting secretion of angiotensinogen directly into the tubule.[121,122] These data suggest that the angiotensinogen produced by proximal tubule cells is secreted, in part, into the proximal tubule. However, it is also possible that intracellularly generated Ang I or Ang II is secreted into the tubular fluid.

One of the major issues related to the generation of Ang I in the proximal tubule has been the source of renin. However, cultured proximal tubule cells produce renin in small quantities and contain low levels of renin mRNA, suggesting that renin may be formed in proximal tubule cells.[123,124] Leyssac[125] reported measurable renin concentrations in proximal tubule fluid and suggested that sufficient renin is filtered to allow generation of Ang I in tubular fluid. Because ACE is abundant on the proximal tubule brush border membranes, tubular Ang I easily can be converted to Ang II.[74,126,127] A recent study by Vio et al.[87] confirmed the abundance of brush border ACE and its marked upregulation in hypertension. Figure 7 provides an overall summary of the intratubular concentrations of angiotensinogen, Ang I, and Ang II and of the possible sources of proximal tubule Ang II. However, important issues are yet to be resolved. It has not been determined how much of the peptide is formed intracellularly and how much within the tubular lumen. In addition, the mechanisms regulating intratubular Ang II levels have not been delineated. Nevertheless, several studies have shown that proximal tubular fluid Ang II concentrations are maintained at

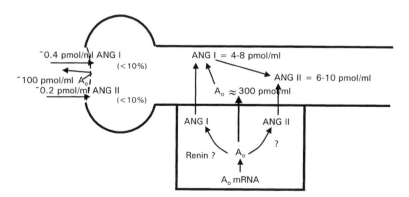

Figure 7. Schematic of proximal tubule depicting proximal tubule fluid Ang I, Ang II, and angiotensinogen (Ao) concentrations and possible sources of the high proximal tubule Ang II concentrations.

the high levels found in normal rats in nonclipped kidneys of 2K1C hypertensive rats, kidneys of Ang II-infused hypertensive rats, and kidneys from hypertensive Ren-2 transgenic rats.[90,128,129] To the extent that these hypertensive models have the same intrarenal and intratubular Ang II concentrations as normotensive rats, they can be considered as inappropriately high for the prevailing elevated blood pressure. Of interest, tubular Ang II concentrations remain at the nanomolar level in experimental models of hypertension, even though the kidneys become renin-depleted.

In addition to luminal secretion of Ang II or its precursors, evidence also suggests that local Ang II production is responsible for the relatively high interstitial fluid concentrations of Ang II. Whereas older studies relied on the analysis of lymph composition,[88] recent studies have used microdialysis probes to study the interstitial Ang II concentrations. Siragy et al.[130] reported concentrations of Ang II in the interstitial fluid that were much higher than plasma concentrations and in the same range reported for proximal tubular fluid.

■ Intrarenal Actions of Angiotensin II

Ang II exerts an important regulatory influence on proximal tubular reabsorption function primarily via activation of AT_1 receptors on both basolateral and luminal membranes. Studies using in vivo micropuncture and isolated perfused tubules have shown dose-dependent biphasic effects of peritubular Ang II on proximal tubular sodium reabsorption. Ang II concentrations in the range of 10^{-12}–10^{-10}M enhance proximal tubular reabsorption rate, whereas concentrations greater than 10^{-7}M inhibit proximal tubular reabsorption rate.[20,131] It is likely, however, that the inhibitory effects of the high interstitial Ang II levels do not occur under normal conditions because of the marked vasoconstrictor actions of such Ang II concentrations, which reduce filtration rate.[20,132] Indeed, when postglomerular interstitial Ang II levels are increased above the normal endogenous levels by either systemic or peritubular administration of Ang II, fractional proximal reabsorption rate is augmented.[20,115] The stimulatory action of Ang II on proximal tubular reabsorptive function also has been shown by the numerous studies using Ang II receptor antagonists or ACE inhibitors to unmask the preexisting influence exerted by Ang II.[20] Studies in chronically sodium-depleted rats demonstrated that both absolute and fractional proximal tubule reabsorption rates were reduced after blockade of Ang II receptors with saralasin.[133] Similarly, ACE inhibition results in marked reductions in both absolute and fractional proximal tubule reabsorption rates in the nonclipped kidney of Goldblatt hypertensive rats.[134,135] Furthermore, systemic administration of either the ACE inhibitor, captopril, or the AT_1 receptor antagonist, losartan, inhibits proximal tubular solute and fluid reabsorption in normal rats.[1,136,137] To the extent that pharmacologic blockade of the renin-angiotensin system unmasks the preexisting influence exerted by Ang II, the results obtained using pharmacologic blockers of the renin-angiotensin system indicate that the endogenous basolateral Ang II concentrations normally exert a tonic stimulatory influence on proximal tubular reabsorptive function.

Ang II also exerts proximal tubule transport effects via activation of luminal membrane AT_1 receptors. The tubular Ang II receptors are interesting because several pharmacologically distinct receptor subtypes have been identified.[138,139]

Although AT_1 receptors are much more abundant than AT_2 receptors in adults,[59] the proximal tubules have high-affinity and low-affinity receptors sensitive to the AT_1 receptor blocker, losartan, and another subtype that binds to the AT_2 receptor blocker, PD122979. Expression and function of proximal tubular Ang II receptors can be regulated in several ways, including desensitization, endocytosis, and production.[139] Chronic salt intake and ACE inhibitors can influence AT_1 receptor expression. In vivo micropuncture experiments demonstrated that intraluminal application of Ang II can enhance proximal tubule sodium and bicarbonate reabsorption through stimulatory actions on the sodium/hydrogen (Na^+/H^+) exchanger.[140] Studies in isolated proximal tubular cells showed that Ang II stimulated Na^+/H^+ exchange via an amiloride-sensitive pathway.[141]

In more recent micropuncture studies, addition of Ang II to proximal tubular fluid of normal rats did not significantly increase proximal reabsorption rate, but intraluminal addition of AT_1 blockers or ACE inhibitors reduced the proximal bicarbonate and volume reabsorption rate.[116,117,142] Proximal reabsorption rate was restored to normal levels when Ang II was added in the presence of an ACE inhibitor.[116,117] After acute volume expansion, proximal reabsorption was decreased and, under the same conditions, addition of losartan decreased proximal reabsorption rate rate to a lesser degree.[142] However, addition of Ang II to the lumen increased net proximal tubule fluid reabsorption to levels seen in control rats. These results indicate that endogenous Ang II concentrations in the proximal tubule fluid of normal anesthetized rats exert a tonic stimulatory influence on proximal reabsorption rate. Of interest, both AT_1 and AT_2 blockers appear to inhibit proximal reabsorption rate. It was recently shown that the inhibitory effects of intraluminal application of an AT_1 and an AT_2 receptor antagonist were additive.[143] These results are consistent with pressure-natriuresis studies indicating that both AT_1 and AT_2 receptor blockers augmented sodium excretion and increased the slope of the pressure-natriuresis relationship.[144] These observations indicate that AT_2 receptors contribute to the stimulatory action of intraluminal Ang II on proximal reabsorptive function and oppose the suggestion that AT_2 receptor activation exerts transport effects opposite to those of AT_1 receptor activation.[145]

Recent micropuncture studies also indicate a role for Ang II in the regulation of distal tubule reabsorption rate.[146–149] Addition of Ang II to both early and late distal tubular fluid enhanced net bicarbonate and fluid reabsorption.[148,149] These effects were blocked by either saralasin or losartan, indicating that the effects on distal tubule reabsorptive function were mediated by activation of luminal AT_1 receptors. These findings, together with the demonstration that Ang II receptors are present on distal nephron segments (see discussion of receptors), suggest an important role for luminal Ang II in the regulation not only of proximal reabsorption rate but also of distal tubule reabsorptive function.

In addition to its modulatory influence on tubular reabsorptive function, intrarenal Ang II exerts pronounced effects on the renal vasculature. Whole kidney clearance studies have demonstrated that Ang II elicits dose-dependent decreases in renal blood flow, smaller decreases in glomerular filtration rate, and increases in filtration fraction.[1,20,76] Similarly, in vivo micropuncture studies clearly demonstrate that Ang II elicits reductions in single nephron filtration rate and glomerular plasma flow.[1,150–153] These renal hemodynamic responses to Ang

II are due primarily to direct constriction of the afferent and efferent arterioles and thus increases in both pre- and postglomerular resistances.[154–157] Although it is often stated that the vasoconstrictor effects of Ang II are exerted predominantly on the efferent arterioles, this conclusion is based on the misconception that increases in filtration fraction reflect predominant efferent arteriolar constriction. However, constriction of both pre- and postglomerular resistances also increases filtration fraction.[158] Indeed, numerous studies using various preparations and methods that allow direct assessment of microvascular responses clearly demonstrate that Ang II receptors are present on afferent arterioles and that Ang II exerts powerful direct constrictor effects on afferent as well as efferent arterioles.[1,76,155] The vasoconstrictor effects are clearly due to AT_1 receptor activation, since losartan completely reversed the Ang II-induced vasoconstriction at both sites.[155] Of interest, the exact mechanisms appear to be different because the afferent vasoconstrictor effects of Ang II are blocked by the L-type calcium channel blockers, whereas the efferent effects are not.[157] Studies in dispersed afferent arteriolar vascular smooth muscle cells and preglomerular vessel segments have shown that Ang II causes most of its increase in intracellular Ca^{2+} via AT_1 receptors and activation of L-type voltage-dependent calcium channels.[159] The decreases in both whole kidney and single nephron filtration rates observed in many experimental studies are also attributable to the effects of Ang II to reduce the glomerular filtration coefficient (K_f).[76,150,153] This effect on K_f commonly has been thought to reflect the actions of the hormone on the contractility of the glomerular mesangial cells; however, the exact mechanism by which mesangial cell contraction reduces K_f remains unclear. As mentioned earlier, AT_1 and AT_2 receptors also have been identified on glomerular epithelial cells,[63] which also may influence K_f.

Previous studies have shown a high density of Ang II receptors in medullary structures as well as in the renal cortex.[61,111] Functional studies also demonstrate medullary hemodynamic responses to Ang II.[76,160] Of interest, medullary responses appear to be counteracted by several vasodilator systems, including nitric oxide, kinins, and prostaglandins.[76,161] Ang II can activate increased nitric oxide levels in the medulla to prevent its vasoconstrictor effect.[160] This finding is particularly significant in view of the high medullary content of Ang II, which is 3–4 times higher per gram of tissue than the cortical content.[3,88]

The results obtained during administration of exogenous Ang II are consistent with those obtained from studies in which inhibitors or antagonists of the renin-angiotensin system have been used to unmask the renal hemodynamic effects of endogenous Ang II. In vivo micropuncture studies demonstrate that pharmacologic blockade of the renin-angiotensin system in both normal kidneys and the nonclipped kidneys of 2K1C Goldblatt hypertensive rats results in decreases in both afferent and efferent arteriolar resistances.[1] When arterial pressure is not markedly reduced, Ang II blockade may increase single nephron filtration rate as well as single nephron plasma flow.[76] Thus, the data obtained from studies using pharmacologic antagonists of the renin-angiotensin system indicate that when the prevailing endogenous Ang II levels are elevated, they exert approximately equivalent vasoconstrictor effects on both the pre- and postglomerular resistance vessels. To date, all of the vasoconstrictor actions of Ang II on the renal vasculature have been demonstrated to be mediated by activation of AT_1 receptors.[76]

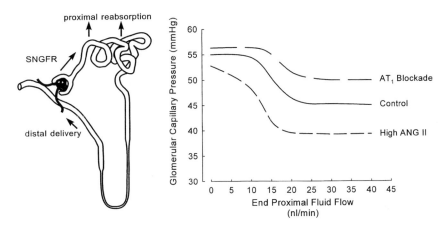

Figure 8. Effects of changes in angiotensin influence on the sensitivity of the tubuloglomerular feedback (TGF) mechanism. High angiotensin states increase and low angiotensin states or AT₁ receptor blockade decreases TGF sensitivity and thus allows modulation of distal volume delivery without major changes in glomerular capillary pressure. SNGR = single nephron glomerular filtration rate.

Intrarenal Ang II also exerts an important modulatory influence on the sensitivity of the tubuloglomerular feedback mechanism (Fig. 8).[162] This mechanism provides a balance between the reabsorption capabilities of the tubules and the filtered load by regulating GFR.[163] When flow-dependent changes in tubular fluid solute concentration at the level of the macula densa in the terminal part of the loop of Henle are sensed, signals are transmitted to the afferent arterioles to constrict or dilate in order to maintain stability of the filtered load. Ang II alters the sensitivity of the tubuloglomerular feedback mechanism.[76,164] Systemic administration of peptide Ang II receptor antagonists, such as saralasin, and ACE inhibitors, markedly attenuate feedback responsiveness as assessed by stop-flow pressure feedback responses to increases in distal nephron perfusion rate.[165,166] In addition, infusion of exogenous Ang II during conditions of converting enzyme blockade results in partial restoration of feedback responsiveness.[167] Furthermore, tubuloglomerular feedback responsiveness in normal rats is enhanced during either systemic or peritubular capillary infusion of exogenous Ang II.[1,162] This issue has been reexamined recently in experiments using mice with deletion of the ACE or AT₁ receptor gene.[168,169] Both AT₁ receptor knockout and ACE-deficient mice have markedly attenuated tubuloglomerular feedback responses to increases in distal nephron perfusion rate. In ACE-deficient mice, infusion of Ang II partially restored the feedback responses, indicating that Ang II is essential for maintaining the sensitivity of the tubuloglomerular feedback mechanism but is not the direct mediator of the response. Collectively, these findings indicate that Ang II enhances the sensitivity of the vascular elements that mediate tubuloglomerular feedback-induced alterations in single nephron hemodynamic function. These effects probably are mediated both by direct actions on the vascular smooth muscle cells and by modulating the Na⁺/H⁺ exchange activity of macula densa cells.[170]

The recent observation that stop-flow pressure tubuloglomerular feedback responses are attenuated after both systemic and peritubular capillary administration of AT₁ receptor antagonists[165] and the loss of feedback responses in AT₁ₐ receptor-deficient mice[168] indicate that Ang II exerts its modulatory influence on tubuloglomerular feedback responsiveness via activation of AT_1 receptors. Such a modulatory influence of Ang II on tubuloglomerular feedback responsiveness shifts the operating point of the system and allows nephron filtration rate to be maintained at a lower distal nephron volume delivery.[1] During conditions of elevated intrarenal Ang II levels the modulatory influence of Ang II on tubuloglomerular feedback responsiveness is of pivotal importance in maintaining the Ang II-mediated stimulation of proximal tubular reabsorption and the consequent decrease in distal nephron volume delivery.[164] In this manner, the interactive effects of Ang II to enhance both proximal tubular reabsorption rate and sensitivity of the tubuloglomerular feedback mechanism increase intrarenal Ang II levels to elicit sustained decreases in distal nephron volume delivery and, thus, urinary sodium and water excretion.

The combined effects of Ang II on tubular and vascular structures are synergistic and provide a powerful influence on sodium excretion and on the pressure natriuresis relationship.[1,2,164] Seeliger et al.[171] demonstrated the power of this system by infusing Ang II plus aldosterone into dogs under conditions in which the renal perfusion pressure was prevented from rising. They observed a substantial increase in sodium balance and elevated systemic arterial pressure, even though no other counteracting systems were blocked. This study indicates that the direct effects of Ang II and the indirect effects caused by aldosterone cannot be overcome by all of the counterbalancing natriuretic influences if the perfusion pressure to the kidney is not allowed to increase.

■ Integrated Renal Responses to AT_1 Receptor Blockade

The development of specific AT_1 receptor blockers has provided a means to obtain a more comprehensive assessment of the specific actions of AT_1 receptors by determining the renal responses to the receptor antagonists. An extensive literature describes the cardiovascular and renal responses to systemic administration of AT_1 receptor blockers. However, the overall renal hemodynamic and excretory responses to AT_1 receptor blockade have been quite variable because of the counteracting influences of the associated decreases in systemic arterial pressure.[165,172,173] Substantial decreases in arterial pressure due to systemic blockade of vascular smooth muscle AT_1 receptors may be associated with compensatory activation of the sympathetic nervous system, which increases renal nerve sympathetic traffic and decreases renal function.[174–176] The increased renal sympathetic nerve activity after AT_1 receptor blockade is due primarily to the associated decreases in arterial pressure because, when blood pressure responses are controlled, AT_1 receptor blockade suppresses sympathetic activity.[175] Decreases in arterial pressure in response to AT_1 receptor blockade are more pronounced during sodium-depleted states because activation of the renin-angiotensin system helps to maintain arterial pressure.[177,178] The large decreases in arterial pressure due to sodium depletion in the presence of AT_1 receptor blockade cause compensatory activation of the sympathetic system, which contributes to the decreases in renal function associated with pronounced hypotension.[177] Direct interstitial infusion or renal arterial infusions of AT_1 receptor blockers that avoid decreases in arterial pressure cause increases in sodium excretion.[128,178]

Until the development of the nonpeptide receptor antagonists that exhibited receptor selectivity, the consequences of Ang II receptor blockade were studied by using peptide analogs with substitutions that blocked receptor activation but allowed receptor binding.[179] Many different studies were performed with these nonspecific receptor antagonists, such as saralasin.[1,76,180,181] Intrarenal arterial infusion of [Sar^1-Ile^8]-Ang II into normal and sodium-depleted dogs demonstrated that the effects of Ang II receptor blockade were greater in sodium-depleted dogs, which have an activated renin-angiotensin system. In sodium-depleted dogs, Ang II receptor blockade led to significant increases in renal blood flow, glomerular filtration rate (GFR), sodium excretion, and fractional sodium excretion.[182] Siragy et al.[183] combined intrarenal infusions of a renin inhibitor, an ACE inhibitor, and saralasin to achieve maximal intrarenal blockade without substantive systemic spillover. When administered to sodium-depleted dogs, this combination caused approximately tenfold increases in sodium excretion and twofold increases in renal blood flow and/or GFR. Likewise, Ang II receptor blockade with saralasin elicited significant increases in renal blood flow, GFR, urine flow, and sodium excretion in normal rats and in nonclipped kidneys of 2K1C Goldblatt hypertensive rats.[180,181] In a comprehensive study by Steiner et al.,[181] saralasin administration to rats maintained on a low sodium diet increased single nephron GFR and renal plasma flow, decreased afferent arteriolar resistance, and inhibited proximal tubule reabsorption rate. Many of these studies, however, raised concerns that the peptide analogs of Ang II also may exert partial agonist effects. The nonspecific antagonists were blocking AT$_2$ receptors as well as AT$_1$ receptors, which may influence the nature and magnitude of the final overall renal responses.[31,32,51,184] The more recent studies using selective receptor blockers suggest that one advantage of AT$_1$ receptor blockers over nonspecific inhibition is that the AT$_2$ receptors can be stimulated by the elevated Ang II concentrations, which may exert compensatory renal vasodilator effects by increasing renal interstitial fluid concentrations of bradykinin, cyclic GMP, and nitric oxide.[31]

The availability of specific AT$_1$ receptor blockers has allowed further evaluation of the renal responses to AT$_1$ receptor blockade in normal and hypertensive animals. As mentioned previously, AT$_1$ receptor blockers administered systemically decrease mean arterial pressure in normal and hypertensive animal models, including 2K1C Goldblatt hypertensive rats and Ang II-infused rats.[91,92,165,172,173] Dose-dependent differences in renal responses occurred with the larger doses that decrease arterial pressure and cause reductions in sodium excretion and variable responses in GFR and renal blood flow. Of interest, doses of AT$_1$ receptor blockers, which did not cause large or immediate decreases in arterial pressure, elicited increases in renal blood flow and/or GFR as well as sodium excretion and led to reductions in renal vascular resistance in both normal and Goldblatt hypertensive rats.[137,172,173,185] Zhuo et al.[137] observed a large increase in GFR but failed to document an increase in renal plasma flow. Some of the effects on GFR and sodium excretion may be mediated indirectly by activation of other associated paracrine systems.[185]

Studies in dogs have reported increases in renal blood flow with variable increases or no changes in GFR along with marked diuresis and natriuresis in response to AT$_1$ receptor blockade at doses that did not acutely reduce arterial pressure.[186–189] Several studies have reported up to 20% increases in renal blood flow and nearly twofold increases in sodium excretion with AT$_1$ receptor blockade, whereas AT_2 receptor blockade with PD123177 or PD123319 failed to elicit significant changes in renal blood flow or sodium excretion.[187,188,190] However, AT_2 blockade did increase urine flow and free water clearance.[188]

The sodium excretory responses to AT_1 receptor blockers appear to involve two phases, as shown in Ang II-infused rats that were treated chronically with losartan.[92] The chronic losartan dose prevented the hypertension that occurs with chronic Ang II infusions as well as the vascular and pressor responses to exogenous Ang II bolus doses. Nevertheless, an acute infusion with losartan superimposed on the chronic dose produced a marked natriuresis, suggesting that the higher concentration of losartan acted on low-affinity receptors or poorly accessible receptors (as described for the proximal tubule).[138]

As in other hypertensive models,[84,86,191] renal Ang II levels in the nonclipped kidneys of 2K1C hypertensive rats remain elevated even though the renal renin content and renin mRNA are markedly suppressed. Recent micropuncture experiments demonstrated that the proximal tubular fluid Ang II concentrations in the nonclipped kidneys of 2K1C Goldblatt hypertensive rats also are maintained in the nanomolar range and are similar to values recently reported for normal rats that have normal renin contents.[128] Thus, the Ang II levels in the nonclipped kidneys of 2K1C hypertensive rats are distributed to the proximal tubular fluid in a manner similar to that observed in normal rats.[90,120,121] Because of the elevated systemic arterial pressure and the marked renin suppression, the failure of the nonclipped kidney to suppress appropriately intrarenal Ang II remains unclear, but inappropriately high intraluminal and intrarenal Ang II levels observed in nonclipped kidneys of 2K1C hypertensive rats presumably continue to stimulate proximal tubular reabsorption rate and exert Ang II-mediated renal vasoconstriction. These effects, combined with an enhancement of tubuloglomerular feedback responsiveness,[165] may be of substantial importance in the development and long-term maintenance of hypertension by sustaining inappropriately elevated sodium reabsorption rates at a time when the elevated arterial pressures should be exerting a pressure natriuresis response.[4] Vascular AT_1 receptor density is not decreased after 2–4 weeks of clipping,[192] and proximal tubular AT_1 receptor mRNA in fact may be increased by elevated Ang II levels.[193] In addition, renal AT_1 receptor mRNA and protein expression are maintained in Ang II-induced hypertensive rats.[194] The failure to downregulate AT_1 receptors, especially in proximal tubules, maintains Ang II dependency in these hypertensive models.

Activation of AT_1 receptors contributes to the enhanced preglomerular vascular tone and blunted microvascular autoregulatory responsiveness to changes in perfusion pressure in hypertensive models.[195–197] The blunted autoregulatory responsiveness of the afferent arteriole in Ang II-dependent hypertension apparently results from chronic elevations of Ang II since acute exposure to tenfold greater concentrations of Ang II does not affect autoregulatory behavior.[198] The compromised renal autoregulatory efficiency and elevation in arterial pressure in Ang II-infused hypertensive rats are prevented by coadministration of AT_1 receptor blockers,[196] suggesting that chronic treatment with AT_1 receptor blockers provides protection against Ang II-mediated increases in arterial pressure and prevents the associated deterioration of renal autoregulatory responsiveness.

In a recent study, the high-affinity nonsurmountable AT$_1$ receptor antagonist, candesartan,[199] was administered directly into the renal artery to avoid the compensatory cardiovascular and sympathetic responses to reductions in systemic arterial pressure that occur with systemic infusions.[200] Intraarterial administration of candesartan led to significant increases in renal blood flow and GFR in the range of 15–25% and proportionately greater increases in sodium excretion (Fig. 9).[128] Sodium excretion and fractional sodium excretion increased four- to fivefold. The proportionately greater increases in sodium excretion reflect the combined effects of both vascular and tubular effects and are consistent with the experimental findings that tubular AT$_1$ receptors contribute to sodium reabsorption. Their blockade thus contributes significantly to the increases in urinary sodium excretion.[1,115] These actions of AT$_1$ receptor blockers contribute significantly to the leftward shift in the pressure natriuresis relation that occurs in hypertensive models after treatment with AT$_1$ receptor blockers.[201,202]

Similar effects of AT$_1$ receptor blockers have been reported in patients with essential hypertension. In particular, several studies have evaluated the effects of AT$_1$ receptor blockers on renal blood flow, GFR, and sodium excretory function. Hypertensive patients given AT$_1$ receptor blockers exhibited renal responses similar to or slightly greater than those observed with ACE inhibitors.[203–207] The general responses include decreases in systolic and diastolic pressures as well as increases in renal blood flow, thus resulting in substantial decreases in renal vascular resistance. In agreement with previous results with ACE inhibitors, AT$_1$ receptor blockers do not usually elicit significant changes in GFR.[76,205,208] It is important to emphasize again that the decreases in filtration fraction obtained with AT$_1$ receptor blockers do not indicate predominant actions on the postglomerular arterioles. The most direct way to explain increases in renal blood flow without changes in GFR is by combined decreases in both pre- and postglomerular resistances.[76,158] If the dilation was predominantly

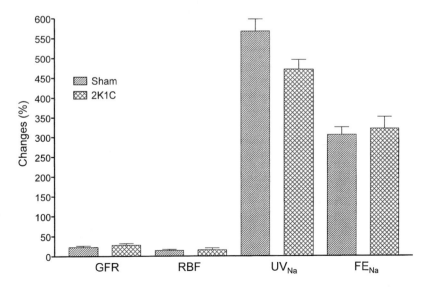

Figure 9. Summary of the renal hemodynamic and sodium excretory responses to intraarterial administration of candesartan in 2K1C Goldblatt hypertensive rats and in normal control (sham) rats.

postglomerular, GFR would decrease instead of remain unchanged.[209] Thus, the ability of AT_1 receptor blockers to elicit combined dilation of pre- and post-glomerular resistances allows renal vasodilation and natriuresis to occur without major changes in glomerular pressure or GFR. In some studies, GFR also has been shown to be increased slightly in response to treatment with AT_1 receptor blockers.[204,210] This finding may be due to slight increases in glomerular pressure or filtration coefficient.

As observed in experimental studies, AT_1 receptor blockers increase sodium excretion rates in humans.[211] Significant increases in sodium and potassium excretion rates were observed. Natriuresis was observed in the absence of an increase in GFR and thus filtered sodium load. These data in humans support the interpretations based on laboratory studies, indicating that AT_1 receptor blockers directly inhibit tubular sodium reabsorption. Thus, it seems likely that an important characteristic of AT_1 receptor blockers is to block AT_1 receptor-mediated stimulation of tubular reabsorption rate.

■ Conclusion

AT_1 receptor blockade has combined effects that increase sodium excretion and reduce Ang II-dependent vascular tone. Whereas the vascular effects are important in counteracting the direct actions of Ang II on peripheral vascular resistance, the natriuretic effects probably contribute to the long-term control of sodium balance, extracellular fluid volume, and blood volume, which is essential for the long-term control of arterial pressure.[4,212]

Acknowledgments

Studies performed in the authors' laboratory were supported by grants from the National Heart, Lung, and Blood Institute and the American Heart Association. The authors thank Agnes C. Buffone for preparation of the figures and manuscript.

References

1. Mitchell KD, Navar LG: Intrarenal actions of angiotensin II in the pathogenesis of experimental hypertension. In Laragh JH, Brenner BM (eds): Hypertension: Pathophysiology, Diagnosis, and Management, 2nd ed. New York, Raven Press, 1995, pp 1437–1450.
2. Navar LG, Hamm LL: The kidney in blood pressure regulation. In Wilcox CS (ed): Atlas of Diseases of the Kidney. Hypertension and the Kidney. Philadelphia, Current Medicine, 1999, pp 1.1–1.22.
3. Navar LG, Imig JD, Zou L, Wang C-T: Intrarenal production of angiotensin II. Semin Nephrol 17:412–422, 1997.
4. Navar LG: The kidney in blood pressure regulation and development of hypertension. Med Clin North Am 81:1165–1198, 1997.
5. Zhuo J, Song K, Abdelrahman A, Mendelsohn FAO: Blockade by intravenous losartan of AT_1 angiotensin II receptors in rat brain, kidney and adrenals demonstrated by in vitro autoradiography. Clin Exp Pharmacol Physiol 21:557–567, 1994.
6. Wexler RR, Greenlee WJ, Irvin JD, et al: Nonpeptide angiotensin II receptor antagonists: The next generation in antihypertensive therapy. J Med Chem 39:625–656, 1996.
7. Yamamoto K, Chappell MC, Broshnihan KB, Ferrario CM: In vivo metabolism of angiotensin I by neutral endopeptidase (EC 3.4.24.11) in spontaneously hypertensive rats. Hypertension 19:692–696, 1992.
8. Harding JW, Wright JW, Swanson GN, et al: AT_4 receptors: Specificity and distribution. Kidney Int 46:1510–1512, 1994.
9. Ferrario CM, Chappell MC, Dean RH, Iyer SN: Novel angiotensin peptides regulate blood pressure, endothelial function, and natriuresis. J Am Soc Nephrol 9:1716–1722, 1998.
10. Handa RK, Krebs LT, Harding JW, Handa SE: Angiotensin IV AT_4-receptor system in the rat kidney. Am J Physiol 274:F290–F299, 1998.

11. Brasier AR, Li J: Mechanisms for inducible control of angiotensinogen gene transcription. Hypertension 27(Pt 2):465–475, 1996.
12. Gomez RA, Lynch KR, Chevalier RL, et al: Renin and angiotensinogen gene expression and intrarenal renin distribution during ACE inhibition. Am J Physiol 254:F900–F906, 1988.
13. Darby IA, Sernia C: In situ hybridization and immunohistochemistry of renal angiotensinogen in neonatal and adult rat kidneys. Cell Tissue Res 281:197–206, 1995.
14. Ingelfinger J, Zuo WM, Fon EA, et al: In situ hybridization evidence for angiotensinogen messenger RNA in the rat proximal tubule. J Clin Invest 85:417–423, 1990.
15. Von Thun AM, El-Dahr SS, Vari RC, Navar LG: Modulation of renin-angiotensin and kallikrein gene expression in experimental hypertension. Hypertension 23(Suppl I):I-131–I-136, 1994.
16. Zou L, Imig JD, Von Thun AM, et al: Receptor-mediated intrarenal ANG II augmentation in ANG II-infused rats. Hypertension 28:669–677, 1996.
17. Campbell DJ, Lawrence AC, Towrie A, et al: Differential regulation of angiotensin peptide levels in plasma and kidney of the rat. Hypertension 18:763–773, 1991.
18. Erdos EG: Angiotensin I converting enzyme and the changes in our concepts through the years. Hypertension 16:363–370, 1990.
19. Luft FC, Wilcox CS, Unger T, et al: Angiotensin-induced hypertension in the rat: Effects on sympathetic nerve activity and the renal excretion of prostaglandins. Hypertension 14:396–403, 1989.
20. Mitchell KD, Navar LG: The renin-angiotensin-aldosterone system in volume control. In Baylis PH (ed): Bailliere's Clinical Endocrinology and Metabolism, 2nd ed. London, Bailliere Tindall, 1989, pp 393–430.
21. Griendling KK, Ushio-Fukai M, Lassègue B, Alexander RW: Angiotensin II signaling in vascular smooth muscle. New concepts. Hypertension 29(Pt 2):366–373, 1997.
22. Ichikawa I, Harris RC: Angiotensin actions in the kidney: Renewed insight into the old hormone. Kidney Int 40:583–596, 1991.
23. Ferrario CM, Flack JM: Pathologic consequences of increased angiotensin II activity. Cardiovasc Drugs Ther 10:511–518, 1996.
24. Corvol P, Jeunemaitre X, Charru A, et al: Role of the renin-angiotensin system in blood pressure regulation and in human hypertension: New insights from molecular genetics. Rec Progr Hormone Res 50:287–308, 1995.
25. Wolf G, Ziyadeh F: The role of angiotensin II in diabetic nephropathy: Emphasis on nonhemodynamic mechanisms. Am J Kidney Dis 29:153–163, 1997.
26. Wolf G, Neilson EG: Angiotensin II as a renal growth factor. J Am Soc Nephrol 3:1531–1540, 1993.
27. Otsuka F, Yamauchi T, Kataoka H, et al: Effects of chronic inhibition of ACE and AT$_1$ receptors on glomerular injury in Dahl salt-sensitive rats. Am J Physiol 274:R1797–R1806, 1998.
28. Tomita H, Egashira K, Ohara Y, et al: Early induction of transforming growth factor-β via angiotensin II type 1 receptors contributes to cardiac fibrosis induced by long-term blockade of nitric oxide synthesis in rats. Hypertension 32:273–279, 1998.
29. Yoo KH, Thornhill BA, Wolstenholme JT, Chevalier RL: Tissue-specific regulation of growth factors and clusterin by angiotensin II. Am J Hypertens 11:715–722, 1998.
30. Siragy HM, Carey RM: The subtype 2 (AT$_2$) angiotensin receptor mediates renal production of nitric oxide in conscious rats. J Clin Invest 100(2):264–269, 1997.
31. Siragy HM, Carey RM: Protective role of the angiotensin AT$_2$ receptor in a renal wrap hypertension model. Hypertension 33:1237–1242, 1999.
32. Siragy HM, Inagami T, Ichiki T, Carey RM: Sustained hypersensitivity to angiotensin II and its mechanism in mice lacking the subtype-2 (AT$_2$) angiotensin receptor. Proc Natl Acad Sci USA 96:6506–6510, 1999.
33. Sasamura H, Hein L, Krieger JE, et al: Cloning, characterization, and expression of two angiotensin receptor (AT-1) isoforms from the mouse genome. Biochem Biophys Res Commun 185:253–259, 1992.
34. Iwai N, Inagami T: Identification of two subtypes in rat type I angiotensin II receptor. FEBS Lett 298:257–260, 1992.
35. Bouby N, Hus-Citharel A, Marchetti J, et al: Expression of type 1 angiotensin II receptor subtypes and angiotensin II-induced calcium mobilization along the rat nephron. J Am Soc Nephrol 8:1658–1667, 1997.
36. Bumpus FM, Catt KJ, Chiu AT, et al: Nomenclature for angiotensin receptors. A report of the Nomenclature Committee of the Council for High Blood Pressure Research. Hypertension 17:720–721, 1991.
37. Iwai N, Yamano Y, Chaki S, et al: Rat angiotensin II receptor: cDNA sequence and regulation of the gene expression. Biochem Biophys Res Commun 177:299–304, 1991.
38. Murphy TJ, Alexander RW, Griendling KK, et al: Isolation of a cDNA encoding the vascular type-1 angiotensin II receptor. Nature (Lond) 351:233–236, 1991.

39. Sasaki K, Yamano Y, Bardhan S, et al: Cloning and expression of a complementary DNA encoding a bovine adrenal angiotensin II type-1 receptor. Nature 351:230–233, 1991.
40. Kambayashi Y, Bardhan S, Takahashi K, et al: Molecular cloning of a novel angiotensin II receptor isoform involved in phosphotyrosine phosphatase inhibition. J Biol Chem 268:24543–24546, 1993.
41. Mukoyama M, Nakajima M, Horiuchi M, et al: Expression cloning of type 2 angiotensin II receptor reveals a unique class of seven-transmembrane receptors. J Biol Chem 268:24539–24542, 1993.
42. Nakajima M, Mukoyama M, Pratt RE, et al: Cloning of cDNA and analysis of the gene for mouse angiotensin II type 2 receptor. Biochem Biophys Res Commun 197:393–399, 1993.
43. Tsuzuki S, Ichiki T, Nakakubo H, et al: Molecular cloning and expression of the gene encoding human angiotensin II type 2 receptor. Biochem Biophys Res Commun 200:1449–1454, 1994.
44. Madhun ZT, Ernsberger P, Ke F-C, et al: Signal transduction mediated by angiotensin II receptor subtypes expressed in rat renal mesangial cells. Regul Pept 44:149–157, 1993.
45. Bernstein KE, Berk BC: Physiology and cell biology update: The biology of angiotensin II receptors. Am J Kid Dis 22:745–754, 1993.
46. Elton T, Stephan C, Taylor S, et al: Isolation of two distinct type 1 angiotensin II receptor genes. Biochem Biophys Res Commun 184:1067–1073, 1992.
47. Kakar S, Seller J, Devor D, et al: Angiotensin II type-1 receptor subtype cDNAs: Differential tissue expression and hormone regulation. Biochem Biophys Res Commun 183:1090–1096, 1992.
48. Sandberg K, Ji H, Clark AJL, et al: Cloning and expression of a novel angiotensin II receptor subtype. J Biol Chem 267:9455–9458, 1992.
49. Ohnishi J, Ishido M, Shibata T, et al: The rat angiotensin II AT_{1A} receptor couples with three different signal transduction pathways. Biochem Biophys Res Commun 186:1094–1101, 1992.
50. Ohyama K, Yamano Y, Chaki S, et al: Domains for G protein coupling in angiotensin II receptor type 1: Studies by site-directed mutagenesis. Biochem Biophys Res Commun 189:677–683, 1992.
51. de Gasparo M, Siragy HM: The AT_2 receptor: Fact, fancy and fantasy. Regul Pept 81:11–24, 1999.
52. Hayashida W, Horiuchi M, Dzau VJ: Intracellular third loop domain of angiotensin II type-2 receptor: Role in mediating signal transduction and cellular function. J Biol Chem 271:21985–21992, 1996.
53. Douglas JG: Angiotensin receptor subtypes of the kidney cortex. Am J Physiol 253:F1–F7, 1987.
54. Mendelsohn FAO, Dunbar M, Allen A, et al: Angiotensin II receptors in the kidney. Fed Proc 45:1420–1425, 1986.
55. Burns KD, Inagami T, Harris RC: Cloning of a rabbit kidney cortex AT_1 angiotensin II receptor that is present in proximal tubule epithelium. Am J Physiol 264:F645–F654, 1993.
56. Paxton WG, Runge M, Horaist C, et al: Immunohistochemical localization of rat angiotensin II AT_1 receptor. Am J Physiol 264:F989–F995, 1993.
57. Zhuo J, Alcorn D, McCausland J, Mendelsohn FAO: Localization and regulation of angiotensin II receptors in renomedullary interstitial cells. Kidney Int 46:1483–1485, 1994.
58. Harrison-Bernard LM, Navar LG, Ho MM, et al: Immunohistochemical localization of ANG II AT_1 receptor in adult rat kidney using a monoclonal antibody. Am J Physiol 273:F170–F177, 1997.
59. Wang Z-Q, Millatt LJ, Heiderstadt NT, et al: Differential regulation of renal angiotensin subtype AT_{1A} and AT_2 receptor protein in rats with angiotensin-dependent hypertension. Hypertension 33:96–101, 1999.
60. Miyata N, Park F, Li Xf, Cowley AW Jr: Distribution of angiotensin AT1 and AT2 receptor subtypes in the rat kidney. Am J Physiol 277:F437–F446, 1999.
61. Zhuo J, Allen AM, Alcorn D, et al: The distribution of angiotensin II receptors. In Laragh JH, Brenner BM (eds): Hypertension: Pathophysiology, Diagnosis and Management, 2nd ed. New York, Raven Press, 1995, pp 1739–1762.
62. DeLeon H, Garcia R: Angiotensin II receptor subtypes in rat renal preglomerular vessels. Receptor 2:253–260, 1993.
63. Sharma M, Sharma R, Greene AS, et al: Documentation of angiotensin II receptors in glomerular epithelial cells. Am J Physiol 274:F623–F627, 1998.
64. Meister B, Lippoldt A, Bunnemann B, et al: Cellular expression of angiotensin type-1 receptor mRNA in the kidney. Kidney Int 44:331–336, 1993.
65. Tufro-McReddie A, Harrison JK, Everett AD, Gomez RA: Ontogeny of type 1 angiotensin II receptor gene expression in the rat. J Clin Invest 91:530–537, 1993.
66. Gasc J-M, Monnot C, Clauser E, Corvol P: Co-expression of type 1 angiotensin II receptor (AT_1R) and renin mRNAs in juxtaglomerular cells of the rat kidney. Endocrinology

132:2723–2725, 1993.

67. Terada Y, Tomita K, Nonoguchi H, Marumo F: PCR localization of angiotensin II receptor and angiotensinogen mRNAs in rat kidney. Kidney Int 43:1251–1259, 1993.

68. Burns KD, Regnier L, Roczniak A, Hébert RL: Immortalized rabbit cortical collecting duct cells express AT₁ angiotensin II receptors. Am J Physiol 271:F1147–F1157, 1996.

69. Du Y, Yao A, Guo D, et al: Differential regulation of angiotensin II receptor subtypes in rat kidney by low dietary sodium. Hypertension 25(Pt 2):872–877, 1995.

70. Ruan XP, Wagner C, Chatziantoniou C, et al: Regulation of angiotensin II receptor AT₁ subtypes in renal afferent arterioles during chronic changes in sodium diet. J Clin Invest 99:1072–1081, 1997.

71. Norwood VF, Craig MR, Harris JM, Gomez RA: Differential expression of angiotensin II receptors during early renal morphogenesis. Am J Physiol 272:R662–R668, 1997.

72. Danser AHJ, Koning MMG, Admiraal PJJ, et al: Production of angiotensins I and II at tissue sites in intact pigs. Am J Physiol 263:H429–H437, 1992.

73. Johnston CI: Tissue angiotensin converting enzyme in cardiac and vascular hypertrophy, repair, and remodeling. Hypertension 23:258–268, 1994.

74. Schulz WW, Hagler HK, Buja LM, Erdos EG: Ultrastructural localization of angiotensin I-converting enzyme (EC 3.4.15.1) and neutral metalloendopeptidase (EC 3.4.24.11) in the proximal tubule of the human kidney. Lab Invest 59:789–797, 1988.

75. Campbell DJ: Differential regulation of angiotensin peptides in plasma and kidney: Effects of adrenalectomy and estrogen treatment. Clin Exp Hypertens 19:687–698, 1997.

76. Navar LG, Inscho EW, Majid DSA, et al: Paracrine regulation of the renal microcirculation. Physiol Rev 76:425–536, 1996.

77. Müller DN, Bohlender J, Hilgers KF, et al: Vascular angiotensin-converting enzyme expression regulates local angiotensin II. Hypertension 29:98–104, 1997.

78. Zimmerman BG, Dunham EW: Tissue renin-angiotensin system: A site of drug action? Annu Rev Pharmacol Toxicol 37:53–69, 1997.

79. De Silva PE, Husain A, Smeby RR, Khairallah PA: Measurement of immunoreactive angiotensin peptides in rat tissues: Some pitfalls in angiotensin II analysis. Analyt Biochem 174:80–87, 1988.

80. Fox J, Guan S, Hymel AA, Navar LG: Dietary Na and ACE inhibition effects on renal tissue angiotensin I and II and ACE activity in rats. Am J Physiol 262:F902–F909, 1992.

81. Rosivall L, Narkates AJ, Oparil S, Navar LG: De novo intrarenal formation of angiotensin II during control and enhanced renin secretion. Am J Physiol 252:F1118–F1123, 1987.

82. Loghman-Adham M, Rohrwasser A, Helin C, et al: A conditionally immortalized cell line from murine proximal tubule. Kidney Int 52:229–239, 1997.

83. Wang L, Lei C, Zhang S-L, et al: Synergistic effect of dexamethasone and isoproterenol on the expression of angiotensinogen in immortalized rat proximal tubular cells. Kidney Int 53:287–295, 1998.

84. Von Thun AM, Vari RC, El-Dahr SS, Navar LG: Augmentation of intrarenal angiotensin II levels by chronic angiotensin II infusion. Am J Physiol 266:F120–F128, 1994.

85. Jin D, Takai S, Shiota N, Miyazaki M: Roles of vascular angiotensin converting enzyme and chymase in two-kidney, one clip hypertensive hamsters. J Hypertens 16:657–664, 1998.

86. Guan S, Fox J, Mitchell KD, Navar LG: Angiotensin and angiotensin converting enzyme tissue levels in two-kidney, one-clip hypertensive rats. Hypertension 20:763–767, 1992.

87. Vio CP, Cordova M, Alhenc-Gelas F: Increased angiotensin I-converting enzyme in epithelial, endothelial and interstitial cells in hypertensive kidneys [abstract]. Hypertension 29:847, 1997.

88. Navar LG, Harrison-Bernard LM, Imig JD: Compartmentalization of intrarenal angiotensin II. In Ulfendahl HR, Aurell M (eds): Renin-Angiotensin. London, Portland Press, 1998, pp 193–208.

89. Zou L, Imig JD, Hymel A, Navar LG: Renal uptake of circulating angiotensin II in Val⁵-angiotensin II infused rats is mediated by AT₁ receptor. Am J Hypertens 11:570–578, 1998.

90. Mitchell KD, Jacinto SM, Mullins JJ: Proximal tubular fluid, kidney, and plasma levels of angiotensin II in hypertensive ren-2 transgenic rats. Am J Physiol 273:F246–F253, 1997.

91. Imamura A, Mackenzie HS, Lacy ER, et al: Effects of chronic treatment with angiotensin converting enzyme inhibitor or angiotensin II receptor antagonist in two-kidney, one-clip hypertensive rats. Kidney Int 47:1394–1402, 1995.

92. Wang C-T, Zou L, Navar LG: Renal responses to AT₁ blockade in angiotensin II-induced hypertensive rats. J Am Soc Nephrol 8:535–542, 1997.

93. Zou L, Hymel A, Imig JD, Navar LG: Renal accumulation of circulating angiotensin II in angiotensin II-infused rats. Hypertension 27(Pt 2):658–662, 1996.

94. Becker BN, Harris RC: A potential mechanism for proximal tubule angiotensin II-mediated sodium flux associated with receptor-mediate endocytosis and arachidonic acid release. Kidney

Int 50(Suppl 57):S-66–S-72, 1996.

95. Linas SL: Role of receptor mediated endocytosis in proximal tubule epithelial function. Kidney Int 52(Suppl 61):S-18–S-21, 1997.

96. Becker BN, Cheng H-F, Harris RC: Apical ANG II-stimulated PLA_2 activity and Na^+ flux: A potential role for Ca^{2+}-independent PLA_2. Am J Physiol 273:F554–F562, 1997.

97. Schelling JR, Hanson AS, Marzec R, Linas SL: Cytoskeleton-dependent endocytosis is required for apical type 1 angiotensin II receptor-mediated phospholipase C activation in cultured rat proximal tubule cells. J Clin Invest 90:2472–2480, 1992.

98. Schelling JR, Linas SL: Angiotensin II-dependent proximal tubule sodium transport requires receptor-mediated endocytosis. Am J Physiol 266:C669–C675, 1994.

99. Thekkumkara TJ, Cookson R, Linas SL: Angiotensin (AT_{1A}) receptor-mediated increases in transcellular sodium transport in proximal tubule cells. Am J Physiol 274:F897–F905, 1998.

100. Becker BN, Cheng HF, Burns KD, Harris RC: Polarized rabbit type 1 angiotensin II receptors manifest differential rates of endocytosis and recycling. Am J Physiol 269:C1048–C1056, 1995.

101. Anderson KM, Peach MJ: Receptor binding and internalization of a unique biologically active angiotensin II-colloidal gold conjugate: Morphological analysis of angiotensin II processing in isolated vascular strips. J Vasc Res 31:10–17, 1994.

102. Hein L, Meinel L, Pratt RE, et al: Intracellular trafficking of angiotensin II and its AT_1 and AT_2 receptors: Evidence for selective sorting of receptor and ligand. Mol Endocrinol 11:1266–1277, 1997.

103. van Kats JP, de Lannoy LM, Danser AHJ, et al: Angiotensin II type 1 (AT_1) receptor-mediated accumulation of angiotensin II in tissues and its intracellular half-life in vivo. Hypertension 30 (Pt 1):42–49, 1997.

104. Imig JD, Navar GL, Zou LX, et al: Renal endosomes contain angiotensin peptides, converting enzyme, and AT_{1A} receptors. Am J Physiol 277:F303–F311, 1999.

105. Allan DR, McKnight JA, Kifor I, et al: Converting enzyme inhibition and renal tissue angiotensin II in the rat. Hypertension 24:516–522, 1994.

106. Thomas WG, Thekkumkara TJ, Baker KM: Molecular mechanisms of angiotensin II (AT_{1A}) receptor endocytosis. Clin Exp Pharmacol Physiol 23:S74–S80, 1996.

107. Pallone TL, Robertson CR, Jamison RL: Renal medullary microcirculation. Physiol Rev 70:885–920, 1990.

108. Pallone TL: Vasoconstriction of outer medullary vasa recta by angiotensin II is modulated by prostaglandin E_2. Am J Physiol 266:F850–F857, 1994.

109. Chou S-Y, Porush JG, Faubert PF: Renal medullary circulation: Hormonal control. Kidney Int 37:1–13, 1990.

110. Mendelsohn FAO, Millan M, Quirion R, et al: Localization of angiotensin II receptors in rat and monkey kidney by in vitro autoradiography. Kidney Int 31(Suppl 20):S-40–S-44, 1987.

111. Zhuo J, Alcorn D, McCausland J, et al: In vivo occupancy of angiotensin II subtype 1 receptors in rat medullary interstitial cells. Hypertension 23(Pt 2):838–843, 1994.

112. Zhuo J, Alcorn D, Allen AM, Mendelsohn FAO: High resolution localization of angiotensin II receptors in rat renal medulla. Kidney Int 42:1372–1380, 1992.

113. Hunt MK, Ramos SP, Geary KM, et al: Colocalization and release of angiotensin and renin in renal cortical cells. Am J Physiol 263:F363–F373, 1992.

114. Ingelfinger JR, Jung F, Diamant D, et al: Rat proximal tubule cell line transformed with origin-defective SV40 DNA: Autocrine ANG II feedback. Am J Physiol 276:F218–F227, 1999.

115. Cogan MG: Angiotensin II: A powerful controller of sodium transport in the early proximal tubule. Hypertension 15:451–458, 1990.

116. Quan A, Baum M: Endogenous production of angiotensin II modulates rat proximal tubule transport. J Clin Invest 97:2878–2882, 1996.

117. Baum M, Quigley R, Quan A: Effect of luminal angiotensin II on rabbit proximal convoluted tubule bicarbonate absorption. Am J Physiol 273:F595–F600, 1997.

118. Li L, Wang Y-P, Capparelli AW, et al: Effect of luminal angiotensin II on proximal tubule fluid transport: Role of apical phospholipase A_2. Am J Physiol 266:F202–F209, 1994.

119. Seikaly MG, Arant BS Jr, Seney FD Jr: Endogenous angiotensin concentrations in specific intrarenal fluid compartments of the rat. J Clin Invest 86:1352–1357, 1990.

120. Braam B, Mitchell KD, Fox J, Navar LG: Proximal tubular secretion of angiotensin II in rats. Am J Physiol 264:F891–F898, 1993.

121. Navar LG, Lewis L, Hymel A, et al: Tubular fluid concentrations and kidney contents of angiotensins I and II in anesthetized rats. J Am Soc Nephrol 5:1153–1158, 1994.

122. Navar LG, Lewis L, Hymel A, Mitchell KD: Proximal tubular fluid levels of angiotensinogen in anesthetized rats [abstract]. FASEB J 10:A22, 1996.

123. Henrich WL, McAllister EA, Eskue A, et al: Renin regulation in cultured proximal tubular cells. Hypertension 27:1337–1340, 1996.

124. Moe OW, Ujiie K, Star RA, et al: Renin expression in renal proximal tubule. J Clin Invest 91:774–779, 1993.

125. Leyssac PP: Changes in single nephron renin release are mediated by tubular fluid flow rate. Kidney Int 30:332–339, 1986.

126. Sibony M, Gasc J-M, Soubrier F, et al: Gene expression and tissue localization of the two isoforms of angiotensin I converting enzyme. Hypertension 21:827–835, 1993.

127. Ikemoto F, Ito S, Song G, et al: Contribution of renal angiotensin converting enzyme (ACE) to blood pressure regulation: Possible role of brush border ace. Clin Exp Theor Pract 9:441–447, 1987.

128. Cervenka L, Wang C-T, Mitchell KD, Navar LG: Proximal tubular angiotensin II levels and renal functional responses to AT$_1$ receptor blockade in nonclipped kidneys of Goldblatt hypertensive rats. Hypertension 33:102–107, 1999.

129. Wang C-T, Mitchell KD, Navar LG: Proximal tubular fluid angiotensin II levels in angiotensin II-infused hypertensive rats [abstract]. J Am Soc Nephrol 8:1428, 1997.

130. Siragy HM, Howell NL, Ragsdale NV, Carey RM: Renal interstitial fluid angiotensin: Modulation by anesthesia, epinephrine, sodium depletion and renin inhibition. Hypertension 25:1021–1024, 1995.

131. Harris PJ, Navar LG: Tubular transport responses to angiotensin. Am J Physiol 248:F621–F630, 1985.

132. Mitchell KD, Navar LG: Superficial nephron responses to peritubular capillary infusions of angiotensins I and II. Am J Physiol 252:F818–F824, 1987.

133. Steiner RW, Blantz RC: Acute reversal by saralasin of multiple intrarenal effects of angiotensin. Am J Physiol 237:F386–F391, 1979.

134. Huang W-C, Ploth DW, Navar LG: Angiotensin mediated alterations in nephron function in Goldblatt hypertensive rats. Am J Physiol 243:F553–F560, 1982.

135. Huang W-C, Jackson CA, Navar LG: Nephron responses to converting enzyme inhibition in non-clipped kidney of Goldblatt hypertensive rat at normotensive pressures. Kidney Int 28:128–134, 1985.

136. Xie MH, Liu FY, Wong PC, et al: Proximal nephron and renal effects of DuP 753, a nonpeptide angiotensin II receptor antagonist. Kidney Int 38:473–479, 1990.

137. Zhuo J, Thomas D, Harris PJ, Skinner SL: The role of endogenous angiotensin II in the regulation of renal haemodynamics and proximal fluid reabsorption in the rat. J Physiol (Lond) 453:1–13, 1992.

138. Dulin NO, Ernsberger P, Suciu DJ, Douglas JG: Rabbit renal epithelial angiotensin II receptors. Am J Physiol 267:F776–F782, 1994.

139. Harris RC, Becker BN, Cheng H-F: Acute and chronic mechanisms for regulating proximal tubule angiotensin II receptor expression. J Am Soc Nephrol 8:306–313, 1997.

140. Liu FY, Cogan MG: Angiotensin II stimulation of hydrogen ion secretion in the rat early proximal tubule: Modes of action, mechanism, and kinetics. J Clin Invest 82:601–607, 1988.

141. Saccomani G, Mitchell KD, Navar LG: Angiotensin II stimulation of Na$^+$-H$^+$ exchange in proximal tubule cells. Am J Physiol 258:F1188–F1195, 1990.

142. Quan A, Baum M: Endogenous angiotensin II modulates rat proximal tubule transport with acute changes in extracellular volume. Am J Physiol 275:F74–F78, 1998.

143. Quan A, Baum M: Effect of luminal angiotensin II receptor antagonists on proximal tubule transport. Am J Hypertens 12:499–503, 1999.

144. Lo M, Liu K-L, Lantelme P, Sassard J: Subtype 2 of angiotensin II receptors controls pressure-natriuresis in rats. J Clin Invest 95:1394–1397, 1995.

145. Millatt LJ, Abdel-Rahman EM, Siragy HM: Angiotensin II and nitric oxide: A question of balance. Regul Pept 81:1–10, 1999.

146. Levine DZ, Iacovitti M, Buckman S, Burns KD: Role of angiotensin II in dietary modulation of rat late distal tubule bicarbonate flux in vivo. J Clin Invest 97:120–125, 1996.

147. Levine DZ, Lacovitti M, Buckman S, Harrison V: In vivo modulation of rat distal tubule net HCO$_3$ flux by VIP, isoproterenol, angiotensin II, and ADH. Am J Physiol 266:F878–F883, 1994.

148. Wang T, Giebisch G: Effects of angiotensin II on electrolyte transport in the early and late distal tubule in rat kidney. Am J Physiol 271:F143–F149, 1996.

149. Barreto-Chaves MLM, Mello-Aires M: Effect of luminal angiotensin II and ANP on early and late cortical distal tubule HCO$_3^-$ reabsorption. Am J Physiol 271:F977–F984, 1996.

150. Blantz RC, Konnen KS, Tucker BJ: Angiotensin II effects upon the glomerular microcirculation and ultrafiltration coefficient of the rat. J Clin Invest 57:419–426, 1976.

151. Baylis C, Brenner BM: Modulation by prostaglandin synthesis inhibitors of the action of exogenous angiotensin II on glomerular ultrafiltration in the rat. Circ Res 43:889–898, 1978.

152. Rosivall L, Navar LG: Effects on renal hemodynamics of intra-arterial infusions of angiotensins I and II. Am J Physiol 245:F181–F187, 1983.

153. Schor N, Ichikawa I, Brenner BM: Glomerular adaptations to chronic dietary salt restriction or excess. Am J Physiol 238:F428–F436, 1980.
154. Casellas D, Carmines PK, Navar LG: Microvascular reactivity of in vitro blood perfused juxtamedullary nephrons from rats. Kidney Int 28:752–759, 1985.
155. Loutzenhiser R, Epstein M, Hayashi K, et al: Characterization of the renal microvascular effects of angiotensin II antagonist, DuP 753: Studies in isolated perfused hydronephrotic kidneys. Am J Hypertens 4:309S–314S, 1991.
156. Carmines PK, Morrison TK, Navar LG: Angiotensin II effects on microvascular diameters of in vitro blood-perfused juxtamedullary nephrons. Am J Physiol 251:F610–F618, 1986.
157. Carmines PK, Navar LG: Disparate effects of Ca channel blockade on afferent and efferent arteriolar responses to ANG II. Am J Physiol 256:F1015–F1020, 1989.
158. Carmines PK, Perry MD, Hazelrig JB, Navar LG: Effects of preglomerular and postglomerular vascular resistance alterations on filtration fraction. Kidney Int 31(Suppl 20):S-229–S-232, 1987.
159. Iversen BM, Arendshorst WJ: ANG II and vasopressin stimulate calcium entry in dispersed smooth muscle cells of preglomerular arterioles. Am J Physiol 274:F498–F508, 1998.
160. Zou A-P, Wu F, Cowley AW Jr: Protective effect of angiotensin II-induced increase in nitric oxide in the renal medullary circulation. Hypertension 31(Pt 2):271–276, 1998.
161. Zhuo J, Dean R, Maric C, et al: Localization and interactions of vasoactive peptide receptors in renomedullary interstitial cells of the kidney. Kidney Int 67:S-22–S-28, 1998.
162. Schnermann J, Briggs J: Role of the renin-angiotensin system in tubuloglomerular feedback. Fed Proc 45:1426–1430, 1986.
163. Braam B, Mitchell KD, Koomans HA, Navar LG: Relevance of the tubuloglomerular feedback mechanism in pathophysiology. J Am Soc Nephrol 4:1257–1274, 1993.
164. Mitchell KD, Braam B, Navar LG: Hypertensinogenic mechanisms mediated by renal actions of renin-angiotensin system. Hypertension 19(Suppl I):I-18–I-27, 1992.
165. Braam B, Navar LG, Mitchell KD: Modulation of tubuloglomerular feedback by angiotensin II type 1 receptors during the development of Goldblatt hypertension. Hypertension 25:1232–1237, 1995.
166. Ploth DW: Angiotensin-dependent renal mechanisms in two-kidney one-clip renal vascular hypertension. Am J Physiol 245:F131–F141, 1983.
167. Huang W-C, Bell PD, Harvey D, et al: Angiotensin influences on tubuloglomerular feedback mechanism in hypertensive rats. Kidney Int 34:631–637, 1988.
168. Schnermann JB, Traynor T, Yang T, et al: Absence of tubuloglomerular feedback responses in AT_{1A} receptor-deficient mice. Am J Physiol 273:F315–F320, 1997.
169. Traynor T, Yang T, Huang YG, et al: Tubuloglomerular feedback in ACE-deficient mice. Am J Physiol 276:F751–F757, 1999.
170. Peti-Peterdi J, Bell PD: Regulation of macula densa Na:H exchange by angiotensin II. Kidney Int 54:2021–2028, 1998.
171. Seeliger E, Boemke W, Corea M, et al: Mechanisms compensating Na and water retention induced by long-term reduction of renal perfusion pressure. Am J Physiol 273:R646–R654, 1997.
172. Cervenka L, Wang C-T, Navar LG: Effects of acute AT_1 receptor blockade by candesartan on arterial pressure and renal function in rats. Am J Physiol 274:F940–F945, 1998.
173. Cervenka L, Navar LG: Renal responses of the nonclipped kidney of two-kidney/one-clip Goldblatt hypertensive rats to type 1 angiotensin II receptor blockade with candesartan. J Am Soc Nephrol 10:S196–S201, 1999.
174. Takishita S, Muratani H, Sesoko S, et al: Short-term effects of angiotensin II blockade on renal blood flow and sympathetic activity in awake rats. Hypertension 24:445–450, 1994.
175. Xu L, Brooks VL: ANG II chronically supports renal and lumbar sympathetic activity in sodium-deprived, conscious rats. Am J Physiol 271:H2591–H2598, 1996.
176. DiBona GF, Jones SY, Sawin LL: Angiotensin receptor antagonist improves cardiac reflex control of renal sodium handling in heart failure. Am J Physiol 274:H636–H641, 1998.
177. Jover B, Saladini D, Nafrialdi N, et al: Effect of losartan and enalapril on renal adaptation to sodium restriction in rat. Am J Physiol 267:F281–F288, 1994.
178. Peng Y, Knox FG: Comparison of systemic and direct intrarenal angiotensin II blockade on sodium excretion in rats. Am J Physiol 269:F40–F46, 1995.
179. Khosla MC, Smeby RC, Bumpus FM: Structure activity relationship in angiotensin II analogs. In Page IH, Bumpus FM (eds): Angiotensin. New York, Springer-Verlag, 1974, pp 126–161.
180. Huang W-C, Ploth DW, Navar LG: Effects of saralasin infusion on bilateral renal function in 2 kidney, 1 clip Goldblatt hypertensive rats. Clin Sci 62:573–579, 1982.
181. Steiner RW, Tucker BJ, Blantz RC: Glomerular hemodynamics in rats with chronic sodium depletion. J Clin Invest 64:503–512, 1979.
182. Hall JE, Guyton AC, Trippodo NC, et al: Intrarenal control of electrolyte excretion by angiotensin II. Am J Physiol 232:F538–F544, 1977.

183. Siragy HM, Howell NL, Peach MJ, Carey RM: Combined intrarenal blockade of the renin-angiotensin system in the conscious dog. Am J Physiol 258:F522–F529, 1990.

184. Liu KL, Lo M, Grouzmann E, et al: The subtype 2 of angiotensin II receptors and pressure-natriuresis in adult rat kidneys. Br J Pharmacol 126:826–832, 1999.

185. Muñoz-García R, Maeso R, Rodrigo E, et al: Acute renal excretory actions of losartan in spontaneously hypertensive rats: Role of AT_2 receptors, prostaglandins, kinins and nitric oxide. J Hypertens 13:1779–1784, 1995.

186. Tamaki T, Nishiyama A, Yoshida H, et al: Effects of EXP3174, a non-peptide angiotensin II receptor antagonist, on renal hemodynamics and renal function in dogs. Eur J Pharmacol 236:15–21, 1993.

187. Clark KL, Robertson MJ, Drew GM: Renal pharmacology of GR138950, a novel non-peptide angiotensin AT_1 receptor antagonist. Eur J Pharmacol 280:193–203, 1995.

188. Keiser JA, Bjork FA, Hodges JC, Taylor DG Jr: Renal hemodynamic and excretory responses to PD 123319 and losartan, nonpeptide AT_1 and AT_2 subtype-specific angiotensin II ligands. J Pharmacol Exp Ther 262:1154–1160, 1992.

189. Chan DP, Sandok EK, Aahrus LL, et al: Renal-specific actions of angiotensin II receptor antagonism in the anesthetized dog. Am J Hypertens 5:354–360, 1992.

190. Clark KL, Robertson MJ, Drew GM: Role of angiotensin AT_1 and AT_2 receptors in mediating the renal effects of angiotensin II in the anaesthetized dog. Br J Pharmacol 109:148–156, 1993.

191. El-Dahr SS, Dipp S, Guan S, Navar LG: Renin, angiotensinogen, and kallikrein gene expression in two-kidney Goldblatt hypertensive rats. Am J Hypertens 6:914–919, 1993.

192. Amiri F, Garcia R: Renal angiotensin II receptor regulation in two-kidney, one clip hypertensive rats. Effect of ACE inhibition. Hypertension 30(Pt 1):337–344, 1997.

193. Cheng H-F, Becker BN, Burns KD, Harris RC: Angiotensin II upregulates type-1 angiotensin II receptors in renal proximal tubule. J Clin Invest 95:2012–2019, 1995.

194. Harrison-Bernard LM, El-Dahr SS, O'Leary DF, Navar LG: Regulation of angiotensin II type 1 receptor mRNA and protein in angiotensin II-induced hypertension. Hypertension 33(Pt II):340–346, 1999.

195. Ichihara A, Inscho EW, Imig JD, et al: Role of renal nerves in afferent arteriolar reactivity in angiotensin-induced hypertension. Hypertension 29(Pt 2):442–449, 1997.

196. Inscho EW, Imig JD, Deichmann PC, Cook AK: Candesartan cilexetil protects against loss of autoregulatory efficiency in angiotensin II-infused rats. J Am Soc Nephrol 10:S178–S183, 1999.

197. Inscho EW, Carmines PK, Cook AK, Navar LG: Afferent arteriolar responsiveness to altered perfusion pressure in renal hypertension. Hypertension 15:748–752, 1990.

198. Inscho EW, Cook AK, Navar LG: Pressure-mediated vasoconstriction of juxtamedullary afferent arterioles involves P_2-purinoceptor activation. Am J Physiol 271:F1077–F1085, 1996.

199. Morsing P, Adler G, Brandt-Eliasson U, et al: Mechanistic differences of various AT_1-receptor blockers in isolated vessels of different origin. Hypertension 33:1406–1413, 1999.

200. Anderson IK, Drew GM: The antihypertensive profile of the angiotensin AT_1 receptor antagonist, GR138950, and the influence of potential homeostatic compensatory mechanisms in renal hypertensive rats. Br J Pharmacol 125:1236–1246, 1998.

201. Mervaala E, Dehmel B, Gross V, et al: Angiotensin-converting enzyme inhibition and AT_1 receptor blockade modify the pressure-natriuresis relationship by additive mechanisms in rats with human renin and angiotensinogen gene. J Am Soc Nephrol 10:1669–1680, 1999.

202. Gross V, Lippoldt A, Schneider W, Luft FC: Effect of captopril and angiotensin II receptor blockade on pressure natriuresis in transgenic TGR(mRen-2)27 rats. Hypertension 26:471–479, 1995.

203. Price DA, De'Oliveira JM, Fisher NDL, Hollenberg NK: Renal hemodynamic response to an angiotensin II antagonist, eprosartan, in healthy men. Hypertension 30(Pt 1):240–246, 1997.

204. Pechère-Bertschi A, Nussberger J, Decosterd L, et al: Renal response to the angiotensin II receptor subtype 1 antagonist irbesartan versus enalapril in hypertensive patients. J Hypertens 16:385–393, 1998.

205. Gansevoort RT, deZeeuw D, deJong PE: Is the antiproteinuric effect of ACE inhibition mediated by interference in the renin-angiotensin system? Kidney Int 45:861–867, 1994.

206. Burnier M, Waeber B, Brunner HR: The advantages of angiotensin II antagonism. J Hypertens 12(Suppl 2):S7–S15, 1994.

207. Kawabata M, Takabatake T, Ohta H, et al: Effects of an angiotensin II receptor antagonist, TCV-116, on renal haemodynamics in essential hypertension. Blood Pressure 3(Suppl 5):117–121, 1994.

208. Buter H, Navis G, de Zeeuw D, de Jong PE: Renal hemodynamic effects of candesartan in normal and impaired renal function in humans. Kidney Int 63:S185–S187, 1997.

209. Arendshorst WJ, Navar LG: Renal circulation and glomerular hemodynamics. In Schrier RW, Gottschalk CW (eds): Diseases of the Kidney, 6th ed. Boston, Little, Brown, 1997, pp 59–106.

210. Fridman K, Andersson OK, Wysocki M, et al: Acute effects of candesartan cilexetil (the new angiotensin II antagonist) on systemic and renal haemodynamics in hypertensive patients. Eur J Pharmacol 54:497–501, 1998.
211. Burnier M, Rutschmann B, Nussberger J, et al: Salt-dependent renal effects of an angiotensin II antagonist in healthy subjects. Hypertension 22:339–347, 1993.
212. Guyton AC: Blood pressure control—special role of the kidneys and body fluids. Science 252:1813–1816, 1991.

CHAPTER 14

Cardiac Effects of Angiotensin II and AT$_1$ Receptor Blockade

IRENE GAVRAS, M.D.
HARALAMBOS GAVRAS, M.D.

For 60 years angiotensin II (Ang II) has been recognized as the effector substance of the renin-angiotensin system (RAS), but for a long time it was viewed mostly as a systemically circulating vasoconstrictor and steroidogenic hormone. In recent years, however, the development and application of cellular and molecular biology techniques have revealed another aspect of Ang II as a tissue hormone or autocoid with paracrine, autocrine, and intracrine actions. These actions differ in various organs and depend on the cell types within tissues. The cardiac effects of Ang II are both direct, exerted via activation of specific receptors on cardiomyocytes, endothelial cells, and fibroblasts; and indirect, resulting from systemic vasoconstriction (pressure/volume overload), particularly coronary artery constriction, as well as from stimulation of other neurohormonal substances (e.g., norepinephrine, endothelin).

■ Cardiac Receptors for Angiotensin II

Renin is the rate-limiting enzymatic step for Ang II synthesis in the RAS cascade[1] and is mostly of renal origin. However, all components of the RAS cascade have been identified in cardiac tissues by biochemical methods. Moreover, molecular biologic techniques have demonstrated the presence of mRNA for renin, angiotensinogen, and angiotensin-converting enzyme (ACE) in cardiac cells, although some are found in embryonic cells only.[2] Therefore, all RAS components appear to be present and regulated at the molecular level in heart tissues, although the synthesis of Ang II in vivo may vary under different circumstances, such as species, age, and pathologic condition of the heart. Nevertheless, the renal renin and circulating components of the RAS are produced in amounts greater by several orders of magnitude than the amounts produced by extrarenal tissues and are mainly or solely responsible for the systemic hormonal and hemodynamic effects of Ang II. On the the hand, the minute amounts of Ang II produced locally may be responsible for its direct paracrine, autocrine, and, possibly, intracrine effects (such as trophic) that persist even in the renoprival state.

Whether blood-borne or locally generated, Ang II exerts its effects on the heart via activation of its type 1 (AT_1) receptor, a G protein-linked receptor identified on cardiac cell membranes.[3] This receptor activates protein kinase C through formation of diacylglycerol and hydrolysis of phosphatidylinositol.[3,4] An AT_2 receptor also has been identified by radioligand-binding studies but has not been clearly linked to biologic responses; it is believed to play a role mostly in fetal growth and development because its density declines sharply in the postnatal period.[5]

Activation of the AT_1 receptors by Ang II elicits a variety of responses, depending on the cellular type. In cardiomyocytes and vascular smooth muscle cells these responses alter the electrophysiologic milieu and the growth and proliferation of cells. Endothelial cells respond by secreting various autacoids, such as nitric oxide (NO) and endothelin, whereas neural cells respond by modulating the release of neurotransmitters, fibroblasts and platelets respond by releasing growth factors. Accordingly, the effects of Ang II on the heart include those exerted directly via activation of AT_1 receptors and mobilization of intracellular messengers of myocardial cells, those mediated by locally released substances from other cells (e.g., endothelial cells, fibroblasts), and those resulting indirectly from the systemic and regional hemodynamic and metabolic actions of Ang II (Table 1).

The AT_2 type receptor appears to be involved in the developmental effects of Ang II in the fetus, but its postnatal function remains elusive. Of interest, about 30% of the Ang II receptors found in normal rat heart are of the AT_2 type, and their percentage increases to 60% in the hypertrophied heart.[6] Reports of their function seem to be contradictory. Some investigators have found evidence suggesting that AT_2 activation sets in motion intracellular events leading to apoptosis (i.e., programmed cell death).[7] Others, however, have attributed to these receptors a cardioprotective effect, possibly mediated via activation of kinins and other autacoids, similar to those participating in the actions of ACE inhibitors.[8] New data may soon reconcile seemingly conflicting pieces of evidence.

■ Angiotensin II Effects Resulting from Activation of AT_1 Receptors on Cardiac Cell Membranes

AT_1 receptors are distributed abundantly on the surface of cardiomyocytes, fibroblasts, and vascular smooth muscle cells and are particularly dense in the conduction system of the heart.[9] Activation of these receptors triggers a series of intracellular reactions that lead to cell hypertrophy and proliferation, increased contractile responses, altered electrophysiologic milieu, and metabolic conditions.

Table 1.   Effects of Angiotensin II on the Heart

Direct Effects	Indirect Effects
1. Trophic/mitogenic (cardiomyocytes, fibroblasts, platelets)	1. Hemodynamic burden (systemic vasoconstriction, left ventricular hypertrophy/stretch, pump failure)
2. Inotropic/contractile (cardiomyocytes, vascular smooth muscle cells)	2. Coronary vasoconstriction (ischemic cardiomyopathy, myocardial infarction)
3. Chronotropic/arrhythmogenic (cardiomyocytes, Purkinje cells)	3. Sympathetic stimulation/neurogenic effects
4. Thrombogenic (platelets, endothelial cells)	4. Endothelin stimulation/paracrine effects
5. Oxidative (endothelial cells, macrophages)	5. Vasopressin stimulation

Activation of AT$_1$ receptors stimulates release of numerous growth factors, such as T-cell growth factor beta$_1$ (TGFβ_1), platelet-derived growth factor (PDGF), beta fibroblast growth factor (βFGF), and insulin-like growth factor-1 (IGF-1) which act in an autocrine fashion to activate enzymes and genes that induce protein and DNA synthesis.[10–13] Ang II per se acts also as a peptide growth factor stimulating expression of genes that regulate cell growth and proliferation, such as *c-fos, c-jun, c-myc,* and *c-myb,*[11,14,15] and generating intracellular second messengers, such as phospholipases and phosphatidic acid, which can increase thymidine incorporation and induce mRNA expression of protooncogenes.[16,17] Activation of AT$_2$ receptors, in contrast, may counteract these effects.[18,19]

The intracellular responses triggered by AT$_1$ receptor activation include mobilization of calcium, stimulation of nitrogen and hydrogen ion exchange, activation of protein kinase (and other kinases), activation of phosphorylation pathways, and alteration in cytoplasmic proteins, including contractile proteins.[2,20] The resulting altered conductance of calcium channels and shortening of cardiac fibers increase the conduction velocity of electrical currents[21,22] and the contractility of cardiomyocytes[23] and account in part for the positive inotropic and chronotropic effects and proarrhythmic properties of Ang II.

The thrombogenic[24] and oxidative[25] properties of Ang II are of particular relevance to cardiovascular ischemic events and myocardial tissue damage. Ang II has been reported to stimulate excessive production of plasminogen activator inhibitor type I (PAI-1) via induction of its mRNA expression in cell cultures,[26] thus increasing the risk of thrombotic events.[27] It is unclear, however, which types of Ang fragments or receptors are involved in this process.[28]

Ang II also has been reported to increase activity of the reduced nicotinamide adenine dinucleotide (NADH) and reduced nicotinamide adenine dinucleotide phosphate (NADPH) oxidases, leading to production of superoxide anions.[29] Reactive oxygen intermediates, which may be part of the normal intracellular signaling responses to AT$_1$ receptor stimulation, cause oxidative damage to various cellular structures and proteins (including DNA sequences and enzymes).[30] Excessive Ang II, therefore, may precipitate myocardial infarcts via multiple mechanisms, including coronary constriction,[31–33] inhibition of NO-dependent vasodilation,[34] prothrombotic alterations in blood rheology,[35] lipid peroxidation promoting atherogenesis,[36] and vascular wall hypertrophy[37] promoting arteriolar obstruction.

■ Cardiac Effects of Angiotensin II Resulting from Its Hemodynamic and Hormonal Actions

Systemically, Ang II produces intense generalized vasoconstriction, which is particularly pronounced in the vital organs, whose vasculature is most sensitive to Ang II, such as the cerebral, cardiac, and renal vasculatures.[32,33] Surges of Ang II of exogenous or endogenous origin cause widespread areas of myocardial necrosis[31,32] attributable to both ischemia and direct cardiotoxicity.[38] Vasoconstriction is further enhanced by Ang II-mediated stimulation of other vasopressor neurohormones, such as vasopressin,[39] catecholamines,[40,41] and endothelin,[42,43] which possess their own trophic, mitogenic, and arrhythmogenic properties. The steroidogenic action of Ang II (i.e., stimulation of aldosterone synthesis and release) not only contributes to the hemodynamic burden via retention of salt and fluid but also may exert an additional cardiotoxic effect.[44]

All of these influences tend to accentuate the pressure-volume overload on the myocardium, resulting in left ventricular stress and cardiomyopathy typical of hypertension and/or congestive heart failure.[45] The mechanical stretching of cardiomyocytes and other cardiac cells triggers release of humoral factors that activate a number of intracellular trophic and mitogenic factors, including protein kinases and protooncogenes.[46,47] Evidence indicates that the humoral factor triggered by stretch may be locally produced Ang II acting in a paracrine or autocrine manner. Left ventricular hypertrophy (LVH) is associated with increased gene expression of some of the RAS components, such as angiotensinogen[48] and ACE,[49] in the hypertrophied myocardium. LVH is independently associated with relative coronary insufficiency (even in the absence of arterial obstruction) as well as diastolic heart dysfunction and electrophysiological instability,[50,51] all of which are aggravated indirectly and directly by excessive Ang II and predispose to increased mortality.[52]

■ Experimental Studies of the Effects of Angiotensin II Blockade on the Heart

The first experimental animal studies with Ang II blockade were conducted in the early 1970s using saralasin[53] and focused mostly on assessing the systemic and regional hemodynamic consequences. In the following years the cardiac effects of the RAS were investigated exhaustively with the help of various ACE inhibitors. When the nonpeptide selective AT_1 receptor blockers became available, interest in the effects of Ang II on the heart was revived. In comparative studies using AT_1 receptor antagonists and ACE inhibitors, investigators attempted to dissect the knowledge accumulated over the past two decades by separating the Ang II-mediated from the bradykinin-mediated effects of ACE inhibition. It soon became apparent that the systemic and regional hemodynamic changes of ACE inhibition are attributable almost solely to withdrawal of Ang II,[54] although bradykinin may account for variations in blood flow within areas of certain organs (e.g., epicardial vs. endocardial layers of the myocardium[55] or cortical vs. papillary areas of the kidney[56]). Bradykinin also may contribute to ACE inhibitor-induced cardioprotection of the injured myocardium via its metabolic properties (i.e., enhancement of insulin-dependent glucose transport and uptake).[57] Nevertheless, withdrawal of the Ang II-mediated effects also accounts to a large extent for these cardioprotective properties, as indicated by the following examples of experimental studies using selective Ang II receptor blockade.

In rats submitted to experimental myocardial infarcts, AT_1 receptor blockade was shown to minimize the area of scarring and extent of myocardial fibrosis and to attenuate the cardiac remodeling and attendant dysfunction.[58] Pretreatment with losartan before coronary artery ligation, followed by removal of the ligature, was found to minimize the myocardial tissue injury from ischemia and reperfusion, with reduced infarct size and decreased incidence of ventricular arrhythmias and overall mortality in comparison with placebo-treated rats.[59] Another acute study of coronary occlusion followed by reperfusion in dogs found that treatment with losartan before occlusion reduced the incidence of ventricular tachyarrhythmias, whereas placebo-treated dogs had more episodes and a lower threshold for induction of arrhythmia.[60] A study of global ischemia followed by reperfusion of isolated rat hearts found that an ACE inhibitor, an

Ang II receptor blocker, and a renin inhibitor were equally effective in diminishing the duration of ventricular fibrillation, although none seemed to affect markers of cellular damage or mechanical function.[61]

In chronic experiments in spontaneously hypertensive rats, various antihypertensive treatments were compared in terms of their effects on electrophysiologic parameters, which are markers of susceptibility to malignant ventricular arrhythmias. Rats treated with ACE inhibitor and rats treated with an Ang II antagonist had significant regression of LVH and indices of electrophysiologic stability similar to those of normotensive rats. In contrast, rats treated with hydralazine had no LVH regression, and their electrophysiologic markers were similar to those of placebo-treated hypertensive rats, despite lowering of blood pressure to the same extent as the groups treated with Ang II inhibition.[62] Another intriguing study, however, suggested that losartan indeed has antiarrhythmic properties, but not via blockade of AT$_1$ receptors.[63] The investigators simulated the conditions of ischemia and reperfusion in an isolated pig heart model and measured changes in a number of electrophysiologic parameters, such as conduction time, action potential duration, and effective refractory period. Surprisingly, they found that exogenous Ang II produced changes that inhibit arrhythmias, whereas losartan had an antiarrhythmic effect that was independent of the presence or absence of Ang II. This finding suggests that the mechanism may not be AT$_1$ receptor blockade.

Despite this isolated report, the experimental evidence overwhelmingly favors AT$_1$-receptor mediated cardioprotective effects, because they can be reproduced by other AT$_1$ antagonists, such as telmisartan and candesartan. For example, transgenic rats harboring the murine Ren-2 gene exhibit fulminant hypertension and marked cardiac hypertrophy. When such rats were treated with telmisartan in various doses over a 9-week period, cardiac hypertrophy was reduced significantly. This reduction was observed even at doses too low to produce an antihypertensive effect, suggesting that the reversal of hypertrophy did not result from hemodynamic improvement but rather was a local effect of AT$_1$ receptor blockade on cardiomyocytes.[64] The same was true for the renal complications of hypertension (i.e., telmisartan at the lowest dosage) that had no hypotensive effect but prevented glomerulosclerosis and proteinuria, although systemic blood pressure remained in the range of 225 mmHg or over.[65] These studies further corroborate the concept that Ang II exerts a detrimental effect on target organs independent of (or in addition to) the hemodynamic burden of systemic hypertension. These results agree with similar findings obtained with other Ang II antagonists as well as ACE inhibitors. To investigate further the cardioprotective properties of telmisartan, a recent study used a porcine model of cardiac arrest obtained by induction of ventricular fibrillation for 4 minutes followed by cardiopulmonary resuscitation. Studies of cardiac function after restoration of spontaneous circulation showed that animals treated with telmisartan, 1 mg/kg, had significantly better left ventricular contractility and right ventricular end-systolic and end-diastolic volumes and right ventricular ejection fraction than control animals treated with saline.[66] These findings appear to be comparable to reports in the literature that ACE inhibitors minimize the effects of myocardial "stunning." Furthermore, chronic treatment with oral telmisartan of genetically hypertensive rats of a stroke-prone strain revealed blood pressure-lowering and renoprotective effects comparable to those of losartan and captopril as well as a marked reduction of cardiac hypertrophy.[67] These studies indicate that all AT_1-receptor antagonists probably possess a cardioprotective potential and that it is a class effect. Clinical trials to test this hypothesis are under way.

Acknowledgment

This paper is supported by NIH grant No. 1P50HL 55001.

References

1. Lee MR: Renin and Hypertension. Baltimore, Williams & Wilkins, 1969.
2. Dostal DE, Baker KM: Biochemistry, molecular biology, and potential roles of the cardiac renin-angiotensin system. In Dhalla NS, Takeda N, Nagano M (eds): The Failing Heart. Philadelphia, Lippincott-Raven, 1995, pp 275–294.
3. Rogers TB, Gaa ST, Allen IS: Identification and characterization of functional angiotensin II receptors on cultured heart myocytes. J Pharm Exp Ther 236:438–444, 1986.
4. Allen IS, Cohen NM, Dhallan RS, et al: Angiotensin II increases spontaneous contractile frequency and stimulates calcium current in cultured neonatal rat heart myocytes: Insights into the underlying biochemical mechanisms. Circ Res 62:524–534, 1988.
5. Urata H, Healy B, Stewart RW, et al: Angiotensin receptors in normal and failing human hearts. J Clin Endocrinol Metab 69:54–66, 1989.
6. Lopez JJ, Lorell BH, Ingelfinger JR, et al: Distribution and function of cardiac angiotensin AT_1 and AT_2 receptor subtypes in hypertrophied rat hearts. Am J Physiol 267:H844–H852, 1994.
7. Yamada T, Horiuchi M, Dzau VJ: Angiotensin II type 2 receptor mediates programmed cell death. Proc Natl Acad Sci 93:156–160, 1996.
8. Liu Y-H, Yang X-P, Sharov VG, et al: Effects of angiotensin-converting enzyme inhibitors and angiotensin II type 1 receptor antagonists in rats with heart failure: Role of kinins and angiotensin II type 2 receptors. J Clin Invest 99:1926–1935, 1997.
9. Saito K, Gutkind JS, Saavedra JM: Angiotensin II binding sites in the conduction system of rat hearts. Am J Physiol 253:H1618–H1622, 1987.
10. Stouffer GA, Owens GK: Angiotensin II-induced mitogenesis of spontaneously hypertensive rat-derived cultured smooth muscle cells is dependent on autocrine production of transforming growth factor-beta. Circ Res 70:820–828, 1992.
11. Naftilan AJ, Pratt RE, Dzau VJ: Induction of platelet-derived growth factor A-chain and *c-myc* gene expression by angiotensin II in cultured rat vascular smooth muscle cell. J Clin Invest 83:1419–1424, 1989.
12. Schorb W, Singer HA, Dostal DE, Baker KM: Angiotensin II is a potent simulator of MAP-kinase activity in neonatal rat cardiac fibroblasts. J Mol Cell Cardiol 27:1151–1160, 1995.
13. Delafontaine P, Lou H: Angiotensin II regulates insulin-like growth factor I gene expression in vascular smooth muscle cells. J Biol Chem 268:16866–16870, 1993.
14. Naftilan AJ, Pratt RE, Eldrige CS, et al: Angiotensin II induces *c-fos* expression in smooth muscle via transcriptional control. Hypertension 13:706–711, 1989.
15. Pauet J-L, Baudouin-Legros M, Brunell G, Meyer P: Angiotensin II-induced proliferation of aortic myocytes in spontaneously hypertensive rats. J Hypertens 8:565–572, 1990.
16. Yu C, Tsai M, Stacey DW: Cellular ras activity and phospholipid metabolism. Cell 52:63–71, 1988.
17. Knauss TC, Jaffer FE, Abboud HE: Phosphatidic acid modulates DNA synthesis, phospholipase C, and platelet-derived growth factor mRNAs in cultured mesangial cells. J Biol Chem 265:14457–14463, 1990.
18. Nakajima M, Hutchinson HG, Fujinaga W: The angiotensin II type 2 (AT_2) receptor antagonizes the growth effects of the AT_1 receptor: Gain-of-function study using gene transfer. Proc Natl Acad Sci USA 92:10663–10667, 1995.
19. Stoll M, Steckelings UM, Paul M, et al: The angiotensin AT_2-receptor mediates inhibition of cell proliferation in coronary endothelial cells. J Clin Invest 95:651–657, 1995.
20. Scott-Burden T, Hahn AWA, Resink TJ, Buhler FR: Modulation of extracellular matrix by angiotensin II: Stimulated glycoconjugate synthesis and growth in vascular smooth muscle cells. J Cardiovasc Pharmacol 16(Suppl 4):36–41, 1990.
21. Kass RS, Blair ML: Effects of angiotensin II on membrane current in cardiac Purkinje fibers. J Mol Cell CArdiol 13:797–809, 1981.
22. De Mello WC: Renin-angiotensin system and cell communication in the failing heart. Hypertension 27:1267–1272, 1996.

23. Kobayashi M, Furukawa Y, Chiba S: Positive chronotropic and inotropic effects of angiotensin II in the dog heart. Eur J Pharmacol 50:17–25, 1978.
24. Ridker PM: An epidemiologic assessment of thrombotic risk factors for cardiovascular disease. Curr Opin Lipid 3:285–290, 1992.
25. Oskarsson HJ, Heistad DD: Oxidative stress produced by angiotensin II: Implications for hypertension and vascular injury. Circulation 95:557–559, 1997.
26. Van Leeuwen RT, Kol A, Andreotti F, et al: Angiotensin II increases plasminogen activator inhibitor type 1 and tissue-type plasminogen activator messenger RNA in culture rat aortic smooth muscle cells. Circulation 62:362–368, 1994.
27. Vaughn DE, Lazos SA, Tong K: Angiotensin II regulates the expression of plasminogen activator inhibitor-1 in cultured endothelial cells. A potential link between the renin-angiotensin system and thrombosis. J Clin Invest 95:995–1001, 1995.
28. Kerins DM, Hao Q, Vaughan DE: Angiotensin induction of PAI-1 expression in endothelial cells is mediated by the hexapeptide angiotensin IV. J Clin Invest 96:2515–2520, 1995.
29. Griendling KK, Minieri CA, Ollerenshaw JD, Alexander RW: Angiotensin II stimulates NADH and NADPH oxidase activity in cultured smooth muscle cells. Circ Res 74:1141–1148, 1994.
30. Ames BN, Shigenaga MK, Hagen TM: Oxidants, antioxidants, and the degenerative disease of aging. Proc Natl Acad Sci USA 90:7915–7922, 1993.
31. Gavras H, Brown JJ, Lever AF, et al: Acute renal failure, tubular necrosis and myocardial infarction induced in the rabbit by intravenous angiotensin II. Lancet ii:19–22, 1971.
32. Gavras H, Kremer D, Brown JJ, et al: Angiotensin and norepinephrine-induced myocardial lesions: Experimental and clinical studies in rabbit and man. Am Heart J 89:321–332, 1975.
33. Liang C, Gavras H, Hood WB Jr: Renin-angiotensin system inhibition in conscious sodium-depleted dogs: Effects on systemic and coronary hemodynamics. J Clin Invest 61:874–883, 1978.
34. Rajagopalan S, Kurz S, Munzel T, et al: Angiotensin II-mediated hypertension in the rat increases vascular superoxide production via membrane NADH/NADPH oxidase activation: Contribution to alterations of vasomotor tone. J Clin Invest 97:1916–1923, 1996.
35. Hamsten A, DeFaire U, Walldius G, et al: Plasminogen activator inhibitor in plasma: Risk factor for recurrent myocardial infarction. Lancet ii:3–9, 1987.
36. Keaney JF, Frei B: Antioxidant protection of low-density lipoprotein and its role in the prevention of atherosclerotic vascular disease. In Frei B (ed): Natural Antioxidants in Human Health and Disease. Orlando, FL, Academic Press, 1994, pp 303–351.
37. Puri PL, Avantaggiati ML, Burgio VL: Reactive oxygen intermediates mediate angiotensin II-induced c-jun c-fos heterodimer DNA binding activity and proliferative hypertropic responses in myogenic cells. J Biol Chem 270:22129–22134, 1995.
38. Tan LB, Jalil JE, Pick R, et al: Cardiac myocyte necrosis induced by angiotensin II. Circ Res 69:1185–1195, 1991.
39. Sladek CD: Regulation of vasopressin release by neurotransmitters, neuropeptides and osmotic stimuli. In Gross BA, Leng C (eds): The Neurophysics: Structure, Function and Control Progress in Brain Research. Amsterdam, Elsevier Science, 1983, pp 71–90.
40. Malik KU, Nasjletti A: Facilitation of adrenergic transmission by locally generated angiotensin II in rat mesenteric arteries. Circ Res 38:26–30, 1976.
41. Newling RP, Fletcher PJ, Coutis M, Shaw J: Noradrenaline and cardiac hypertrophy in the rat: Changes in morphology, blood pressure and ventricular performance. J Hypertens 7:561–567, 1989.
42. Chua BH, Chua CC, Diglio CA, Siu BB: Regulation of endothelin-1 mRNA by angiotensin II in rat heart endothelial cells. Biochim Biophys Acta 1178:201–206, 1993.
43. Rajagopalan S, Laursen JB, Borthayre A: Role for endothelin-1 in angiotensin II-mediated hypertension. Hypertension 30(Part 1):29–34, 1997.
44. Weber KT, Brilla CG, Campbell SE, Reddy HK: Myocardial fibrosis and the concepts of cardioprotection and cardioreparation. J Hypertens 10(Suppl 5):S87–S94, 1992.
45. Katz AM: Cardiomyopathy of overload. A major determinant of prognosis in congestive heart failure. N Engl J Med 322:100–110, 1990.
46. Yamazaki T, Tobe K, Hoh E, et al: Mechanical loading activates mitogen-activated protein kinase and S6 peptide kinase in cultured rat cardiac myocytes. J Biol Chem 268:12069–12076, 1993.
47. Komuro I, Katoh Y, Kaida T, et al: Mechanical loading stimulates cell hypertrophy and specific gene expression in cultured rat cardiac myocytes. J Biol Chem 266:1265–1268, 1991.
48. Lindpaintner K, Ganten D: The cardiac renin-angiotensin system. Circ Res 68:905–921, 1991.
49. Fabris B, Jackson B, Kohzuki M, et al: Increased cardiac angiotensin-converting enzyme in rats with chronic heart failure. Clin Exp Pharmacol Physiol 17:309–314, 1990.
50. TenEick RE, Houser SR, Bassett AL: Cardiac hypertrophy and altered cellular electrical activity of the myocardium: Possible electrophysiological basis for myocardial contractility changes. In Sperelakis N (ed): Physiology and Pathophysiology of the Heart, 2nd ed. Boston, Kluwer Academic, 1989, pp 57–94.

51. Manolis AJ, Beldekos D, Hatzissavas J, et al: Hemodynamic and humoral correlates in essential hypertension. Relationship between patterns of LVH and myocardial ischemia. Hypertension 30(Part 2):730–734, 1997.

52. Kannel WB, Doyle JT, McNamara PM, et al: Precursors of sudden death: Factors related to the incidence of sudden death. Circulation 51:606–613, 1975.

53. Gavras H, Gavras I, Brunner HR, Liang C: Physiologic studies with saralasin in animals. Kidney Int 15:S-20–S-28, 1979.

54. Wang Y-X, Gavras I, Wierzba T, Gavras H: Comparison of systemic and regional hemodynamic effects of a diuretic, an angiotensin-II receptor antagonist, and an angiotensin-converting enzyme inhibitor. J Lab Clin Med 119:267–272, 1992.

55. Ruocco NA Jr, Bergelson BA, Yu T-K, et al: Augmentation of coronary blood flow by ACE inhibition: Role of angiotensin and bradykinin. Clin Exp Hypertens 17:1059–1072, 1995.

56. Fenoy FJ, Scicli AG, Carretero O, Roman RJ: Effect of an angiotensin II and a kinin receptor antagonist on the renal hemodynamic response to captopril. Hypertension 17:1038–1044, 1991.

57. Kohlman O Jr, De Assis Rocha Neves F, Ginoza M, et al: Role of bradykinin in insulin sensitivity and blood pressure regulation during hyperinsulinemia. Hypertension 25:1003–1007, 1995.

58. De Carvalho FC, Sun Y, Weber KT: Angiotensin II receptor blockade and myocardial fibrosis of the infarcted rat heart. J Lab Clin Med 129:439–446, 1997.

59. Lee Y-M, Peng Y-Y, Ding Y-A, Yen M-H: Losartan attenuates myocardial ischemia-induced ventricular arrhythmias and reperfusion injury in spontaneously hypertensive rats. Am J Hypertens 10:852–858, 1997.

60. Matsuo K, Kumagai K, Annoura M, et al: Effects of an angiotensin II antagonist on reperfusion arrhythmias in dogs. Pacing Clin Electrophysiol 20:938–945, 1997.

61. Fleetwood G, Boutinet S, Meier M, Wood JM: Involvement of the renin-angiotensin system in ischemic damage and reperfusion arrhythmias in the isolated perfused rat heart. J Cardiovasc Pharmacol 17:351–356, 1991.

62. Kohya T, Yokoshiki H, Tohse N, et al: Regression of left ventricular hypertrophy prevents ischemia-induced lethal arrhythmias: Beneficial effect of angiotensin II blockade. Circ Res 76:892–899, 1995.

63. Thomas GP, Gerrier GR, Howlett SE: Losartan exerts antiarrhythmic activity independent of angiotensin II receptor blockade in simulated ventricular ischemia and reperfusion. J Pharmacol Exp Ther 278:1090–1097, 1996.

64. Bohn M, Lippoldt A, Wienen W, et al: Reduction of cardiac hypertrophy in TGR (mREN2) 27 by angiotensin II receptor blockade. Mol Cell Biochem 163–164:217–221, 1996.

65. Bohn M, Lee M, Kreutz R, et al: Angiotensin II receptor blockade in TGR (mREN2) 27: Effects of renin-angiotensin system gene expression and cardiovascular functions. J Hypertens 13:891–899, 1995.

66. Strohmenger HU, Lindner KH, Wienen W, Vogt J: Effects of the AT1-selective angiotensin II antagonist, telmisartan, on hemodynamics and ventricular function after cardiopulmonary resuscitation in pigs. Resuscitation 35:61–68, 1997.

67. Wagner J, Drab M, Bohlender J, et al: Effects of AT1 receptor blockade on blood pressure and the renin-angiotensin system in spontaneously hypertensive rats of the stroke-prone strain. Clin Exper Hypertens 20:205–221, 1998.

CHAPTER 15

Wall Stress, Angiotensin II, and Left Ventricular Hypertrophy

TREFOR O. MORGAN, M.B.B.S., B.Sc., M.D.
CORY D. GRIFFITHS, Ph.D.
LEA M. D. DELBRIDGE, Ph.D.

Cardiac hypertrophy is common in people with hypertension and is associated with increased morbidity and mortality independently of the level of blood pressure.[1,2,3] Increased mortality is due to sudden death from arrhythmias, development of cardiac failure and associated coronary artery disease. Cardiac arrhythmias and cardiac failure are a direct consequence of left ventricular hypertrophy (LVH), whereas coronary artery disease is linked more closely to etiologic factors that compound the hypertrophy-related risk factors.

Despite the commonness of LVH, considerable debate surrounds its cause. The simplest explanation is that cardiac hypertrophy occurs in response to the increased workload caused by higher blood pressure. However, the correlation between clinical blood pressure and LVH is weak (r value < 0.2 in most studies).[3,4] The correlation is improved but still relatively weak when LVH is compared with the mean 24-hour arterial blood pressure, which is a better measure of workload.[5,6] Other factors clearly must contribute to LVH. As further evidence, LVH is more pronounced in people with similar blood pressure if they have diabetes, renal disease, or high sodium intake.[7-9] Thus, people have looked for factors apart from workload that may precipitate LVH. In particular, attention has focused on angiotensin II (Ang II) and wall stress.[10-12] Wall stress increases when blood pressure is high, but despite a correlation with workload, they are not equivalent indices. It has been claimed that Ang II is the preeminent factor in LVH. This chapter proposes that workload and acute wall stress provide qualitatively different triggers that activate the signal which will cause cardiac hypertrophy. LVH results only if an appropriate hormonal and cellular environment allows this signal to be translated into increased cell growth (Fig. 1). Although increased cell size is an important contributor to LVH, it also may result from increased interstitial and fibrous tissue, and different triggers may affect these factors differently.[13]

Hemodynamic Stimuli

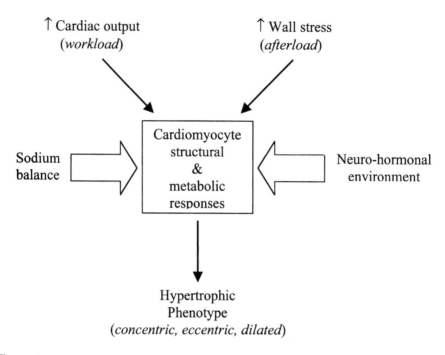

Figure 1.   A hypothetical outline of the interactions that occur between the signal that may trigger the hypertrophic process and the humoral environment critical for the phenotype development. Workload or pressure load may not result in a large heart without an appropriate neurohormonal and cellular environment.

■ *What Is Meant by Cardiac Hypertrophy?*

From radiologic and pathologic studies cardiac hypertrophy has been divided into two types: concentric hypertrophy, which is associated with hypertension and other states of pressure load (e.g., aortic stenosis), and eccentric hypertrophy, which results from volume overload. Volume overload may occur in athletes or in pathologic states as a result of arteriovenous fistulas. Concentric hypertrophy is more likely to be associated with sudden death or diastolic dysfunction and may progress to output failure. Eccentric hypertrophy in athletes probably has no adverse consequences because of the intermittent nature of the load, but when associated with pathologic high output states, eccentric hypertrophy also may lead to cardiac failure.

Our concept related to cell type is summarized in Fig. 2, but the data are inconclusive. We propose that so-called physiologic hypertrophy is characterized by a predominant increase in cell length as sarcomeres are laid down in series, although in some situations the cross sectional area and length may increase in proportion, maintaining the normal relationship. Aortic banding and hypertension are the prototypes of pressure load (Table 1). If the stimulus is a pressure load due to aortic banding, the response is a modest increase in cardiac size and a proportional increase in cell length and width (see Fig. 2). The effect is present

Table 1. Cellular Remodeling of Left Ventricular Cells in Different Forms
of Cardiac Hypertrophy

	Length Increase(%)	Width Increase (%)
Aortic arch stenosis (2 wk)	5.5	6.0*
Abdominal aortic stenosis (12 wk)	6.6	5.4
SHR[†]	16.4	28.4
Ang II infusion 4 weeks	5.9	14.3
SHHF—early failure[‡] 12 mo	16.8	10.1
SHHF—late failure[∞] 24 mo	29.3	0.9

* Calculated.
[†] Compared with Donryu control.
[‡] Compared with 9 mo.
[∞] Compared with 12 mo.
SHHF = spontaneous hypertensive heart failure, SHR = spontaneously hypertensive rat.

within 2 weeks and maintains a similar size.[14,15] However, if a similar level of aortic pressure is achieved in a genetic hypertensive model (e.g., spontaneously hypertensive rats), the result is concentric hypertrophy. The cells increase disproportionately in width (cross-sectional area) as sarcomeres are laid down in parallel (unpublished observation by Delbridge). This process may be due to an inappropriate increase in Ang II levels. Our studies indicate that acute pressure loading without an elevated Ang level produces a qualitative difference in cellular remodeling (Fig. 3). We propose that Ang II is associated with the laying down of sarcomeres in parallel.

As compensated hypertrophy progresses to cardiac failure, the myocytes elongate with no increase in cross-sectional area.[16,17] The nature of this elongation may be substantially different from that observed with physiologic hypertrophy. The hormone cardiotrophin causes sarcomeres to be added in series, and this

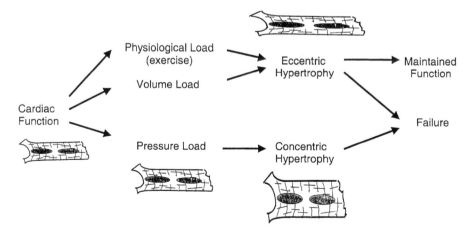

Figure 2. An outline of the relationship of cardiac hypertrophy to various signals and an indication of the cell morphology that may be associated. Pressure load causes an initial proportional increase in cell length and width, and a more severe or Ang II-dependent response produces pronounced increase in cross-sectional area with concentric hypertrophy. Transition to failure is associated with marked cell lengthening. Initial response to physiologic volume load may involve cell lengthening with minimal alteration in cross-sectional area.

hormone may be an important signalling factor in the transition to failure-associated chamber dilation.[18] In hypertensive models, angiotensin-converting enzyme (ACE) inhibitors cause resolution of LVH when blood pressure decreases. In aortic stenosis, ACE inhibitors have no effect on cardiac size.

■ *Problems and Questions Related to Cardiac Hypertrophy*

Cardiac hypertrophy is associated most commonly with elevated blood pressure, but other factors can influence cardiac size. In humans a genetic component has been clearly defined.[19] A strain of rats has been bred with marked cardiac hypertrophy but normal blood pressure.[20] When additional copies of the angiotensinogen gene are inserted into cardiac tissue, mice develop marked cardiac hypertrophy in both right and left ventricles without an elevation of blood pressure.[21] Thus, hemodynamic loading is not an absolute prerequisite for development of cardiac hypertrophy.

In both humans and rats a high salt intake is associated with or can cause cardiac hypertrophy without an effect on blood pressure.[22] In this setting, levels of renin, Ang II, and aldosterone are low. Aldosterone also can cause cardiac hypertrophy and cardiac fibrosis[23] with low levels of renin and angiotensin. Whether aldosterone works via retention of sodium or some other mechanism is not clear.

Various rat models have been used to study the relationship between hypertension, Ang II, and cardiac hypertrophy. Both the continuous angiotensin infusion model[24-26] and the two-kidney, one-clip (2K-1C) Goldblatt hypertension model (believed to be Ang II-dependent) lead to LVH, but it is not as pronounced

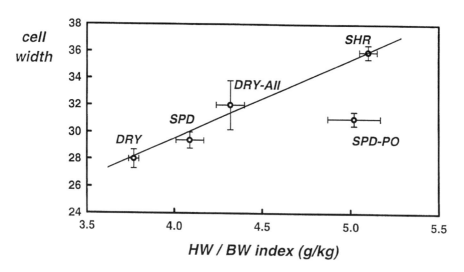

Figure 3. Myocyte width is plotted against cardiac index (heart weight/body weight). The cardiac index is higher than usual because (1) hearts were weighed before Langendorff perfusion to isolate the myocytes and (2) blood vessels were attached. All data are from 20–22-week-old rats, with 8–40 rats in each group and 50 myocytes from each rat. The aortic pressures in SHR and SPD-PO rats were similar. Normotensive rat strains: Donryu (DRY) and Sprague-Dawley (SPD). Hypertensive models: Sprague-Dawley pressure overload induced by suprarenal abdominal aortic clip (SPD-PO), Ang II infused Donryu (DRY-AII, 200 μg/kg/day) and spontaneously hypertensive rats (SHR).(Data from reference 15. Also included are unpublished data from Delbridge and Hart.)

as in the 1K-1C model (which is believed to be associated with low levels of Ang II), despite similar blood pressures.[27,28] All three models develop hypertrophy only of the left ventricle, suggesting that the hemodynamic signal is important. This suggestion appears to be confirmed by studies in the aorta-caval fistula model, in which both right and left ventricular hypertrophy develop.[29,30] Finally, it has been claimed that bradykinin may reverse LVH in the renin-dependent Goldblatt model.[31]

These associations and questions indicate the complexity of the interaction between a variety of factors. Many of the above factors may have independent effects on blood pressure, cardiac growth, and also on each other. Likewise, various factors may affect the myocyte and cardiac fibroblast in different ways, causing different types of cardiac hypertrophy.

■ Role of Angiotensin II in Left Ventricular Hypertrophy

In Vitro

Various experimental approaches, both in vivo and in vitro, have been used to investigate the relationship between Ang II levels and stress or stretch in the hypertrophic response. In neonatal cultured cardiomyocyte systems, acute Ang II exposure increases protein synthesis.[32] In these myocytes Ang II release also has been shown to mediate the hypertrophic response to stretch. In short-term cultures of adult cardiomyocytes, however, the increased protein synthesis that occurs in response to stretch is not Ang II-dependent, although induction of expression of some proto-oncogenes is blocked in the presence of an Ang II receptor antagonist.[33] It is difficult to interpret data obtained from cultured cell systems, because the Ang II hypertrophic signalling pathways may be altered by culture and may differ in adult and neonatal cardiomyocytes.

In Vivo

When Ang II is administered to rats, a series of molecular events is activated.[10,25] Because blood pressure also is elevated, it is difficult to determine whether blood pressure elevation or Ang II is the signal. Hydralazine has been administered concomitantly with Ang II to prevent the rise in blood pressure. In one study cardiac hypertrophy did not result, although vascular hypertrophy persisted.[24] In a similar study by a different group, however, treatment with hydralazine did not prevent LVH.[25] Both Ang II infusion studies and 2K-1C hypertension involve an independent, internal control. If Ang II has a direct effect on cardiocytes, increasing cell growth, it would be expected to affect the myocytes in the right and left ventricles to a similar extent. No studies have reported right ventricular enlargement.[26]

The results in two other models of severe LVH are also of interest.[27,28] In the 1K-1C model of hypertension with high salt intake, the renin (Ang II) level is low. Administration of a large dose of captopril (75 mg/kg/day) lowers blood pressure slightly but has no effect on left ventricle size (Table 2).[28] Combined administration in the same situation of an ACE inhibitor and an AT$_1$ receptor blocker also results in no reduction in size.[30] Thus, cardiac hypertrophy clearly can persist independently of the action of Ang II. If in the same model captopril

Table 2. Effect of Sodium, Angiotensin II, and Blood Pressure on Cardiac Size in the One-kidney, One-clip Goldblatt Model[28,29]

	Bradykinin	Ang II AT$_1$	Ang II AT$_2$	Blood Pressure	Cardiac Hypertrophy
1K-1C – ACE inhibitor	↑	↓	↓	0	0
1K-1C—losartan	0	↓	↑	0	0
1K-1C—low Salt + ACE inhibitor	↑	↓	↓	↓	↓
1K-1C–low salt + losartan	0	↓	↑*	↓	↓
1K-1C—low salt	0	↑	↑*	0	0

1K-1C = one kidney, one-clip rat model, ACE = angiotensin-converting enzyme, 0 = no effect, ↓ = decreased, ↑ = increased.
* Uncertain what will happen. Ang II may or may not rise; AT$_2$ receptor may be altered. With resolution of LVH the common feature was a fall in blood pressure.

is given to rats on a reduced salt intake, blood pressure decreases and cardiac hypertrophy resolves.[28]

In other experiments[34] we have demonstrated that if rats with different sodium intakes are given Ang I, cardiac hypertrophy is greatest in rats with high salt intake. Rats with low sodium intake show little difference in cardiac size (Table 3). Thus, there is an important interaction between Ang II level (in plasma or tissue) and sodium status. Clear evidence, however, indicates that Ang II is important. In the aorto-caval model, hypertrophy of both left and right ventricles develops, probably as a result of direct work hypertrophy.[29,30] If the effect of Ang II is prevented by either an AT$_1$ receptor blocker or an ACE inhibitor, hypertrophy of both ventricles resolves.[29,30] Thus, Ang II clearly has an effect on cardiac cell growth, but expression of this effect requires an initiating signal. This finding also explains why Ang II infusion into rats causes hypertrophy only of the left ventricle. Although right ventricular myocytes are exposed to Ang II, no signal triggers the hypertrophic process because right ventricular pressure (wall stress) is not altered.

■ *Wall Stress or Cardiac Work*

Increased stretch of myocytes in culture can cause release of Ang II and activate molecular markers that may lead to hypertrophy.[35] Wall stress is increased when the heart contracts against a higher aortic systolic blood pressure. Cardiac

Table 3. Effect of Intermittent Angiotensin II on Cardiac Size and the Influence of Sodium Intake[28]

Diet	Ang II	24-hr BP Elevation	% Increase in Cardiac Size
Normal	Continuous	↑↑↑	(14)*
Normal	4 hr	↑	10 (13)*
High Salt	—	0	9
High Salt	4 hr	↑	18
Low Salt	—	0	− 1
Low Salt	4 hr	↑	7

BP = blood pressure.
( )* = Wistar rats. Others = Sprague-Dawley rats.

hypertrophy is a physical response to increased blood pressure to normalize wall stress. The increase in tissue mass presents an oxygenation challenge, and oxygen supply to the myocardium may become limiting if angiogenesis does not occur to an appropriate extent.

Although it clearly has been established that workload increases, such as those in the aorto-caval fistula model, can cause cardiac hypertrophy, evidence indicates that the wall stress characteristic of hypertension is the more powerful hypertrophic signal. In experimental animals, when blood pressure is elevated for short periods (4 hr/day) by intermittent administration of Ang II, the extent of cardiac hypertrophy is equivalent to that seen when blood pressure elevation is maintained over a 24-hour period by continuous infusion (see Table 3).[34] The short period of Ang II administration had only a slight effect on mean blood pressure for the 24-hour period.[34] Thus, it appears that a period of severe wall stress (or severe increased cardiac work over a short period) is more important than cardiac workload over 24 hours.

The opposite approach of hemodynamic unloading has been adopted by two groups. Battle et al.[36] and Morgan et al.[37] demonstrated in the 2K-1C model that normalizing blood pressure for 12 hours and 4 hours/day led to a resolution of cardiac hypertrophy similar to that achieved with 24-hour control (Table 4). Thus, a period of normal blood pressure appears to interrupt the hypertensive process.

Such findings appear to be paradoxical. On one hand, high blood pressure (wall stress) for 4 hours with normal blood pressure for 20 hours caused cardiac hypertrophy, whereas normal blood pressure for 4 hours with high blood pressure for 20 hours allowed resolution of cardiac hypertrophy. This apparent paradox may be explained as follows: In studies in which blood pressure was elevated, pharmacologic normalization during the rats' normal sleeping hours was associated with LVH. During sleep, growth hormone and renin are secreted, and renin reaches up to 4 times its basal value.[38,39] If a signal is initiated by wall stress (or severe cardiac workload) at this time, cardiac hypertrophy results. If wall stress is normal at this time, the process leading to hypertrophy is not activated (or it is inactivated). If blood pressure is elevated during the awake hours, the level of circulating growth hormone and Ang II is much lower; thus, although the trigger is present, it does not translate into cardiac hypertrophy.

■ Cellular Mechanism of Response

The intracellular signal that leads to cardiomyocyte hypertrophy is unproved, but almost certainly it is a subtle alteration in calcium handling.[40] Several studies have shown that variations in calcium homeostasis are implicated in load-related cardiac hypertrophy.[41,42] Calcium (Ca) and sodium (Na)

Table 4. Cardiac Hypertrophy and Its Resolution in Two-kidney, One-clip Goldblatt Rats

Hours of Normal Blood Pressure	% Involution
24 hr[36]	22
12 hr (sleep)[36]	16
24 hr[37]	16
4–8 hr (sleep)[37]	17

levels in the cardiomyocyte are coregulated via the electrogenic Na/Ca exchanger (Fig. 4). In addition, cellular pH regulation is tightly linked to Na flux by the operations of transporters, some of which are subject to Ang II modulation: the sodium/hydrogen exchanger (NHE1), the Na^+-$2HCO_3^-$ cotransporter (NBC), and sodium-potassium adenosine triphosphatase (Na,K-ATPase).[43–45] The manner in which hemodynamic, dietary and endocrinologic interventions affect cellular Na (and thus pH) handling is not well understood. Indeed, the fundamental question of whether intracellular or interstitial free Na levels may be shifted by dietary and/or pharmacologic manipulation is not resolved.

We postulate that in cardiac muscle the signal to initiate hypertrophy is similar to that which leads to calcium overload and cell death. When cardiomyocytes become ischemic (i.e., when the oxygen supply is not sufficient to meet the metabolic needs), calcium accumulates in the cell and cell death may ensue. In the normal working cardiomyocyte, hydrogen ions accumulate as a result of the metabolic process, and the modes of correction are Na^+-H^+ countertransport and Na^+-$2HCO_3^-$ cotransport. In most circumstances this correction creates a sufficient balance to prevent accumulation of sodium; thus, calcium levels are not altered. However, if cardiac work is markedly increased by either gross volume overload (aorto-caval model) or acute blood pressure elevation (wall stress and acute increase in workload), the amount of sodium that enters the cell to correct the acidosis becomes excessive. The consequence is a change in activity of the Na^+-Ca^{2+} countertransport, and calcium is not removed as effectively. Thus, calcium homeostasis is altered. The elevated cellular calcium is thought to be a control signal that reinforces the programmed growth response triggered by altered

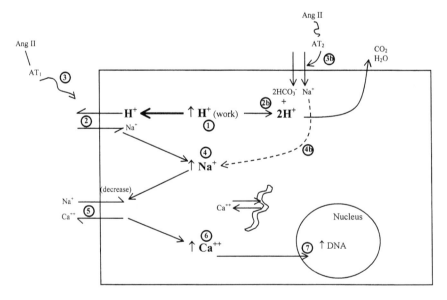

Figure 4.   When a cell contracts, hydrogen ions (H^+) are produced (1). Their production is greater with increased workload. H^+ is removed predominantly by sodium-hydrogen exchange (2), which is stimulated by Ang II via the AT_1 receptor (3). This process leads to increased cellular sodium (4) and decreased removal of calcium during relaxation (5). An increased amount of Ca^+ complex (6) may enter the nucleus, initiating cardiac hypertrophy (7). If proton-loading can be corrected by the Na^+-$2HCO_3^-$ cotransporter, this effect is reduced due to a different pathway (2b) (3b) (4b).

trophic or load conditions in the myocardium.[41] Many studies report that even in conditions of major perturbations in Na status, the levels of intracellular Na are defended by alterations in kinetic properties of membrane transporters.[46–48] This Na maintenance must occur at the expense of elevated intracellular Ca.

Ang II working via the AT_1 receptor increases the activity of the Na^+-H^+ countertransport system.[43] If the renin and Ang II levels are high, correction of the cellular acidosis is predominantly through Na^+-H^+ countertransport (with 1:1 stoichiometry). The resultant calcium loading promotes hypertrophic growth. However, if the correction of the acidosis can be shifted to the Na^+-$2HCO_3^-$ cotransport system, less Na^+ would enter the cell, and the sequence of events would be interrupted. It is postulated that a number of factors may increase the activity of the Na^+-$2HCO_3^-$ cotransport, including a reduced or low sodium diet, bradykinin, and Ang II acting via the AT_2 receptor. This postulate explains why Ang II does not cause cardiac hypertrophy in rats on a low sodium diet; the inferred effects of bradykinin on cardiac hypertrophy; and why AT_1 receptor blockers reverse cardiac hypertrophy via the shift from Na^+-H^+ countertransport to Na^+-$2HCO_3^-$ cotransport.

Other subtle interactions also take place. Thus, in people with high salt intake plasma renin and Ang II are decreased, and the AT_1 receptor may be upregulated, leading to excessive response to exogenous Ang II (or intracardiac release of Ang II). In people with low sodium intake Ang II levels are elevated, and the AT_1 receptor is downregulated. Thus, cardiac hypertrophy may not result from Ang II administration. Whether through regulation of the AT_1 receptor, changes in the AT_2 receptor, or both, the balance of forces correcting the proton load is shifted. If the cell clearance capacity is exceeded, sodium and then calcium may accumulate and cause cardiac hypertrophy.

■ *Correlates of Left Ventricular Hypertrophy*

LVH is an important physiologic response that enables the heart to adjust to altered hemodynamic conditions. When the hypertrophic response is driven by a requirement for increased cardiac output due to aerobic exercise (e.g., marathon runners) or an aorta-caval fistula, cardiocyte enlargement occurs with a predominant increase in cell length as sarcomeres are laid down in series. Minimal increase in interstitial tissue appears to preserve the juxtaposition of capillaries and myocytes, facilitating optimal oxygenation. In contrast, when hypertrophic remodeling is due to pressure loading associated with hypertension (wall stress and/or an acute increase in cardiac work), much of the hypertrophy is due to increased cell thickness as the sarcomeres in the myocytes are laid down in parallel.[15] Thus, the individual myocytes become thicker. At the same time the wall stress (or tissue damage) activates fibroblasts to increase collagen formation.[49,50] Elevated levels of Ang II promote myocardial fibrosis.[51] Increased extracellular matrix deposition increases the diffusional distance and impedes oxygen delivery to the cardiomyocytes as well as contributes to increased chamber stiffness. When oxygen demand is elevated as a consequence of workload, limited capacity for oxygen delivery at the tissues may become critical. Oxidative energy shortage in the myocyte contributes to diastolic dysfunction because complete resequestration of activator Ca is prevented and relaxation impaired.

This setting is vulnerable to arrhythmogenesis.[42] The influence of Ang II on cardiomyocyte growth patterns in the absence of coincident stress stimulus has been difficult to study. Whether the direct trophic effect of Ang II alone promotes balanced cellular growth—with sarcomeres laid down in series and parallel and with appropriate angiogenic support—remains to be investigated.

■ Conclusion

Cardiac hypertrophy in hypertension is an important complication leading to sudden death and diastolic cardiac failure. The cause is multifactorial. In addition to the factors discussed in this chapter, catecholamines, growth hormone, and other growth factors are also important. Workload, wall stress, sodium intake, Ang II levels, and other variables are clearly important in determining the outcome. The signals that initiate the sequence of events leading to cardiac hypertrophy are wall stress and excessive workload. Both alter the metabolism of the cell and result in a disturbance in calcium homeostasis, which is the cellular signal leading to LVH. However, the outcome is influenced by the way in which the cell corrects the acidosis produced by excessive cardiac work. The corrective mechanism is altered by the neurohumoral environment. Such alterations may enable greater work with less likelihood of hypertrophy. Once the signal has been provided to the cell, the final outcome is decided by the presence of various growth factors, of which Ang II and growth hormone are two important examples. Thus, development of cardiac hypertrophy requires the trigger signal and the appropriate hormonal environment. The most appropriate hormonal environment is activated during sleep and at the time of awakening. If wall stress or workload increases at either time, cardiac hypertrophy is more likely.

Acknowledgment

The graphical contributions of Ms. Petcharat Trongtorsak are much appreciated.

References

1. Levy D, Garrison RJ, Savage DD, et al: Prognostic implications of echocardiographically determined left ventricular mass in the Framingham Heart Study. N Engl J Med 322:1561–1566, 1990.
2. Cooper RS, Simmons BE, Castaner A, et al: Left ventricular hypertrophy is associated with increased mortality independent of ventricular function and number of coronary arteries severely narrowed. Am J Cardiol 65:441–445, 1990.
3. Muiesan ML, Salvetti M, Rizzoni D, et al: Association of change in left ventricular mass with prognosis during long term antihypertensive treatment. J Hypertens 113:1091–1095, 1995.
4. Verdecchia P, Porcellati C, Schillaci G, et al: Ambulatory blood pressure: An independent predicter of prognosis in essential hypertension. Hypertens 24:793–801, 1994.
5. Fagard RH, Staessen JA, Thijs L: Prediction of cardiac structure and function by repeated clinic and ambulatory blood pressure. Hypertens 29:22–29, 1997.
6. White WB, Dey HM, Shulman P: Assessment of daily blood pressure load as a determinant of cardiac function in patients with mild to moderate hypertension. Am Heart J 118:782–795, 1989.
7. Fields NG, Yuan BX, Leenen FH: Sodium-induced cardiac hypertrophy. Circ Res 68(3):745–755, 1999.
8. Heimann JC, Drumond S, Alves ATR, et al: Left ventricular hypertrophy is more marked in salt-sensitive than in salt-resistant hypertensive patients. J Cardiovasc Pharmacol 17(Suppl 2):S122–S124, 1991.
9. Fields NG, Yuan BX, Leenen FH: Sodium-induced cardiac hypertrophy. Circ Res 68:745–755, 1991.
10. Everett AD, Tufro-McReddie A, Fisher A, Gomez RA: Angiotensin receptor regulates cardiac hypertrophy and transforming growth factor-β1 expression. Hypertension 23:587–592, 1994.

11. Sadoshima J, Xu Y, Slayter HS, Izumo S: Autocrine release of angiotensin II mediates stretch induced hypertrophy of cardiac myocytes. Cell 75:977–984, 1993.
12. Yamazaki T, Komuro I, Kudoh S: Angiotensin II partly mediates mechanical stress induced cardiac hypertrophy. Circ Res 77:258–265, 1995.
13. Brilla CG, Pick R, Tan LB, et al: Remodeling of the rat right and left ventricles in experimental hypertension. Circ Res 67:1355–1364, 1990.
14. Zierhut W, Zimmer H-G, Gerdes AM: Effect of angiotensin convertering enzyme inhibition on pressure-induced left ventricular hypertrophy in rats. Circ Res 69:609–617, 1991.
15. Delbridge LMD, Satoh H, Yuan W, et al: Cardiac myocyte volume, Ca^{2+} fluxes, and sarcoplasmic reticulum loading in pressure-overload hypertrophy. Am J Physiol 272:H2425–2435, 1997.
16. Gerdes AM, Onodera T, Wang X, McCune SA: Myocyte remodeling during the progression to failure in rats with hypertension. Hypertension 28:609–614, 1996.
17. Onodera T, Tamura T, Said S, et al: Maladaptive remodeling of cardiac myocyte shape begins long before failure in hypertension. Hypertension 32:753–757, 1998.
18. Wollert KC, Taga T, Saito M, et al: Cardiotrophin-1 activates a distinct form of cardiac muscle cell hypertrophy. J Biol Chem 271:9535–9545, 1996.
19. Wollert KC, Taga T, Saito M, et al: Cardiotrophin-1 activates a distinct form of cardiac muscle cell hypertrophy. J Biol Chem 271:9535–9545, 1996.
20. Danes VR, Harrap SB, Jones EF, Delbridge LMD: Characterization of a new experimental genetic model of primary cardiac hypertrophy. J Mol Cell Cardiol [in press].
21. Mazzolai L, Nussberger J, Aubert J-F, et al: Blood pressure independent cardiac hypertrophy induced by locally activated renin-angiotensin system. Hypertension 31:1324–1330, 1998.
22. Yuan BX, Leenen FH: Dietary sodium intake and left ventricular hypertrophy in normotensive rats. Am J Physiol 261:H1397–H1401, 1991.
23. Brilla CG, Pick R, Tan LB, et al: Remodeling of the rat right and left ventricles in experimental hypertension. Circ Res 67:883–890, 1990.
24. Griffin SA, Brown WC, MacPherson F, et al: Angiotensin II causes vascular hypertrophy in part by a non-pressor mechanism. Hypertension 17:626–635, 1991.
25. Kim S, Ohta K, Hamaguchi A, et al: Angiotensin II induces cardiac phenotypic modulation and remodeling in vivo in rats. Hypertension 25:1252–1259, 1995.
26. Dostal DE, Baker KM: Angiotensin II stimulation of left ventricular hypertrophy in adult rat heart. Mediation by the AT1 receptor. Am J Hypertens 5:276–280, 1992.
27. Morgan TO, Aubert JF, Wang Q, Brunner HR: Importance of BP, NaCl, angiotensin II (Ang II) or bradykinin in resolution of cardiac hypertrophy [abstract]. J Hypertens 16(Suppl. 2):S337, 1998.
28. Morgan TO, Aubert J-F, Wang Q: Sodium, angiotensin II, blood pressure and cardiac hypertrophy. Kidney Int 54(Suppl 67):S213–S215, 1998.
29. Ruzicka M, Yuan B, Harmsen E, Leenen FH: The renin-angiotensin system and volume overload-induced cardiac hypertrophy in rats: Effects of angiotensin converting enzyme inhibitors versus angiotensin II receptor blocker. Circulation 87:921–930, 1993.
30. Iwai N, Shimoike H, Kinoshita M: Cardiac renin-angiotensin system in the hypertrophied heart. Circulation 92:2690–2696, 1996.
31. Linz W, Schölkens BA: A specific B_2-bradykinin receptor antagonist HOE 140 abolishes the antihypertrophic effect of ramipril. Br J Pharmacol 105:771–772, 1992.
32. Sadoshima J, Izumo S: Molecular characterization of angiotensin II-induced hypertrophy of cardiac myocytes and hyperplasia of cardiac fibroblasts: Critical role of the AT_1 receptor subtype. Circ Res 73:413–423, 1993.
33. Kent RL, McDermott PJ: Passive load and angiotensin II evoke differential response of gene expression and protein synthesis in cardiac myocytes. Circ Res 78:829–838, 1996.
34. Morgan T, Brunner H, Aubert J-F, Connell P: The relationship of blood pressure to cardiac hypertrophy: Experimental studies in rats. Clin Exp Hypertens 19:827–841, 1997.
35. Kijima K, Matsubara H, Murasawa S, et al: Mechanical stretch induces enhanced expression of angiotensin II receptor subtypes in neonatal rat cardiac myocytes. Circ Res 79:887–897, 1996.
36. Battle T, Schnell C, Bunkenburg B, et al: Continuous versus intermittent angiotensin converting enzyme inhibition in renal hypertensive rats. Hypertension 22:188–196, 1993.
37. Morgan TO, Brunner HR, Aubert J-F, et al: Cardiac hypertrophy depends upon sleep blood pressure: A study in rats. J Hypertens [in press].
38. Golstein J, Van Cauter E, Désir D, et al: Effect of "jet lag" on hormonal patterns. IV: Time shifts increase growth hormone release. J Clin Endocrinol Metab 56:433–440, 1983.
39. Brandenberger G, Follenius M, Goichot B, et al: Twenty-four hour profiles of plasma renin activity in relation to the sleep-wake cycle. J Hypertens 12:277–283, 1994.
40. Marban E, Korestsune Y: Cell calcium, oncogenes and hypertrophy. Hypertension 15:652–658, 1990.

41. Molkentin JD, Lu JT, Antos CL, et al: A calcinerurin-dependent transcriptional pathway for cardiac hypertrophy. Cell 93:215–228, 1998.
42. Tomaselli GF, Marban E: Electrophysiological remodeling in hypertrophy and heart failure. Cardiovas Res 42:270–283, 1999.
43. Matsui H, Barry WH, Livsey V, Spitzer KW: Angiotensin II stimulates sodium-hydrogen exchange in adult rabbit ventricular myocytes. Cardiovas Res 29:215–221, 1995.
44. Yu MH, Sandmann ST, Unger T: Differential roles of AT-1 and AT-2 receptor subtypes in the expression of Na-HCO_3 symporter and Na-H exchanger in rat myocardium after myocardial infarction. J Hypertens 17:S153, 1999.
45. Hool LC, Gray DF, Robinson BG, Rasmussen HH: Angiotensin-converting enzyme inhibitors regulate the Na^+-K^+ pump via effects on angiotensin metabolism. Am J Physiol 271:C172–C180, 1996.
46. Zicha J, Kronauer J, Duhm J: Effects of chronic high salt intake on blood pressure and the kinetics of sodium and potassium transport in erythrocytes of young and adult subtotally nephrectomized Sprague-Dawley rats. J Hypertens 8:207–217, 1990.
47. Quintanilla AP, Weffer MI, Koh H, et al: Effect of high salt intake on sodium, potassium-dependent adenosine triphosphatase activity in the erythrocytes of normotensive men. Clin Sci 75:167–170, 1988.
48. Magargal WW, Overbeck HW: Effect of hypertension rat plasma on ion transport of cultured vascular smooth muscle. Am J Physiol 251(5 Pt 2):H984–H990, 1986.
49. Villareal FJ, Dillmann WH. Cardiac hypertrophy-induced changes in mRNA levels for TGF-β1, fibronectin, and collagen. Am J Physiol 262:H1861–H1866, 1992.
50. Crawford DC, Chobanian AV, Brecher P: Angiotensin II induces fibronectin expression associated with cardiac fibrosis in the rat. Circ Res 74:727–739, 1994.
51. Tan LB, Jalil JE, Janicki JS, Weber KT: Cardiac myocyte necrosis induced by angiotensin II. Circ Res 69:1185–1195, 1991.

CHAPTER 16

Vascular Effects of Angiotensin II and AT$_1$ Receptor Blockade

SHARON L. GRANT, Ph.D.
KATHY K. GRIENDLING, Ph.D.

The hormone angiotensin II (Ang II) is one of the most potent and multifactorial vasoactive agents ever identified. The physiologic effect of Ang II on the vessel wall depends on the cellular phenotype and environment and ranges from vasoconstriction to modulation of growth and regulation of the inflammatory process. Ang II acts on virtually all vascular cells—endothelial cells, smooth muscle cells, fibroblasts, and monocytes/macrophages—resulting in an integrated response that can be physiologic or pathophysiologic. Most of the vascular effects of Ang II are mediated by AT$_1$ receptors. This chapter addresses both molecular and in vivo effects of Ang II on the vasculature.

■ AT$_1$ Receptor Coupling in Vascular Cells

In vascular smooth muscle cells (VSMCs), the seven-transmembrane AT$_1$ receptor mediates most of the prominent and well-characterized responses to Ang II. AT$_1$ receptors couple to multiple effectors and initiate a myriad of signaling cascades that not only cause vessel contraction but also modulate cell growth and vessel remodeling. It has been shown recently that Ang II does not act in isolation, but rather it cross-talks with signaling molecules activated by other receptors and in fact utilizes these receptors to mediate its responses. In turn, these receptors interact with the AT$_1$ receptor, providing multifaceted and complex signaling cascades in VSMCs (Fig. 1). These pathways can be roughly divided into two classifications that are becoming less distinct as the various linkages are explored. The first involves classic AT$_1$ receptor signaling, including G-protein activation, phospholipase C (PLC), protein kinase C (PKC), and an increase in cytosolic calcium from both intrinsic and extracellular sources. The other signaling cascades are not so clearly defined and involve not only receptor tyrosine kinases but also reactive oxygen species. Finally, AT$_1$ receptor-mediated effects can be regulated by modulation of the expression of the various signaling components and by the physical location of the receptor as it internalizes and degrades.

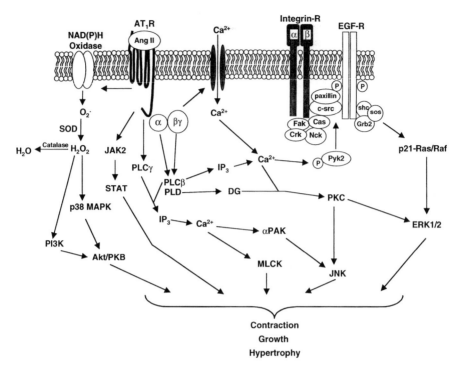

Figure 1.   Signaling pathways activated by Ang II in vascular smooth muscle. Ang II activates multiple signaling pathways in vascular smooth muscle that interact to regulate contraction and growth. See text for description of interaction. PLC, phospholipase C; PLD, phospholipase D; PKC, protein kinase C; EGF-R, epidermal growth factor receptor; SOD, superoxide dismutase; PI3K, phosphatidylinositol 3-kinase; MLCK, myosin light chain kinase; ERK1/2, extracellular signal regulated kinase; Ang II, angiotensin II; AT_1R, angiotensin type 1 receptor; PKB, protein kinase B; p38MAPK, p38 mitogen-activated protein kinase; DG, diacylglycerol; Fak, focal adhesion kinase; Cas, p-130[Cas]; JAK2, janus associated kinase 2; Pyk2, proline-rich tyrosine kinase 2; crk and Nck, adapter proteins; shc, src homology complex; sos, son of sevenless; JNK, c-jun N-terminal kinase; STAT, signal transducers and activators of transcription; H_2O_2, hydrogen peroxide.

Classic AT_1 Receptor Signaling Cascades

The AT_1 receptor in VSMCs interacts with both $G\alpha_{q/11}$ and $G\alpha_{12}$ heterotrimeric G-proteins.[1,2] Targeted deletion studies have determined that G-protein coupling involves all three intracellular loops and the C-terminus of the AT_1 receptor.[3] The three distinct phases of the Ang II classic signaling cascade involve activation of PLCβ, PLCγ, and phospholipase D (PLD). Immediately upon activation of the AT_1 receptor, PLCβ is activated, hydrolyzing membrane phospholipids (PIP$_2$) to release inositol trisphosphate (IP$_3$) and diacylglycerol (DG).[1,4] This response is transient and has abated by 1 minute. Approximately 30 seconds after Ang II binds to its receptor, PLCγ becomes activated and remains so for up to 5 minutes.[5] The activation mechanism of these two PLC isoforms is vastly different: PLCβ is activated through the G-protein alpha subunits $G\alpha_{q/11}$ and $G\alpha_{12}$ and their βγ subunits,[1] whereas PLCγ binds to the AT_1 receptor by interaction of its C-terminal SH2 domain with phosphorylated tyrosine 319 in the cytoplasmic domain of the receptor.[6] The third phase of the Ang II response involves activation of PLD, which occurs within 1 minute and is a sustained response (hours).[7,8] PLD hydrolyzes phosphatidylcholine to phosphatidic acid and choline. Phosphatidic acid is rapidly dephosphorylated to DG. The mediators of this response are complex. Electroporation of $G\alpha_{12}$, $G\beta\gamma$, and c-Src antibodies block Ang II-mediated PLD stimulation, whereas overexpression of a $G\beta\gamma$-binding protein suppresses Ang II-induced PLD activation.[2] PLD stimulation by Ang II also depends on extracellular calcium levels, PKC, and sequestration into caveolae.[7,9,10] These classic signaling pathways are important for the acute responses to Ang II, including VSMC contraction.

In addition to these acute responses, Ang II also exerts longer-term responses, including hypertrophy and hyperplasia of VSMCs. Although classic signaling pathways contribute to these responses, other, less defined pathways involving tyrosine and serine/threonine kinases are important as well. In addition, recent work by our laboratory has shown that AT₁ receptor activation increases intracellular reactive oxygen species (ROS), which serve as second messengers for specific pathways.[11-13]

Nonclassical AT₁ Receptor Signaling

Tyrosine Kinases

AT₁ receptor activation induces tyrosine phosphorylation of several cellular proteins. Many of these proteins are the upstream mediators of the mitogen-activated protein kinase (MAPK) pathway. These proteins include c-Src, receptor tyrosine kinases (including the EGF receptor), focal adhesion kinases, and calcium-dependent kinases.

MAPKs are serine/threonine kinases that transduce signals from the cell membrane to the nucleus in response to classic growth factors and G-protein coupled receptor agonists.[14-16] Four groups of MAPKs have been identified in mammalian cells: the extracellular signal-regulated kinases 1 and 2 (ERK1/2, also termed p42/44 MAPK); the c-Jun NH_2-terminal kinases (JNK), also termed stress-activated protein kinase (SAPK); p38MAPK, also termed CSBP; and Big MAPK 1 (BMK1), also termed ERK5.[15-17] Although the MAPK families are structurally related, they generally are activated by distinct extracellular stimuli and phosphorylate different molecular substrates.[14-16] ERK1/2 are stimulated by growth factors and mitogenic stimuli and play pivotal roles in cell growth and differentiation.[15,16] ERK1/2 stimulation initiates phosphorylation events, leading to activation of transcription factors, such as Elk-1 and c-fos, and stimulation of p90[rsk] ribosomal S6 kinase.[15] In contrast, p38MAPK and JNK are primarily activated by cellular stresses, including heat and osmotic shock, ultraviolet irradiation, proinflammatory cytokines, and hypoxia/reoxygenation in other systems.[18,19] JNKs phosphorylate and activate transcription factors such as c-Jun, ATF-2, and Elk-1,[20-23] whereas p38MAPK phosphorylates ATF-2 and C/EPT-homologous protein (CHOP).[24,25] In addition, p38MAPK phosphorylates and activates MAPKAP kinase 2/3 and phosphorylates the heat shock proteins HSP25/27,[26,27] which enhance its protective properties.

Ang II has been shown to activate ERK1/2,[28,29] p38MAPK,[11] and JNK,[30] but only weakly BMK-1[17] (see Fig. 1). Not surprisingly, the upstream activators of each of these kinases are unique. Eguchi et al.[29] observed that Ang II activates ERK1/2 through a PLC-mediated increase in calcium and activation of p21-Ras.

They found no role for PKC. Liao et al.,[31] however, found that PKC-ζ interacts with Ras to activate ERK1/2. More recent work provides evidence for a role of the epidermal growth factor (EGF) receptor in ERK1/2 phosphorylation. Eguchi et al.[32] demonstrated that EGF receptor kinase inhibitors blocked Ang II activation of ERK1/2. Further work suggested that phosphorylation of the EGF receptor by Ang II provides a docking site for the Shc/Grb2/Sos complex, which in turn activates p21-Ras/Raf. It also was demonstrated that EGF receptor activation by Ang II is calcium-dependent.[32] Insight into the relationship between increased intracellular calcium and EGF receptor phosphorylation has been gained from studies focusing on the calcium-sensitive tyrosine kinase, proline rich tyrosine kinase 2 (Pyk2), or calcium-dependent tyrosine kinase (CADTK). Pyk2 is a nonreceptor tyrosine kinase that has sequence homology with the p125 focal adhesion kinase (FAK). Ang II stimulates calcium-dependent phosphorylation of Pyk2 and initiates an interaction between Pyk2 and c-Src, which is required for EGF receptor phosphorylation.[33]

The upstream activators of JNK and p38MAPK have been less well studied. Ang II activation of JNK is less robust than stimulation of ERK1/2. JNK activation by Ang II is calcium-dependent and involves a nonclassic PKC isoform.[30] It has been clearly established that the p21-activated kinase α-PAK is upstream of JNK, and evidence suggests that an unidentified non-Src tyrosine kinase is upstream of α-PAK. The specific kinases that mediate p38MAPK activation by Ang II have not been investigated, although it has been demonstrated that ROS are involved in this process.[11] One target of p38MAPK is the sodium/hydrogen (Na+/H+) exchanger, which appears to be phosphorylated by both p38MAPK and ERK1/2.[34]

Another important tyrosine kinase activated by Ang II is JAK2.[35] JAK2 initiates activation of the transcription factors STAT-1 and STAT-3. Ang II treatment activates JAK2 and TYK2, which stimulate tyrosine phosphorylation of STAT-1.[35] STAT-1 translocates to the nucleus and binds to the serum-inducible elements in the promoters of the early growth response genes c-fos and c-jun, initiating transcription. Immunoprecipitation studies demonstrated that the AT$_1$ receptor binds JAK2 through the YIPP sequence in the tail of the AT$_1$ receptor.[36] Marrero et al.[37] also showed that Ang II-mediated ERK1/2 activation and cell growth are dependent on JAK2.

Focal Adhesion Kinases

The predominant effects of Ang II on VSMCs involve cellular shape, volume, and migration; for these events to occur, there must be communication with the cytoskeleton. Recent evidence indicates that focal adhesion complexes act as mediators for signaling cascades to interact with the cellular matrix. Smilenov et al.[38] demonstrated that in fibroblasts focal adhesion complexes are highly motile within the plane of the membrane; however, once an activator is added, these complexes become stationary and perform a ratchet-like function to perpetuate directional migration. Focal adhesions contain a set of tyrosine kinases and related proteins that form the signaling complex, including p125FAK, p130Cas, Crk, c-Src, and paxillin. One of the best-studied focal adhesion kinases is p125FAK. There have been conflicting reports about the involvement of FAK in Ang II signaling in VSMCs. Early studies showed that FAK was phosphorylated by Ang II in VSMCs.[39]; however, several later reports failed to confirm this finding.[33,40] As noted above, c-Src is also activated by Ang II and plays an important role in phosphorylation of the cytoskeletal protein paxillin.[41–43] Finally, the docking protein p130Cas is rapidly phosphorylated by Ang II in a Src-dependent manner.[44] Phosphorylation of p130Cas by Ang II promotes its interaction with the adapter proteins Crk[45] and Nck, which is phosphorylated by Ang II.[46]

Reactive Oxygen Species

ROS such as superoxide ($O_2^{\bullet-}$) and hydrogen peroxide (H_2O_2), which once were known only as toxic byproducts, have now been shown to act as signaling molecules for Ang II. In VSMCs, Ang II stimulates production of both $O_2^{\bullet-}$ and H_2O_2.[12,47,48] These ROS are derived from a membrane-associated NAD(P)H oxidase that transfers electrons from NADPH or NADH to oxygen to form $O_2^{\bullet-}$.[47] H_2O_2 is then produced by metabolism of $O_2^{\bullet-}$ by superoxide dismutase. Both $O_2^{\bullet-}$ and H_2O_2 stimulate specific signaling pathways, although for Ang II the evidence is strongest for a role of H_2O_2. As noted above, H_2O_2 mediates the activation of p38MAPK by Ang II. Activation of p38MAPK is inhibited in VSMCs that overexpress catalase, and enzyme that catabolizes H_2O_2, or by incubation with the NAD(P)H oxidase inhibitor diphenylene iodonium (DPI).[11] Stimulation of Akt/protein kinase B, another serine kinase that is downstream of phosphatidylinositol 3-kinase, is also redox-sensitive in VSMCs.[13] In these cells, Ang II stimulation of Akt is blocked by catalase overexpression and antioxidants, suggesting that it is a redox-sensitive kinase or that activation of an upstream kinase such as p38MAPK is mediated by ROS. Others have shown that ERK1/2 activation by Ang II is sensitive to antioxidants,[49] and Baas and Berk[50] found that $O_2^{\bullet-}$, but not H_2O_2, activated ERK1/2. These discrepancies may be due to differences in cell culture conditions, such as serum content or glucose concentration or the phenotype of the cells. Many other signaling molecules are sensitive to oxidant stress, including PKC[51] and protein tyrosine phosphatases,[52] but the redox-sensitivity of these pathways with respect to Ang II signaling has not been investigated.

Another area in which Ang II functions in a redox-sensitive manner is gene expression. Certain transcription factors, including NF-κB and AP-1, are activated by ROS.[53] In at least one case, MCP-1, induction of the gene by Ang II in VSMCs is inhibited by DPI.[54] Other genes, such as IL-6, are activated by Ang II in an NF-κB-dependent fashion,[55] indicating that they, too, may be mediated by ROS. These data strongly suggest that ROS are second messengers regulating gene expression by Ang II in VSMCs. The universality of this concept remains to be tested as more redox-sensitive genes are identified.

AT$_1$ Receptor Desensitization and Internalization

There are three distinct mechanisms through which receptor signaling has been shown to terminate. First, receptors can be phosphorylated and thus inactivated within seconds.[56] Second, they become desensitized by rapid inactivation of signaling components[57] and internalization (seconds to minutes).[58] Finally, over minutes to hours, receptors can be downregulated, thus limiting the number of surface receptors available to respond to the agonist.[8]

Ang II phosphorylates the AT$_1$ receptor on both serine/threonine and tyrosine residues.[59] Serine/threonine residues are by far the most heavily phosphorylated.

As is the case for β-adrenergic receptors, G protein receptor kinases phosphorylate the AT_1 receptor within minutes of stimulation.[60] This receptor is a substrate for GRK-1, GRK-2 and GRK-5,[60] but only GRK-5 is in turn regulated by Ang II.[61] The phosphorylation of the receptor usually enhances binding of β-arrestin and targets it for movement to coated pits, which are invaginations of the membrane coated with clathrin. Coated pits pinch off into coated vesicles by dynamin activation, and the acidic pH found within these vesicles facilitates receptor and ligand dissociation. The receptor is recycled and sent back to the membrane, whereas the ligand is sent to the lysozyme where it is degraded. However, recent studies using overexpression of dominant negative dynamin and β-arrestin showed that internalization of the AT_1 receptor was not dependent on this pathway.[62]

Internalization of the AT_1 receptor does occur, however, possibly via caveolae. Anderson et al.[63,64] showed that upon Ang II binding, AT_1 receptors coalesce and are internalized through both noncoated as well as coated pits. This concept of agonist-induced AT_1 receptor sequestration or internalization by a caveolae-dependent mechanism is supported by the observations that Ang II induces movement of a portion of AT_1 receptors into caveolin-enriched membrane fractions and that caveolin-1 co-immunoprecipitates with the AT_1 receptor.[10] Furthermore, interventions that interfere with agonist-induced AT_1 receptor sequestration (and tonic phase signaling), such as low temperature and treatment with phenylarsine oxide, impair movement of the receptor to the caveolin-enriched membrane fraction. Thus, the available data suggest a model in which the AT_1 receptors in VSMC are dispersed on the cell surface and, after agonist occupation, aggregate in and are internalized with specialized membrane domains represented, at least in part, by caveolae.

Receptor internalization is not solely responsible for the rapid termination of early signaling mechanisms. PKC activation inhibits IP_3 generation by Ang II.[57] The target of PKC has been variously proposed to be the receptor itself,[60] the coupling G protein,[65] or PLC.[66] Recently, a new class of proteins, regulators of G-protein signaling (RGS proteins), have been identified that act as GTPase activating proteins (GAPs) for heterotrimeric G protein alpha subunits. RGS2, one of the members of the RGS family, is a selective and potent inhibitor of Gαq.[67,68] Furthermore, when RGS2 is reconstituted with phospholipid vesicles, it inhibits Gq activation of PLCβ1.[68] These proteins may provide a potential target for PKC-mediated termination of Ang II signaling. Indeed, we have recently shown that Ang II can regulate the expression of RGS2 in VSMCs.[69]

■ *Physiologic Effects of Angiotensin II on Vascular Smooth Muscle*

Ang II has multiple effects on VSMCs, depending on the phenotype of the cell, the ratio of expressed receptor sybtypes, and the environmental influences impinging upon the cell. AT_1 receptors mediate contraction, hypertrophy, and hyperplasia, and some evidence suggests that AT_2 receptors are growth inhibitory.[70] Although Ang II causes contraction of differentiated VSMCs,[71] in VSMCs that are phenotypically modulated, Ang II can lead to hypertrophy[72,73] or hyperplasia.[74] Each of these responses is associated with shared and unique signaling pathways.

Contraction

The ability of Ang II to cause arterial contraction has been known for over 30 years and, upon cloning of the Ang II receptors, was shown to be mediated by the AT$_1$ receptor subtype.[75] Upon activation of these receptors, blood vessels contract transiently. This initial, rapid phase of force development is directly attributable to the increase in intracellular calcium (Ca^{2+}) that results from PLC-mediated generation of inositol trisphosphate (IP$_3$). IP$_3$ induces calcium release from intracellular stores by binding to its receptor on the sarcoplasmic reticulum, whereas calcium and DG activate PKC, which in turn phosphorylates target proteins, including calponin,[76] caldesmon,[77] and phosphatase-1 inhibitor protein[78] (see Fig. 1). Ca^{2+} binds to calmodulin, which then associates with the enzyme myosin light-chain kinase, converting it from an inactive to an active form. This enzyme phosphorylates the myosin light chain, permitting actin activation of the Mg^{2+}-adenosine triphosphatase and resulting in attachment of the phosphorylated myosin heads (or cross-bridges) to the actin filaments. The catalysis of adenosine triphosphate hydrolysis to generate tension occurs in a cyclic manner for the duration of contraction. Thus, the calcium/calmodulin signaling pathway is a predominate mediator of contraction in arterial smooth muscle. In addition, Ang II stimulates calcium influx through receptor-operated calcium channels that are activated by free G$\beta\gamma$ subunits,[79] which most likely play a role in contraction in vessels that respond to Ang II tonically.

Growth of Vascular Smooth Muscle Cells

In cultured VSMCs and in large vessels of hypertensive animals, Ang II stimulates an increase in protein synthesis and thus hypertrophy.[72,73,80] Because it develops over days (culture) to weeks (in vivo), the hypertrophic response is complex and in part depends on gene transcription.[72] It was demonstrated earlier that Ang II-induced hypertrophy is Ca^{2+}-dependent and PKC-independent,[72] but recently further insights have been made into hypertrophic pathways. Emerging evidence indicates that Ang II-induced hypertrophy is mediated by intracellularly produced H$_2$O$_2$ that is derived, at least in part, from a membrane-associated NADH/NADPH oxidase.[12,47,48] This conclusion is based on three lines of evidence. Ang II-induced hypertrophy is attenuated by DPI, an inhibitor of flavin-containing enzymes such as the NADH/NADPH oxidase.[47] In addition, decreasing NADH/NADPH oxidase activity by transfection of antisense p22phox (a major component of the oxidase enzyme complex) inhibits hypertrophy.[12] NADH/NADPH oxidase activation produces both O$_2$$^{\bullet-}$ and H$_2$O$_2$; thus inhibition of this enzyme system results in a decrease in both of these potential second messengers.[12,48] However, H$_2$O$_2$ appears to mediate the hypertrophic effects, because overexpression of catalase, one of the major enzymes that catabolizes H$_2$O$_2$, attenuates Ang II-induced hypertrophy.[48]

The effects of Ang II to modify the growth response of VSMCs are complex, because Ang II stimulates both proliferative and antiproliferative signals.[81] Incubation of VSMCs with Ang II leads to induction of PDGF,[82] IGF-1,[83] FGF,[70] and TGF-β[84] as well as the protooncogenes c-fos and c-jun.[85,86] Although PDGF and FGF are clearly growth-promoting, TGF-β inhibits VSMC growth. Based on a gene-transfer, gain-of-function study, it has been suggested that AT$_2$ receptors counteract the growth effects of AT_1 receptor stimulation and are in fact antiproliferative.[81] When AT_2 receptor levels are increased by transfection, the proliferative effects of Ang II are attenuated. The molecular mechanisms activated by AT_2 receptors remain unclear but may include activation of phosphatases,[87] which would inhibit the phosphorylation of growth-regulatory proteins activated by the AT_1 receptor.

■ Angiotensin II Effects on Endothelial Cells

Expression of AT_1 receptors in endothelial cells is controversial. Patel et al.[88] first described the existence of Ang II receptors in pulmonary arterial and aortic endothelial cells. A single population of binding sites also was identified on bovine brain microvessel endothelial cells[89]; however, in neither study was the receptor subtype identified. Biochemical experiments in pulmonary artery endothelial cells indicated that Ang II and Ang III activate typical AT_1 receptor signaling pathways (PLC and PLD),[90] which are blocked by both an angiotensin-converting enzyme (ACE) inhibitor and an Ang II receptor antagonist. With the development of specific Ang II receptor antagonists, Mineo et al.[91] demonstrated that Ang II binding on porcine aortic endothelial cells is not mediated by typical AT_1 or AT_2 receptors. Later it was shown that bovine aortic endothelial cells contain an angiotensin-(1-7) receptor[92] and that bovine coronary microvascular endothelial cells contain a functional Ang IV receptor.[93] It is difficult to reconcile these studies, although it is likely that expression of Ang receptor subtypes differs according to the vascular bed from which the endothelial cells are derived.

Ang II has multiple effects on endothelial cells, ranging from activation of apoptotic signaling pathways,[94] induction of nitric oxide (NO),[95,96] and activation of plasminogen activating factor.[97-99] However, all of these effects are not mediated solely by the AT_1 receptor. The AT_2 receptor is also responsible for some of the responses on endothelial cells to Ang II.

Angiotensin II and Nitric Oxide

One of the most far-reaching effects of Ang II on endothelial cells is regulation of production of NO, the endothelium-derived relaxing factor. NO plays a diverse role in the vessel. It is formed from L-arginine by nitric oxide synthase (NOS), which is present in several isoforms. Endothelial cells express both the constitutive calcium-dependent isoform (eNOS) and the cytokine-inducible and calcium-independent isoform (iNOS).[96] More than three years ago, Saito et al.[95] demonstrated that in bovine endothelial cells Ang II stimulation resulted in a dose-dependent increase in NO formation. This increase was abolished both by a NOS inhibitor and an AT_1 receptor antagonist (DuP 753), but not by an AT_2 receptor antagonist (PD 123177). They also showed that a calcium chelator and calmodulin inhibitor abolished the Ang II increase in NO formation, as did PKC inhibition. Later it was reported that Ang II induces both eNOS mRNA and NO production in human umbilical vein endothelial cells,[96] eNOS protein and mRNA in bovine pulmonary artery endothelial cells,[100] and NO production in rat aortic endothelial cells.[101] The latter study also found that NO was produced through the AT_1 receptor. However, Ang II did not increase eNOS protein or mRNA in bovine coronary artery endothelial cells,[100] whereas in porcine pulmonary and aortic endothelial cells Ang II-stimulated release of NO was mediated through the AT_4 receptor rather than the AT_1 receptor.[102]

Angiotensin II and Endothelial Cell Growth or Apoptosis

It has been proposed that Ang II simultaneously stimulates both proliferative and antiproliferative autocrine factors in VSMCs,[70] possibly by activating opposing pathways in an AT$_1$- or AT$_2$-receptor–specific manner. A similar paradigm has been proposed in endothelial cells;[103] however, most studies find that Ang II is growth-inhibitory in endothelial cells. For example, in the HUVEC study, Ang II exposure induced apoptosis in a dose dependent manner[94] without causing necrosis. This increase in apoptosis by Ang II was not blocked by AT$_1$ receptor or AT$_2$ receptor antagonism but was blocked by a combination of both antagonists. The specific AT$_2$ receptor agonist CGP42112 and Ang II both increased caspase-3 activity, whereas caspase-3 inhibition decreased the apoptotic effects of Ang II on endothelial cells. This finding demonstrates that although Ang II-induced apoptosis requires activation of AT$_2$ receptors, AT$_1$ receptor activation also must occur. The proapoptotic pathways downstream of AT$_1$ receptors remain to be defined. Thus, in endothelial cells, both AT$_1$ and AT$_2$ receptors may work together rather than in opposition to regulate growth.

Effects of Angiotensin II on Thrombosis and Adhesion

Endothelial cells also maintain a balance between hemostatic and prothrombotic factors. Ang II can alter this balance by increasing plasminogen activator inhibitor (PAI)-1 and PAI-2[97–99] and tissue factor[97] without affecting tissue plasminogen activator and tissue factor pathway inhibitor,[97] thereby acting as a prothrombotic agent. There is some controversy as to which receptor mediates these effects. In rat microvessel endothelial cells, Ang II-mediated PAI-1 and PAI-2 upregulation was inhibited by losartan but not PD123319.[98] Similar results were found in rat aortic endothelial cells for Ang II effects on PAI-1 and tissue factor.[97] However, in bovine aortic endothelial cells, stimulation of PAI-1 release by Ang II was not mediated by AT$_1$ or AT$_2$ receptors, but rather by Ang IV.[99]

Ang II also exerts proinflammatory effects by promoting leukocyte adhesion. In human aortic endothelial cells, Ang II induces adhesion of monocytes via activation of both AT$_1$ and AT$_2$ receptors.[104] Gräfe et al.[105] found that Ang II induced E-selectin expression and leukocyte adhesion to human coronary and microvascular endothelial cells, although it was much less potent than TNF-α. These effects were mediated by the AT$_1$ receptor. The ability of Ang II to activate prothrombotic and proinflammatory pathways probably contributes to its proatherosclerotic effects (see below).

■ *In Vivo Studies of the Vascular Effects of Angiotensin II*

The renin-angiotensin system is an important regulator of blood pressure and fluid and electrolyte homeostasis. Ang II, the hormone responsible for these physiologic functions, interacts with multiple targets, including the adrenal cortex, myocardium, vascular smooth muscle, kidney, and brain. Among its more important effects are the modulation of vascular tone, aldosterone release, heart rate and contractility, glomerular filtration and sodium reabsorption, and pituitary secretion of vasopressin. These functions of Ang II have been known for many years and are mediated mainly by the AT$_1$ receptor. However, the renin-angiotensin system also contributes to vascular diseases such as hypertension and atherosclerosis. Ang II promotes growth and hypertrophy of cardiac

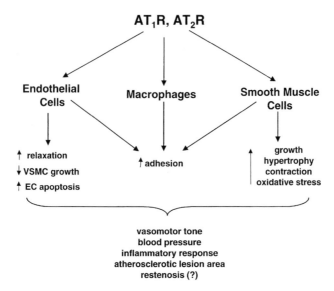

Figure 2.   Potential interactions between the renin angiotensin system and vascular cells. Ang II has effects on many types of vascular cells. It modulates growth and contraction of cells and changes the pattern of expression of adhesion molecules and the paracrine factors secreted by cells. These events combine to modulate vasomotor tone and blood pressure and contribute to the inflammatory response and abnormal growth/hypertrophy that are hallmarks of hypertension and atherosclerosis.

and smooth muscle, increases oxidative stress, modifies the inflammatory response, and influences endothelial function (Fig. 2).

Hypertension

Antihypertensive Effects of AT_1 Receptor Blockers and ACE Inhibitors

When given subcutaneously, Ang II induces a chronic elevation in blood pressure that is reversed upon termination of infusion. The increase in blood pressure induced by Ang II is due not only to its vasopressor actions but also to its effects on the renal microcirculation and natriuresis. ACE inhibitors have been the most commonly used method of blocking the renin-angiotensin system and have been highly successful in attenuating mild, moderate, and severe forms of hypertension.[106] However, with the advent of the AT_1 receptor inhibitors it is now possible to block just one arm of the renin-angiotensin cascade. AT_1 receptor blockers have been as successful as ACE inhibitors in reducing blood pressure for all levels of hypertension.[106] Unfortunately, a major side effect of the AT_1 receptor blockers is an increase in circulating levels of Ang II,[107] thus potentially enhancing AT_2 receptor-mediated events. Relatively little is known about the effects of the AT_2 receptor in vivo. Recent studies have shown that AT_2 receptor knockout mice have a slightly elevated baseline systolic blood pressure and an enhanced response to subpressor doses of Ang II.[108] Systolic blood pressure is increased by approximately 80 mmHg in response to Ang II infusion, whereas when control mice are given Ang II, their blood pressure increases by less than 20 mmHg.[108] Recently it has been shown that AT_2 receptor knockout mice have an increased number of AT_1 receptors, an observation that may explain these puzzling results.[109]

High plasma renin levels have been correlated with an increased risk of cardiovascular complications in humans with essential hypertension.[110] These complications may influence the course of the disease. ACE inhibitors, which block signaling through both AT_1 and AT_2 receptors, have beneficial effects beyond their antihypertensive effects; in particular, they have a marked effect on regression of left ventricular hypertrophy.[111] Blockade of the renin-angiotensin system probably also has effects on vascular hypertrophy, which may contribute to its therapeutic benefit.[112] ACE inhibitors delay the progression of diabetic nephropathy and may even delay the onset of diabetes.[113] In addition, they decrease the incidence of stroke in high-risk patients.[113]

AT₁ Receptor Antisense Delivery as an Antihypertensive Therapy

Antisense gene technology is currently being tested in a wide variety of settings as an alternative to drug therapy. Recent studies delivering antisense AT_1 receptor, either as an oligonucleotide or cloned into a retroviral- or adenoviral-based vector, have suggested that this technology may provide the same advantages as the AT_1 receptor blockers without the same side effects.[114] In addition, it avoids the peaks and troughs associated with oral administration of ACE inhibitors or AT_1 receptor inhibitors. In cultured VSMCs, adeno-associated virus expressing antisense AT_1 receptor DNA significantly reduced AT_1 receptor expression and Ang II-induced calcium mobilization.[115] A single injection of retrovirally packaged antisense AT_1 receptor DNA to 5-day-old spontaneously hypertensive rats (SHRs) decreased blood pressure for up to 3 months.[116] Intracardiac delivery of this construct reduced blood pressure in adult SHRs and reversed renovascular pathophysiology.[117] Further studies showed that injection of antisense virus into neonatal heart of SHR prevented the development of hypertension as well as the changes in renovascular calcium homeostasis associated with hypertension for at least 210 days.[118] Surprisingly, the F1 and F2 generation offspring of antisense-treated SHRs also had a persistently lower blood pressure, decreased cardiac hypertrophy and fibrosis, decreased medial thickness, and normalization of renal artery excitation-contraction coupling.[119] This finding suggests that the antisense sequence has been integrated into the genome, raising the possibility of permanent cardiovascular protection. Much additional work is required to test this therapeutic approach and its potential side effects.

Angiotensin II, Oxidative Stress, and Hypertension

As noted above, Ang II is prooxidant for both VSMCs and endothelial cells. Recently, it has become clear that oxidative stress plays an important role in hypertension. Nakazono and coworkers[120] originally showed that a form of superoxide dismutase modified to bind to the extracellular matrix acutely lowered blood pressure in SHRs, but had no effect on blood pressure in normal rats. In the past few years, similar results have been found in Ang II-induced hypertension.[121–123] Using osmotic minipumps to infuse Ang II subcutaneously (0.6 mg/kg/day) in Sprague-Dawley rats, Rajagopalan et al.[121] showed that Ang II increased blood pressure with a peak at 5–7 days. A model of hypertension associated with low levels of Ang II (infusion of norepinephrine) also was used. Of interest, $O_2^{\bullet-}$ production in the vessel wall was increased in rats infused with Ang II but not epinephrine. When the endothelium was intentionally removed, the increase in $O_2^{\bullet-}$ persisted, suggesting that the source of the increase in O_2·⁻ was VSMCs. Subsequent studies indicated that the oxidase involved in the increase in O_2·⁻ production was the membrane-associated NAD(P)H oxidase.[122] It also has been shown that Ang II can increase O_2·⁻ production in the adventitia[124] and thus inactivate NO.[125]

The increase in VSMC production of O_2·⁻ caused by Ang II was associated with an impairment of endothelium-dependent vascular relaxation as well as relaxations to nitroglycerin,[121,126] presumably due to the inactivation of NO by O_2·⁻. These responses may be normalized by treatment with liposome-encapsulated SOD.[121] Because loss of NO reduces vasodilation, an increase in O_2·⁻ in the resistance circulation may contribute to the hypertension caused by Ang II infusion. Bech-Laursen et al.[123] used in vivo administration of liposome-encapsulated SOD to lower endogenous steady-state levels of vascular O_2·⁻ and to prevent the increase in response to Ang II. They found that this treatment had no effect on blood pressure in either control or norepinephrine-infused rats but significantly lowered blood pressure in rats infused with Ang II. These data imply that a portion of the blood pressure response to elevated Ang II results from an increase in vascular O_2·⁻ production and presumably inactivation of NO. Of note, expression of p22phox mRNA in aortas from Ang II-treated rats accompanied the increase in oxidase activity and the onset of hypertension, suggesting that they are closely related.[122] Based on these findings, it is possible to speculate that patients with hypertension associated with elevated levels of Ang II may exhibit greater alterations of endothelium-dependent vascular relaxation than do hypertensives with low-renin states. Studies of endothelium-dependent vascular relaxation in humans should consider renin/angiotensin profiles.

These findings may provide some insight into why forms of hypertension associated with elevated plasma renin activity are associated with increased cardiovascular events. Of interest, infusion of lower doses of Ang II, which had minimal effects on blood pressure, also increased NAD(P)H oxidase activity. This finding suggests that hypertension itself is not a stimulus for increased O_2·⁻ production and that Ang II may have unique effects on the vessel wall independent of elevating blood pressure. However, both oxidase activity and p22phox expression were blocked by the antihypertensive agent hydralazine, raising the possibility that blood pressure may contribute to oxidase upregulation in the setting of elevated Ang II.[122] These results provide a potential molecular mechanism by which Ang II can affect vascular function at multiple levels.

Angiotensin II and Endothelin

Another mediator of hypertension caused by Ang II is endothelin production by VSMCs. Ang II increases endothelin-1 gene expression in the vessel wall.[127,128] Of importance, endothelin-1 antagonists can prevent hypertension caused by Ang II infusion,[129,130] and expression of ET-1 protein is markedly increased in vessels from these rats.[129] The interactions between oxidative stress, loss of NO bioactivity, and Ang II that lead to enhanced ET-1 protein production in vivo are unclear, but they are likely to contribute to the pathogenesis of hypertension and probably other vascular diseases.

Atherosclerosis

The concept of Ang II as a proatherogenic factor originally came from the observation that patients with high-renin hypertension had a high incidence of atherosclerotic heart disease.[131] ACE has been found in fibroproliferative lesions of human atherosclerotic plaques, suggesting an involvement of the renin-angiotensin system in atherosclerosis.[132] Recently, it has been shown that in patients at risk for cardiovascular disease the ACE inhibitor ramapril decreases the risk of myocardial infarction, all causes of cardiovascular mortality, stroke, and death from congestive heart failure.[113] Animal studies have been directed toward understanding the cellular mechanisms by which Ang II mediates these events.

In an elegant study using apoE-/- mice, Weiss et al.[133] clearly demonstrated that Ang II accelerates plaque formation. Infusion of ApoE-deficient mice with Ang II induced hypertension and dramatically increased atherosclerotic lesion area by over 800% at 8 weeks. Animals on a high-fat diet had a similar marked increase in lesion area in response to Ang II. By 12 weeks, lesion-associated mortality was extremely high. In the absence of Ang II, lesions of this severity do not develop until 16 weeks.[133] Although the mechanisms responsible for this enhancement of lesion formation are not known, Ang II activates several potential proatherogenic pathways, including induction of adhesion molecules,[134] enhanced uptake of oxidized low-density lipoprotein (LDL)[135] and increased oxidative stress.[47] These events in particular contribute to monocyte infiltration into the vessel wall, endothelial dysfunction, and abnormal smooth muscle cell proliferation.

Ang II leads to the induction of both adhesion molecules and chemotactic factors. Infusion of rats with Ang II or stimulation of VSMCs increases VCAM-1 expression,[134] presumably leading to increased leukocyte adhesion. Ang II also increases monocyte binding to endothelial cells independent of induction of known adhesion molecules.[104] Furthermore, Ang II stimulates monocyte chemotaxis by increasing expression of monocyte chemotactic factor (MCP-1) in smooth muscle cells.[54,136] Recently it has been shown that human monocytes[137] as well as macrophages in atherosclerotic lesions[138] contain Ang II and are thus a potential local source of Ang II in plaques. Moreover, Ang II induces an AT₁ receptor-dependent increase in intracellular peroxide production,[139] enhances lipid peroxidation,[140] and increases oxidation and uptake of LDL into macrophages, possibly by increasing the activity of the macrophage-oxidized LDL receptors.[135] Thus, both adhesion and migration of monocytes can be stimulated by Ang II, and once the cells become resident in the vessel wall, they too respond to Ang II.

Studies of hypercholesterolemic rabbits support the concept that Ang II is involved in the pathogenesis of atherosclerosis. Many years ago, Chobanian et al.[141] showed that chronic administration of captopril to Watanabe rabbits (in which hypercholesterolemia is secondary to a LDL-receptor defect) reduced aortic lesion area. Of interest, AT₁ receptor expression is strikingly increased in the media of hypercholesterolemic rabbit aortas[142] and Cynomolgus monkeys fed a high-cholesterol diet.[143] Insight into the mechanisms responsible for this increase comes from a study by Nickenig et al.,[144] who showed that oxidized LDL causes an upregulation of AT₁ receptors in VSMCs. Furthermore, Ang II may be produced locally in atherosclerotic lesions, because chymase, an enzyme that cleaves Ang I to Ang II, is present in atherosclerotic monkey aortas and the intima of human atheromatous plaques.[145–147]

Increased Ang II activity and AT₁ receptor expression lead to increased oxidative stress in the vessel wall. Recently, it was shown that in Watanabe rabbits vascular NADH-driven $O_2^{\bullet-}$ is increased twofold compared with controls after 8 weeks.[148] The excess $O_2{}^{\bullet-}$ production was localized to the intima, because endothelial denudation normalized the differences in $O_2{}^{\bullet-}$. Of importance, the AT_1 receptor antagonist BAY 10-6734 normalized $O_2{}^{\bullet-}$ and endothelial function and reduced early atherosclerotic lesion formation, indicating a role for Ang II in this hypercholesterolemic model of early atherosclerosis. In more advanced atherosclerotic lesions, Ang II stimulation of NAD(P)H oxidase-derived ROS may play a crucial role in progression and biologic activity. Ang II probably increases ROS in the atherosclerotic lesion by stimulating the local vascular myocytes to produce ROS, as they do in culture. Subsequently ROS may contribute to LDL oxidation, local MCP-1 production, upregulation of adhesion molecules, macrophage recruitment, endothelial dysfunction, and extracellular matrix remodeling.

Vascular Remodeling

Restenosis or an angiographic loss/gain ratio greater than 50% is a major regulator of vessel patency after percutaneous transluminal coronary angioplasty (PTCA). In the United States alone, restenosis occurs in 30–50% of cases within 6 months of PTCA.[149] The three stages of restenosis include (1) thrombus formation, inflammation, and secretion of growth factors (i.e., PDGF, FGF-β, and IL-1β); (2) migration of smooth muscle cells and myofibroblasts to the injured area, where they proliferate and secrete extracellular matrix; and (3) remodeling, in which the smooth muscle cells organize the extracellular matrix and the endothelium reforms.

Studies of the involvement of the renin-angiotensin system in restenosis have focused predominantly on the role of Ang II in neointimal thickening and remodeling. Two of the main features of the restenotic lesion are proliferation of smooth muscle cells and production of extracellular matrix. In culture, Ang II induces DNA synthesis and hypertrophy of VSMCs,[150] whereas in vivo Ang II infusion induces vessel hypertrophy after 7 days of treatment.[74] These results suggest that the renin-angiotensin system may play a crucial role in restenosis.

To test this hypothesis, early studies were performed in the rat carotid balloon injury model of restenosis. ACE, renin, angiotensinogen, and AT_1 receptor levels were regulated after vascular injury.[151–153] AT_1 receptor expression was elevated not only at early stages of lesion formation (3 days), but also at later stages (14–15 days).[151,152] Furthermore, neointimal AT_1 receptor binding was increased considerably compared with medial binding in both injured and uninjured vessels.[154] If Ang II was administered for 14 days 3 weeks after balloon injury, DNA synthesis was increased in both the media and the neointima. Ang II administration at later points still increased neointimal DNA synthesis but had little effect on DNA synthesis in the media.[154] These studies suggest not only that the necessary components of the renin-angiotensin system are upregulated in the vessel wall after injury, but also that inhibition of this system may provide therapeutic benefits.

ACE inhibitors were used to assess the role of the renin-angiotensin system in the progression of lesion formation in a rat model of vessel injury. Quinapril given before injury to the vessel inhibited blood pressure, tissue and serum ACE levels, AT_1 receptor expression, and neointimal formation in a dose-dependent manner.[149,151] With the advent of the AT_1 receptor inhibitors, it became possible to analyze the direct effects of AT_1 receptor activation on the progression of neointimal formation after vascular injury. Nozawa et al.[155] recently reported that TH-142177, a novel selective AT₁ receptor inhibitor, blocked not only Ang II-induced DNA synthesis and migration but also neointimal thickening after balloon injury in rats. Taken together, these results indicate that the Ang II-producing, rather than the bradykinin-degrading, activity of ACE is involved in neointimal formation.

The theory that the renin-angiotensin system is involved in restenosis has been tested in an AT₁ receptor knockout mouse by Harada et al.[156] with unexpected results. Similar to previously reported data, 14 days after balloon injury AT₁ and AT₂ receptor expression was elevated in wild-type mice. As predicted, knockout mice only had elevated AT₂ receptor expression. However, in contrast to the studies using pharmacologic inhibition, balloon injury still induced intimal thickening in the AT₁ receptor knockout mouse. Ang II administration in subpressor doses elevated growth of the neointima in wild-type mice but not knockout mice. AT₁ receptor antagonism attenuated neointimal growth only in wild-type mice, and AT₂ receptor antagonism had no effect on either mouse. It is possible that these transgenic animals have upregulated another aspect of the growth program to compensate for the loss of the Ang II system, but the identity of this putative signaling system remains unknown. It is clear from these studies, however, that the progression of the smooth muscle proliferation and vessel remodeling after vessel injury is a complicated process to which the renin-angiotensin system may contribute, but for which it is not a sufficient component.

Although small animal studies have shown that Ang II may play a role in restenosis, large animal studies and clinical trials have not confirmed this conclusion. Administration of Ang II receptor antagonists (L-158,809, AT₁ receptor; L-163,082, AT₁/AT₂ receptor; and L-164,282, AT₂ receptor) in a porcine model of coronary artery restenosis had no effect on neointimal thickness.[157] Similar results were found in a baboon model of restenosis using the ACE inhibitor cilazapril[158] and in human trials. The MERCATOR[159] and the MARCATOR[160] trials examined the ability of cilazapril to prevent restenosis after angioplasty injury. Three doses of cilazapril were used (1, 5, or 10 mg orally twice daily), and patients were analyzed 6 months after successful coronary angioplasty. In the follow-up analysis it was determined that ACE inhibition did nothing to prevent restenosis of the coronary artery.

The differences between the human, porcine, and baboon studies and the rat studies, are not easy to explain. After the release of the MERCATOR trial results, the study design was criticized.[161] Were the appropriate doses used? The doses used in the trials were those routinely used to lower blood pressure; however, whether this dose is enough to inhibit the tissue angiotensin system is debatable. The route of administration and the initiation of treatment also were questioned, in part because ACE inhibitors were not given before injury, as they were in rats. Thus, more information is clearly needed to define the exact role of the renin-angiotensin system in the multitude of factors contributing to restenosis.

■ Conclusion

Recent work has provided exciting new insights into the molecular pathways activated by Ang II in the vasculature. Clearly, more work is needed to assess fully the role of oxidative stress in mediating the functions of Ang II and to define the relationship between the multitude of tyrosine kinases activated by

Ang II. The role of the AT_2 receptor also requires further investigation. In addition, it is necessary to clarify the effect of Ang II on endothelial cells and to determine definitively the predominant endothelial Ang II receptors. Furthermore, the far-reaching pathophysiologic effects of Ang II, its role in hypertension and atherosclerosis, and the vast therapeutic potential of AT_1 receptor blockers are only beginning to be fully understood. Clarifying the role of Ang II in the cellular events that contribute to vascular disease is an important undertaking that is likely to provide new breakthroughs in therapy for vascular disorders.

Acknowledgments

This review was supported by NIH grants HL38206, HL58000, and HL58863. The authors thank Carolyn Morris for excellent secretarial assistance.

References

1. Ushio-Fukai M, Griendling KK, Akers M, et al: Temporal dispersion of activation of phospholipase C-β1 and -γ isoforms by angiotensin II in vascular smooth muscle cells: Role of $α_{q/11}$, $α_{12}$, and βγ G protein subunits. J Biol Chem 273:19772–19777, 1998.
2. Ushio-Fukai M, Alexander RW, Akers M, et al: Angiotensin II receptor coupling to phospholipase D is mediated by the βγ subunits of heterotrimeric G proteins in vascular smooth muscle cells. Mol Pharmacol 55:142–149, 1999.
3. Kai H, Alexander RW, Ushio-Fukai M, et al: G-Protein binding domains of the angiotensin II AT_{1A} receptors mapped with synthetic peptides selected from the receptor sequence. Biochem J 332:781–787, 1998.
4. Griendling KK, Rittenhouse SE, Brock TA, et al: Sustained diacylglycerol formation from inositol phospholipids in angiotensin II-stimulated vascular smooth muscle cells. J Biol Chem 261:5901–5906, 1986.
5. Marrero MB, Paxton WG, Duff JL, et al: Angiotensin II stimulates tyrosine phosphorylation of phospholipase C-gamma 1 in vascular smooth muscle cells. J Biol Chem 269:10935–10939, 1994.
6. Venema RC, Ju H, Venema VJ, et al: Angiotensin II-induced association of phospholipase Cgamma1 with the G-protein-coupled AT1 receptor. J Biol Chem 273:7703–7708, 1998.
7. Lassègue B, Alexander RW, Clark M, et al: Phosphatidylcholine is a major source of phosphatidic acid and diacylglycerol in angiotensin II-stimulated vascular smooth muscle cells. Biochem J 292:509–517, 1993.
8. Lassègue B, Alexander RW, Nickenig G, et al: Angiotensin II down-regulates the vascular AT_1 receptor by transcriptional and post-transcriptional mechanisms: Evidence for homologous and heterologous regulation. Mol Pharmacol 48:601–609, 1995.
9. Lassègue B, Alexander RW, Clark M, Griendling KK: Angiotensin II-induced phosphatidylcholine hydrolysis in cultured vascular smooth-muscle cells. Regulation and localization. Biochem J 276:19–25, 1991.
10. Ishizaka N, Griendling KK, Lassègue B, Alexander RW: Type 1 angiotensin II receptor: Relationship with caveolae and caveolin after initial agonist stimulation. Hypertension 32:459–466, 1998.
11. Ushio-Fukai M, Alexander RW, Akers M, Griendling KK: p38MAP kinase is a critical component of the redox-sensitive signaling pathways by angiotensin II: Role in vascular smooth muscle cell hypertrophy. J Biol Chem 273:15022–15029, 1998.
12. Ushio-Fukai M, Zafari AM, Fukui T, et al: p22phox is a critical component of the superoxide-generating NADH/NADPH oxidase system and regulates angiotensin II-induced hypertrophy in vascular smooth muscle cells. J Biol Chem 271:23317–23321, 1996.
13. Ushio-Fukai M, Alexander RW, Akers M, et al: Reactive oxygen species mediate the activation of Akt/Protein kinase B by angiotensin II in vascular smooth muscle cells. J Biol Chem 274:22699–22704, 1999.
14. Davis RJ: MAPKs: New JNK expands the group. Trends Biochem Sci 19:470–473, 1994.
15. Cano E, Mahadevan LC: Parallel signal processing among mammalian MAPKs. Trends Biochem Sci 20:117–122, 1995.
16. Cobb MH, Goldsmith EJ: How MAP kinases are regulated. J Biol Chem 25:14843–14846, 1995.
17. Abe J, Kusuhara M, Ulevitch RJ, et al: Big mitogen-activated protein kinase 1 (BMK1) is a redox-sensitive kinase. J Biol Chem 271:16586–16590, 1996.
18. Kyriakis JM, Avruch J: Sounding the alarm: Protein kinase cascades activated by stress and inflammation. J Biol Chem 271:24313–24316, 1996.

19. Paul A, Wilson S, Belham CM, et al: Stress-activated protein kinases: Activation, regulation and function. Cell Signal 9:403–410, 1997.

20. Derijard B, Hibi M, Wu IH, et al: JNK1: A protein kinase stimulated by UV light and Ha-Ras that binds and phosphorylates the c-Jun activation domain. Cell 76:1025–1037, 1994.

21. Kyriakis JM, Banerjee P, Nikolakaki E, et al: The stress-activated protein kinase subfamily of c-Jun kinases. Nature 369:156–160, 1994.

22. Gupta S, Campbell D, Derijard B, Davis RJ: Transcription factor ATF2 regulation by the JNK signal transduction pathway. Science 267:389–393, 1995.

23. Whitmarsh AJ, Shore P, Sharrocks AD, Davis RJ: Integration of MAP kinase signal transduction pathways at the serum response element. Science 269:403–407, 1995.

24. Raingeaud J, Gupta S, Rogers JS, et al: Pro-inflammatory cytokines and environmental stress cause p38 mitogen-activated protein kinase activation by dual phosphorylation on tyrosine and threonine. J Biol Chem 270:7420–7426, 1995.

25. Wang XZ, Ron D: Stress-induced phosphorylation and activation of the transcription factor CHOP (GADD153) by p38 MAP kinase. Science 272:1347–1349, 1996.

26. Rouse J, Cohen P, Trigon S, et al: A novel kinase cascade triggered by stress and heat shock that stimulates MAPKAP kinase-2 and phosphorylation of the small heat shock proteins. Cell 78:1027–1037, 1994.

27. McLaughlin MM, Kumar S, McDonnell PC, et al: Identification of mitogen-activated protein (MAP) kinase-activated protein kinase-3, a novel substrate of CSBP p38 MAP kinase. J Biol Chem 271:8488–8492, 1996.

28. Mii S, Ware JA, Mallette SA, Kent KC: Effect of angiotensin II on human vascular smooth muscle cell growth. J Surg Res 57:174–178, 1994.

29. Eguchi S, Matsumoto T, Motley ED, et al: Identification of an essential signaling cascade for mitogen-activated protein kinase activation by angiotensin II in cultured rat vascular smooth muscle cells. J Biol Chem 271:14169–14175, 1996.

30. Schmitz U, Ishida T, Ishida M, et al: Angiotensin II stimulates p21-activated kinase in vascular smooth muscle cells: Role in activation of JNK. Circ Res 82:1272–1278, 1998.

31. Liao D-F, Monia B, Dean N, Berk BC: Protein kinase C-ζ mediates angiotensin II activation of ERK1/2 in vascular smooth muscle cells. J Biol Chem 272:6146–6150, 1997.

32. Eguchi S, Numaguchi K, Iwasaki H, et al: Calcium-dependent epidermal growth factor receptor transactivation mediates the angiotensin II-induced mitogen-activated protein kinase activation in vascular smooth muscle cells. J Biol Chem 273:8890–8896, 1998.

33. Eguchi S, Iwasaki H, Inagami I, et al: Involvement of PYK2 in angiotensin II signaling of vascular smooth muscle cells. Hypertension 33:201–206, 1999.

34. Kushuhara M, Takahashi E, Peterson TE, et al: p38 Kinase is a negative regulator of angiotensin II signal transduction in vascular smooth muscle cells: Effects on Na+/H+ exchange and ERK1/2. Circ Res 83:824–831, 1998.

35. Marrero MB, Schieffer B, Paxton WG, et al: Direct stimulation of Jak/STAT pathway by the angiotensin II AT1 receptor. Nature 375:247–250, 1995.

36. Ali MS, Sayeski PP, Dirksen LB, et al: Dependence on the motif YIPP for the physical association of Jak2 kinase with the intracellular carboxyl tail of the angiotensin II AT1 receptor. J Biol Chem 272:23382–23388, 1997.

37. Marrero MB, Schieffer B, Li B, et al: Role of Janus kinase/signal transducer and activator of transcription and mitogen-activated protein kinase cascades in angiotensin II- and platelet-derived growth factor-induced vascular smooth muscle cell proliferation. J Biol Chem 272:24684–24690, 1997.

38. Smilenov LB, Mikhailov A, Pelham RJ, et al: Focal adhesion motility revealed in stationary fibroblasts. Science 286:1172–1174, 1999.

39. Polte TR, Naftilan AJ, Hanks SK: Focal adhesion kinase is abundant in developing blood vessels and elevation of its phosphotyrosine content in vascular smooth muscle cells is a rapid response to angiotensin II. J Cell Biochem 55:106–119, 1994.

40. Berk BC: Angiotensin II signal transduction in vascular smooth muscle: Pathways activated by specific tyrosine kinases. J Am Soc Nephrol 10(Suppl 11):S62–68, 1999.

41. Ishida T, Ishida M, Suero J, et al: Agonist-stimulated cytoskeletal reorganization and signal transduction at focal adhesions in vascular smooth muscle cells require c-Src. J Clin Invest 103:789–797, 1999.

42. Ishida M, Marrero MB, Schieffer B, et al: Angiotensin II activates pp60c-src in vascular smooth muscle cells. Circ Res 77:1053–1059, 1995.

43. Brinson AE, Harding T, Diliberto PA, et al: Regulation of a calcium-dependent tyrosine kinase in vascular smooth muscle cells by angiotensin II and platelet-derived growth factor. Dependence on calcium and the actin cytoskeleton. J Biol Chem 273:1711–1718, 1998.

44. Sayeski PP, Ali MS, Harp JB, et al: Phosphorylation of p130Cas by angiotensin II is dependent on c-Src, intracellular Ca2+, and protein kinase C, Circ Res 82:1279–1288, 1998.

45. Takahashi T, Kawahara Y, Taniguchi T, Yokoyama M: Tyrosine phosphorylation and association of p130Cas and c-Crk II by Ang II in vascular smooth muscle cells. Am J Physiol 274:H1059–1065, 1998.

46. Voisin L, Larose L, Meloche S: Angiotensin II stimulates serine phosphorylation of the adaptor protein Nck: Physical association with the serine/threonine kinases Pak1 and casein kinase I. Biochem J 341:217–223, 1999.

47. Griendling KK, Minieri CA, Ollerenshaw JD, Alexander RW: Angiotensin II stimulates NADH and NADPH oxidase activity in cultured vascular smooth muscle cells. Circ Res 74:1141–1148, 1994.

48. Zafari AM, Ushio-Fukai M, Akers M, et al: Novel role of NADH/NADPH oxidase-derived hydrogen peroxide in angiotensin II-induced hypertrophy of rat vascular smooth muscle cells. Hypertension 32:488–495, 1998.

49. Wang D, Yu X, Brecher P: Nitric oxide and N-acetylcysteine inhibit the activation of mitogen-activated protein kinases by angiotensin II in rat cardiac fibroblasts [published erratum appears in J Biol Chem 274:1180, 1999]. J Biol Chem 273:33027–33034, 1998.

50. Baas AS, Berk BC: Differential activation of mitogen-activated protein kinases by H_2O_2 and O_2^- in vascular smooth muscle cells. Circ Res 77:29–36, 1995.

51. Konishi H, Tanaka M, Takemura Y, et al: Activation of protein kinase C by tyrosine phosphorylation in response to H_2O_2. Proc Natl Acad Sci USA 94:11233–11237, 1997.

52. Hecht D, Zick Y: Selective inhibition of protein tyrosine phosphatase activities by H_2O_2 and vanadate in vitro. Biochem Biophys Res Commun 188:773–779, 1992.

53. Sen CK, Packer L: Antioxidant and redox regulation of gene transcription. FASEB J 10:709–720, 1996.

54. Chen XL, Tummala PE, Olbrych MT, et al: Angiotensin II induces monocyte chemoattractant protein-1 gene expression in rat vascular smooth muscle cells. Circ Res 83:952–959, 1998.

55. Han Y, Runge MS, Brasier AR: Angiotensin II induces interleukin-6 transcription in vascular smooth muscle cells through pleiotropic activation of nuclear factor-kappa B transcription factors. Circ Res 84:695–703, 1999.

56. Freedman NJ, Liggett SB, Drachman DE, et al: Phosphorylation and desensitization of the human beta 1-adrenergic receptor. Involvement of G protein-coupled receptor kinases and cAMP-dependent protein kinase. J Biol Chem 270:17953–17961, 1995.

57. Brock TA, Rittenhouse SE, Powers CW, et al: Phorbol ester and 1-oleoyl-2-acetylglycerol inhibit angiotensin activation of phospholipase C in cultured vascular smooth muscle cells. J Biol Chem 260:14158–14162, 1985.

58. Griendling KK, Delafontaine P, Rittenhouse SE, et al: Correlation of receptor sequestration with sustained diacylglycerol accumulation in angiotensin II-stimulated cultured vascular smooth muscle cells. J Biol Chem 262:14555–14562, 1987.

59. Kai H, Griendling KK, Lassegue B, et al: Agonist-induced phosphorylation of the vascular type 1 angiotensin II receptor. Hypertension 24:523–527, 1994.

60. Oppermann M, Freedman NJ, Alexander RW, Lefkowitz RJ: Phosphorylation of the type 1A angiotensin II receptor by G protein-coupled receptor kinases and protein kinase C. J Biol Chem 271:13266–13272, 1996.

61. Ishizaka N, Alexander RW, Laursen JB, et al: G protein-coupled receptor kinase 5 in cultured vascular smooth muscle cells and rat aorta: Regulation by angiotensin II and hypertension. J Biol Chem 272:32482–32488, 1997.

62. Zhang J, Ferguson SSG, Barak LS, et al: Dynamin and beta-arrestin reveal distinct mechanisms for G-protein coupled receptor internalization. J Biol Chem 271:18302–18305, 1996.

63. Anderson KM, Murahashi T, Dostal DE, Peach MJ: Morphological and biochemical analysis of angiotensin II internalization in cultured rat aortic smooth muscle cells. Am J Physiol 264:C179–C188, 1993.

64. Anderson KM, Peach MJ: Receptor binding and internalization of a unique biologically active angiotensin II-colloidal gold conjugate: Morphological analysis of angiotensin II processing in isolated vascular strips. J Vasc Res 31:10–17, 1994.

65. Morishita R, Nakayama H, Isobe T, et al: Primary structure of a gamma subunit of G protein, gamma12, and its phosphorylation by protein kinase C. J Biol Chem 270:29469–29475, 1995.

66. Ryu SH, Kim UH, Wahl MI, et al: Feedback regulation of phospholipase C-beta by protein kinase C. J Biol Chem 265:17941–17945, 1990.

67. Heximer SP, Srinivasa SP, Bernstein LS, et al: G Protein selectivity is a determinant of RGS2 function. J Biol Chem 274:34253–34259, 1999.

68. Heximer SP, Watson N, Linder ME, et al: RGS2/G0S8 is a selective inhibitor of G-alpha function. Proc Natl Acad Sci USA 94:14389–14393, 1997.

69. Grant SL, Lassègue B, Griendling KK, et al: Specific regulation of RGS2 mRNA by angiotensin II in cultured vascular smooth muscle cells. Mol Pharmacol 2000 [in press].

70. Itoh H, Mukoyama M, Pratt RE, et al: Multiple autocrine growth factors modulate vascular smooth muscle cell growth response to angiotensin II. J Clin Invest 91:2268–2274, 1993.

71. Peach MJ: Renin-angiotensin system: Biochemistry and mechanisms of action. Physiol Rev 57:313–370, 1977.

72. Berk BC, Vekshtein V, Gordon HM, Tsuda T: Angiotensin II-stimulated protein synthesis in cultured vascular smooth muscle cells. Hypertension 13:305–314, 1989.

73. Geisterfer A, Peach MJ, Owens GK: Angiotensin II induces hypertrophy, not hyperplasia of cultured rat aortic smooth muscle cells. Circ Res 62:749–756, 1988.

74. Daemen MJAP, Lombardi DM, Bosman FT, Schwartz SM: Angiotensin II induces smooth muscle cell proliferation in the normal and injured rat arterial wall. Circ Res 68:450–456, 1991.

75. Dudley DT, Panek RL, Major TC, et al: Subclasses of angiotensin II binding sites and their functional significance. Mol Pharmacol 38:370–377, 1990.

76. Rokolya A, Walsh MP, Singer HA, Moreland RS: Protein kinase C-catalyzed calponin phosphorylation in swine carotid arterial homogenate. J Cell Physiol 176:545–552, 1998.

77. Throckmorton DC, Packer CS, Brophy CM: Protein kinase C activation during Ca²⁺-independent vascular smooth muscle contraction. J Surg Res 78:48–53, 1998.

78. Kitazawa T, Takizawa N, Ikebe M, et al: Reconstitution of protein kinase C-induced contractile Ca²⁺ sensitization in triton X-100-demembranated rabbit arterial smooth muscle. J Physiol (Lond) 520(Pt 1):139–152, 1999.

79. Macrez N, Morel J-L, Kalkbrenner F, et al: A βγ dimer derived from G₁₃ transduces the angiotensin AT₁ receptor signal to stimulation of Ca²⁺ channels in rat portal vein myocytes. J Biol Chem 272:23180–23185, 1997.

80. Owens GK, Rabinovitch PS, Schwartz SM: Smooth muscle cell hypertrophy versus hyperplasia in hypertension. Proc Natl Acad Sci USA 78:7759–7763, 1981.

81. Nakajima M, Hutchinson HG, Fujinaga M, et al: The angiotensin II type 2 (AT2) receptor antagonizes the growth effects of the AT1 receptor: Gain-of-function study using gene transfer. Proc Natl Acad Sci USA 92:10663–10667, 1995.

82. Berk BC, Rao GN: Angiotensin II-induced vascular smooth muscle cell hypertrophy: PDGF A-chain mediates the increase in cell size. J Cell Physiol 154:368–380, 1993.

83. Delafontaine P, Lou H: Angiotensin II regulates insulin-like growth factor I gene expression in vascular smooth muscle cells. J Biol Chem 268:16866–16870, 1993.

84. Gibbons GH, Pratt RE, Dzau VJ: Vascular smooth muscle cell hypertrophy vs. hyperplasia. Autocrine transforming growth factor-beta 1 expression determines growth response to angiotensin II. J Clin Invest 90:456–461, 1992.

85. Taubman MB, Berk BC, Izumo S, et al: Angiotensin II induces c-fos mRNA in aortic smooth muscle. Role of Ca²⁺ mobilization and protein kinase C activation. J Biol Chem 264:526–530, 1989.

86. Naftilan AJ, Gilliland GK, Eldridge CS, Kraft AS: Induction of the proto-oncogene c-jun by angiotensin II. Mol Cell Biol 10:5536–5540, 1990.

87. Kambayashi Y, Bardhan S, Takahashi K, et al: Molecular cloning of a novel angiotensin II receptor isoform involved in phosphotyrosine phosphatase inhibition. J Biol Chem 268:24543–24546, 1993.

88. Patel JM, Yarid FR, Block ER, Raizada MK: Angiotensin receptors in pulmonary arterial and aortic endothelial cells. Am J Physiol 256:C987–C993, 1989.

89. Guillot FL, Audus KL: Some characteristics of specific angiotensin II binding sites on bovine brain microvessel endothelial cell monolayers. Peptides 12:535–540, 1991.

90. Patel JM, Sekharam KM, Block ER: Angiotensin receptor-mediated stimulation of diacylglycerol production in pulmonary artery endothelial cells. Am J Respir Cell Mol Biol 5:321–327, 1991.

91. Mineo C, Shimizu H, Takada K, et al: Angiotensin II binding activity in cultured porcine arterial endothelial cells. Biochem Pharmacol 48:1993–1995, 1994.

92. Tallant EA, Lu X, Weiss RB, et al: Bovine aortic endothelial cells contain an angiotensin-(1-7) receptor. Hypertension 29:388–393, 1997.

93. Hall KL, Venkateswaran S, Hanesworth JM, et al: Characterization of a functional angiotensin IV receptor on coronary microvascular endothelial cells. Regul Pept 58:107–115, 1995.

94. Dimmeler S, Rippmann V, Weiland U, et al: Angiotensin II induces apoptosis of human endothelial cells. Protective effect of nitric oxide. Circ Res 81:970–976, 1997.

95. Saito S, Hirata Y, Emori T, et al: Angiotensin II activates endothelial constitutive nitric oxide synthase via AT1 receptors. Hypertens Res 19:201–206, 1996.

96. Schena M, Mulatero P, Schiavone D, et al: Vasoactive hormones induce nitric oxide synthase mRNA expression and nitric oxide production in human endothelial cells and monocytes. Am J Hypertens 12:388–397, 1999.

97. Nishimura H, Tsuji H, Masuda H, et al: Angiotensin II increases plasminogen activator inhibitor-1 and tissue factor mRNA expression without changing that of tissue type plasminogen activator or tissue factor pathway inhibitor in cultured rat aortic endothelial cells. Thromb Haemost 77:1189–1195, 1997.

98. Feener EP, Northrup JM, Aiello LP, King GL: Angiotensin II induces plasminogen activator inhibitor-1 and -2 expression in vascular endothelial and smooth muscle cells. J Clin Invest 95:1353–1362, 1995.

99. Kerins DM, Hao Q, Vaughan DE: Angiotensin induction of PAI-1 expression in endothelial cells is mediated by the hexapeptide angiotensin IV. J Clin Invest 96:2515–2520, 1995.

100. Olson SC, Dowds TA, Pino PA, et al: Ang II stimulates endothelial nitric oxide synthase expression in bovine pulmonary artery endothelium. Am J Physiol 273:L315–L321, 1997.

101. Pueyo ME, Arnal JF, Rami J, Michel JB: Angiotensin II stimulates the production of NO and peroxynitrite in endothelial cells. Am J Physiol 274:C214–C220, 1998.

102. Hill-Kapturczak N, Kapturczak MH, Block ER, et al: Angiotensin II-stimulated nitric oxide release from porcine pulmonary endothelium is mediated by angiotensin IV. J Am Soc Nephrol 10:481–491, 1999.

103. Stoll M, Meffert S, Stroth U, Unger T: Growth or antigrowth: Angiotensin and the endothelium. J Hypertens 13:1529–1534, 1995.

104. Kim JA, Berliner JA, Nadler JL: Angiotensin II increases monocyte binding to endothelial cells. Biochem Biophys Res Commun 226:862–868, 1996.

105. Grafe M, Auch-Schwelk W, Zakrzewicz A, et al: Angiotensin II-induced leukocyte adhesion on human coronary endothelial cells is mediated by E-selectin. Circ Res 81:804–811, 1997.

106. Burnier M, Brunner HR: Comparative antihypertensive effects of angiotensin II receptor antagonists. J Am Soc Nephrol 10(Suppl 12):S278–282, 1999.

107. Birkenhager WH, de Leeuw PW: Non-peptide angiotensin type 1 receptor antagonists in the treatment of hypertension. J Hypertens 17:873–881, 1999.

108. Siragy HM, Inagami T, Ichiki T, Carey RM: Sustained hypersensitivity to angiotensin II and its mechanism in mice lacking the subtype-2 (AT2) angiotensin receptor. Proc Natl Acad Sci USA 96:6506–6510, 1999.

109. Tanaka M, Tsuchida S, Imai T, et al: Vascular response to angiotensin II is exaggerated through an upregulation of AT1 receptor in AT2 knockout mice. Biochem Biophys Res Commun 258:194–198, 1999.

110. Allikmets K, Parik T, Viigimaa M: The renin-angiotensin system in essential hypertension: Associations with cardiovascular risk. Blood Press 8:70–78, 1999.

111. Mallion JM, Baguet JP, Siche JP, et al: Cardiac and vascular remodelling: Effect of antihypertensive agents. J Hum Hypertens 13(Suppl 1):S35–S41; discussion, S49–S50, 1999.

112. Lee AF, Struthers AD: The impact of angiotensin converting enzyme inhibitors on the arterial wall. Vasc Med 1:109–113, 1996.

113. Yusuf S, Sleight P, Pogue J, et al: Effects of an angiotensin-converting-enzyme inhibitor, ramapril, on death from cardiovascular causes, myocardial infarction, and stroke in high risk patients. N Engl J Med 342:145–153, 2000.

114. Wang H, Lu D, Reaves PY, et al: Retrovirally mediated delivery of angiotensin II type 1 receptor antisense in vitro and in vivo. Methods Enzymol 314:581–590, 2000.

115. Mohuczy D, Gelband CH, Phillips MI: Antisense inhibition of AT1 receptor in vascular smooth muscle cells using adeno-associated virus-based vector. Hypertension 33:354–359, 1999.

116. Iyer SN, Lu D, Katovich MJ, Raizada MK: Chronic control of high blood pressure in the spontaneously hypertensive rat by delivery of angiotensin type 1 receptor antisense. Proc Natl Acad Sci USA 93:9960–9965, 1996.

117. Katovich MJ, Gelband GH, Reaves P, et al: Reversal of hypertension by angiotensin II type 1 receptor antisense gene therapy in the adult SHR. Am J Physiol 277:H1260–1264, 1999.

118. Gelband CH, Reaves PY, Evans J, et al: Angiotensin II type 1 receptor antisense gene therapy prevents altered renal vascular calcium homeostasis in hypertension. Hypertension 33:360–365, 1999.

119. Reaves PY, Gelband CH, Wang H, et al: Permanent cardiovascular protection from hypertension by the AT(1) receptor antisense gene therapy in hypertensive rat offspring. Circ Res 85:44–50, 1999.

120. Nakazono K, Watanabe N, Matsuno K, et al: Does superoxide underlie the pathogenesis of hypertension? Proc Natl Acad Sci USA 88:10045–10048, 1991.

121. Rajagopalan S, Kurz S, Münzel T, et al: Angiotensin II mediated hypertension in the rat increases vascular superoxide production via membrane NADH/NADPH oxidase activation: Contribution to alterations of vasomotor tone. J Clin Invest 97:1916–1923, 1996.

122. Fukui T, Ishizaka N, Rajagopalan S, et al: p22phox mRNA expression and NADPH oxidase activity are increased in aortas from hypertensive rats. Circ Res 80:45–51, 1997.

123. Bech-Laursen J, Rajagopalan S, Galis Z, et al: Role of superoxide in angiotensin II-induced but not catecholamine-induced hypertension. Circulation 95:588–593, 1997.

124. Pagano PJ, Clark JK, Cifuentes-Pagano ME, et al: Localization of a constitutively active, phagocyte-like NADPH oxidase in rabbit aortic adventitia: Enhancement by angiotensin II. Proc Natl Acad Sci USA 94:14438–14488, 1997.

125. Wang HD, Pagano PJ, Du Y, et al: Superoxide anion from the adventitia of the rat thoracic aorta inactivates nitric oxide. Circ Res 82:810–818, 1998.

126. Munzel T, Sayegh H, Freeman BA, et al: Evidence for enhanced vascular superoxide anion production in nitrate tolerance. A novel mechanism underlying tolerance and cross-tolerance. J Clin Invest 95:187–194, 1995.

127. Chua BH, Chua CC, Diglio CA, Siu BB: Regulation of endothelin-1 mRNA by angiotensin II in rat heart endothelial cells. Biochim Biophys Acta 1178:201–206, 1993.

128. Imai T, Hirata Y, Emori T, et al: Induction of endothelin-1 gene by angiotensin and vasopressin in endothelial cells. Hypertension 19:753–757, 1992.

129. Rajagopalan S, Bech-Laursen J, Borthayre A, et al: A role for endothelin-1 in angiotensin II mediated hypertension. Hypertension 24:29–34, 1997.

130. d'Uscio LV, Moreau P, Shaw S, et al: Effects of chronic ET_A-receptor blockade in angiotensin II-induced hypertension. Hypertension 29:435–441, 1997.

131. Laragh JH, Sealy JE: The renin-angiotensin-aldosterone system in hypertensive disorders: A key to two forms of arteriolar vasoconstriction and a possible clue to risk of vascular injury (heart attack and stroke) and prognosis. In Laragh JH, Brenner BM (eds): Hypertension: Pathophysiology, Diagnosis, and Management. New York, Raven Press, 1990, pp 1329–1348.

132. Dzau VJ: Cell biology and genetics of angiotensin in cardiovascular disease. J Hypertens Suppl 12:S3–S10, 1994.

133. Weiss D, Kools JJ, Taylor WR: Angiotensin II-induced hypertension accelerates the development of atherosclerosis in ApoE-deficient mice. Circulation 100:I-474, 1999.

134. Tummala PE, Chen XL, Sundell CL, et al: Angiotensin II induces vascular cell adhesion molecule-1 expression in rat vasculature: A potential link between the renin-angiotensin system and atherosclerosis. Circulation 100:1223–1229, 1999.

135. Keidar S, Attias J: Angiotensin II injection into mice increases the uptake of oxidized LDL by their macrophages via a proteoglycan-mediated pathway. Biochem Biophys Res Commun 239:63–67, 1997.

136. Capers QT, Alexander RW, Lou P, et al: Monocyte chemoattractant protein-1 expression in aortic tissues of hypertensive rats. Hypertension 30:1397–1402, 1997.

137. Kitazono T, Padgett RC, Armstrong ML, et al: Evidence that angiotensin II is present in human monocytes. Circulation 91:1129–1134, 1995.

138. Potter DD, Sobey CG, Tompkins PK, et al: Evidence that macrophages in atherosclerotic lesions contain angiotensin II. Circulation 98:800–807, 1998.

139. Yanagitani Y, Rakugi H, Okamura A, et al: Angiotensin II type 1 receptor-mediated peroxide production in human macrophages. Hypertension 33:335–339, 1999.

140. Keidar S: Angiotensin, LDL peroxidation and atherosclerosis. Life Sci 63:1–11, 1998.

141. Chobanian AV, Haudenschild CC, Nickerson C, Drago R: Antiatherogenic effect of captopril in the Watanabe heritable hyperlipidemic rabbit. Hypertension 15:327–331, 1990.

142. Yang BC, Phillips MI, Mohuczy D, et al; Increased angiotensin II type 1 receptor expression in hypercholesterolemic atherosclerosis in rabbits. Arterioscler Thromb Vasc Biol 18:1433–1439, 1998.

143. Song K, Shiota N, Takai S, et al: Induction of angiotensin converting enzyme and angiotensin II receptors in the atherosclerotic aorta of high-cholesterol fed Cynomolgus monkeys. Atherosclerosis 138:171–182, 1998.

144. Nickenig G, Sachinidis A, Michaelsen F, et al: Upregulation of vascular angiotensin II receptor gene expression by low-density lipoprotein in vascular smooth muscle cells. Circulation 95:473–478, 1997.

145. Ohishi M, Ueda M, Rakugi H, et al: Relative localization of angiotensin-converting enzyme, chymase and angiotensin II in human coronary atherosclerotic lesions. J Hypertens 17:547–553, 1999.

146. Ihara M, Urata H, Kinoshita A, et al: Increased chymase-dependent angiotensin II formation in human atherosclerotic aorta. Hypertension 33:1399–1405, 1999.

147. Takai S, Shiota N, Kobayashi S, et al: Induction of chymase that forms angiotensin II in the monkey atherosclerotic aorta. FEBS Lett 412:86–90, 1997.

148. Warnholtz A, Nickenig G, Schulz E, et al: Increased NADH-oxidase-mediated superoxide production in the early stages of atherosclerosis: Evidence for involvement of the renin-angiotensin system. Circulation 99:2027–2033, 1999.

149. Rakugi H, Wang DS, Dzau VJ, Pratt RE: Potential importance of tissue angiotensin-converting enzyme inhibition in preventing neointima formation. Circulation 90:449–455, 1994.

150. Touyz RM, Deng LY, He G, et al: Angiotensin II stimulates DNA and protein synthesis in vascular smooth muscle cells from human arteries: Role of extracellular signal-regulated kinases. J Hypertens 17:907–916, 1999.

151. Iwai N, Izumi M, Inagami T, Kinoshita M: Induction of renin in medial smooth muscle cells by balloon injury. Hypertension 29:1044–1050, 1997.

152. Viswanathan M, Stromberg C, Seltzer A, Saavedra JM: Balloon angioplasty enhances the expression of angiotensin II AT1 receptors in neointima of rat aorta. J Clin Invest 90:1707–1712, 1992.

153. Rakugi H, Jacob HJ, Krieger JE, et al: Vascular injury induces angiotensinogen gene expression in the media and neointima. Circulation 87:283–290, 1993.

154. deBlois D, Viswanathan M, Su JE, et al: Smooth muscle DNA replication in response to angiotensin II is regulated differently in the neointima and media at different times after balloon injury in the rat carotid artery. Role of AT1 receptor expression. Arterioscler Thromb Vasc Biol 16:1130–1137, 1996.

155. Nozawa Y, Matsuura N, Miyake H, et al: Effects of TH-142177 on angiotensin II-induced proliferation, migration and intracellular signaling in vascular smooth muscle cells and on neointimal thickening after balloon injury. Life Sci 64:2061–2070, 1999.

156. Harada K, Komuro I, Sugaya T, et al: Vascular injury causes neointimal formation in angiotensin II type 1a receptor knockout mice. Circ Res 84:179–185, 1999.

157. Huckle WR, Drag MD, Acker WR, et al: Effects of subtype-selective and balanced angiotensin II receptor antagonists in a porcine coronary artery model of vascular restenosis. Circulation 93:1009–1019, 1996.

158. Hanson SR, Powell JS, Dodson T, et al: Effects of angiotensin converting enzyme inhibition with cilazapril on intimal hyperplasia in injured arteries and vascular grafts in the baboon. Hypertension 18(Suppl II):II-70–II-76, 1991.

159. Mercator-Study-Group: The multicenter European research trial with cilazapril after angioplasty to prevent transluminal coronary obstruction and restenosis. Circulation 86:100–110, 1992.

160. Faxon DP: Effect of high dose angiotensin-converting enzyme inhibition on restenosis: Final results of the MARCATOR Study, a multicenter, double-blind, placebo-controlled trial of cilazapril. The Multicenter American Research Trial With Cilazapril After Angioplasty to Prevent Transluminal Coronary Obstruction and Restenosis (MARCATOR) Study Group. J Am Coll Cardiol 25:362–369, 1995.

161. Pratt RE, Dzau VJ: Pharmacological strategies to prevent restenosis: Lessons learned from blockade of the renin-angiotensin system [editorial]. Circulation 93:848–852, 1996.

CHAPTER 17

Angiotensin II Receptor Antagonists: Current Status

MURRAY EPSTEIN, M.D., FACP

During the past several years, several new, nonpeptide, orally active angiotensin II (Ang II) receptor antagonists have been approved for clinical use. As detailed in chapters 1, 3, and 7, these agents represent the most specific way to block the renin-angiotensin system (RAS) by terminal blockade of the RAS cascade. Ang II receptor antagonists are assuming an important role in the treatment of patients with hypertension and various cardiovascular disorders in the United States and elsewhere, and their availability constitutes an important advance in the management of hypertension.

Since the first Ang II receptor antagonist, losartan, was introduced a few years ago, numerous clinical trials have demonstrated the efficacy of these agents in patients with essential hypertension. Clinical trials also have investigated their potential use in patients with congestive heart failure. Several Ang II receptor antagonists have been approved for use in hypertension by the U.S. Food and Drug Administration (FDA), including losartan (Cozaar), valsartan (Diovan), irbesartan (Avapro), candesartan (Atacand), telmisartan (Micardis), and, most recently, eprosartan (Teveten). Other Ang II receptor antagonists, such as zolasartan and saprisartan, are currently under investigation and development. Recently the development of tasosartan (Verdia) was discontinued.

Tables 1–3 compare salient features of the Ang II receptor blockers currently available for clinical use. Table 1 summarizes their chemical classification; Table 2, their phamacokinetic properties; and Table 3, dosage information. The antihypertensive effects should become apparent within 2 or 4 weeks after the initiation of therapy. Such effects are enhanced by adding a low-dose diuretic, such as hydrochlorothiazide, rather than by increasing the Ang II receptor antagonist dosage.

■ Efficacy and Tolerability

Numerous studies have demonstrated that Ang II antagonists are as effective as angiotensin-converting enzyme (ACE) inhibitors, calcium antagonists, beta blockers, or diuretics in lowering blood pressure in patients with hypertension. In general, the effects of currently approved Ang II receptor antagonists do not

Table 1. Chemical Classification of Major Angiotensin II Receptor Blockers

Drug	Code	Pharmaceutical Company
Biphenyl tetrazoles		
Losartan	DUP753/MK954	Merck/DuPont
	EXP-3174	
Candesartan	H 212/92	AstraZeneca/Takeda
	CV-11974	
Irbesartan	SR 47436	BMS/Sanofi
	BMS 186295	
Tasosartan	ANA 756	Ayerst/Wyeth
Nonbiphenyl tetrazoles		
Eprosartan	SKF108566	SmithKline Beecham/Unimed
Telmisartan	BIBR 277	Boehringer Ingelheim/Abbott
Nonheterocyclic		
Valsartan	CGP 48933	Novartis

Adapted from Birkenhager WH, de Leeuw PS: Non-peptide angiotensin type I receptor antagonists in the treatment of hypertension. J Hypertens 17:873–881, 1999.

differ substantially; all are alleged to have a somewhat flat dose-response curve, although this notion may be due to flawed methodology during clinical development. However, blood pressure-lowering effects are improved when the dosage of the Ang II receptor antagonist is increased. First-dose hypotension seldom occurs. The Ang II receptor antagonists do not change average heart rate, and no rebound hypertension occurs after they are discontinued.

The advantages of Ang II receptor antagonists include good efficacy with once-daily dosing and a safety and tolerability profile that generally is similar to that of placebo, independent of age and race. As detailed in chapter 23, the safety, tolerability, and efficacy of Ang II receptor antagonists were carefully evaluated as a function of patients' gender, age, and race. None of these factors influenced the incidence of adverse effects. In particular, Ang II receptor antagonists are tolerated equally well by younger (< 65 years) and elderly (> 65 years) patients, including patients > 75 years.

■ Metabolic Effects

· Hypertension often is accompanied by impaired glucose tolerance, insulin resistance, clinically evident type II diabetes mellitus, and dyslipidemia. Thus, the metabolic effects of antihypertensive agents and their effect on cardiovascular risk reduction are important concerns. In contrast to the metabolic abnormalities associated with diuretics and beta blockers, such as hypokalemia, hypercalcemia, and hyperuricemia, Ang II receptor antagonists are metabolically neutral. Losartan has a neutral effect on glucose metabolism, insulin sensitivity, and serum lipid concentrations in patients with mild hypertension. In clinical studies in diabetic patients, candesartan does not appreciably alter hemoglobin A_{1c} level, serum glucose concentration, or lipid profile. Of note, losartan has a unique uricosuric effect, resulting in a reduction in plasma levels of uric acid.

■ Therapeutic Utility in Treating Cardiovascular and Renal Disease: Future Prospects

Ang II has been linked to the development of cardiovascular hypertrophy through hemodynamic and nonhemodynamic mechanisms. In addition to raising

Table 2. Pharmacokinetic Parameters of Angiotensin II Receptor Antagonists

Drug	Time to Peak Concentration	Absolute Bioavailability	Administration with Food: Area Under the Curve	Elimination Half-life	Elimination Altered Renally	Elimination Altered Hepatically	Protein Binding
Losartan (Cozaar)	1 hr for losartan, 3–4 hr for its active metabolite*	Approximately 33%	Decreased 10%	2 hr for losartan, 6–9 hr for its active metabolite*	No	Yes	98.7%
Valsartan (Diovan)	2–4 hr	Approximately 25%	Decreased 40%	6 hr	No	Yes**	95%
Irbesartan (Avapro)	1.5–2 hr	60–80%	No effect	11–15 hr	No	No	96–99%
Candesartan (Atacand)†	3–4 hr	Approximately 15%	No effect	9 hr	No	No	> 99%
Telmisartan (Micardis)	0.5–1 hr	Approximately 42–58%	Decreased 6–20%	24 hr	No	Yes	99.5%

* Losartan's active metabolite, EXP3174, comprises two-thirds of the active drug.
† Candesartan cilexitil, the prodrug, is completely converted to candesartan during absorption in the gastrointestinal tract.
** No initial dosage adjustment required in mild to moderate hepatic insufficiency.

Table 3. Dosing Considerations with Angiotensin II Receptor Antagonists

Drug	Dosage Range	Recommended Initial Dosage	Strengths Available	Tablet/ Capsule
Losartan (Cozaar)	25–50 mg once or twice daily, 100 mg once daily	50 mg once daily	25, 50, 100 mg	Unscored tablet
Valsartan (Diovan)	80–320 mg once daily	80 mg once daily	80, 160 mg	Capsule
Irbesartan (Avapro)	75–300 mg once daily	150 mg once daily	75, 150, 300 mg	Unscored tablet
Candesartan (Atacand)	8–16 mg once or twice daily 32 mg once daily	16 mg once daily	4, 8, 16, 32 mg	Unscored tablet
Telmisartan (Micardis)	40–160 mg once daily	40 mg once daily	40, 80 mg	Unscored tablet*

* Tablets have decorative score.

blood pressure by its vasoconstrictor action, Ang II also affects cardiac structure and function by stimulating cell proliferation and growth as well as fibrosis. Several studies consistently have demonstrated that ACE inhibitors produce greater reductions in left ventricular hypertrophy (LVH) than beta blockers, calcium antagonists, or diuretics, despite similar reductions in blood pressure. This finding indicates that the RAS is involved in the development of LVH. Recently several small clinical studies have suggested that Ang II antagonists have similar beneficial effects on LVH. In addition, several large randomized trials, including the Losartan Intervention for End-point (LIFE) study, also are examining the long-term effects of Ang II receptor blockade on cardiovascular morbidity and mortality in hypertensive patients with LVH.

Ang II also plays an important role in the pathophysiology of renal disease and the progression to end-stage renal failure. ACE inhibitors slow the progression of both diabetic and nondiabetic renal disease. Because the detrimental effects of Ang II are mediated by the AT1 receptor, Ang II antagonists may exert renoprotective effects similar to those of ACE inhibitors. Whether this theoretical extrapolation holds true remains a contentious issue. Chapter 20 reviews the status of ongoing studies designed to test this hypothesis in patients with nondiabetic renal disease. Chapter 21 reviews the rationale for treatment with Ang II receptor antagonists in diabetic patients and provides an update on several large randomized trials designed to evaluate the renoprotective effects of losartan and irbesartan in diabetic patients.

References

1. Goodfriend TL, Elliot ME, Catt KJ: Angiotensin receptors and their antagonists. N Engl J Med 334:1649–1654, 1996.
2. Griendling KK, Lassegue B, Alexander RW: Angiotensin receptors and their therapeutic implications. Annu Rev Pharmacol Toxicol 36:281–306, 1996.
3. Birkenhager WH, de Leeuw PS: Non-peptide angiotensin type 1 receptor antagonists in the treatment of hypertension. J Hypertens 17:873–881, 1999.
4. Burnier M, Brunner HR: Angiotensin II receptor antagonists in hypertension. Kidney Int 68(Suppl):S107–S111, 1998.

5. Johnston CI, Naitoh M, Burrell LM: Rationale and pharmacology of angiotensin II receptor antagonists: Current status and future issues. J Hypertens 15(Suppl):S3–S6, 1997.

6. Oparil S, Guthrie R, Lewin AJ, on behalf of the Irbesartan/Losartan Study Investigators: An elective-titration study of the comparative effectiveness of two angiotensin II-receptor blockers, irbesartan and losartan. Clin Ther 20:398–409, 1998.

7. Andersson OK, Neldam S: The antihypertensive effect and tolerability of candesartan cilexetil, a new generation angiotensin II antagonist, in comparison with losartan. Blood Pressure 7:53–59, 1998.

8. Hedner T, Oparil S, Rasmussen K, et al: A comparison of the angiotensin II antagonists valsartan and losartan in the treatment of essential hypertension. Am J Hypertens 12:414–417, 1999.

9. Mallion JM, Siche JP, Lacourciere Y, and the Telmisartan Blood Pressure Monitoring Group: ABPM comparison of the antihypertensive profiles of the selective angiotensin II receptor antagonists telmisartan and losartan in patients with mild-to-moderate hypertension. J Hum Hypertens 13:657–664, 1999.

10. Markham A, Goa KL: Valsartan: A review of its pharmacology and therapeutic use in essential hypertension. Drugs: 54:299–311, 1997.

11. McClellan KJ, Goa KL: Candesartan cilexetil: A review of its use in essential hypertension. Drugs 56:847–869, 1998.

12. Townsend R, Haggert B, Liss C, Edelman JM: Efficacy and tolerability of losartan versus enalapril alone or in combination with hydorchlorathizide in patients with essential hypertension. Clin Ther 17:911–923, 1995.

13. Chan JC, Critchley JA, Lappe JT, et al: Randomized, double-blind, parallel study of the anti-hypertensive efficacy and safety of losartan potassium compared with felodipine ER in elderly patients with mild to moderate hypertension. J Hum Hypertens 9:765–771, 1995.

CHAPTER 18

AT_1 Receptor Antagonists as Antihypertensive Agents

MAURICE E. FABIANI, M.D.
COLIN I. JOHNSTON, M.D.

The renin-angiotensin system (RAS) plays a major role in the regulation of blood pressure and maintenance of fluid and electrolyte balance. Angiotensin II (Ang II) is the primary effector molecule of the RAS and exerts a variety of physiologic effects that support blood pressure and cardiovascular function and structure. On the other hand, hyperactivity of the RAS, resulting in excessive generation of Ang II, has been linked to the pathophysiology of hypertension and other cardiovascular diseases. Blockade of the RAS is, therefore, a logical and effective means of treating hypertension and related disorders. Angiotensin-converting enzyme (ACE) inhibitors were the first class of drugs to interfere with the RAS and have proved remarkably successful in the treatment of hypertension, congestive heart failure, and diabetic nephropathy. ACE inhibitors exert their beneficial effects by inhibiting the formation of Ang II; however, they have certain shortcomings that limit their therapeutic utility.

Ang II receptor antagonists are a new class of antihypertensive agents that allow more specific and complete blockade of the RAS than ACE inhibitors. They antagonize the detrimental effects of Ang II selectively at its receptor site, regardless of how it is generated. The enhanced specificity of action of the Ang II receptor antagonists may overcome limitations posed by ACE inhibitors and offer clear advantages and benefits over other currently available antihypertensive agents. Ang II receptor antagonists thus represent a new and important advance in cardiovascular medicine and undoubtedly will become an established part of the arsenal of cardiovascular drugs. This chapter reviews current knowledge of Ang II antagonists and discusses the rationale for their use as antihypertensive agents.

◼ Renin-Angiotensin System and Angiotensin Receptors

The RAS is a biochemical cascade that results in the production of the principal effector peptide, Ang II.[1] The biosynthesis of Ang II involves the cleavage of the precursor macromolecule angiotensinogen by renin to the inactive decapeptide

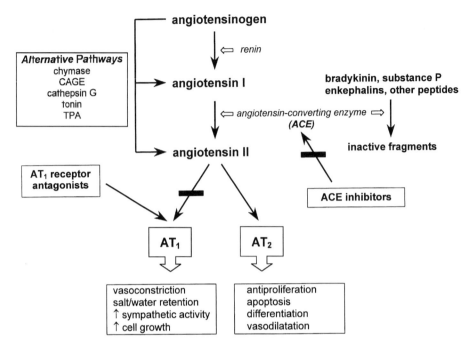

Figure 1.   Bioenzymatic cascade of the renin-angiotensin system and sites of inhibition by AT_1 receptor antagonists and ACE inhibitors.

Ang I, which is then metabolized by ACE to generate the active octapeptide Ang II (Fig. 1).

In addition to its formation within the systemic circulation, Ang II also can be formed at local tissue sites, such as the kidney, brain, heart, and blood vessels, and thus may mediate autocrine, paracrine, and intracrine effects.[2-4] The concept of a tissue-based (local) RAS in addition to the well-known circulating (systemic) RAS is reinforced by the presence of all requisite components of a complete local RAS, such as renin, angiotensinogen, ACE, and angiotensin receptors, in many cardiovascular organs. Furthermore, Ang II also can be generated by alternative pathways independent of renin or ACE, such as chymase, chymostatin-sensitive angiotensin II-generating enzyme (CAGE), cathepsin G, tissue plasminogen activator (tPA), and tonin.[5-7] The functional role of these alternative non-ACE, nonrenin pathways for the formation of Ang II in vivo is not known but may have important implications in cardiovascular disease states. For instance, chymase, the major Ang II-forming enzyme in the human heart, is not susceptible to blockade by ACE inhibitors.[8-10]

Ang II exerts its biologic effects by interacting with at least two Ang receptor subtypes, denoted type 1 (AT_1) and type 2 (AT_2).[11-13] The classification of Ang II receptor subtypes into two major classes was made possible by the advent of selective nonpeptide Ang antagonists. AT_1 receptors were defined as binding sites sensitive to inhibition by losartan, whereas AT_2 receptors are sensitive to PD123177 or PD123319.[14] Additional subtypes of the AT_1 receptor have been identified (i.e., AT_{1A} and AT_{1B}), but they are present only in rodents—not in humans.[15,16]

Although other Ang receptor subtypes also have been proposed, such as AT_4, which recognizes the peptide fragment Ang IV,[17] the AT_1 and AT_2 receptors are the only Ang receptors that have been cloned in humans or animals.[18–23]

Ang II exerts various effects, including vasoconstriction, stimulation of aldosterone release, facilitation of sympathetic activity, and stimulation of cellular growth, all of which are mediated by activation of AT_1 receptors.[13,24] Much less is known about the function of the AT_2 receptor, but recent studies suggest that it may play a role in mediating antiproliferation and inhibition of cell growth, apoptosis, differentiation, and possibly vasodilatation.[13,24,25] In this regard, the AT_2 receptor may oppose the action of the AT_1 receptor.

■ *Pharmacologic Blockade of the Renin-Angiotensin System by Angiotensin II Receptor Antagonists*

Ang II receptor antagonists are a novel class of antihypertensive agents that inhibit the RAS by selectively antagonizing the action of Ang II at the AT_1 receptor subtype.[14,26,27] Losartan was the first orally active, nonpeptide AT_1 receptor antagonist developed clinically for the treatment of hypertension. It was followed by a spate of Ang II receptor antagonists developed by various drug companies. AT_1 receptor antagonists currently available for clinical use are summarized in Table 1.

Losartan per se is a competitive antagonist, but it is converted in vivo to the more potent active metabolite, EXP3174, which displays noncompetitive antagonism. EXP3174 has a 10-fold higher affinity for the AT_1 receptor and longer duration of action and, therefore, is mainly responsible for the antihypertensive effect of losartan in vivo. Valsartan, the second AT_1 receptor antagonist released on the market, is also a competitive antagonist, but it is not converted to an active metabolite to sustain its antihypertensive activity. Irbesartan is a new long-acting AT_1 receptor antagonist that also does not require biologic transformation to manifest its antihypertensive action. Candesartan appears to be the most potent orally active AT_1 receptor antagonist yet developed. It is administered as an inactive prodrug (candesartan cilexetil) that is converted rapidly and completely to the active compound candesartan during gastrointestinal absorption. Both candesartan and irbesartan display noncompetitive insurmountable antagonism. The insurmountable nature of antagonism afforded by these drugs may offer advantages over competitive surmountable agents by providing persistent AT_1 receptor blockade in the face of high Ang II levels.

By virtue of their mechanism of action, Ang II receptor antagonists provide improved specificity and selectivity and more complete blockade of the RAS than ACE inhibitors. Whereas ACE inhibitors interfere with Ang II synthesis, AT_1 receptor antagonists block the actions of Ang II at its receptor site, regardless of its synthetic pathway. Although ACE inhibitors have proved successful in the treatment of hypertension and other cardiovascular diseases, they possess certain limitations. For instance, ACE inhibitors interfere with the breakdown of bradykinin and possibly other peptides. Although the bradykinin-potentiating action of ACE inhibitors may contribute to the their antihypertensive effect, it also has been associated with the troublesome side effect of cough and the serious condition of angioedema.[28–30] Furthermore, ACE inhibitors produce competitive blockade that, over the long term, may be overcome by an increase in the

TABLE 1. Nonpeptide AT_1 Receptor Antagonists Currently Available for Clinical Use

Generic Name	Trade Name	Prodrug	Oral Dose Range (mg)	Active Metabolite	Half-life (hr)	Drug Company
Losartan (DuP-753, MK-954)	Cozaar	Yes	50–100	EXP-3174	2 (6–9)	Merck/DuPont
Valsartan (CGP-48933)	Diovan	No	80–320	—	6–7	Novartis
Irbesartan (SR-47436, BMS-186295)	Avapro, Aprovel Karvea	No	150–300	—	11–15	Bristol-Myers Squibb Sanofi Winthrop
Candesartan cilexetil (TCV-116)	Atacand, Amias Blopress	Yes	8–32	Candesartan (CV-11974)	9	AstraZeneca Takeda
Eprosartan (SKF-108566)	Teveten	No	400–800	—	5–9	SmithKline Beecham
Telmisartan (BIBR-0277)	Pritor Micardis	No	20–160	—	20	Glaxo Wellcome Boehringer Ingelheim
Tasosartan (ANA-756)	Verdia	No	100–1200	—	1–6	Wyeth-Ayerst

availability of the substrate Ang I. Plasma levels of Ang II tend to return toward predrug levels after long-term therapy with ACE inhibitors. As mentioned previously, Ang II also can be generated by non-ACE pathways, as demonstrated in the heart[8–10] and blood vessels[31,32]; thus, ACE inhibitors may not provide total blockade of Ang II synthesis. Because AT_1 receptors mediate all of the well-known cardiovascular effects of Ang II, blockade of AT_1 receptors should provide more specific and complete blockade of the RAS. Ang II antagonists have been shown to reduce elevated blood pressure and to inhibit a variety of Ang II-mediated effects, such as vasoconstriction; sodium reabsorption; release of aldosterone, catecholamine, renin, and vasopressin; and thirst.[13,33,34]

Ang II antagonists cause an increase in the circulating levels of Ang II, which is driven by the rise in plasma renin activity as a result of removal of negative feedback. The high levels of Ang II in the face of AT_1 receptor blockade may lead to hyperstimulation of the unopposed AT_2 receptors. The consequence of indirect hyperstimulation of AT_2 receptors with AT_1 receptor blockade is not known. However, it is possible that activation of exposed AT_2 receptors may counteract the effects mediated by AT_1 receptors and, thus, contribute to the antihypertensive action and beneficial effects of AT_1 receptor antagonists. For example, it was shown recently that the AT_2 antagonist PD123319 offset the blood pressure-lowering effect of the AT_1 receptor antagonist losartan in salt-depleted and bilateral nephrectomized rats.[35]

■ Antihypertensive Efficacy

Hypertension remains a major cause of cardiovascular morbidity and mortality globally. Hence, safe and effective antihypertensive pharmacotherapy is a principal objective in the treatment of hypertension and related cardiovascular disorders. Ang II receptor antagonists are a new class of therapeutic agents for the treatment of hypertension. Most clinical experience lies with the prototype AT_1 receptor antagonist, losartan, although an abundance of recently published data is also available for irbesartan, candesartan, valsartan, telmisartan, and other AT_1 receptor antagonists. In numerous double-blind, placebo-controlled studies, all drugs of the Ang II receptor antagonist class have been shown to lower elevated blood pressure effectively and safely in patients with essential hypertension.[36–41] The blood pressure-lowering effect of AT_1 antagonists is akin to other classes of antihypertensive agents, including ACE inhibitors, calcium channel blockers, and beta-adrenoceptor antagonists. Losartan, for example, possesses similar antihypertensive efficacy but greater tolerability compared with enalapril, amlodipine, nifedipine, felodipine, and atenolol in patients with essential hypertension.[42–48]

Losartan and valsartan have a relatively flat dose-response curve, which initially made it difficult to establish dose-dependency with respect to antihypertensive action.[49–51] In contrast, the newer AT_1 receptor antagonists, such as candesartan and irbesartan, significantly lower blood pressure in a clear dose-dependent manner.[52–54]

AT_1 receptor antagonists have been shown to reduce blood pressure in mild, moderate, and severe hypertension regardless of age, gender, or race.[36–41] They have a slow and gradual onset of action and thereby avoid first-dose hypotension, which is commonly observed with other antihypertensive drugs. The maximal blood pressure-lowering effect of AT_1 receptor antagonists typically takes

4–6 weeks to become fully manifest. AT_1 receptor antagonists provide effective blood pressure control over a 24-hour period with a high trough-to-peak ratio, as determined by ambulatory blood pressure monitoring, and do not affect the normal circadian pattern of blood pressure.[55–57] Thus, AT_1 receptor antagonists are suitable for administration on a once-daily basis. The antihypertensive efficacy of AT_1 receptor antagonists is maintained in the long term. Candesartan, for example, produces significant reductions in mean systolic and diastolic blood pressure after 12 months.[58]

The antihypertensive effect of AT_1 receptor antagonists can be enhanced by the addition of a diuretic. For instance, the blood pressure-lowering effect of losartan or candesartan can be potentiated by the addition of hydrochlorothiazide.[59–62] AT_1 receptor antagonists also tend to reduce the adverse metabolic effects of diuretics. Of interest, losartan has a unique uricosuric action that is not displayed by its active metabolite, EXP3174, or other AT_1 receptor antagonists.[63–65] It is not clear, however, whether this uricosuric effect confers additional benefits over other Ang II antagonists.

Direct comparative studies among the different AT_1 receptor antagonists are still quite limited. However, recent data suggest that differences may exist among AT_1 receptor antagonists in relation to antihypertensive efficacy. Valsartan and losartan produce comparatively similar reductions in blood pressure, but valsartan (160 mg once daily) was associated with a higher rate of responders than losartan (100 mg once daily).[66] On the other hand, at maximally effective once-daily doses irbesartan (300 mg) lowers blood pressure to a significantly greater extent than losartan (100 mg) in patients with mild-to-moderate hypertension.[67,68] In another study, candesartan cilexetil (16 mg once daily) was shown to exert a significantly greater antihypertensive effect than losartan (50 mg once daily) in patients with essential hypertension.[69] The dosing regimens in this study, however, may not have been therapeutically equivalent. In a more recent study, candesartan cilexetil (16 mg) was shown to produce a significantly greater reduction in blood pressure than losartan (100 mg) at 8 weeks in patients with mild-to-moderate hypertension.[70] Of interest, after a missed dose the antihypertensive effect of candesartan cilexetil (16 mg) was maintained, whereas after a missed dose of losartan (100 mg) systolic and diastolic blood pressure returned toward baseline.[70] The enhanced antihypertensive efficacy of candesartan cilexetil and irbesartan may be linked to the fact that both agents have a long duration of action and display insurmountable antagonism of AT_1 receptors.

■ *Clinical Trials with Cardiovascular Outcomes*

Although Ang II antagonists display the desirable qualities of ideal antihypertensive agents, their effects on hard clinical end-points are still largely unknown. Several large-scale clinical trials are ongoing to examine the impact of AT_1 receptor antagonists on morbidity and mortality (Table 2). The LIFE (Losartan Intervention For End-point reduction in hypertension) trial is a large double-blind, randomized study comparing the effects of losartan and the beta blocker atenolol on cardiovascular mortality and morbidity in patients with hypertension and left ventricular hypertrophy (LVH).[71] The VALUE (Valsartan Antihypertensive Long-term Use Evaluation) trial is another large-scale, double blind study comparing the effects of valsartan and the calcium channel blocker

Table 2. Clinical Trials of AT$_1$ Receptor Antagonists with Morbidity and Mortality Outcomes

Trial	Patient Group	Drugs
LIFE	Hypertension/LVH	Losartan vs. atenolol
VALUE	Hypertension + risk factors	Valsartan vs. amlodipine
ACCESS	Stroke	Candesartan vs. placebo
ELITE II	Congestive heart failure	Losartan vs. captopril
VAL-HEFT	Congestive heart failure	Valsartan + ACEI vs. ACEI alone
CHARM	Congestive heart failure	Candesartan + ACEI vs. ACEI alone
		Candesartan vs. placebo
VALIANT	Post-AMI LV dysfunction	Valsartan vs. captopril vs. valsartan + captopril
OPTIMAAL	Post-AMI LV dysfunction	Losartan vs.captopril
RENAAL	Diabetic nephropathy	Losartan vs. placebo

ACCESS = Acute Candesartan Cilexetil Evaluation in Stroke Survivors, CHARM = Candesartan in Heart failure Assessment of Reduction in Mortality and morbidity, ELITE = Evaluation of Losartan In The Elderly, LIFE = Losartan Intervention For Endpoint reduction, OPTIMAAL = OPtimal Therapy In Myocardial infarction with Angiotensin II Antagonist Losartan, RENAAL = Reduction of Endpoints in NIDDM with the Angiotensin II Antagonist Losartan, VAL-HEFT = VALsartan HEart Failure Trial, VALIANT = VALsartan In Acute myocardial iNfarction Trial, VALUE = Valsartan Antihypertensive Long-term Use Evaluation, ACEI = angiotensin-converting enzyme inhibitor, LV = left ventricular, LVH = left ventricular hypertrophy, and AMI = acute myocardial infarction.

amlodipine on morbidity and mortality in high-risk hypertensive patients with other known cardiovascular risk factors.[72] The ACCESS (Acute Candesartan Cilexetil Evaluation in Stroke Survivors) study examines the effects of candesartan on morbidity and mortality in hypertensive patients with acute stroke.[73] Other clinical studies with cardiovascular outcomes in the setting of cardiac and renal disease are discussed below. The outcome data from these large clinical trials will help to define the role of AT$_1$ receptor antagonists as first-line antihypertensive agents.

■ *Beyond Blood Pressure Reduction*

Modern antihypertensive agents must do more than simply lower elevated blood pressure. They also should prevent or reverse end-organ damage, reduce other cardiovascular risk factors, and, ultimately, reduce cardiovascular morbidity and mortality without interfering with the patient's quality of life. In this respect, AT$_1$ receptor antagonists may confer benefits beyond merely lowering blood pressure.

Cardioprotective Effects

LVH is a major independent risk factor for cardiovascular morbidity and mortality. The RAS has been implicated in the development of cardiovascular hypertrophy via hemodynamic and nonhemodynamic actions.[74,75] The effects of Ang II on cardiac structure are due not only to elevation of blood pressure (vasoconstriction) but also to promotion of cardiac cell growth and fibrosis. The central involvement of the RAS in the development of LVH is supported by data analysis showing that, although they produce similar falls in blood pressure, ACE inhibitors reduce LVH to a greater extent than beta blockers, calcium antagonists, or diuretics.[76–78] AT$_1$ receptor antagonists may have similar beneficial effects on LVH. In clinical studies, losartan, valsartan, and candesartan cilexetil significantly reduce LVH in patients with essential hypertension.[79–81] Although exerting similar antihypertensive effects, irbesartan produces a greater reduction in LVH than the beta blocker atenolol in hypertensive patients.[82,83] The SILVER (Study of Irbesartan in Left VEntricular hypertrophy Regression) trial assesses whether irbesartan reduces LVH to a greater extent than the extended-release calcium channel antagonist felodipine in patients with hypertension.[84] As mentioned previously, the LIFE trial assesses the long-term outcome effects of losartan on cardiovascular morbidity and mortality in hypertensive patients with LVH.[71,85]

ACE inhibitors dramatically reduce morbidity and mortality in patients with congestive heart failure.[86–89] AT$_1$ receptor antagonists also may have beneficial effects in the clinical setting of heart failure. Losartan and valsartan exert favorable hemodynamic effects; they reduce afterload, decrease pulmonary capillary wedge pressure, and increase cardiac output in patients with symptomatic congestive heart failure and left ventricular dysfunction.[90,91] Furthermore, losartan recently was shown to be well tolerated and to possess similar beneficial effects as enalapril on exercise tolerance and left ejection fractions in patients with heart failure.[92] Moreover, losartan further reduces afterload in patients with heart failure already maximally treated with ACE inhibitors,[93] suggesting that additional benefit may be obtained by the use of an AT$_1$ receptor antagonist in combination with an ACE inhibitor.

Initial findings from the ELITE (Evaluation of Losartan In The Elderly) study suggest that AT$_1$ receptor antagonists may provide greater therapeutic benefit than ACE inhibitors.[94] The ELITE study compared the effects of losartan with captopril, primarily on renal function in elderly patients with symptomatic heart failure. Although there was no difference in renal dysfunction, the losartan group had a lower all-cause mortality rate than the captopril group, reflected mainly in the incidence of sudden cardiac deaths.[94]

The RESOLVD (Randomised Evaluation of Strategies fOr Left Ventricular Dysfunction) study compared the effects of candesartan cilexetil and enalapril, alone or in combination, on exercise tolerance and left ventricular function in patients with heart failure.[95–97] The two drugs had similar effects on exercise capacity, left ventricular function, and neurohormones, and the combination of both drugs had a greater effect on left ventricular remodeling than either alone. The study, however, was stopped prematurely because of a nonsignificant trend of increased deaths in candesartan-treated groups.

The mortality data from the ELITE and RESOLVD studies should be interpreted cautiously. Both studies were small-scale trials in which mortality was not the primary end-point. The ELITE II trial is a properly designed, randomized, double-blind mortality study to examine specifically the effects of losartan in comparison with captopril on all-cause mortality in patients with symptomatic heart failure.[98] Recent data from the ELITE II study, presented at the 72nd Scientific Meeting of the American Heart Association (7–10 November 1999)[99] showed no significant difference between losartan and captopril in mortality rates in patients with heart failure, although losartan was better tolerated. The findings from the ELITE II study do not support the hypothesis that losartan provides superior survival benefit to captopril in patients with heart failure. This scenario highlights the pitfalls of extrapolating or interpreting too readily outcome data from small-scale, low-powered clinical studies. The CHARM

(Candesartan cilexetil in Heart failure Assessment of Reduction in Mortality and morbidity) and VALHEFT (VALsartan HEart Failure Trial) studies are currently under way to examine the effects of candesartan and valsartan, respectively, compared with an ACE inhibitor, alone or in combination, on morbidity and mortality in patients with congestive heart failure.[100,101] The outcome of the CHARM and VALHEFT trials will help to establish the place of AT$_1$ receptor antagonists in treatment of heart failure.

Acute myocardial infarction (AMI) combined with evidence of heart failure or left ventricular dysfunction is associated with a high mortality risk. ACE inhibitors reduce morbidity and mortality in this high-risk patient group.[87] The OPTIMAAL (OPtimal Trial In Myocardial infarction with the Angiotensin II Antagonist Losartan) and VALIANT (VALsartan In Acute myocardial iNfarction Trial) studies are large-scale, double-blind, randomized trials undertaken to determine the effects of losartan and valsartan, respectively, in comparison with captopril on morbidity and mortality in patients with AMI and heart failure or left ventricular dysfunction.[102]

Renoprotective Effects

Ang II plays a pathologic role in the development of renal disease and the progression to end-stage renal failure.[103] Inhibition of the RAS with ACE inhibitors slows the progression of both diabetic and nondiabetic renal disease.[104–106] Because the deleterious actions of Ang II are mediated by the AT$_1$ receptor, Ang II antagonists should offer similar renoprotective effects. It should be emphasized that blockade of the RAS with ACE inhibitors is contraindicated in patients with renal artery stenosis. Under these conditions, renal blood flow is critically dependent on Ang II; thus, administration of ACE inhibitors or AT$_1$ receptor antagonists may worsen renal function in lead to acute renal failure.[107]

The place of AT$_1$ receptor antagonists in treatment of renal disease is currently being assessed. Losartan has been reported to lower blood pressure and albuminuria significantly more than captopril in hypertensive patients with renal disease.[108] In addition, losartan reduced blood pressure and albuminuria to a greater extent than amlodipine in renally impaired hypertensive patients.[109] Candesartan cilexetil also exerts favorable effects on renal hemodynamics in patients with renal function impairment.[110] In renally impaired patients, candesartan cilexetil reduced mean arterial pressure and increased renal blood flow, whereas glomerular filtration rate was unaffected.[110] Recently valsartan also has been shown to reduce proteinuria and albuminuria in patients with chronic renal disease.[111] Moreover, in the ELITE study, losartan and captopril had similar effects on renal function in patients with congestive heart failure.[94] These data suggest that AT$_1$ receptor antagonists may have similar efficacy to ACE inhibitors in retarding the development and progression of organ damage in patients with renal disease. However, it remains to be determined whether the beneficial effects of AT$_1$ receptor antagonists on renal hemodynamics and proteinuria translate into long-term renoprotection and prevention of end-stage renal disease. The RENAAL (Reduction of End-points in Non–insulin-dependent diabetes mellitus with the Angiotensin II Antagonist Losartan) and CALM (Candesartan And Lisinopril in Microalbuminuria) studies are currently under way to assess the effects of AT$_1$ receptor antagonists in the setting of renal disease. These clinical studies are investigating whether losartan and candesartan, respectively, exert renoprotective effects by delaying the progression to end-stage renal failure in patients with diabetic nephropathy.

Safety and Tolerability

Although a wide array of antihypertensive agents is available on the market, their therapeutic utility is limited by adverse effects, tolerability, and patient compliance. Ang II antagonists are superior to existing antihypertensive agents in this respect (Table 3). They possess an excellent safety and tolerability profile. AT_1 receptor antagonists as a class have a low incidence of adverse effects and low rates of withdrawal comparable to placebo but far superior to other classes of antihypertensive agents.[112–115] A constant dry cough is the most frequent adverse effect associated with ACE inhibitors, probably as a result of the levels of bradykinin and possibly other peptides.[28–30] AT_1 receptor antagonists, on the other hand, do not affect peptide metabolism and thus should not induce cough. Indeed, in recent controlled clinical trials the incidence, severity, and frequency of dry cough in patients with a prior history of ACE inhibitor-induced cough was significantly lower in patients receiving losartan compared with lisinopril but similar to placebo.[116] Similar findings also have been obtained with other AT_1 receptor antagonists, such as valsartan, irbesartan, and candesartan.[115] Angioedema, a rare but nonetheless life-threatening side effect associated with ACE inhibitors, also is thought to be due to bradykinin accumulation. Theoretically, AT_1 receptor antagonists should not cause angioedema; however, some cases of angioedema have been reported in patients taking losartan or valsartan.[117–120] At this stage, it is not clear whether AT_1 antagonists as a class cause angioedema. Hence, it is judicious not to administer AT_1 antagonists to patients with a known history of angioedema or known sensitivity to ACE inhibitors and angioedema.

The RAS plays a critical role in fetal development during pregnancy. Blockade of the RAS with ACE inhibitors is fetotoxic; thus, Ang II antagonists should be avoided during all stages of pregnancy.[121] Furthermore, as mentioned above, AT_1 receptor antagonists, like ACE inhibitors, should not be used in patients with renal artery stenosis because they may worsen renal function and lead to renal collapse.[107]

■ *Conclusion*

Nonpeptide Ang II antagonists are a new class of orally active agents for the treatment of hypertension. They manifest antihypertensive effects by interfering with the RAS at the AT_1 receptor level. Ang II antagonists provide more specific and complete blockade of the RAS by preventing the detrimental actions of Ang II at its site of action, regardless of the synthetic pathway by which it is generated. Ang II receptor antagonists do not affect peptide metabolism; their improved specificity of action also may help to avoid untoward side effects, such as cough, which are commonly associated with ACE inhibitors. AT_1 receptor antagonists indirectly stimulate unopposed AT_2 receptors because of the prevailing levels of Ang II, which may enhance their beneficial effects by counterbalancing the effects of AT_1 receptor stimulation.

Ang II antagonists display tremendous therapeutic potential in the management of hypertension and other cardiovascular diseases. AT_1 receptor antagonists

TABLE 3. Percentage Incidence of Reported Adverse Effects in Randomized, Double-Blind Clinical Trials with Antihyperensive Agents

Adverse Effect	Placebo (n = 535)	Losartan (n = 2085)	Losartan + HCTZ (n = 858)	ACE Inhibitors (n = 239)	Beta Blockers (n = 68)	Calcium Channel Blockers (n = 43)	HCTZ (n = 217)
Any adverse experience	52.0	46.8	45.0	50.6	57.4	53.5	48.3
Any drug-related adverse experience	15.5	15.3	14.8	24.7	26.5	23.3	18.1
Withdrawals	3.7	2.3	2.8	2.5	8.8	9.3	3.0
Dizziness	2.4	4.1	5.7	6.3	7.4	2.3	4.1
Asthenia/fatigue	3.9	3.8	2.9	6.7	5.9	0.0	5.5
Cough	2.6	3.1	2.6	8.8	0.0	2.3	4.1
Diarrhea	1.9	1.9	1.5	2.9	0.0	4.7	0.4
Edema	1.9	1.7	1.3	1.7	1.5	14.0	1.8
Headache	17.2	14.1	7.7	10.9	19.1	14.0	14.0
Insomnia	0.7	1.1	0.5	0.8	4.4	2.3	1.1
Upper respiratory tract infection	5.6	6.5	6.1	5.4	1.5	7.0	5.5

ACE = angiotensin-converting enzyme, HCTZ = hydrochlorothiazide.
Adapted from Goldberg AI, Dunlay MC, Sweet CS: Safety and tolerability of losartan potassium, an angiotensin II receptor antagonist, compared with hydrochlorothiazide, atenolol, felodipine ER, and angiotensin-converting enzyme inhibitors for the treatment of systemic hypertension. Am J Cardiol 75:793–795, 1995.

possess the hallmarks of an ideal antihypertensive agent: they effectively lower blood pressure and have an unparalleled safety and tolerability profile. Ang II antagonists no doubt will become part of the repertoire of drugs for the treatment of hypertension and other cardiovascular disorders. The outcome of several large intervention trials with cardiovascular end-points will place in proper prospective the use of AT_1 receptor antagonists as first-line antihypertensive agents.

Acknowledgments

We gratefully acknowledge the financial support of the National Health and Medical Research Council of Australia, Commonwealth Department of Veterans' Affairs, Sir Edward Dunlop Medical Research Foundation, and Ramaciotti Medical Research Foundation.

References

1. Johnston CI: Biochemistry and pharmacology of the renin-angiotensin system. Drugs 39(Suppl 1):21–31, 1990.
2. Campbell DJ: Circulating and tissue angiotensin systems. J Clin Invest 79:1–6, 1987.
3. Dzau VJ: Circulating versus local renin-angiotensin system in cardiovascular homeostasis. Circulation 77(6 Pt 2):14–13, 1988.
4. Johnson CI: Renin-angiotensin system: A dual tissue and hormonal system for cardiovascular control. J Hypertens 10(Suppl):S13–S26, 1992.
5. Urata H, Nishimura H, Ganten D: Mechanisms of angiotensin II formation in humans. Eur Heart J 16(Suppl N):79–85, 1995.
6. Urata H, Nishimura H, Ganten D, Arakawa K: Angiotensin-converting enzyme-independent pathways of angiotensin II formation in human tissues and cardiovascular diseases. Blood Pressure 2(Suppl):22–28, 1996.
7. Hollenberg NK, Fisher ND, Price DA: Pathways for angiotensin II generation in intact human tissue: Evidence from comparative pharmacological interruption of the renin system. Hypertension 32:387–392, 1998.
8. Urata H, Kinoshita A, Misono KS, et al: Identification of a highly specific chymase as the major angiotensin II-forming enzyme in the human heart. J Biol Chem 265:22348–22357, 1990 [published erratum appears in J Biol Chem 266:12114, 1991).
9. Urata H, Kinoshita A, Perez DM, et al: Cloning of the gene and cDNA for human heart chymase. J Biol Chem 266:17173–17179, 1991.
10. Urata H, Ganten D: Cardiac angiotensin II formation: The angiotensin-I converting enzyme and human chymase. Eur Heart J 14(Suppl 1):177–182, 1993.
11. Unger T, Chung O, Csikos T, et al: Angiotensin receptors. J Hypertens 14(Suppl):S95–S103, 1996.
12. Griendling KK, Lassegue B, Alexander RW: Angiotensin receptors and their therapeutic implications. Annu Rev Pharmacol Toxicol 36:281–306, 1996.
13. Fabiani ME: Angiotensin receptor subtypes: Novel targets for cardiovascular therapy. Drug News Perspect 12:207–215, 1999.
14. Timmermans PB, Wong PC, Chiu AT, et al: Angiotensin II receptors and angiotensin II receptor antagonists. Pharmacol Rev 45:205–251, 1993.
15. Iwai N, Inagami T: Identification of two subtypes in the rat type I angiotensin II receptor. FEBS Lett 298:257–260, 1992.
16. Yoshida H, Kakuchi J, Guo DF, et al: Analysis of the evolution of angiotensin II type 1 receptor gene in mammals (mouse, rat, bovine and human). Biochem Biophys Res Commun 186:1042–1049, 1992.
17. Wright JW, Krebs LT, Stobb JW, Harding JW: The angiotensin IV system: Functional implications. Front Neuroendocrinol 16:23–52, 1995.
18. Furuta H, Guo DF, Inagami T: Molecular cloning and sequencing of the gene encoding human angiotensin II type 1 receptor. Biochem Biophys Res Commun 183:8–13, 1992.
19. Takayanagi R, Ohnaka K, Sakai Y, et al: Molecular cloning, sequence analysis and expression of a cDNA encoding human type-1 angiotensin II receptor. Biochem Biophys Res Commun 183:910–916, 1992.
20. Bergsma DJ, Ellis C, Kumar C, et al: Cloning and characterization of a human angiotensin II type 1 receptor. Biochem Biophys Res Commun 183:989–995, 1992.
21. Martin MM, Su B, Elton TS: Molecular cloning of the human angiotensin II type 2 receptor cDNA. Biochem Biophys Res Commun 205:645–651, 1994.

22. Koike G, Horiuchi M, Yamada T, et al: Human type 2 angiotensin II receptor gene: Cloned, mapped to the X chromosome, and its mRNA is expressed in the human lung. Biochem Biophys Res Commun 203:1842–1850, 1994.

23. Mukoyama M, Nakajima M, Horiuchi M, et al: Expression cloning of type 2 angiotensin II receptor reveals a unique class of seven-transmembrane receptors. J Biol Chem 268:24539–24542, 1993.

24. Chung O, Kuhl H, Stoll M, Unger T: Physiological and pharmacological implications of AT1 versus AT2 receptors. Kidney Int 67(Suppl):S95–S99, 1998.

25. Csikos T, Chung O, Unger T: Receptors and their classification: Focus on angiotensin II and the AT2 receptor. J Hum Hypertens 12:311–318, 1998.

26. Johnston CI: Angiotensin receptor antagonists: Focus on losartan. Lancet 346:1403–1407, 1995.

27. Mimran A, Ribstein J: Angiotensin receptor blockers: Pharmacology and clinical significance. J Am Soc Nephrol 10(Suppl 12):S273–S277, 1999.

28. Semple PF: Putative mechanisms of cough after treatment with angiotensin converting enzyme inhibitors. J Hypertens 13(Suppl 3):S17–S21, 1995.

29. Overlack A: ACE inhibitor-induced cough and bronchospasm: Incidence, mechanisms and management. Drug Safety 15:72–78, 1996.

30. Pylypchuk GB: ACE inhibitor- versus angiotensin II blocker-induced cough and angioedema. Ann Pharmacother 32:1060–1066, 1998.

31. Voors AA, Pinto YM, Buikema H, et al: Dual pathway for angiotensin II formation in human internal mammary arteries. Br J Pharmacol 125:1028–1032, 1998.

32. Ihara M, Urata H, Kinoshita A, et al: Increased chymase-dependent angiotensin II formation in human atherosclerotic aorta. Hypertension 33:1399–1405, 1999.

33. Johnston CI, Naitoh M, Burrell LM: Rationale and pharmacology of angiotensin II receptor antagonists: Current status and future issues. J Hypertens 15(Suppl):S3–S6, 1997.

34. Johnston CI, Risvanis J: Preclinical pharmacology of angiotensin II receptor antagonists: Update and outstanding issues. Am J Hypertens 10(12 Pt 2):306S–310S, 1997.

35. Gigante B, Piras O, De Paolis P, et al: Role of the angiotensin II AT2-subtype receptors in the blood pressure-lowering effect of losartan in salt-restricted rats. J Hypertens 16(12 Pt 2):2039–2043, 1998.

36. McIntyre M, Caffe SE, Michalak RA, Reid JL: Losartan, an orally active angiotensin (AT₁) receptor antagonist: A review of its efficacy and safety in essential hypertension. Pharmacol Ther 74:181–194, ;1997.

37. Markham A, Goa KL: Valsartan: A review of its pharmacology and therapeutic use in essential hypertension. Drugs 54:299–311, 1997.

38. Brown MJ: Irbesartan treatment in hypertension. Hosp Med 59:808–811, 1998.

39. McClellan KJ, Goa KL: Candesartan cilexetil: A review of its use in essential hypertension. Drugs 56:847–869, 1998.

40. McClellan KJ, Markham A: Telmisartan. Drugs 56:1039–1044, 1998; discussion, 1045–1046.

41. McClellan KJ, Balfour JA: Eprosartan. Drugs 55:713–718, 1998; discussion, 719–720.

42. Tikkanen I, Omvik P, Jensen HA: Comparison of the angiotensin II antagonist losartan with the angiotensin converting enzyme inhibitor enalapril in patients with essential hypertension. J Hypertens 13:1343–1351, 1995.

43. Townsend R, Haggert B, Liss C, Edelman JM: Efficacy and tolerability of losartan versus enalapril alone or in combination with hydrochlorothiazide in patients with essential hypertension. Clin Ther 17:911–923, 1995.

44. Oparil S, Barr E, Elkins M, et al: Efficacy, tolerability, and effects on quality of life of losartan, alone or with hydrochlorothiazide, versus amlodipine, alone or with hydrochlorothiazide, in patients with essential hypertension. Clin Ther 18:608–625, 1996.

45. Weir MR, Elkins M, Liss C, et al: Efficacy, tolerability, and quality of life of losartan, alone or with hydrochlorothiazide, versus nifedipine GITS in patients with essential hypertension. Clin Ther 18:411–428, 1996.

46. Conlin PR, Elkins M:, Liss C, et al: A study of losartan, alone or with hydrochlorothiazide vs. nifedipine GITS in elderly patients with diastolic hypertension. J Hum Hypertens 12:693–699, 1998.

47. Chan JC, Critchley JA, Lappe JT, et al: Randomised, double-blind, parallel study of the anti-hypertensive efficacy and safety of losartan potassium compared with felodipine ER in elderly patients with mild to moderate hypertension. J Hum Hypertens 9:765–771, 1995.

48. Dahlof B, Keller SE, Makris L, et al: Efficacy and tolerability of losartan potassium and atenolol in patients with mild to moderate essential hypertension. Am J Hypertens 8:578–583, 1995.

49. Ikeda LS, Harm SC, Arcuri KE, et al: Comparative antihypertensive effects of losartan 50 mg and losartan 50 mg titrated to 100 mg in patients with essential hypertension. Blood Pressure 6:35–43, 1997.

50. Pool J, Oparil S, Hedner T, et al: Dose-responsive antihypertensive efficacy of valsartan, a new angiotensin II-receptor blocker. Clin Ther 20:1106–1114, 1998.

51. Pool JL, Glazer R, Chiang YT, Gatlin M: Dose-response efficacy of valsartan, a new angiotensin II receptor blocker. J Hum Hypertens 13:275–281, 1999.

52. Elmfeldt D, George M, Hubner R, Olofsson B: Candesartan cilexetil, a new generation angiotensin II antagonist, provides dose dependent antihypertensive effect. J Hum Hypertens 11(Suppl 2):S49–S53, 1997.

53. Pool JL, Guthrie RM, Littlejohn TW III, et al: Dose-related antihypertensive effects of irbesartan in patients with mild-to-moderate hypertension. Am J Hypertens 11(4 Pt 1):462–470, 1998.

54. Reeves RA, Lin CS, Kassler-Taub K, Pouleur H: Dose-related efficacy of irbesartan for hypertension: An intregrated analysis. Hypertension 31:1311–1316, 1998.

55. Weber MA, Neutel JM, Smith DH: Controlling blood pressure throughout the day: Issues in testing a new anti-hypertensive agent. J Hum Hypertens 9(Suppl 5):S29–S35, 1995.

56. Heuer HJ, Schondorfer G, Hogemann AM: Twenty-four hour blood pressure profile of different doses of candesartan cilexetil in patients with mild to moderate hypertension. J Hum Hypertens 11(Suppl 2):S55–S56, 1997.

57. Mallion J, Siche J, Locourciere Y: ABPM comparison of the antihypertensive profiles of the selective angiotensin II receptor antagonists telmisartan and losartan in patients with mild-to-moderate hypertension. J Hum Hypertens 13:657–664, 1999.

58. Sever P, Holzgreve H: Long-term efficacy and tolerability of candesartan cilexetil in patients with mild to moderate hypertension. J Hum Hypertens 11(Suppl 2):S69–S73, 1997.

59. MacKay JH, Arcuri KE, Goldberg AI, et al: Losartan and low-dose hydrochlorothiazide in patients with essential hypertension. A double-blind, placebo-controlled trial of concomitant administration compared with individual components. Arch Intern Med 156:278–285, 1996.

60. Ruilope LM, Simpson RL, Toh J, et al: Controlled trial of losartan given concomitantly with different doses of hydrochlorothiazide in hypertensive patients. Blood Pressure 5:32–40, 1996.

61. Plouin PF: Combination therapy with candesartan cilexetil plus hydrochlorothiazide in patients unresponsive to low-dose hydrochlorothiazide. J Hum Hypertens 11(Suppl 2):S65–S66, 1997.

62. Philipp T, Letzel H, Arens HJ: Dose-finding study of candesartan cilexetil plus hydrochlorothiazide in patients with mild to moderate hypertension. J Hum Hypertens 11(Suppl 2):S67–S68, 1997.

63. Nakashima M, Uematsu T, Kosuge K, Kanamaru M: Pilot study of the uricosuric effect of DuP-753, a new angiotensin II receptor antagonist, in healthy subjects. Eur J Clin Pharmacol 42:333–335, 1992.

64. Burnier M, Rutschmann B, Nussberger J, et al: Salt-dependent renal effects of an angiotensin II antagonist in healthy subjects. Hypertension 22:339–347, 1993.

65. Minghelli G, Seydoux C, Goy JJ, Burnier M: Urisosuric effect of the angiotensin II receptor antagonist losartan in heart transplant recipients. Transplantation 66:268–271, 1998.

66. Hedner T, Oparil S, Rasmussen K, et al: A comparison of the angiotensin II antagonists valsartan and losartan in the treatment of essential hypertension. Am J Hypertens 12 (4 Pt 1):414–417, 1999.

67. Kassler-Taub K, Littlejohn T, Elliott W, et al: Comparative efficacy of two angiotensin II receptor antagonists, irbesartan and losartan, in mild-to-moderate hypertension. Irbesartan/Losartan Study Investigators. Am J Hypertens 11(1 Pt 1):445–453, 1998 [published erratum appears in Am J Hypertens 11(6 Pt 1):736, 1998].

68. Oparil S, Guthrie R, Lewin AJ, et al: An elective-titration study of the comparative effectiveness of two angiotensin II-receptor blockers, irbesartan and losartan. Irbesarta/Losartan Study Investigators. Clin Ther 20:398–409, 1998.

69. Andersson OK, Neldam S: The antihypertensive effect and tolerability of candesartan cilexetil, a new generation angiotensin II antagonist, in comparsion with losartan. Blood Pressure 7:53–59, 1998.

70. Mancia G, Dell'Oro R, Turri C, Grassi C: Comparison of angiotensin II receptor blockers: Impact of missed doses of candesartan cilexetil and losartan in systemic hypertension. Am J Cardiol 84(10A):28S–34S, 1999.

71. Dahlof B, Devereux R, de Faire U, et al: The Losartan Intervention For Endpoint reduction (LIFE) in hypertension study: Rationale, design, and methods. The LIFE Study Group. Am J Hypertens 10(7 Pt 1):705–713, 1997.

72. Mann J, Julius S: The Valsartan Antihypertensive Long-term Use Evaluation (VALUE) trial of cardiovascular events in hypertension. Rationale and design. Blood Pressure 7:176–183, 1998.

73. Schrader J, Rothemeyer M, Luders S, Kollmann K: Hypertension and stroke—rationale behind the ACCESS trial. Acute Candesartan Cilexetil Evaluation in Stroke Survivors. Basic Res Cardiol 93(Suppl 2):69–78, 1998.

74. Dahlof B: The importance of the renin-angiotensin system in reversal of left ventricular hypertrophy. J Hypertens 11(Suppl):S29–S35, 1993.

75. Jacobi J, Schlaich MP, Delles C, et al: Angiotensin II stimulates left ventricular hypertrophy in hypertensive patients independently of blood pressure. Am J Hypertens 12(4 Pt 1):418–422, 1999.

76. Dahlof B: Angiotensin-converting enzyme inhibitors and effects on left ventricular hypertrophy. Blood Pressure 2(Suppl):35–40, 1994.

77. Schmeider RE, Martus P, Klingbeil A: Reversal of left ventricular hypertrophy in essential hypertension. A meta-analysis of randomized double-blind studies. JAMA 275:1507–1513, 1996.

78. Schmeider RE, Schlaich MP, Klingbeil AU, Martus P: Update on reversal of left ventricular hypertrophy in essential hypertension (a meta-analysis of all randomized double-blind studies until December 1996). Neprhol Dial Transplant 13:564–569, 1998.

79. Tedesco MA, Ratti G, Aquino D, et al: Effects of losartan on hypertension and left ventricular mass: A long-term study. J Hum Hypertens 12:505–510, 1998.

80. Thurmann PA, Kenedi P, Schmidt A, et al: Influence of the angiotensin II antagonist valsartan on left ventricular hypertrophy in patients with essential hypertension. Circulation 98:2037–2042, 1998.

81. Mitsunami K, Inoue S, Maeda K, et al: Three-month effects of candesartan cilexetil, an angiotensin II type 1 (AT1) receptor antagonist, on left ventricular mass and hemodynamics in patients with essential hypertension. Cardiovasc Drugs Ther 12:469–474, 1998.

82. Kahan T: The importance of left ventricular hypertrophy in human hypertension. J Hypertens 16 (Suppl 7):S23-S29, 1998.

83. Kahan T, Malmqvist K, Edner M, et al: Rate and extent of left ventricular hypertrophy regression: A comparison of angiotensin II blockade with irbesartan and beta-blockade. J Am Coll Cardiol 31:212A, 1998 [abstract].

84. Cohen A, Bregman B, Ababiti Rosei E, et al: Comparison of irbesartan vs felodipine in the regression after 1 year of left ventricular hypertrophy in hypertensive patients (the SILVER trial). Study of Irbesartan in Left VEntricular hypertrophy Regression). J Hum Hypertens 12:479–483, 1998.

85. Dahlof B, Devereux RB, Julius S, et al: Characteristics of 9194 patients with left ventricular hypertrophy: The LIFE Study. Losartan Intervention For Endpoint reduction in hypertension. Hypertension 32:989–997, 1998.

86. CONSENSUS Trial Study Group: Effects of enalapril on mortality in severe congestive heart failure. Results of the Cooperative North Scandinavian Enalapril Survival Study (CONSENSUS. N Engl J Med 316:1429–1435, 1987.

87. Pfeffer MA, Braunwald E, Moye LA, et al: Effect of captopril on mortality and morbidity in patients with left ventricular dysfunction afeer myocardial infarction. Results of the Survival and Ventricular Enlargement trial. The SAVE Investigators. N Engl J Med 327:669–677, 1992.

88. SOLVD Investigators: Effect of enalapril on survival in patients with reduced left ventricular ejection fractions and congestive heart failure. N Engl J Med 325:293–302, 1991.

89. SOLVD Investigators: Effect of enalapril on mortality and the development of heart failure in asymptomatic patients with reduced left ventricular ejection fractions. N Engl J Med 327: 685–691, 1992 [published erratum appears in N Engl J Med 327:1768, 1992].

90. Crozier I, Ikram H, Awan N, et al: Losartan in heart failure: Hemodynamic effects and tolerability. Losartan Hemodynamic Study Group. Circulation 91:691–697, 1995.

91. Mazayev VP, Fomina IG, Kazakov EN, et al: Valsartan in heart failure patients previously untreated with an ACE inhibitor. Int J Cardiol 65:239–246, 1998.

92. Lang RM, Elkayam U, Yellen LG, et al: Comparative effects of losartan and enalapril on exercise capacity and clinical status in patients with heart failure. The Losartan Pilot Exercise Study Investigators. J Am Coll Cardiol 30:983–991, 1997.

93. Hamroff G, Blaufarb I, Mancini D, et al: Angiotensin II-receptor blockade further reduces afterload safely in patients maximally treated with angiotensin-converting enzyme inhibitors for heart failure. J Cardiovasc Pharmacol 30:533–536, 1997.

94. Pitt B, Segal R, Martinez FA, et al: Randomised trial of losartan versus captopril in patients over 65 with heart failure (Evaluation of Losartan In The Elderly study, ELITE). Lancet 349:747–752, 1997.

95. Tsuyuki RT, Yusuf S, Rouleau JL, et al: Combination neurohormonal blockade with ACE inhibitors, angiotensin II antagonists and beta blockers in patients with congestive heart failure: Design of the Randomized Evaluation of Strategies for Left Ventricular Dysfunction (RESOLVD) Pilot Study. Can J Cardiol 13:1166–1174, 1997.

96. Yusuf S, Maggioni AP, Held P, Rouleau JL: Effects of candesartan, enalapril, or their combination on exercise capacity, ventricular function, clinical deterioration and quality of life in heart failure: Randomized Evaluation of Strategies for Left Ventricular Dysfunction (RESOLVD) Pilot Study. Circulation 96:2527, 1997 [abstract].

97. McKelvie RS, Yusuf S, Pericak D, et al: Comparison of candesartan, enalparil, and their combination in congestive heart failure: Randomized Evaluation of Strategies for Left Ventricular Dysfunction (RESOLVD) Pilot Study: The RESOLVD Pilot Study Investigators. Circulation 100:1056–1064, 1999.

98. Pitt B, Poole-Wilson P, Segal R, et al: Effects of losartan versus captopril on mortality in patients with symptomatic heart failure: Rationale, design, and baseline characteristics of patients in the Losartan Heart Failure Survival Study—ELITE II. J Card Fail 5:146–154, 1999.

99. Pitt B, Poole-Wilson PA, Segal R, et al: Losartan Heart Failure Survival Study—ELITE II. Circulation 100(18 Suppl 1):1826, 1999 [abstract].

100. Swedberg K, Pfeffer M, Granger C, et al: Candesartan in heart failure—assessment of reduction in mortality and morbidity (CHARM): Rationale and design. Charm-Programme Investigators. J Card Fail 5:276–282, 1999.

101. Cohn JN, Tognoni G, Glazer RD, et al: Rationale and design of the Valsartan Heart Failure Trial: A large multinational trial to assess the effects of valsartan, an angiotensin-receptor blocker, on morbidity and mortality in chronic congestive heart failure. J Card Fail 5:155–160, 1999.

102. Dickstein K, Kjekshus J: Comparison of the effects of losaratn and captopril on mortality in patients after acute myocardial infarction: The OPTIMAAL trial design. Optimal Therapy in Myocardial Infarctions with the Angiotensin II Antagonist Losartan. Am J Cardiol 83:477–481, 1999.

103. Wolf G: Angiotensin II: A pivotal factor in the progression of renal diseases. Nephrol Dial Transplant 14(Suppl 1):42–44, 1999.

104. Lewis EJ, Hunsicker LG, Bain RP, Rohde RD: The effect of angiotensin-converting enzyme inhibition on diabetic nephropathy. The Collaborative Study Group. N Engl J Med 329:1456–1462, 1993 [published erratum appears in N Engl J Med 330:152, 1993].

105. GISEN Group: Randomised placebo-controlled trial of effect of ramipril on decline in glomerular filtration rate and risk of terminal renal failure in proteinuric, non-diabetic nephropathy. Lancet 349:1857–1863, 1997.

106. Maschio G, Alberti D, Janin G, et al: Effect of the angiotensin-converting enzyme inhibitor benazepril on the progression of chronic renal insufficiency. N Engl J Med 334:939–945, 1996.

107. Antonios TF, MacGregor GA: Angiotensin converting enzyme inhibitors in hypertension: Potential problems. J Hypertens 13(Suppl 3):S11–S16, 1995.

108. Nielsen S, Dollerup J, Nielsen B, et al: Losartan reduces albuminuria in patients with essential hypertension. An enalapril controlled 3 months study. Nephrol Dial Transplant 12(Suppl 2):19–23, 1997.

109. Fernandez-Andrade C, Russo D, Iversen B, et al: Comparison of losartan and amlodipine in renally impaired hypertensive patients. Kidney Int 68(Suppl):S120–S124, 1998.

110. Buter H, Navis G, de Zeeuw D, de Jong PE: Renal hemodynamic effects of candesartan in normal and impaired renal function in humans. Kidney Int 63(Suppl):S185–S187, 1997.

111. Plum J, Bunten B, Nemeth R, Grabensee B: Effects of the angiotensin II antagonist valsartan on blood pressure, proteinuria, and renal hemodynamics in patients with chronic renal failure and hypertension. J Am Soc Nephrol 9:2223–2234, 1998.

112. Goldberg AI, Dunlay MC, Sweet CS: Safety and tolerability of losartan potassium, an angiotensin II receptor antagonist, compared with hydrochlorothiazide, atenoleo, felodipine ER, and angiotensin-converting enzyme inhibitors for the treatment of systemic hypertension. Am J Cardiol 75:793–795, 1995.

113. Belcher G, Hubner R, George M, et al: Candesartan cilexetil: Safety and tolerability in healthy volunteers and patients with hypertension. J Hum Hypertens 11(Suppl 2):S85–S89, 1997.

114. Simon TA, Gelarden RT, Freitag SA, et al: Safety of irbesartan in the treatment of mild to moderate systemic hypertension. Am J Cardiol 82:179–182, 1998.

115. Mazzolai L, Burnier M: Comparative safety and tolerability of angiotensin II receptor antagonists. Drug Safety 21:23–33, 1999.

116. Paster RZ, Snavely DB, Sweet AR, et al: Use of losartan in the treatment of hypertensive patients with a history of cough induced by angiotensin-converting enzyme inhibitors. Clin Ther 20:978–989, 1998.

117. van Rijnsoever EW, Kwee-Zuiderwijk WJ, Feenstra J: Angioneurotic edema attributed to the use of losartan. Arch Intern Med 158:2063–2065, 1998.

118. Frye CB, Pettigrew TJ: Angioedema and photosensitive rash induced by valsartan. Pharmacotherapy 18:866–868, 1998.

119. Sharma PK, Yium JJ: Angioedema associated with angiotensin II receptor antagonist losartan. South Med J 90:552–553, 1997.

120. Acker CG, Greenberg A: Angioedema induced by the angiotensin II blocker losartan. N Engl J Med 333:1572, 1995.

121. Mastrobattista JM: Angiotensin converting enzyme inhibitors in pregnancy. Semin Perinatol 21:124–134, 1997.

CHAPTER 19

Role of AT_1 Angiotensin Receptors in Vascular Remodeling in Hypertension

ERNESTO L. SCHIFFRIN, M.D., Ph.D., FRCPC, FACP
DANIEL HAYOZ, M.D.

The participation of alterations in structure and function of blood vessels in the pathogenesis and pathophysiology of hypertension in experimental animals and humans is today still unclear.[1-4] The arterial vascular tree comprises large or conduit arteries, which can be elastic (proximal) and muscular (more distal), and resistance arteries, which measure less than 350 μm in lumen diameter, and which include small arteries and arterioles. The participation of these different vessels in the mechanisms and complications of hypertension are different.

Large arteries in humans are the site of atherosclerotic complications, which are accelerated by hypertension.[5] Large arteries are also the part of the arterial tree which determines pulse pressure, increasingly identified as an important cardiovascular risk factor.[6,7] When these vessels become stiffer and are invaded by atherosclerotic plaques, their "windkessel" function is blunted, and they may then contribute critically to elevation of systolic blood pressure (in the elderly for example), and to isolated systolic or predominantly systolic hypertension. Atheromatous infiltration of the wall of large elastic arteries is also involved in the atherothromboembolic long-term complications of hypertension. Large muscular arteries such as the brachial or radial and other similar vessels may develop thickening of the intima-media layer, and could contribute to enhanced vascular impedance.[8] Although free of atherosclerotic lesions, the radial artery undergoes remodeling when exposed to elevated blood pressure.

It is as yet unclear to what degree small arteries contribute to mechanisms of hypertension[9-11] or its complications. Although the role of small arteries or arterioles in mechanisms of elevation of blood pressure may as yet be unknown, small artery remodeling contributes to stroke[12] and nephroangiosclerosis.[13] Small artery disease may also contribute to myocardial ischemia, by itself,[14] or as a result of downstream modulation of the effects of epicardial coronary artery occlusion or plaque rupture.[15] This role is the result of alterations in structure, or a consequence of endothelial dysfunction.[16] Some of the improvement in the complications of hypertension or lack thereof in multicenter clinical trials with older antihypertensive agents[17-21] may result from effects on vascular structure or function rather than lowering of blood pressure by itself. Treatment of hypertension[17-21] reduces the incidence of stroke and heart or renal failure as would be expected from cohort studies for the degree of blood pressure lowering (5–6 mmHg) in clinical trials. Nevertheless, it appears to be less effective in decreasing coronary ischemic events and mortality thereof.[22,23] This smaller benefit in protection from cardiac ischemia derived from lower blood pressure in comparison to stroke could be due to the role of persistent alterations in coronary small vessel structure and function in patients treated with the older antihypertensive drugs, the ones employed in multicenter randomized clinical trials.[17-21] To improve outcome in hypertensive patients, it may indeed be necessary to induce a regression of vascular remodeling and functional changes, particularly endothelial dysfunction, not only lower blood pressure.

In this chapter we examine the actions of antihypertensive agents on the changes of the vascular wall of hypertensive humans and experimental animals in both small arteries and conduit vessels, with a particular emphasis on the effects of interrupting the renin-angiotensin system, and a particular focus on actions of AT_1 angiotensin receptor antagonists.

■ *Remodeling of Conduit Arteries in Hypertension*

Direct and indirect vascular complications due to arterial hypertension affect both conduit and resistance arteries. Small arteries determine the resistance to blood flow that is abnormally elevated in essential hypertension.[1] They contribute in part to conduit vessel remodeling by modifying the timing of pressure wave reflection generated by peripheral resistance.[24] Here, we focus on the direct mechanical consequences of hypertension on conduit arteries, and on atherosclerosis development as an indirect consequence. The hypertension-induced arterial wall hypertrophy with stiffening of its constituents is in part responsible for increased pulse pressure, for left ventricular hypertrophy, and possibly for aortic aneurysm and dissection. A consequence of these functional and structural vascular alterations is to facilitate an acceleration of development of atherosclerosis, and to precipitate hypertensive complications: i.e., coronary artery disease, ischemic stroke, and peripheral arterial occlusive disease. The assessment of modifications of the geometry and of elastic properties of conduit arteries undergoing hypertrophic remodeling has been a subject of debate over the last decades.[25-28] It is generally accepted that systemic vascular compliance and/or distensibility are reduced in the presence of chronic essential hypertension.[24] Stiffening of the arterial wall is not only a direct consequence of elevated blood pressure because of the inverse curvilinear relationship between arterial compliance and blood pressure, but represents a genuine alteration of the elastic properties of vascular wall material. These intrinsic material properties are best expressed both in animal experiments and in clinical studies by assessment of Young's modulus (E_{inc}), which is not affected by the geometry of the thickened artery wall components.[29,30] However, the arterial tree is not homogeneous and differences in the local elastic properties of conduit vessels have been reported. High resolution methods such as echotracking techniques have demonstrated quite consistently both in animal experiments[31-33] and in human studies[34-36] that large artery wall thickness is increased in hypertension, and that a certain degree of autoregulation of their elastic properties develops to maintain circumferential wall stress constant.[31,37] A parallel cardiac adaptation is also observed in hypertension.[37]

Under isobaric conditions, conduit arteries tend to be slightly more distensible in the presence of hypertension than under normal blood pressure conditions. This was first demonstrated in the radial artery of newly diagnosed and untreated hypertensive patients. In these subjects, radial artery isobaric compliance and distensibility are higher than in control subjects, although the radial wall thickness is increased.[8] Similar results were found for the common carotid artery.[38] Whether the same is true with long duration of uncontrolled hypertension remains to be demonstrated. In experimental conditions the distensibility of elastic arteries remained constant or slightly higher in hypertensive animals under isobaric conditions, whereas Young's modulus increased with time for a similar level of circumferential stress.[32] However, determination of the systemic elastic function of conduit arteries by pulse wave velocity measurement[39] or by diastolic decay curve analysis[40,41] supports a stiffening of the central vascular tree due to reduction in arterial compliance or distensibility. Reduced systemic arterial compliance results in an augmentation of pulse pressure and in an increased energy cost to the heart in order to maintain adequate flow.[42] For a given stroke volume, systolic pressure increases, whereas storage capacity for blood and energy to be released during the diastole is reduced. Therefore, the lower buffering potential of the central capacitance system causes a decrease in diastolic pressure. Thus, the reduction of the dampening capacity of conduit arteries adversely affects myocardial energy efficiency and contributes to myocardial ischemic events. Recent data confirm that systolic hypertension and the magnitude of pulse pressure are stronger predictors of adverse cardiovascular events than diastolic blood pressure.[6,7,43,44] However, diastolic blood pressure has served over the years as the chief inclusion criteria for most of the large antihypertensive trials because it predicts cardiovascular events in younger patients.[45] One may speculate that a proportion of patients at the highest risk of adverse cardiovascular events were not enrolled in these trials and may also have been undertreated. Future studies will have to define the relationship between dose and efficacy of the different classes of antihypertensive treatment on systolic and pulse pressures.

Increased pulse pressure generates a greater cyclic strain on smooth muscle cells, leading to accelerated growth rate and greater migration potential.[46,47] This may represent a critical mechanical trigger for hypertrophic remodeling of conduit arteries. In animal models of hypertension, pulse pressure has also been shown to contribute to changes in small vessel structure, since a positive correlation between pulse pressure reduction and reduction of wall to lumen ratio has been reported.[48,49] This may partly explain how structural modifications of the vascular bed perpetuate the vicious circle that maintains a high blood pressure level. Interestingly, in young and middle-aged hypertensive patients, systolic, diastolic and mean blood pressure correlated with media-to-lumen ratio of small arteries, whereas pulse pressure did not.[50] This may indicate that as hypertensive patients age, they evolve from a disease in which the vasculature both affects and is affected by diastolic blood pressure, to one in which risk is conferred and vascular damage induced by pulse pressure, as systolic pressure rises disproportionately, and diastolic blood pressure falls as a result of changes in vascular stiffness.[45]

The contribution of the peripheral versus the central compliance remains to be more precisely determined. One possible explanation for an increased isobaric distensibility is a partial transfer of the central buffering capacity toward the periphery. At least in the initial phase, an increased elasticity of the conduit arteries seems to temper the effects of the hypertrophic remodeling encountered in hypertension. The possible time-limited beneficial effect of conduit artery remodeling may be counterbalanced by negative functional consequences. Indeed, thickening of the arterial intima-media has been associated with metabolic changes that contribute to endothelial dysfunction and progression of atherosclerosis.[51] In this setting, the renin-angiotensin system seems to play a crucial role. In animal models of angiotensin II-dependent hypertension, oxidative stress-dependent hypertrophy of vascular smooth muscle cells has been demonstrated, contributing to amplify the trophic effect of mechanical load.[52] Furthermore, macrophages trapped into the vessel wall show an upregulation of the expression of AT_1 receptors that may contribute in part to up-regulation of peroxide production.[53] Not only does this increased oxidative stress favor hypertrophy, but it may also contribute to development of atherosclerosis via the NO pathway. A reduction in NO bioavailability through production of excessive oxidative stress could represent an important mechanism by which a dysfunctional endothelium potentiates atherosclerosis and thrombosis in essential hypertension. Additionally, angiotensin II may also promote atherosclerosis by modifying extracellular matrix deposition,[54-56] by interacting with the fibrinolytic system,[57] and by inducing the release of cytokines and chemotactic factors.[58-60] Thus, activation of the renin-angiotensin system is involved in many of the different pathways leading to atherosclerosis.

■ *Effect of AT_1 Antagonism Antihypertensive Therapy on Conduit Arteries in Hypertension*

There are presently limited data on the effect of blockade of the renin-angiotensin system on remodeling of large arteries in humans. Most of the available data concern animal models of hypertension. As discussed above, functional alterations of large artery function occur with and most likely precede vascular wall remodeling. Endothelial dysfunction appears to be an initial defect promoting vascular wall remodeling and development of atherosclerosis; it may be reversible, at least to some extent. Angiotensin-converting enzyme (ACE) inhibition and more recently AT_1 receptor antagonists have proved efficient in reversing endothelial dysfunction in different conduit vessels both in genetic as well as in renin-dependent hypertension.[61,62]

Therapeutic interventions to increase NO availability interfere favorably on the paradoxical vasoconstriction and loss of endothelial antithrombotic activity. Furthermore, AT_1 blockade has been shown to interfere with the growth promoting action of angiotensin II independently of the blood pressure–lowering effects. Indeed, doses that did not change blood pressure were able to suppress cardiovascular hypertrophy and prevent aortic collagen accumulation.[63,64] In cell culture experiments, AT_1 receptor antagonists are able to suppress cytokine and growth factor release from smooth muscle cells treated with angiotensin II.[59,65] These experimental data strongly support the beneficial role of angiotensin II suppression and/or blockade in the early stream of events that participate in vascular wall remodeling, in disturbance of local homeostasis, and in cytokine release. Angiotensin II suppression and/or blockade are thus appealing therapeutic aims that must be confirmed by demonstration of improvement of patient outcomes.

Numerous studies have reported that chronic blockade of the renin-angiotensin system prevents and/or reverses structural alterations of conduit vessels in experimental and clinical hypertension. Most of the experimental studies have dealt with the rat aorta or the common carotid artery.[66,67] Both prevention and regression of vascular wall hypertrophy with concomitant improvement of the buffering capacity of the vessel have been reported with ACE inhibitors and AT₁ receptor antagonists. However, the great diversity of methods and of animal models of hypertension precludes a comparison of experimental data. Nevertheless, it appears that both converting enzyme inhibition and AT₁ receptor blockade, when decreasing blood pressure with equivalent efficacy, can reduce vascular wall thickness and stiffness as demonstrated by an upward shift of the compliance-pressure curves.[67,68] However, it has been reported that chronic blockade of the AT₁ receptor in rats infused with angiotensin II prevented blood pressure elevation but was unable to block aortic hypertrophy,[69] although other investigators have reported different results.[70] There are data suggesting that blockade of the AT₁ receptor in association with activation of the AT₂ receptor subtype may induce apoptosis of smooth muscle cells that could prevent vascular hypertrophy.[71,72] Other antihypertensive agents such as ACE inhibitors and calcium antagonists may also induce apoptosis in spontaneously hypertensive rats, possibly contributing to regression of vessel wall hypertrophy.[73]

In clinical studies, noninvasive detection of the increased vascular thickness has permitted prospective studies to assess the potential of long-term antihypertensive treatment on regression of vascular hypertrophy. The thickness of the intima-media of the artery is often measured as a marker of vascular hypertrophy. But one should bear in mind that when assessing the dimensions of the vascular wall, the vessel diameter should be taken into account. Indeed, a reduced distention of the vessel due to a blood pressure–lowering effect is accompanied by a thickening of the vessel wall due to dynamic remodeling. Determination of the vascular wall thickness should ideally be performed under constant diameter conditions. Furthermore, using noninvasive techniques, it is still impossible to differentiate intimal thickening from hypertrophy of the media. The two types of vascular remodeling may present quite different risk profiles. Indeed, hypertrophy of the media as a result of adaptation to increased circumferential wall stress may have a different potential as an atherosclerosis risk factor than intimal lipid accumulation.

The Multicenter Isradipine Diuretic Atherosclerosis Study (MIDAS) was the first clinical trial to show a slower progression of intima-media thickness in hypertensive patients following reduction of blood pressure levels, although no differences in the geometrical characteristics of the carotid arteries were observed between the two treatment groups.[74] This study was followed shortly after by the VHAS trial (verapamil or chlorthalidone on carotid intima-media thickness), which showed that small differences in carotid wall changes were paralleled by differences in the incidence of cardiovascular events.[75] The effect of an ACE inhibitor (perindopril) on the geometry and function of conduit arteries has recently been published. When compared to a diuretic (hydrochlorothiazide), the ACE inhibitor induced similar blood pressure reduction, and both drugs reduced radial artery hypertrophy and improved carotid artery compliance.[76]

In addition to the report by the Framingham group that systolic pressure is a better determinant of cardiovascular complications than mean blood pressure in persons over 50 years of age,[43,77] new data have demonstrated, as discussed above, that pulse pressure is a stronger independent determinant of elastic artery hypertrophy than mean blood pressure.[44] These results suggest that local stretch is a key determinant for the induction of vascular growth. We recently tested how antihypertensive drugs with theoretical differences in local pulse pressure reduction potential (celiprolol, a beta blocker with vasodilator properties, vs. the ACE inhibitor enalapril) might affect intima-media thickness of both an elastic (common carotid artery) and a muscular artery (radial artery). No differences were observed between the two treatment groups. The reduction in intima-media thickness was apparent at the carotid and the radial arteries after the nine month treatment period with either agent. The regression of carotid vascular mass was related to the reduction in local pulse pressure, and not to the reduction in mean arterial pressure. This was not observed at the radial artery, in which the relative circumferential stretch is an order of magnitude lower than at the level of the elastic artery such as the carotid. However, there are no data today showing unequivocally that one class of antihypertensive drugs confers a particular advantage on prevention and/or regression of vascular hypertrophy in conduit arteries.

Concerning modifications of the mechanical properties of large arteries in chronic hypertension, there exists today indirect evidence both from animal experiments as well as from human studies that ACE inhibitors or AT_1 receptor antagonists improve the elastic properties of large arteries by reducing pulse wave velocity. Beyond the antihypertensive effects of blocking the renin-angiotensin system, there is a clear potential for reversing structural and functional alterations of large arteries, contributing to vascular protection and interruption of a vicious circle that sustains high blood pressure.

■ Remodeling of Resistance Arteries in Hypertension

Small or resistance arteries, vessels with a lumen diameter of 100 to 350 μm,[1–3] are a major site of resistance to blood flow.[78] Since elevated peripheral resistance is the hallmark of essential hypertension, alterations of small arteries probably participate in mechanisms of elevation of blood pressure. Abnormalities of these small arteries also play an important role in the complications of hypertension such as cerebral infarction[12] and renal failure.[13] Myocardial ischemic events in hypertensive patients result like in normotensive subjects from plaque fissure or rupture, and coronary artery obstruction of the larger epicardial arteries.[15] However, in hypertensive patients the extent and consequences of ischemia may be influenced importantly by disease of the coronary microcirculation.[14] Endothelial dysfunction[16] or structural changes of small arteries modulate the myocardial consequences of upstream events (plaque rupture and epicardial artery obstruction).[14] Treatment of hypertension is not as effective as expected in decreasing coronary ischemic events as it is on stroke,[22,23] which could in part be due to persistent coronary small vessel disease in patients treated with the older antihypertensive drugs.[17–21] We believe that to improve outcome in hypertensive patients, lowering of blood pressure may not suffice; it may indeed be necessary to also induce a regression of small artery remodeling and functional changes.

■ Structural Remodeling and Functional Changes in Small Arteries in Hypertension

The first manifestation of target organ damage present in mild hypertension in humans before development of cardiac hypertrophy, increased carotid intima-media thickness or microalbuminuria and nephroangiosclerosis, is the remodeling of small arteries. Small arteries of hypertensive patients exhibit a reduction in the lumen and external diameter, normal or increased media thickness, and increased media-to-lumen ratio, but normal media cross-section (or volume of the media per unit length),[50,79,80] a change recently defined as "eutrophic remodeling."[81] Vessels have the same number of smooth muscle cells and little evidence of cell hypertrophy.[79] Cells are rearranged around a smaller vessel lumen but it is unknown how this restructuring occurs. It may in part result from changes in cell adhesion molecules,[82] extracellular matrix deposition, or spatial arrangement of fibrillar material. We have recently shown in both spontaneously hypertensive rats (SHR)[82,83] and in human resistance arteries from hypertensive patients[84] that collagen deposition is enhanced. In more severe forms of hypertension, eutrophic remodeling may evolve toward "hypertrophic remodeling,"[81] as other mechanisms are triggered and perhaps growth predominates over apoptosis.[73]

The function of small blood vessels is also altered in hypertensive patients. The media stress developed in response to angiotensin II is usually increased, although sometimes it may be normal, whereas responses to most other vasoconstrictors are reduced.[80,85,86] The structural abnormalities of resistance arteries, however, amplify responses and result in enhanced vasoconstrictor responses,[1] contributing to elevated vascular tone. Endothelial function is impaired in hypertension: vasodilatory responses to acetylcholine in precontracted vessels are blunted both in hypertensive animals[87] and humans.[88,89] Endothelial dysfunction may be due to a deficient generation of nitric oxide or its increased degradation, the latter perhaps a consequence of enhanced oxidative stress in the vascular wall.[90] Endothelium-derived endoperoxides (endothelium-derived contracting factor, EDCF) have also been implicated.[88,91]

■ Mechanism of Small Artery Changes in Hypertension

Smooth muscle cell hyperplasia or hypertrophy in response to angiotensin II,[92] to endothelin or other vasoactive peptides, or to catecholamines may be involved in growth contributing to remodeling of small arteries. This may be combined with collagen deposition in the media.[92,93] There is significant in vivo evidence that angiotensin II plays a pivotal role in small artery remodeling to induce growth,[93] acting via AT₁ receptors,[70] although a role has also been suggested for AT₂ receptors.[69,94] Angiotensin II acts via a complex array of signaling mechanisms inside the cell, including mitogen-activated protein (MAP) kinases and other molecular steps that interact with intracellular calcium at different levels, as shown both in vascular smooth muscle cells from experimental animals[95] and humans.[96] Cellular mechanisms that may contribute to growth include paracrine or autocrine stimulation of growth factors[92] or of endothelin-1[97,98] by angiotensin II, and oxidative stress triggered by angiotensin II via the NADH/NADPH oxidase systems of smooth muscle cells.[99–101] It is possible that apoptosis offsets the growth to result in eutrophic remodeling. Indeed, angiotensin II-induced growth may be associated with secondarily enhanced apoptotic rates in the muscular media.[102] Another potential mechanism modulating growth and remodeling of vessels is AT_1 antagonist-elicited reflex elevation of plasma angiotensin II, which may stimulate unblocked AT_2 receptors. Renal AT_2 receptor stimulation induces nitric oxide production and antagonizes AT_1 receptor-mediated effects.[103] The anti-growth[71] and proapoptotic actions[72] of AT_2 receptors may involve as well stimulation of nitric oxide production, directly or indirectly modulating vascular remodeling.

■ *Effects of Blockade of the Renin-Angiotensin System on Small Arteries in Hypertensive Rats*

The structure and function of small arteries of the heart and kidney,[104–106] and the brain of SHR[106,107] resemble those described in subcutaneous gluteal small arteries of hypertensive humans,[79,80,85] and present eutrophic or hypertrophic remodeling.[4] Endothelium-dependent relaxation is blunted because acetylcholine induces contractions via generation of EDCF.[88,91] SHR treated with ACE inhibitors[105,106,108–112] or angiotensin II receptor antagonists[112,113] showed correction of abnormal endothelial function and regression of vascular remodeling, including the excess collagen deposition.[82,83] Effects of ACE inhibitors may be the result of inhibition of angiotensin II generation or of accumulation of bradykinin, both of which could also beneficially influence endothelial function (angiotensin II reduction by attenuation of oxidative stress, bradykinin via stimulation of nitric oxide). Angiotensin AT_1 receptor antagonists like losartan or others probably act via blockade of angiotensin II-induced growth. The absence of blockade of AT_2 receptors stimulated by the elevated angiotensin II concentrations found under treatment with AT_1 antagonists may stimulate nitric oxide production,[103] which has anti-growth[71] and proapoptotic effects,[72] and would also correct the nitric oxide deficiency by reducing oxidative stress.

■ *Effect of Blockade of the Renin-Angiotensin System Compared to Beta Blockade on Small Artery Structure and Function in Hypertensive Patients*

Based on the previously reported results in experimental animals, a randomized prospective comparison of treatment with an ACE inhibitor compared to a beta blocker was performed to assess whether in essential hypertensive patients small artery structure would be corrected by interrupting the renin-angiotensin system. Patients were treated with the ACE inhibitor cilazapril or the beta blocker atenolol for 1 and 2 years[114,115] or by other investigators with perindopril in a 1-year trial,[116] and small arteries obtained from gluteal subcutaneous biopsies were evaluated. The structure of small arteries under the action of the ACE inhibitors cilazapril for 1 year[114] or 2 years[115] and perindopril for 1 year[116] was corrected, whereas under the beta blocker atenolol there was no improvement. Endothelial function measured by acetylcholine-induced relaxation improved under the ACE inhibitor cilazapril but not with atenolol.[114,117] In a study in which biopsies were performed after treatment with lisinopril for 3 years, structure and endothelial-dependent relaxation of small subcutaneous arteries of hypertensive patients were improved relative to untreated hypertensive subjects.[118] It is of interest that in normotensive subjects with coronary artery disease, treatment for 6 months with another ACE inhibitor, quinapril, resulted in improvement of endothelial function of coronary arteries as shown by coronary angiography in the TREND study.[119]

More recently, the results of interruption of the renin-angiotensin system have been extended to the use of AT$_1$ receptor antagonists.[120] This study was performed in essential hypertensive patients who were treated with losartan for one year in comparison to atenolol. The media width to lumen diameter ratio (M/L) of arteries from losartan-treated patients was reduced following treatment from 8.4 ± 0.4% to 6.9 ± 0.3% (p < 0.01). In contrast, arteries from atenolol-treated patients exhibited no significant change in M/L with treatment, as in previous studies.[114–116] Endothelium-dependent relaxation was normalized by losartan (p < 0.01) but not by atenolol treatment, as observed previously in the comparison of an ACE inhibitor and atenolol.[117] The effects of treatment with losartan or atenolol were unchanged by addition of the diuretic hydrochlorothiazide to achieve goal blood pressure. Selective AT$_1$ receptor blockade may be specifically effective at interrupting vascular effects of angiotensin II, particularly in light of the recent report that dual pathways for generation of angiotensin II, mediated by angiotensin-converting enzyme and by a chymostatin-sensitive enzyme, presumably chymase, exist in human resistance arteries.[121]

■ Discussion

Reversal of structural and functional abnormalities of large and small arteries under antihypertensive treatment in SHR and other models of hypertension in the rat correlates with lowering of blood pressure.[87,88] Correction of structure in hypertensive rat models may be independent of the antihypertensive agent used. However, endothelial function may be normalized, particularly when hypertensive rats are treated with ACE inhibitors or AT$_1$ receptor antagonists.[105,112] In hypertensive patients, in contrast, structural or functional remodeling of small arteries regresses differently according to the agent used to normalize blood pressure. In equally well-controlled hypertensive patients, atenolol-treated patients show persistent abnormalities of small artery structure and function, whereas ACE inhibitor, AT$_1$ receptor, or calcium channel antagonist-treated patients exhibit normalized structure and reversal of altered endothelial and smooth muscle cell responses toward normal.[114–117,120,122]

The media-to-lumen ratio of small arteries is independent of lumen diameter within the range examined in these studies (150–350 μm) and is highly reproducible within and between patients in this type of study.[115,123] It also has major hemodynamic significance.[1–3] Moreover, media-to-lumen ratio of gluteal subcutaneous small arteries correlates closely with forearm minimal vascular resistance at maximal vasodilatation in normotensive and hypertensive subjects.[124] Finally, the changes detected on gluteal subcutaneous small arteries in hypertensive humans are the same ones found in hypertensive rats in more pathophysiologically critical vascular beds, such as in coronary and renal small arteries.[104–106,112] Hypertensive patients show abnormalities of the coronary microcirculation.[14] Treatment with the ACE inhibitor enalapril was recently shown to improve coronary reserve, a manifestation of the regression of structural and functional (possibly endothelial) changes in the coronary microcirculation.[125,126] Thus, small arteries from gluteal subcutaneous tissue appear to be representative of systemic resistance arteries, and as the structure and function of subcutaneous small arteries is normalized, a similar improvement may occur in coronary small arteries in hypertensive patients treated with ACE inhibitors or AT_1 receptor antagonists, which could potentially have a major favorable impact on cardiovascular morbidity in hypertension.

The mechanism of action whereby ACE inhibitors and AT_1 receptor antagonists result in correction of structural and functional changes in small arteries has not been elucidated. The effects of ACE inhibitors may result from inhibition of generation of angiotensin II, but inhibition of degradation of kinins or even hemodynamic effects may also play a role. AT_1 receptor antagonists may act via blockade of AT_1 receptors or via the stimulation of unblocked AT_2 receptors. Both ACE inhibitors and AT_1 receptor antagonists are vasodilators, whereas beta blockers induce a vasoconstrictor effect,[127] which could contribute in part to the differential effects of these antihypertensive agents.

Our enthusiasm for these newer therapies and the potential advantage conferred by their vascular protective effects must, however, be tempered by our knowledge of the results of two recent trials. In the UK Prospective Diabetes Study Group (UKPDS),[128] captopril and atenolol equally reduced the risk of macrovascular endpoints. In the Captopril Prevention Project (CAPPP)[129] comparing captopril and conventional therapy, cardiovascular mortality was lower with captopril than with conventional therapy, the rate of fatal and non-fatal infarction was similar, but fatal and non-fatal strokes were more common with captopril. These studies suggested that ACE inhibitors provide no specific benefit in preventing cardiovascular morbidity and mortality, and that blood pressure reduction itself may be more important than the treatment used. However, in one of the studies, captopril was taken once daily by half the patients, which may lower blood pressure but be insufficient to adequately block the renin-angiotensin system throughout the day, thus limiting the potential benefits of complete inhibition of angiotensin II generation on target organ damage. Randomization problems (patients allocated to captopril had higher blood pressure before and during the study) and the unusual dose of captopril in CAPPP only allow the conclusion that ACE inhibitors are as effective as beta blockers or conventional therapy. They do not exclude the possibility that complete interruption of the renin-angiotensin system will result in vascular protection and improved outcomes. Moreover, selective AT_1 receptor antagonists may be superior to ACE inhibitors regarding target organ protection.[120] In relation to UKPDS, atenolol and perhaps other beta blockers may have particularly beneficial effects in diabetic individuals that compensate for the absence of vascular protective properties, resulting in equal benefit when compared at least with the ACE inhibitor captopril. The recent publication of the HOPE study suggests that indeed interruption of the renin-angiotensin system, in that study with the ACE inhibitor ramipril, in part via vascular protection, may reduce cardiovascular morbidity and mortality.[130]

■ Conclusion

Treatment with specific antihypertensive drugs such as some of the newer antihypertensive agents (angiotensin converting enzyme inhibitors, AT_1 receptor antagonists, and calcium channel antagonists), but not beta blockers like atenolol, may result in reversal of the structural and functional alterations of vessels in essential hypertensive patients. Today we know that this occurs in small arteries, but knowledge of large arteries is more sparse. How structure, function and elastic properties of conduit arteries are modified, and to what extent pulse pressure and cyclic strain are reduced by antihypertensive agents, particularly in older hypertensives, remains to be clearly defined. Whether one class of antihypertensive agents affects large arteries, conferring advantages over other agents in regression of growth and stiffness, is presently being investigated. In the case of small, resistance-size arteries, the protective effect on the vasculature of ACE inhibitors and AT₁ receptor antagonists and extended release or long-acting calcium channel antagonists may result in improved clinical outcomes. This may be particularly true with respect to cardiac events, and could produce benefits in addition to those attributable to blood pressure lowering itself, with a reduction of hypertension-induced morbidity and mortality. However, the latter still remains to be demonstrated, particularly in view of results of recent trials which have suggested the absence of specific benefits independent of blood pressure reduction.[128,129] The HOPE study may be the first to provide evidence of such specific benefits.[130]

Acknowledgments

The authors' work was supported by a group grant from the Medical Research Council of Canada to the Multidisciplinary Research Group on Hypertension; grants from Hoffmann-LaRoche Canada, Bayer Canada, and Merck-Frosst Canada to ELS; and grants from the Swiss National Research Foundation to D.H..

References

1. Folkow B: Physiological aspects of primary hypertension. Physiol Rev 62:347–504, 1982.
2. Mulvany MJ, Aalkjaer C: Structure and function of small arteries. Physiol Rev 70:921–971, 1990.
3. Schiffrin EL: Reactivity of small blood vessels in hypertension. Relationship with structural changes. Hypertension 19 (Suppl. II):II-1–II-9, 1992.
4. Heagerty AM, Aalkjaer C, Bund SJ, et al: Small artery structure in hypertension: Dual processes of remodelling and growth. Hypertension 21:391–397, 1993.
5. Chobanian A: Adaptive and maladaptive responses of the arterial wall to hypertension. Hypertension 15:666–674, 1990.
6. Fang J, Madhavan S, Cohen H, Alderman MH: Measures of blood pressure and myocardial infarction in treated hypertensive patients. J Hypertens 13:413–419, 1995.
7. Benetos A, Rudnichi A, Safar M, Guize L: Pulse pressure and cardiovascular mortality in normotensive and hypertensive subjects. Hypertension 32:560–564, 1998.
8. Hayoz D, Rutschmann B, Perret F, et al: Conduit artery compliance and distensibility are not necessarily reduced in hypertension. Hypertension 20:1–6, 1992.
9. Christensen KL, Mulvany MJ: Mesenteric arcade arteries contribute substantially to vascular resistance in conscious rats. J Vasc Res 30:73–79, 1993.
10. Folkow B: Hypertensive structural changes in systemic precapillary resistance vessels: How important are they for in vivo haemodynamics? J Hypertens 13:1546–1559, 1995.
11. Izzard AS, Heagerty AM: Hypertension and the vasculature: arterioles and the myogenic response. J Hypertens 13:1–4, 1995.
12. Spence JD: Cerebral consequences of hypertension. In Laragh JH, Brenner BM (eds): Hypertension: Pathophysiology, Diagnosis and Management, 2nd ed. New York, Raven Press, 1995, pp 741–753.
13. Ruilope LM, Alcázar JM, Rodicio JL: Renal consequences of hypertension. J Hypertens 10 (Suppl 7):S85–S90, 1992.
14. Brush JE, Cannon RO, Schenke WH, et al: Angina due to coronary microvascular disease in hypertensive patients without left ventricular hypertrophy. N Engl J Med 319:1302–1307, 1988.
15. Fuster V, Badimon L, Badimon JJ, Chesebro JH: The pathogenesis of acute coronary syndromes. N Engl J Med 326:242–250, 310–318, 1992.
16. Hasdai D, Gibbons RJ, Holmes DR Jr, et al: Coronary endothelial dysfunction is associated with myocardial perfusion defects. Circulation 96:3390–3395, 1997.
17. Veterans Administration Cooperative Study Group on Antihypertensive Agents: Effects of treatment on morbidity in hypertension. II: Results in patients with diastolic blood pressure averaging 90 through 114 mmHg. JAMA 202:1143–1152, 1970.

18. Australian National Blood Pressure Study Management Committee: Australian Therapeutic Trial in Mild Hypertension. Lancet 1:1262–1267, 1980.
19. Hypertension Detection and Follow-up Program Cooperative Group: The effect of treatment on mortality in mild hypertension. N Engl J Med 307:976–980, 1982.
20. Medical Research Council Working Party: MRC trial of treatment of mild hypertension: Principal results. BMJ 291:97–104, 1985.
21. Medical Research Council Working Party: MRC trial of treatment of hypertension in older adults: Principal results. BMJ 304:405–412, 1992.
22. Collins R, Peto R, MacMahon S, et al: Blood pressure, stroke, and coronary heart disease. II: Short term reductions in blood pressure: Overview of randomized drug trials in their epidemiological context. Lancet 335:827–838, 1990.
23. MacMahon SW, Cutler JA, Stamler J: Antihypertensive drug treatment. Potential, expected, and observed effects on stroke and on coronary heart disease. Hypertension 13(Suppl I):I-45–I-50, 1989.
24. O'Rourke S: Arterial stiffness, systolic blood pressure, and logical treatment of arterial hypertension. Hypertension 15:339–347, 1990.
25. Armentano R, Megnien JL, Simon A, et al: Effects of hypertension on viscoelasticity of carotid and femoral arteries in humans. Hypertension 26:48–54, 1995.
26. London GM, Guerin AP, Marchais SJ, et al: Cardiac and arterial interactions in end-stage renal disease. Kidney Int 50:600–608, 1996.
27. Hoeks AP, Brands PJ, Smeets FA, Reneman RS: Assessment of the distensibility of superficial arteries. Ultrasound Med Biol 16:121–128, 1990.
28. Bank AJ, Kaiser DR: Smooth muscle relaxation: effects on arterial compliance, distensibility, elastic modulus, and pulse wave velocity. Hypertension 32:356–359, 1998.
29. Laurent S, Girerd X, Mourad JJ, et al: Elastic modulus of the radial artery wall material is not increased in patients with essential hypertension. Arterioscler Thromb 14:1223–1231, 1994.
30. Weber R, Stergiopulos N, Brunner HR, Hayoz D: Contributions of vascular tone and structure to elastic properties of a medium-sized artery. Hypertension 27(Pt 2):816–822, 1996.
31. Zanchi A, Wiesel P, Aubert JF, et al: Time course changes of the mechanical properties of the carotid artery in renal hypertensive rats. Hypertension 29:1199–1203, 1997.
32. van Gorp AW, van Ingen Schenau DS, Hoeks AP, et al: Aortic wall properties in normotensive and hypertensive rats of various ages in vivo. Hypertension 26:363–368, 1995.
33. Lacolley P, Bezie Y, Girerd X, et al: Aortic distensibility and structural changes in sinoaortic-denervated rats. Hypertension 26:337–340, 1995.
34. Gariepy J, Massonneau M, Levenson J, et al: Evidence for in vivo carotid and femoral wall thickening in human hypertension. Groupe de Prevention Cardio-vasculaire en Medecine du Travail. Hypertension 22:111–118, 1993.
35. Girerd X, Giannattasio C, Moulin C, et al: Regression of radial artery wall hypertrophy and improvement of carotid artery compliance after long-term antihypertensive treatment in elderly patients. J Am Coll Cardiol 31:1064–1073, 1998.
36. Laurent S: Arterial wall hypertrophy and stiffness in essential hypertensive patients. Hypertension 26:355–362, 1995.
37. Roman MJ, Saba PS, Pini R, et al: Parallel cardiac and vascular adaptation in hypertension. Circulation 86:1909–1918, 1992.
38. Laurent S, Caviezel B, Beck L, et al: Carotid artery distensibility and distending pressure in hypertensive humans. Hypertension 23(Pt 2):878–883, 1994.
39. Asmar R, Benetos A, Topouchian J, et al: Assessment of arterial distensibility by automatic pulse wave velocity measurement. Validation and clinical application studies. Hypertension 26:485–490, 1995.
40. Watt TB Jr, Burrus CS: Arterial pressure contour analysis for estimating human vascular properties. J Appl Physiol 40:171–176, 1976.
41. McVeigh GE, Bratteli CW, Morgan DJ, et al: Age-related abnormalities in arterial compliance identified by pressure pulse contour analysis: Aging and arterial compliance. Hypertension 33:1392–1398, 1999.
42. Kelly RP, Tunin R, Kass DA: Effect of reduced aortic compliance on cardiac efficiency and contractile function of in situ canine left ventricle. Circ Res 71:490–502, 1992.
43. Sytkowski PA, D'Agostino RB, Belanger AJ, Kannel WB: Secular trends in long-term sustained hypertension, long-term treatment, and cardiovascular mortality. The Framingham Heart Study 1950 to 1990. Circulation 93:697–703, 1996.
44. Boutouyrie P, Bussy C, Lacolley P, et al: Association between local pulse pressure, mean blood pressure, and large-artery remodeling. Circulation 100:1387–1393, 1999.
45. O'Rourke M, Frohlich ED: Pulse pressure: Is this a clinically useful risk factor? Hypertension 34:372–374, 1999.

46. Leung DY, Glagov S, Mathews MB: Cyclic stretching stimulates synthesis of matrix components by arterial smooth muscle cells in vitro. Science 191:475–477, 1976.

47. Reusch P, Wagdy H, Reusch R, et al: Mechanical strain increases smooth muscle and decreases nonmuscule myosin expression in rat vascular smooth muscle cells. Circ Res 79:1046–1053, 1996.

48. Baumbach G: Effects of increased pulse pressure on cerebral arterioles. Hypertension 27:159–167, 1996.

49. Christensen KL: Reducing pulse pressure in hypertension may normalize small artery structure. Hypertension 18:722–727, 1991.

50. Schiffrin EL, Deng LY: Relationship of small artery structure with systolic, diastolic and pulse pressure in essential hypertension. J Hypertens 17:381–387, 1999.

51. Griendling KK, Ushio-Fukai M: Redox control of vascular smooth muscle proliferation. J Lab Clin Med 132:9–15, 1998.

52. Fukai T, Siegfried MR, Ushio-Fukai M, et al: Modulation of extracellular superoxide dismutase expression by angiotensin II and hypertension. Circ Res 85:23–28, 1999.

53. Yanagitani Y, Rakugi H, Okamura A, et al: Angiotensin II type 1 receptor-mediated peroxide production in human macrophages. Hypertension 33 (Pt 2):335–339, 1999.

54. Tamura K, Chiba E, Yokoyama N, et al: Renin-angiotensin system and fibronectin gene expression in Dahl Iwai salt-sensitive and salt-resistant rats. J Hypertens 17:81–89, 1999.

55. Li S, Sims S, Jiao Y, et al: Evidence from a novel human cell clone that adult vascular smooth muscle cells can convert reversibly between noncontractile and contractile phenotypes. Circ Res 85:338–348, 1999.

56. Larsson PT, Schwieler JH, Wallen NH, Hjemdahl P: Acute effects of angiotensin II on fibrinolysis in healthy volunteers. Blood Coagul Fibrinol 10:19–24, 1999.

57. Vaughan DE, Lazos SA, Tong K: Angiotensin II regulates the expression of plasminogen activator inhibitor-1 in cultured endothelial cells. A potential link between the renin-angiotensin system and thrombosis. J Clin Invest 95:995–1001, 1995.

58. Kranzhofer R, Schmidt J, Pfeiffer CA, et al: Angiotensin induces inflammatory activation of human vascular smooth muscle cells. Arterioscler Thromb Vasc Biol 19:1623–1629, 1999.

59. Funakoshi Y, Ichiki T, Ito K, Takeshita A: Induction of interleukin-6 expression by angiotensin II in rat vascular smooth muscle cells. Hypertension 34:118–125, 1999.

60. Han Y, Runge MS, Brasier AR: Angiotensin II induces interleukin-6 transcription in vascular smooth muscle cells through pleiotropic activation of nuclear factor-kappa B transcription factors. Circ Res 84:695–703, 1999.

61. Hoshino J, Nakamura T, Kurashina T, et al: Antagonism of ANG II type 1 receptors protects the endothelium during the early stages of renal hypertension in rats. Am J Physiol 275 (Pt 2):R1950–1957, 1998.

62. Mancini GB: Role of angiotensin-converting enzyme inhibition in reversal of endothelial dysfunction in coronary artery disease. Am J Med 105:40S–47S, 1998.

63. Benetos A, Levy BI, Lacolley P, et al: Role of angiotensin II and bradykinin on aortic collagen following converting enzyme inhibition in spontaneously hypertensive rats. Arterioscler Thromb Vasc Biol 17:3196–3201, 1997.

64. Nishikawa K: Angiotensin AT1 receptor antagonism and protection against cardiovascular end-organ damage. J Hum Hypertens 12:301–309, 1998.

65. Hamaguchi A, Kim S, Izumi Y, et al: Contribution of extracellular signal-regulated kinase to angiotensin II-induced transforming growth factor-beta1 expression in vascular smooth muscle cells. Hypertension 34:126–131, 1999.

66. Koffi I, Lacolley P, Kirchengaast M, et al: Prevention of arterial structural alterations with verapamil and trandolapril and consequences for mechanical properties in spontaneously hypertensive rats. Eur J Pharmacol 361:51–60, 1998.

67. Ceiler DL, Nelissen-Vrancken HJ, De Mey JG, Smits JF: Effect of chronic blockade of angiotensin II-receptor subtypes on aortic compliance in rats with myocardial infarction. J Cardiovasc Pharmacol 31:630–637, 1998.

68. Makki T, Talom RT, Niederhoffer N, et al: Increased arterial distensibility induced by the angiotensin-converting enzyme inhibitor, lisinopril, in normotensive rats. Br J Pharmacol 111:555-560, 1994.

69. Levy BI, Benessiano J, Henrion D, et al: Chronic blockade of AT2-subtype receptors prevents the effect of angiotensin II on the rat vascular structure. J Clin Invest 98:418–425, 1996.

70. Li JS, Touyz RM, Schiffrin EL: Effect of AT$_1$ and AT$_2$ angiotensin receptor antagonists in angiotensin II-infused rats. Hypertension 31[Pt 2]:487–492, 1998.

71. Stoll M, Steckelings UM, Paul M, et al: The angiotensin AT2 receptor mediates inhibition of cell proliferation in coronary endothelial cells. J Clin Invest. 95:651–657, 1995.

72. Yamada T, Horiuchi M, Dzau VJ: Angiotensin II type 2 receptor mediates programmed cell death. Proc Natl Acad Sci USA 93:156–160, 1996.

73. Sharifi AM, Schiffrin EL: Apoptosis in vasculature of spontaneously hypertensive rats: effect of an angiotensin converting enzyme inhibitor and a calcium channel antagonist. Am J Hypertens 11:1108–1116, 1998.

74. Borhani NO, Mercuri M, Borhani PA, et al: Final outcome results of the Multicenter Isradipine Diuretic Atherosclerosis Study (MIDAS). A randomized controlled trial. JAMA 276:785–791, 1996.

75. Zanchetti A, Rosei EA, Dal Palu C,et al: The Verapamil in Hypertension and Atherosclerosis Study (VHAS): Results of long-term randomized treatment with either verapamil or chlorthalidone on carotid intima-media thickness. J Hypertens 16:1667–1676, 1998.

76. Girerd X, Giannattasio C, Moulin C, et al: Regression of radial artery wall hypertrophy and improvement of carotid artery compliance after long-term antihypertensive treatment in elderly patients. J Am Coll Cardiol 31:1064–1073, 1998.

77. Domanski MJ, Davis BR, Pfeffer MA, et al: Isolated systolic hypertension: Prognostic information provided by pulse pressure. Hypertension 34: 375–380, 1999.

78. Bohlen HG: Localization of vascular resistance changes during hypertension. Hypertension 8:181–183, 1986.

79. Korsgaard N, Aalkjær C, Heagerty AM, et al: Histology of subcutaneous small arteries from patients with essential hypertension. Hypertension 22: 523–526, 1993.

80. Schiffrin EL, Deng LY, Larochelle P: Morphology of resistance arteries and comparison of effects of vasoconstrictors in mild essential hypertensive patients. Clin Invest Med 16:177–186, 1993.

81. Mulvany MJ, Baumbach GL, Aalkjaer C, et al: Vascular remodeling [letter to the editor]. Hypertension 27:505–506, 1996.

82. Intengan HD, Thibault G, Li JS, Schiffrin EL: Resistance artery mechanics, structure, and extracellular components in spontaneously hypertensive rats: Effects of angiotensin receptor antagonism and converting enzyme inhibition. Circulation 100:2267–2275, 1999.

83. Sharifi AM, Li JS, Endemann D, Schiffrin EL: Comparison of effects of the angiotensin converting enzyme inhibitor enalapril and the calcium channel antagonist amlodipine on small artery structure and composition, and on endothelial dysfunction in SHR. J Hypertens 16: 457–466, 1998.

84. Intengan HD, Deng LY, Li JS, Schiffrin EL: Mechanics and composition of human subcutaneous resistance arteries in essential hypertension. Hypertension 33 (Pt II):366–372, 1999.

85. Aalkjaer C, Heagerty AM, Petersen KK, et al: Evidence for increased media thickness, increased neuronal amine uptake, and depressed excitation-contraction coupling in isolated resistance vessels from essential hypertensives. Circ Res 61:181–186, 1987.

86. Schiffrin EL, Deng LY, Larochelle P: Blunted effects of endothelin upon small subcutaneous resistance arteries of mild essential hypertensive patients. J Hypertens 10:437–444, 1992.

87. Lockette W, Otsuka Y, Carretero O: The loss of endothelium-dependent vascular relaxation in hypertension. Hypertension 8(Suppl. 2):II-61–II-66, 1986.

88. Deng LY, Li J-S, Schiffrin EL: Endothelium-dependent relaxation of small arteries from essential hypertensive patients. Clin Sci 88:611–622, 1995.

89. Panza JA, Quyyumi AA, Brush JE, Epstein SE: Abnormal endothelium dependent vascular relaxation in patients with essential hypertension. N Engl J Med 323:22–27, 1990.

90. Tschudi MR, Mesaros S, Lüscher TF, Malinski T: Direct in situ measurement of nitric oxide in mesenteric resistance arteries. Hypertension 27:32–35, 1996.

91. Diedrich DA, Yang Z, Bühler FR, Lüscher TF: Impaired endothelium-dependent relaxations in hypertensive small arteries involve the cyclooxygenase pathway. Am J Physiol 258:H445–H451, 1990.

92. Gibbons GH, Pratt RE, Dzau VJ: Vascular smooth muscle cell hypertrophy vs. hyperplasia: Autocrine transforming growth factor-ß1 expression determines growth response to angiotensin II. J Clin Invest 90:456–461, 1992.

93. Griffin SA, Brown WCB, Macpherson F, et al: Angiotensin II causes vascular hypertrophy in part by a non-pressor mechanism. Hypertension 17:626–635, 1991.

94. Sabri A, Lévy BI, Poitevin P, et al: Differential roles of AT_1 and AT_2 receptor subtypes in vascular trophic and phenotypic changes in response to stimulation with angiotensin II. Arterioscler Thromb Vasc Biol 17:257–264, 1997.

95. Touyz RM, Schiffrin EL: Angiotensin II regulates vascular smooth muscle cell pH, contraction, and growth via tyrosine kinase-dependent signaling pathways. Hypertension 30[Pt 1]:222–229, 1997.

96. Touyz RM, He G, Deng LY, Schiffrin EL: Role of extracellular signal-regulated kinases in angiotensin II-stimulated contraction of smooth muscle cells from human resistance arteries. Circulation 99:392–399, 1999.

97. Rajagopalan S, Laursen JB, Borthayre A, et al: Role for endothelin-1 in angiotensin II-mediated hypertension. Hypertension 30:29–34, 1997.

98. D'Uscio LV, Moreau P, Shaw S, et al: Effects of chronic ETA-receptor blockade in angiotensin II-induced hypertension. Hypertension 29:435–441, 1997.

99. Griendling KK, Minieri CA, Ollerenshaw JD, et al: Angiotensin II stimulates NADH and NADPH oxidase activity in cultured vascular smooth muscle cells. Circ Res 74:1141–1148, 1994.

100. Huraux C, Makita T, Kurz S, et al: Superoxide production, risk factors, and endothelium-dependent relaxations in human internal mammary arteries. Circulation 99:53–59, 1999.

101. Laursen JB, Rajagopalan S, Galis Z, et al: Role of superoxide in angiotensin II-induced but not catecholamine-induced hypertension. Circulation 95:588–593, 1997.

102. Diep Q, Li JS, Schiffrin EL: In vivo study of the role of AT₁ and AT₂ angiotensin receptors in apoptosis in rat blood vessels. Hypertension 34:617–624, 1999.

103. Siragy HM, Carey RM: The subtype-2 (AT₂) angiotensin receptor regulates renal cyclic guanosine 3',5'-monophosphate and AT₁ receptor-mediated prostaglandin E₂ production in conscious rats. J Clin Invest 97:1978–1982, 1996.

104. Li J-S, Schiffrin EL: Chronic endothelin receptor antagonist treatment of young spontaneously hypertensive rats. J Hypertens 13:647–652, 1995.

105. Li J-S, Schiffrin EL: Effect of calcium channel blockade or angiotensin converting enzyme inhibition on structure of coronary, renal and other small arteries in SHR. J Cardiovasc Pharmacol 28:68–74, 1996.

106. Thybo NK, Korsgaard N, Eriksen S, et al: Dose-dependent effects of perindopril on blood pressure and small-artery structure. Hypertension 23:659–666, 1994.

107. Baumbach GL, Heistad DD: Remodeling of cerebral arterioles in chronic hypertension. Hypertension 13:968–972, 1989.

108. Dohi Y, Criscione L, Pfeiffer K, Lüscher TF: Angiotensin blockade or calcium antagonists improve endothelial dysfunction in hypertension: Studies in perfused mesenteric resistance arteries. J Cardiovasc Pharmacol 24:372–379, 1994.

109. Rizzoni D, Castellano M, Porteri E, et al: Effects of low and high doses of fosinopril on the structure and function of resistance arteries. Hypertension 26:118–123, 1995.

110. Deng LY, Schiffrin EL: Effect of antihypertensive treatment on response to endothelin of resistance arteries of hypertensive rats. J Cardiovasc Pharmacol 21:725–731, 1993.

111. Harrap SB, Van der Merwe WM, Griffin SA, et al: Brief angiotensin converting enzyme inhibitor treatment in young spontaneously hypertensive rats reduces blood pressure long-term. Hypertension 16:603–614, 1990.

112. Shaw LM, George PR, Oldham AA, Heagerty AM: A comparison of the effect of angiotensin converting enzyme inhibition and angiotensin II receptor antagonism on the structural changes associated with hypertension in rat small arteries. J Hypertens 13:1135–1143, 1995.

113. Li J-S, Sharifi MA, Schiffrin EL: Effect of AT₁ angiotensin receptor blockade on structure and function of small arteries in SHR. J Cardiovasc Pharmacol 30:75–83, 1997.

114. Schiffrin EL, Deng LY, Larochelle P: Effects of a beta blocker or a converting enzyme inhibitor on resistance arteries in essential hypertension. Hypertension 23:83–91, 1994.

115. Schiffrin EL, Deng LY, Larochelle P: Progressive improvement in the structure of resistance arteries of hypertensive patients after 2 years of treatment with an angiotensin converting enzyme inhibitor. Comparison with effects of a beta blocker. Am J Hypertens 8:229–236, 1995.

116. Thybo NK, Stephens N, Cooper A, et al: Effect of antihypertensive treatment on small arteries of patients with previously untreated essential hypertension. Hypertension 25 [Pt 1]:474–481, 1995.

117. Schiffrin EL, Deng LY: Comparison of effects of angiotensin converting enzyme inhibition and beta blockade on function of small arteries from hypertensive patients. Hypertension 25 [Pt 2]:699–703, 1995.

118. Rizzoni D, Muiesan ML, Porteri E, et al: Effects of long-term antihypertensive treatment with lisinopril on resistance arteries in hypertensive patients with left ventricular hypertrophy. J Hypertens 15:197–204, 1997.

119. Mancini GBJ, Henry GC, Macaya C, et al: Angiotensin-converting enzyme inhibition with quinapril improves endothelial vasomotor dysfunction in patients with coronary artery disease—The TREND (Trial on Reversing ENdothelial Dysfunction) study. Circulation 94:258–265, 1996.

120. Schiffrin EL, Park JB, Intengan HD, Touyz RM: Correction of arterial structure and endothelial dysfunction in human essential hypertension by the angiotensin antagonist losartan. Circulation 101, 2000 [in press].

121. Padmanabhan N, Jardine AG, McGrath JC, Connell JMC: Angiotensin-converting enzyme-independent contraction to angiotensin I in human resistance arteries. Circulation 99:2914–2920, 1999.

122. Schiffrin EL, Deng LY: Structure and function of resistance arteries of hypertensive patients treated with a b-blocker or a calcium channel antagonist. J Hypertens 14:1247–1255, 1996.

123. Schiffrin EL: Effect of antihypertensive therapy on small artery structure in hypertensive patients [letter]. Hypertension 26:716–717, 1995.

124. Agabiti Rosei E, Rizzoni D, Castellano M, et al: Media:lumen ratio in human small resistance arteries is related to forearm minimal vascular resistance. J Hypertens 13:349–355, 1995.

125. Motz W, Strauer BE: Improvement of coronary flow reserve after long-term therapy with enalapril. Hypertension 27:1031–1038, 1996.

126. Virdis A, Ghiadoni L, Lucarini A, et al: Presence of cardiovascular structural changes in essential hypertensive patients with coronary microvascular disease and effects of long-term treatment. Am J Hypertens 9:361–369, 1996.

127. Lund-Johansen P, Omvik P: Acute and chronic effects of drugs with different actions on adrenergic receptors: a comparison between alpha blockers and different types of beta blockers with and without vasodilating effect. Cardiovasc Drugs Ther 5:605–615, 1991.

128. UK Prospective Diabetes Study Group: Efficacy of atenolol and captopril in reducing riskof macrovascular and microvascular complicqations in type 2 diabetes: UKPDS 39. BMJ 317:713–720, 1998.

129. Hanson L, Lindholm LH, Niskanen L, et al: Effect of angiotensin converting enzyme inhibition compared with conventional therapy on cardiovascular morbidity and mortality in hypertension: The Captopril Prevention Project (CAPPP) randomised trial. Lancet 353:611–616, 1999.

130. Heart Outcomes Prevention Evaluation Study Investigators: Effects of an angiotensin-converting-enzyme inhibitor, ramipril, on cardiovascular events in high-risk patients.N Engl J Med 342:145–153, 2000.

CHAPTER 20

AT_1 Receptor Antagonists and the Kidney

R.T. GANSEVOORT, M.D., Ph.D.

A. MIMRAN, M.D., Ph.D.

D. DE ZEEUW, M.D., Ph.D.

BERNARD JOVER, Ph.D.

The renin-angiotensin-aldosterone system (RAAS) is of great importance for the primary function of the kidneys: to maintain near-constancy of the volume and composition of extracellular fluid. The main effector hormone of this system is angiotensin II (Ang II). This chapter discusses the pathophysiology of progressive renal disease and the effects of various therapeutic interventions in the RAAS, with special emphasis on the renal effects of AT_1 receptor antagonists.

■ Pathophysiology of Progressive Renal Disease

If the kidney sustains damage, from whatever cause, progressive deterioration of renal function generally follows. The rate of deterioration of renal function varies widely among patients but seems remarkably constant in each individual, regardless of the original renal disorder. Figure 1 summarizes the factors hypothesized to cause this deterioration.

Brenner et al. argue that after renal damage a portion of nephrons is destroyed. In the remaining nephrons, blood flow and filtration rate increase to compensate for the loss of renal function. This process exposes the remnant nephrons to an elevated intraglomerular pressure, which leads to mechanical damage of the glomerular capillary wall, glomerulosclerosis, and further nephron loss.[1] In specific conditions, such as diabetes, the rise in intraglomerular pressure may result from a maladaptation of the preglomerular vessels to the prevailing systemic blood pressure, resulting in a relatively dilated vas afferens. Consistent with this hypothesis is the finding in clinical trials that high blood pressure is associated with an increased rate of renal disease progression and that lowering blood pressure results in improved renal prognosis.

Remuzzi and Bertani offer another approach to explain renal disease progression. They argue that the first step is disruption of glomerular permselectivity,[2]

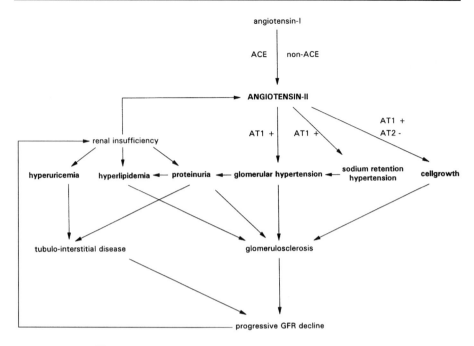

Figure 1.   Factors contributing to renal disease progression.

which may be mediated by mechanical injury to the glomerular capillary wall or, in the absence of increased glomerular capillary pressure toxins or immune reactants. Once glomerular permselectivity has been disrupted, the progression to end-stage renal failure is triggered by the exposure of glomerular, mesangial and tubulointerstitial cells to an abnormal protein load. Indeed, in numerous clinical studies that tried to identify risk factors for progressive loss of renal function, the severity of proteinuria correlated best with the rate of renal function decline.[3] Furthermore, studies with various renoprotective strategies (low-protein diets and various classes of blood pressure-lowering agents) have shown that the decrease in proteinuria correlates better with renal function outcome than the decrease in blood pressure. The more proteinuria is lowered, the better renal outcome will be.

Other factors possibly involved in the progressive decline of renal function include hyperlipidemia, which may be primary or secondary to renal disease. Clinical evidence suggests that hyperlipidemia modifies the rate of renal deterioration.[4,5] This relationship, however, was found in only a few of the many clinical studies that tried to establish an association between the rate of renal function decline and various lipoproteins. Thus, the influence of lipoproteins may be either small or limited to particular disease conditions. Of interest, Kasiske et al. showed in a recent meta-analysis that although lipid reduction in most individual trials had no significant effect on the rate of renal function decline, it did have a statistically significant overall impact.[6]

Finally, many patients with renal disease have increased serum levels of uric acid. An elevated uric acid level has been hypothesized to cause cardiovascular disease[7-9] as well as chronic tubulointerstitial disease (so-called gouty nephropathy).[10] Some investigators, however, argue that gouty nephropathy is a nonentity. Nickeleit et al., for example, concluded on the basis of an investigation of more than 11,000 autopsy cases that chronic uric acid deposits in the kidney rarely cause terminal renal failure.[11] In almost all cases, deterioration of renal function could be better explained by other well-known risk factors, and in a significant number of cases renal tophi were found without evidence of renal malfunction. The authors could not exclude, however, the possibility that renal tophi in association with an underlying renal disease may lead to more rapid deterioration of renal function. Clearly, further studies are needed to confirm a possible pathogenic role for uric acid in the development of renal disease and a possible beneficial effect of lowering serum uric acid levels.

■ Pathophysiologic Role of Angiotensin II in Progressive Renal Disease

Ang II has a central role in the pathophysiologic mechanisms that lead to progression of renal disease (see Fig. 1). Ang II increases systemic blood pressure via direct vasoconstricting actions and release of aldosterone, which in turn leads to water and salt retention. The increased systemic blood pressure is transmitted into the glomerulus, where the elevated intraglomerular pressure may lead to mechanical damage of the glomerular capillary wall. In addition, Ang II has specific effects on renal hemodynamics. Infusion of Ang II in experimental models indicates that the efferent arteriole is more sensitive than the afferent arteriole to the vasoconstrictor effects of Ang II.[12] Because of efferent vasoconstriction during Ang II infusion, intraglomerular pressure increases more than might be expected from the Ang II-induced rise in systemic blood pressure alone.[13] Finally, several experiments have shown that Ang II modulates growth of both vascular smooth muscle cells and mesangial cells, supposedly leading to hypertrophy and glomerulosclerosis.[14–16] For a detailed description of the renal effects of Ang II refer to chapters 13 and 20.

■ Angiotensin-converting Enzyme Inhibitors and Renal Disease Progression

Because of the various pathophysiologic renal actions of Ang II, one may expect beneficial results from agents that modulate the renin-angiotensin system. Angiotensin-converting enzyme (ACE) inhibitors were the first class of pharmaceutical agents available in clinical practice for this purpose. They lower systemic blood pressure through vasodilation and inhibition of aldosterone release, which leads to diminished retention of water and salt. In numerous experimental studies ACE inhibitors have been shown to lower intraglomerular pressure more than conventional antihypertensives.[17] Although in clinical studies intraglomerular pressure cannot be measured directly, ACE inhibitors showed a renal hemodynamic profile (increase in renal plasma flow with maintenance of or slight decrease in glomerular filtration rate) that suggests reduction of intraglomerular pressure by means of postglomerular vasodilation. Furthermore, ACE inhibitors have superior antiproteinuric efficacy compared with other classes of antihypertensives, even at doses that induce similar systemic blood pressure reduction.[18] Lastly, as a consequence of their antiproteinuric effect, ACE inhibitors ameliorate the deranged lipid profile in patients with nephrotic range proteinuria.[19,20] As a result of these beneficial short-term effects on intermediate parameters, one would expect these agents to have renoprotective effects. In a number of recent clinical trials, ACE inhibitors slowed the rate of renal decline in both diabetic and nondiabetic renal disease, and this effect appears to be greater than the effect obtained by lowering blood pressure alone.[21,22] Because of their superior renoprotective effect, ACE inhibitors have become the agents of choice for the symptomatic treatment of patients with renal disease. Several agents in this class have been approved for renoprotection by regulatory authorities.

Treatment Resistance to ACE Inhibitors

Unfortunately, the renoprotective effect of ACE inhibition varies greatly. In some patients ACE inhibition shows little or no effect on the rate of renal decline. The variability in the renoprotective effect of ACE inhibition may be explained by several factors:

1. In patients with water and/or salt retention, the activity of the renin-angiotensin system is decreased. In such patients ACE inhibitors have low efficacy as antihypertensive or antiproteinuric agents.[23] This specific reason for treatment resistance to ACE inhibitors may be overcome by prescription of a salt-restricted diet or diuretics.

2. Several investigators have shown that during chronic ACE inhibition the concentration of plasma Ang II does not fall to zero. This so-called escape phenomenon may be caused by the fact that during ACE inhibitor treatment plasma renin activity rises as a result of negative feedback mechanisms. In at least some patients, substantial production of Ang II, with diminished efficacy of ACE inhibitors, may occur because ACE inhibitors do not induce 100% inhibition of ACE and because non-ACE pathways can convert Ang I into Ang II (for further details, see chapter 1).

3. Differences in genotype among patients may play a role. The ACE gene exists in two isoforms, a D (deletion) and an I (insertion) allele. Patients with a DD genotype have higher serum ACE concentrations than patients with an ID or II genotype.[24] Ueda et al. reported that healthy subjects with a DD genotype displayed more Ang I pressor responsiveness after an intravenous dose of enalapril than subjects with an II or ID genotype.[25] Van der Kleij et al. found smaller short-term effects of ACE inhibitors on blood pressure, renal hemodynamics, and proteinuria in patients with nondiabetic renal disease and the DD genotype, especially when they were on a high sodium diet.[26] Finally, during long-term ACE inhibition patients with the DD genotype have a worse long-term outcome in renal function than patients with the II or ID genotype in both diabetic[27] and nondiabetic renal disease.[28] These data indicate that ACE polymorphism may identify a subgroup of patients who fail to benefit from standard ACE inhibition therapy. In DD patients, because of their higher ACE levels, a standard dose of an ACE inhibitor may be insufficient to inhibit all effects mediated by the renin-angiotensin system.

4. Ang II mediates its effects by binding to receptors. In humans the Ang II receptor appears to exist in at least two subtypes, AT_1 and AT_2. The AT_1 receptor mediates most of the known renal actions of Ang II (see Fig. 1). By binding to the AT_1 receptor, Ang II elicits the release of aldosterone in the kidney, leading to water and salt retention and thus to hypertension. The AT_1 receptor also is

engaged in the regulation of vascular tone of the afferent and especially the efferent glomerular arteriole. Furthermore, the AT$_1$ receptor has been involved in cellular proliferation. The role of the AT$_2$ receptor in the kidney has not been fully clarified. Knowledge so far indicates that blockade of this receptor subtype induces a mild diuretic effect.[29] In vitro studies also have shown that stimulation of the AT$_2$ receptor induces an antiproliferative effect opposite to that of AT$_1$ receptor stimulation (see Fig. 1).[30] Of interest, Klahr et al. reported that AT$_2$ receptor blockade exacerbated the fibrosis of the tubulointerstitium in a model of obstructive nephropathy.[31] A comparable finding was reported by Ma and coworkers, who showed accelerated fibrosis and collagen disposition in the renal interstitium in AT$_2$ receptor-null mutant mice with ureteral obstruction.[32] This AT$_2$ receptor-mediated antifibrotic effect of Ang II may participate in the beneficial effect of AT$_1$ receptor blockade. However, AT$_2$ receptor-mediated effects also may be deleterious. Ito and associates demonstrated AT$_2$ receptor afferent vasodilatation in an in-vitro study.[33] ACE inhibitors, in general, decrease serum and tissue concentrations of Ang II. Their net effect thus depends on the balance between a beneficial effect mediated via the AT$_1$ receptor and a possible deleterious effect mediated by the AT$_2$ receptor. In general, this balance may be shifted toward the beneficial side during ACE inhibition, but in some patients deleterious effects may play a significant role.

5. ACE appears not to be specific. Besides cleaving Ang I to Ang II, it also degrades bradykinin (among other effects). During ACE inhibition, therefore, bradykinin accumulates. Several authors found in experimental studies that bradykinin antagonists may counteract, at least partially, the antiproteinuric effect of ACE inhibitors.[34–36] These studies, however, can be criticized methodologically. In contrast, Wapstra et al. recently showed that the antiproteinuric and blood pressure-lowering effect of ACE inhibitors in the adriamycin rat model can be fully explained by Ang II-related effects. The bradykinin system appeared not to be involved.[37] The bradykinin-accumulating effect of ACE inhibitors also is thought to be important in the genesis of side effects such as cough and angioedema. The fact that these side effects do not occur in every patient implies perhaps that the effect of ACE inhibitors on the kinin system may vary substantially among individuals. This variation also may hold true for the beneficial effects.

■ *AT$_1$ Antagonists and Progression of Renal Disease*

The resistance of a substantial percentage of patients to treatment with ACE inhibitors has led to a growing interest in other agents that modulate the renin-angiotensin system. Recently, another class of agents has become available for clinical use, the AT$_1$ receptor antagonists. These drugs, which specifically block the AT$_1$ receptor-mediated effects of Ang II, have been shown to lower blood pressure and to induce mild natriuretic and diuretic effects (see chapter 13). The U.S. Food and Drug Administration and European regulatory authorities have approved these drugs for the indication of essential hypertension. A renal indication has not yet been granted but is likely to follow. The following sections discuss the results obtained with AT$_1$ receptor antagonists in experimental renal disease, their clinical effects on intermediate parameters for renal disease progression in short-term studies, and their effect on long-term outcome in patients with renal disease.

Experimental Evidence in Models of Progressive Renal Disease

Many experimental studies have assessed the role of AT_1 receptor antagonists in various models of progressive renal disease. These studies uniformly showed the superior efficacy of AT_1 receptor antagonists in retarding the development of proteinuria and glomerulosclerosis compared with antihypertensives that do not interfere with the renin-angiotensin system, even in doses that induce a similar blood pressure reduction.[38–40]

Clinical Evidence Based on Intermediate Parameters for Progression of Renal Disease

The clinical effects of AT_1 receptor antagonists on intermediate parameters for progression of renal disease (blood pressure, renal hemodynamics, proteinuria, uric acid, and lipid profile) have been reported in several short-term studies of healthy volunteers, patients with essential hypertension, and patients with renal disease.

Healthy Volunteers

Studies performed in healthy volunteers are summarized in Table 1.[41–46] The general impression from these short-term trials is that AT_1 antagonists lower blood pressure, and increase renal plasma flow but have no effect on glomerular filtration rate. However, the response to AT_1 antagonists varies remarkably.

Doig et al. examined the response to an oral dose of 100 mg losartan or placebo in volunteers studied in salt-replete and salt-depleted states.[43] Salt depletion was achieved by 4 days of dietary salt restriction (40 mmol sodium/day) and oral diuretic therapy (furosemide, 40 mg twice daily). In the salt-replete state no changes were observed with the AT_1 antagonist in blood pressure or creatinine clearance (Fig. 2). In the salt-depleted state, as expected, the renin-angiotensin

Table 1. Studies with AT_1 Receptor Antagonists of Intermediate Endpoints for Renal Function Deterioration in Healthy Volunteers

Author	n	Agent (mg/day)	DT (days)	Salt Intake*	Water Load†	DBP (%)	GFR (%)	ERPF (%)	UAE/Uprot (%)
Burnier[41] (1993)	23	Losartan (100)	1	50	12	–6	+3	–2	ND
				200	12	+1	+1	+3	ND
Burnier[42] (1995)	24	Irbesartan (50)	8	100	5	–7	–9	+11	ND
Doig[43] (1995)	8	Losartan (100)	1	40‡	NS	–20§	–64§	ND	ND
				100	NS	–4	0	ND	ND
Schmitt[44] (1996)	10	Losartan (50)	1	100	NS	–1	+5	+13§	ND
Price[45] (1997)	10	Eprosartan (400)	1	100	NS	–13§	+2	+16§	ND
Fumeron[46] (1998)	12	Valsartan (80)	4	200	NS	–2	–2	+14§	ND

* mmol/day   † ml/kg   ‡ Plus furosemide   § $p < 0.05$

DT = duration of treatment, DBP = diastolic blood pressure, GFR = glomerular filtration rate, ERPF = effective renal plasma flow, UAE = urinary albumin excretion, Uprot = proteinuria, NS = not stated, ND = not done.

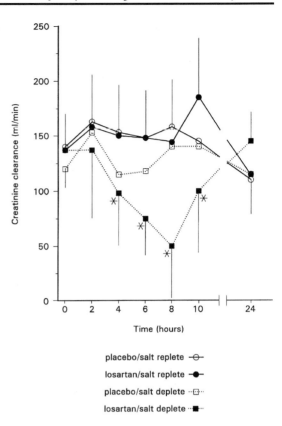

Figure 2. Mean (± SD) creatinine clearance after placebo *(open symbols)* or the AT₁ receptor antagonist losartan *(solid symbols)* in 8 salt-replete *(circles)* or salt-depleted *(squares)* normal volunteers. * p < 0.05 vs. placebo in volunteers of the same salt status. (From Doig JK, MacFayden RJ, Sweet CS, Reid JL: Haemodynamic and renal responses to oral losartan potassium during salt depletion or salt repletion in normal human volunteers. J Cardiovasc Pharmacol 25:511–517, 1995, with permission.)

placebo/salt replete —○—
losartan/salt replete —●—
placebo/salt deplete ··□··
losartan/salt deplete ··■··

system was activated, as reflected by a significant increase in plasma renin. In this setting the AT₁ receptor antagonist showed marked effects. After correction for placebo effect, a fall in blood pressure of 14 mmHg was observed, as well as a decrease in creatinine clearance of 90 ml/min. These data imply that assessment of the clinical effects of AT₁ receptor antagonists requires an awareness of the patient's dietary salt status. These effects are mitigated when the renin-angiotensin system is deactivated by sodium repletion.

Dietary salt intake appears not to be the only factor that influences the activity of the renin-angiotensin system. Burnier et al. reported the effects of losartan (100 mg orally) in subjects maintained on a high-sodium (200 mmol/day) or low-sodium (50 mmol/day) diet.[41] Compared with placebo, losartan increased urinary sodium excretion and urine volume. Surprisingly, no changes were observed in blood pressure, renal plasma flow, or glomerular filtration rate, not even in subjects on the low-salt diet. In contrast, in another study two years later, the same authors found that irbesartan, another AT₁ antagonist, was associated with significant changes in blood pressure and renal hemodynamics in subjects on a similar sodium-restricted diet.[42] These conflicting observations drew attention to a possible confounding factor.[47] Except for the drug, the only difference between the two protocols was the amount of water load. In the first study, subjects received a water load of 12 ml/kg to ensure adequate urine flow rate for renal function studies. A clear decrease in plasma levels of Ang II was observed. In the second study, the water load was less than half that amount, and no decrease in plasma Ang II levels was observed. These results demonstrate that acute water loading is an important consideration because it may change the level of activity of the renin-angiotensin system and diminish the renal effects of AT_1 antagonists.

In conclusion, AT_1 antagonists lower systemic blood pressure and increase renal plasma flow in non–sodium-replete, non–water-replete healthy volunteers.

Patients with Essential Hypertension

Studies that report the renal effects of AT_1 antagonists in patients with essential hypertension are summarized in Table 2.[48–53] In general, a decrease in systemic blood pressure is observed, whereas renal plasma flow increases and glomerular filtration rate remains stable. Several studies show effects on urinary albumin excretion rates.[49–52] The urinary loss of albumin decreases with a range from –29% through –59%. As in healthy volunteers, the renal response to AT_1 antagonism varies widely. As explained above, this variation may be due to differences in salt intake and water loading in the various studies. Unfortunately, however, not all studies in patients with essential hypertension provide detailed information about salt intake or the exact amount of water loading.

Of interest, Pechere-Bertschi et al. drew attention to a third possible confounding factor in the assessment of the renal effects of AT_1 antagonists.[53] They compared the renal response to the AT_1 receptor antagonist irbesartan with the renal response to the ACE inhibitor enalapril. Each agent induced renal vasodilatation with no significant change in glomerular filtration rate. However, the time course of the renal effects appeared to differ markedly between the two drugs. Irbesartan had no significant acute effect after the first dose, but during chronic administration a renal vasodilatory response was found both 12 and 24 hours after dosing (Fig. 3). In contrast, enalapril was effective acutely. During

Table 2.   Studies with AT_1 Receptor Antagonists of Intermediate Endpoints for Renal Function Deterioration in Patients with Essential Hypertension

Author	n	Agent (mg/day)	DT (days)	Salt Intake*	Water Load†	DBP (%)	GFR (%)	ERPF (%)	UAE/Uprot (%)
Kawabata[48] (1994)	12	Candesartan (4/8)	14	NS	800	–8‡	–2	+12‡	ND
Erley[49] (1995)	9	Losartan (50)	28	110	NS	–5	0	+7	–59‡
Fauvel[50] (1996)	10	Losartan (50)	28	200	120	–9‡	–4	–1	–30‡
Nielsen[51] (1997)	47	Losartan (50)	84	NS	0	–9‡	ND	ND	–30‡
Chan[52] (1997)	12	Losartan (50/100)	84	125	0	–14‡	ND	ND	–29‡
Pechere[53] (1998)	10	Irbesartan	84	200	NS	–11‡	+7	+22	ND

* mmol/day   † ml   ‡ p < 0.05
DT = duration of treatment, DBP = diastolic blod pressure, GFR = glomerular filtration rate, ERPF = effective renal plasma flow, UAE = urinary albumin excretion, Uprot = proteinuria, NS = not stated, ND = not done.

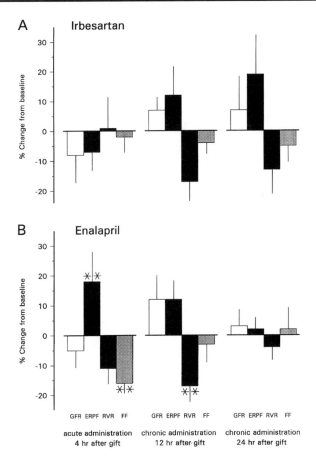

Figure 3.   Effects of administration of the AT₁ receptor antagonist irbesartan *(panel a)* and the ACE inhibitor enalapril *(panel b)* on glomerular filtration rate (GFR), effective renal plasma flow (ERPF), renal vascular resistance (RVR,) and filtration fraction (FF) in hypertensive patients. Bars are means ± SEM. ** p < 0.01 vs. baseline. (From Pechere-Bertschi A, Nussberger J, Decosterd L, et al: Renal response to the angiotensin II receptor subtype 1 antagonist irbesartan versus enalapril in hypertensive patients. J Hypertens 16:385–393, 1998, with permission).

chronic treatment a similar renal hemodynamic profile was observed 12 hours after the last dose as with the AT₁ antagonist. However, no residual effect was found after 24 hours. Both the AT₁ antagonist and the ACE inhibitor lowered mean ambulatory blood pressure effectively, with no significant differences between treatments at any time point. Clearly, duration of treatment and time of day at which effects are measured are important factors in assessing the renal efficacy of irbesartan. The full effect of irbesartan—and perhaps of all AT₁ antagonists—is established only after several days of treatment, but at that point irbesartan shows better 24-hour coverage than enalapril.

Patients with Renal Disease

Table 3 summarizes the 11 studies performed in patients with renal disease.[52,54–63] Again, the response varies widely. As discussed above, this variability may be explained in part by differences in salt intake and water load during

Table 2.   Studies with AT_1 Receptor Antagonists of Intermediate Endpoints for Renal Function Deterioration in Patients with Renal Disease

Author	n	Agent (mg/day)	DT (days)	Salt Intake*	Water Load†	DBP (%)	GFR (%)	ERPF (%)	UAE/Uprot (%)
Gansevoort[54] (1994)	11 nonDM	Losartan (100)	56	120	NS	−15‡	−6	13‡	−46‡
Chan[52] (1995)	7 DM 2	Losartan (50/100)	84	125	0	−10‡	ND	ND	−24‡
Perico[55] (1997)	94 nonDM	Valsartan (40/80)	63	NS	NS	−8‡	−2	ND	−4‡
Buter[56] (1997)	17 nonDM	Candesartan (8)	5	75	NS	−9‡	0	+4‡	ND
Perico[57] (1998)	9 nonDM	Irbesartan (100)	28	170	NS	−2	+2	+28‡	−38‡
Plum[58] (1998)	5 nonDM	Valsartan (80)	180	250	0	−5‡	−15	+1	−55‡
Holdaas[59] (1998)	15 nonDM	Losartan (50/100)	28	NS	2500	−9‡	−3	+6	−24
Fernandez[60] (1998)	24 nonDM	Losartan (50)	84	NS	0	−18‡	0	ND	−19‡
Toto[61] (1998)	24 DM 60 nonDM	Losartan (50/100)	84	150	NS	−11‡	−1	+6	−23‡
Russo[62] 1999	8 nonDM	Losartan (50)	84	140	0	−5	−5	ND	−27‡
Andersen[63] (1999)	16 DM 1	Losartan (100)	56	170	0	−9‡	−1	ND	−45‡

* mmol/day   † ml   ‡ $p < 0.05$

DT = duration of treatment, DBP = diastolic blood pressure, GFR = glomerular filtration rate, ERPF = effective renal plasma flow, UAE = urinary albumin excretion, Uprot = proteinuria, NS = not stated, ND = not done.

renal function measurement. But in patients with renal disease, duration of treatment also seems to be important. We demonstrated that in 11 patients with proteinuric, nondiabetic renal disease the time-course of the antiproteinuric effect of AT_1 receptor antagonism has a slow onset (Fig. 4).[54] A maximal effect is reached 3–4 weeks after start of treatment. Of interest, after the dose of losartan was increased from 50 to 100 mg/day, blood pressure remained stable, whereas a statistically significant fall in proteinuria was seen. The nadir was reached after 3–4 weeks. These findings have implications for clinical practice as well as for the design of future trials. At least 4 weeks should elapse before the antiproteinuric efficacy of AT_1 receptor antagonists is evaluated. In addition, our data suggest that the dose-response curves of AT_1 antagonists for the parameter of proteinuria (and thus, perhaps, for renoprotection) may differ from the dose-response curves for the parameter of blood pressure.

During the course of clinical testing with AT_1 antagonists, losartan produced a transient uricosuric effect and a concomitant decrease in serum uric acid concentration in normal volunteers,[64] hypertensive patients,[65] and patients with renal disease.[66] Curiously, EXP 3174, the active metabolite of losartan,[67] and

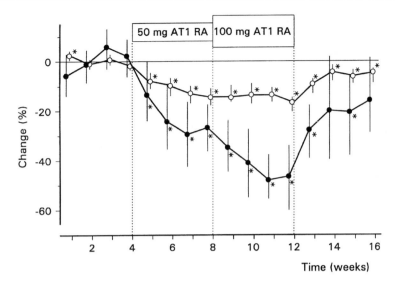

Figure 4.   The course of the effect (median ± 95% confidence interval) of AT₁ receptor antagonism (50 and 100 mg losartan, respectively) on blood pressure *(open symbols)* and urinary protein
excretion *(solid symbols)* in 11 patients with proteinuria due to nondiabetic renal disease. Before
and after the AT₁ receptor antagonist placebo was administered. * p < 0.05 vs. mean of the 4 baseline values. (From Gansevoort RT, de Zeeuw D, de Jong PE: Is the antiproteinuric effect of ACE inhibition mediated by interference in the renin angiotensin system? Kidney Int 45:861–867, 1994,
with permission.)

other AT₁ antagonists did not increase the urinary excretion of uric acid.[68–70] In a
direct comparative study, only losartan reduced serum uric acid levels, whereas
no effects were found with the ACE inhibitor enalapril.[71] These results suggest
that the uricosuric effect induced by losartan is not related to the renin-angiotensin system but is a unique property of losartan itself. Indeed, Edwards et
al. showed in an in-vitro study that the uricosuric effect of losartan is due to the
inhibition of urate reabsorption in the proximal tubule and is unrelated to AT₁
receptor activity.[72] It appears that losartan has far greater affinity for the
urate/anion exchanger than other AT₁ antagonists tested. The clinical implications of the uricosuric effect of losartan are difficult to appreciate. Because many
patients with renal disease have an increased serum level of uric acid and serum
uric acid has been mentioned as a possible causal factor in renal disease progression, the uricosuric effect of losartan may be beneficial. Negative effects, however, are also possible. For example, it has been hypothesized that, in extreme
situations, uric acid stones may develop if supersaturation concentrations of urinary uric acid are reached.[73] However, the current database on losartan shows
no such effect. Clearly larger experience is needed to draw any conclusions.

Several clinical trials in patients with essential hypertension have proved that
AT₁ antagonists have no effect on serum lipid profile.[74,75] In patients with renal
disease, however, the situation may be different. Hyperlipidemia is a well-recognized characteristic of patients with proteinuric renal disease. Increases in serum
total cholesterol, VLDL and LDL cholesterol, and triglycerides are common features of this form of secondary hyperlipidemia.[76] Recent studies also have shown
that lipoprotein (a) is elevated.[77–79] Such a profile is considered highly atherogenic

and may play a role in the progression of renal disease. Of interest, it recently was shown that various forms of symptomatic antiproteinuric treatment positively change the abnormal lipoprotein profile in patients with proteinuric renal disease.[19,20,79] A close correlation was found between the changes in proteinuria and the changes in the various parameters of the lipid profile.[20,79] In proteinuric patients, therefore, antiproteinuric agents, such as AT_1 receptor antagonists, may decrease the risk for atherosclerosis by improving the derangements in lipid profile and also slow the progression of renal disease.

Clinical Evidence in Long-term Renal Outcome Studies

No studies describe the long-term effects of AT_1 receptor antagonists on the decline of renal function in patients with renal disease. A number of such studies are under way, however, and their results are expected in the near future. The RENAAL study, for example, includes 1520 patients with diabetes mellitus type 2 and overt nephropathy, defined as serum creatinine of 133–265 mmol/L and proteinuria of more than 0.5 gm/day. Patients were randomized to either losartan (50 mg) or placebo, given in addition to another antihypertensive medication that does not interfere with the renin-angiotensin system. Target blood pressures are diastolic pressure below 90 and systolic pressure below 140 mmHg. This trial is powered to show a 20% decrease in the incidence of the combined end-points of doubling of serum creatinine and end-stage renal disease or death. Results are expected in November 2000. Table 4 summarizes the details of other long-term renal outcome studies. Several remarkable shortcomings are apparent in the present pursuit for renal indications. First, all studies are performed in patients with nephropathy due to diabetes mellitus type 2. Studies in patients with type 1 diabetic renal disease and nondiabetic populations have not been planned. Of greater importance, the effects of AT_1 antagonists are compared with the effects of placebo and calcium channel antagonists but not with the effects of ACE inhibitors. The present trials, therefore, cannot answer the most clinically relevant question: Are AT_1 antagonists as effective, less effective, or more effective than ACE inhibitors?

Until data from these long-term renal outcome studies become available, we must settle for what we can learn from the effects of AT_1 antagonists in experimental renal disease and short-term clinical studies that report on intermediate parameters for renal function outcome. Although the response to AT_1 receptor antagonism varies among the different studies, the general picture suggests a renal profile characterized by a decrease in blood pressure and proteinuria, an increase in renal plasma flow, and a fairly stable glomerular filtration rate. Agents with such a profile are expected to be renoprotective.

■ Are There Differences between AT_1 Antagonists and ACE Inhibitors?

AT_1 antagonists specifically block the AT_1 receptor-mediated effects of Ang II, whereas, in contrast to ACE inhibition, the AT_2 receptor continues to be exposed to Ang II. If the AT_2-mediated effects are indeed beneficial to the kidney, as presently assumed, AT_1 antagonists may have greater renoprotective effects than ACE inhibitors. Another theoretical advantage of AT_1 antagonists is avoidance of the "escape phenomenon" via non-ACE pathways or suboptimal ACE inhibition.

Table 4. Ongoing Long-term Trials of the Effect of AT_1 Receptor Antagonists on Renal Function Outcome in Patients with Renal Disease

Acronym	n	Diagnosis	Design	Randomization	Primary Endpoints	Duration (End of Study)
RENAAL	1520	DM 2 SBP > 100 mmHg 1.5 < sCreat < 3 mg/dl Uprot > 0.5 gm/day	DB-RCT	Losartan vs. placebo on top of normal AHT	1 Doubling sCreat 2 ESRD 3 Death	3 yr (2000)
IDNT	1650	DM 2 DBP > 85 mmHg or SBP > 135 mmHg 1 < sCreat < 3 mgdl Uprot > 1 gm/day	DB-RCT	Irbesartan vs. amlodipine vs. placebo on top of normal AHT	1 Doubling sCreat 2 ESRD 3 Death	3 yr (2001)
IRMA II	550	DM 2 DBP > 85 mmHg or SBP > 135 mmHg sCreat < 1.5 mg/dl 30 < UAE < 300 µg/day	DB-RCT	Irbesartan (150 mg) vs. irbesartan (300 mg) vs. placebo on top of normal AHT	1 UAE > 300 µg/day 2 Change in GFR	2 yr (2000)
ABCD-2V	722	DM 2 DBP > 75 mmHg	RCT	Moderate blood pressure lowering with valsartan vs. intensive blood pressure lowering with valsartan	1 CVM/M 2 DM-related micro-angiopathy (among which change in GFR)	5 yr (2003)

DM = diabetes mellitus, DBP = diastolic blood pressure, SBP = systolic blood pressure, sCreat = serum creatinine, Uprot = proteinuria, DB-RCT = double-blind randomized, controlled trial, AHT = antihypertensive therapy, CVM/M = cardiovascular morbidity and mortality, UAE = urinary albumin excretion rate.

On the other hand, the fact that AT_1 antagonists have no effect on bradykinin metabolism may be a disadvantage. Because of the various possibilities, great interest has arisen in studies that compare the renal effects of the two classes of drugs.

Experimental Evidence in Models of Progressive Renal Disease

Twenty-eight studies have compared the renal effects of AT_1 receptor antagonists and ACE inhibitors.[38–40,80–105] Of the various experimental models for progressive renal disease, the stroke-prone spontaneously hypertensive rat (n = 8) and the subtotally nephrectomized rat (n = 9) were used most frequently. In 21 of the 28 studies AT_1 receptor antagonists and ACE inhibitors showed similar benefits. One study found a statistically significantly superior renoprotective effect with an ACE inhibitor,[83] whereas six studies showed a superior effect with an AT_1 receptor antagonist.[85,86,92,95,98,99] In only one of the six studies, however, did the difference in favor of the AT_1 receptor antagonist reach statistical significance.[92] Remarkably, all of the studies favoring the AT_1 receptor antagonist were performed with candesartan. This finding may indicate possible differences among the various AT_1 receptor antagonists, but it also may be merely a matter of dosing. With candesartan a clear dose-response relationship was shown for renal end-points. In some studies only the 1- and 10-mg/kg/day doses had more effect than ACE inhibitors. In these particular studies, however, only one dose of the ACE inhibitor was applied. Higher dosages of the ACE inhibitor may have had a greater effect on the development of proteinuria and/or glomerulosclerosis. In conclusion, although data provided by comparative experimental studies are not unequivocal, the vast majority shows that the two classes of agents have similar renoprotective efficacy.

Although similar efficacy is highly suggestive, it does not necessarily mean that the two classes of agents exert their renoprotective action via the same mechanism. The net effect of the two classes of drugs may be equal but achieved via different mechanisms. This question can be investigated in studies that compare the effects of an AT_1 receptor antagonist and an ACE inhibitor, given at optimal doses, with the effects of combination therapy. To our knowledge, in experimental renal disease, only two such combination studies have been published. Neither Kohzuki et al. nor Ots et al. found a greater effect on the development of proteinuria and glomerulosclerosis with combination therapy than with an AT_1 receptor antagonist or an ACE inhibitor alone.[88,94] Unfortunately, interpretation of their findings is seriously hampered by the fact that with monotherapy alone a nearly maximal response was obtained. The amounts of proteinuria and glomerulosclerosis after monotherapy were in the range of values obtained in a control group with no renal disease. In this context a possible additive effect of combined treatment is difficult to prove. The question can be investigated only in the context of an insufficient antiproteinuric response on monotherapy. In our department Bos et al.[81] performed a study in rats with stable adriamycin nephrosis. The most important finding was that animals with a poor antiproteinuric response to initial lisinopril treatment did not improve with cotreatment with an AT_1 receptor antagonist or with an increased dose of the ACE inhibitor. Based on these findings, we conclude that no evidence from experimental models for renal disease progression indicates that the renoprotective effects of ACE inhibition or AT_1 receptor antagonism are caused by different mechanisms, such as the alleged beneficial effect of bradykinin accumulation during ACE inhibition.[106] This conclusion is further supported by the fact that in the comparative studies, the renoprotective effect of ACE inhibition was not attenuated by coadministration of the bradykinin antagonist HOE-140.[80,88,91]

Clinical Evidence Based on Intermediate Parameters for Progression of Renal Disease

The clinical renal profile of AT_1 antagonists in short-term studies closely mimics that of ACE inhibitors. The similarity becomes even clearer from direct comparative studies with the two classes of agents. In 11 patients with proteinuric nondiabetic renal disease, we demonstrated that the effects of losartan and enalapril were qualitatively and quantitatively similar (Fig. 5).[54] This principle applies to both renal hemodynamic and antiproteinuric effects. Our findings were corroborated by Nielsen et al. in a study in patients with essential hypertension and by Andersen et al. in patients with diabetic nephropathy.[51,63]

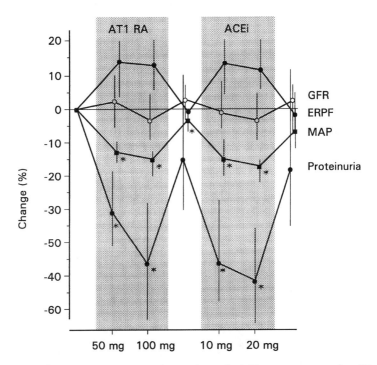

Figure 5. The effects (median ± 95% confidence interval) of AT_1 receptor antagonism (50 and 100 mg losartan, respectively) and ACE inhibition (10 and 20 mg enalapril, respectively) in 11 patients with proteinuria due to nondiabetic renal disease. Shaded areas represent study periods in which active treatment was given; non-shaded areas represent study periods in which placebo was given. Changes in blood pressure *(solid squares)* and urinary protein excretion *(solid circles)* are depicted in the upper panel; changes in glomerular filtration rate *(open circles)* and effective renal plasma flow *(solid circles)* are depicted in the lower panel. Parameters are expressed as percentage change from baseline. * p < 0.05 vs. baseline. (From Gansevoort RT, de Zeeuw D, de Jong PE: Is the antiproteinuric effect of ACE inhibition mediated by interference in the renin angiotensin system? Kidney Int 45:861–867, 1994, with permission.)

Unfortunately, all three studies failed to show the top of the dose-response curve with regard to the antiproteinuric effect achieved with AT_1 antagonists. Thus, proper dose-response research must be carried out (using higher dosages than customary in hypertension treatment) before we can reliably answer the question whether ACE inhibitors and AT_1 antagonists indeed have equal antiproteinuric efficacy. Such studies are currently ongoing.

Three publications report the effect of combining AT_1 receptor antagonists and ACE inhibitors in humans. Schmitt et al. found that in healthy volunteers a single dose of enalapril lowered blood pressure and increased renal plasma flow.[44] When losartan was added, no further changes were observed in these hemodynamic parameters, although an additive effect on plasma renin activity was observed. In patients with type 2 diabetic nephropathy, Hebert and coworkers showed that addition of losartan, 50 or 100 mg, during 1 week to long-term ACE inhibition did not result in an extra effect on blood pressure or proteinuria.[107] This study confirmed that plasma renin activity rose significantly during combined therapy compared with monotherapy, suggesting that with combined treatment a better inhibition of renin-angiotensin system activity can be obtained. Unfortunately, the rather short duration of the losartan treatment periods in both studies (single-dose administration and 1-week daily administration, respectively) seriously limits the conclusions that can be drawn. As discussed earlier, it takes at least 3–4 weeks for the antiproteinuric and hemodynamic effects of losartan to become fully established (see Fig. 4).

This drawback was eliminated in the third study. Russo et al. studied 8 normotensive patients with IgA nephropathy during five study phases (Fig. 6).[62] In the first phase, ACE inhibition was instituted for 12 weeks, resulting in a decrease in proteinuria of approximately 40%. In the second phase, losartan, 50

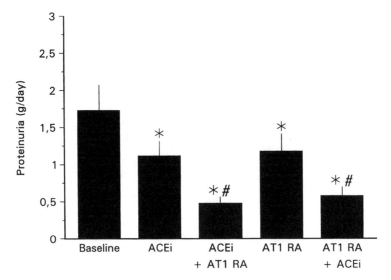

Figure 6. Urinary protein excretion in 8 normotensive patients with IgA nephropathy in basal conditions and after ACE inhibition, AT_1 receptor antagonism, and their combination. * $p < 0.05$ vs. baseline. # $p < 0.05$ vs. other study periods. (From Russo D, Pisani A, Balletta MM, et al: Additive antiproteinuric effect of converting enzyme inhibitor and losartan in normotensive patients with IgA nephropathy. Am J Kidney Dis 33:851–856, 1999, with permission.)

mg/day, was added for 4 weeks, resulting in a further decrease in proteinuria, totalling 70%! In the third phase, ACE inhibition was withdrawn, and patients remained on monotherapy with losartan for 12 weeks. Proteinuria increased to a value comparable to the value obtained during ACE inhibition monotherapy. In the fourth phase, an ACE inhibitor and AT_1 receptor antagonist were again combined for 4 weeks. Proteinuria decreased to –63%. The authors checked whether a similar additional effect on urinary protein loss could have been obtained with a further increase of either AT_1 antagonist or ACE inhibitor monotherapy. In the fifth phase, therefore, the ACE inhibitor was doubled in one-half of patients and the AT_1 antagonist in the other half. In neither subgroup was a further decrease in proteinuria observed compared with the lower dose of monotherapy. This preliminary study suggests that ACE inhibition and AT_1 receptor antagonism have additive effects and thus exert their action via different mechanisms. Of interest, in the different study phases there were no essential changes in blood pressure or creatinine clearance, indicating that the additive antiproteinuric effect of combination therapy was not dependent on changes in (renal) hemodynamics. Although these findings are intriguing, it should be kept in mind that the study involved only a small number of patients; the results obviously must be confirmed in larger-scale trials.

■ *Conclusion*

This chapter discussed the pathophysiology of progressive renal disease, especially the central role of Ang II. With the pivotal role of Ang II in mind, it is not surprising that ACE inhibitors have been shown to possess unique renoprotective effects. As a result, they have become the agents of choice for the symptomatic treatment of patients with nondiabetic as well as diabetic renal disease. Unfortunately, the renoprotective effect of ACE inhibitors varies considerably from patient to patient. This variability has led to growing interest in other agents that modulate the renin-angiotensin system, such as the recently approved AT_1 receptor antagonists.

Currently no studies describe the long-term effects of AT_1 receptor antagonists on the course of renal function decline in patients with renal disease. Until such data become available, we must rely on what we can learn from their effects in experimental renal disease and short-term clinical studies of intermediate end-points. Experimental evidence in models for renal disease progression shows superior efficacy of AT_1 receptor antagonists in retarding the development of proteinuria and glomerulosclerosis compared with antihypertensive agents that do not interfere with the renin-angiotensin system. In experimental models AT_1 receptor antagonists and ACE inhibitors appear to be equally effective. With respect to human data about intermediate parameters for renal disease progression, the various trials show remarkably varied results. This variability may be explained, at least partially, by the setting in which the experiments took place. Salt restriction ameliorates, whereas water loading attenuates, the renal effects of AT_1 antagonists. Furthermore, it takes at least 4–6 weeks for the renal effects of AT_1 antagonists to become fully developed. Lastly, the peak of the dose-response curve in terms of proteinuria seems to be reached at higher dosages of AT_1 antagonists than the peak of the dose-response curve in terms of blood pressure. These findings have implications for clinical practice: to achieve an optimal renal response, AT_1 antagonists should be prescribed at higher dosages than customary for hypertension treatment. Furthermore, patients also should be treated with a salt-restricted diet and/or diuretics, and at least 4 weeks must pass before the renal effects of AT1 receptor antagonists can be reliably assessed.

Despite the variability in results among trials, the general picture indicates that AT_1 receptor antagonists have a short-term renal profile characterized by a decrease in blood pressure and proteinuria and an increase in renal plasma flow, whereas glomerular filtration rate remains fairly stable or slightly decreases. This profile closely mimics that of ACE inhibitors. Indeed, in direct comparative trials AT_1 receptor antagonists have been shown to be equally effective as ACE inhibitors and to be superior to antihypertensive agents that do not modulate the renin-angiotensin system. Thus, AT_1 receptor antagonists are expected to be renoprotective. However, we must await the results of long-term outcome trials before we can prescribe these drugs as initial treatment for renal indications. Once renoprotective efficacy has been proved in clinical trials, AT_1 receptor antagonists may be preferable to ACE inhibitors because of their better side-effect profile. For now, AT_1 receptor antagonists should be reserved for patients who do not tolerate ACE inhibitors because of adverse side effects such as cough and angioedema.

Although similar efficacy is highly suggestive, it does not necessarily mean that AT_1 receptor antagonists and ACE inhibitors exert renal actions via the same mechanism. If the two classes of drugs induce renal actions via different mechanisms, a combination regimen may act additively. Although no evidence yet supports this theory in experimental renal disease, a preliminary study in patients with nondiabetic renal disease suggests that AT_1 receptor antagonists and ACE inhibitors may have an additive effect. This issue clearly needs further study before we conclude that the two classes of drugs are interchangeable or can be prescribed in combination.

References

1. Brenner BM, Meyer TW, Hostetter TH: Dietary protein and the progressive nature of kidney disease. The role of hemodynamically mediated glomerular injury in the pathogenesis of progressive glomerular sclerosis in aging, renal ablation, and intrinsic renal disease. N Engl J Med 307:652–659, 1982
2. Remuzzi G, Bertani T: Is glomerulosclerosis a consequence of altered glomerular permeability to macromolecules? Kidney Int 38:384–394, 1990.
3. Gansevoort RT, Navis GJ, Wapstra FH, et al: Proteinuria and progression of renal disease: Therapeutic implications. Curr Opinion Nephrol Hypertens 6:133–140, 1997.
4. Manttari M, Tiula E, Alikoski T, Manninen V: Effects of hypertension and dyslipidemia on the decline in renal function. Hypertension 26:670–675, 1995.
5. Schreiner GF: Renal toxicity of albumin and other lipoproteins. Curr Opin Nephrol Hypertens 4:369–373, 1995.
6. Fried L, Orchard T, Kasiske B: The effect of lipid reduction on renal disease progression [abstract]. J Am Soc Nephrol 10:A0374, 1999.
7. Freedman DS, Williamson DF, Gunter EW, Byers T: Relation of serum uric acid to mortality and ischemic heart disease. The NHANES I Epidemiologic Follow-up Study. Am J Epidemiol 141:637–644, 1995.
8. Puig JG, Ruilope LM: Uric acid as a cardiovascular risk factor in arterial hypertension. J Hypertens 17:869–872, 1999.
9. Alderman MH, Cohen H, Madhavan S, Kivlighn S: Serum uric acid and cardiovascular events in successfully treated hypertensive patients. Hypertension 34;144–150, 1999.
10. Johnson RJ, Kivlighn SD, Kim YG, et al: Reappraisal of the pathogenesis and consequences of hypertension, cardiovascular disease, and renal disease. Am J Kidney Dis 33:225–234, 1999.
11. Nickeleit V, Mihatsch MG: Uric acid nephropathy and end-stage, renal disease—review of a non-disease. Nephrol Dial Transplant 12:1832–1838, 1997.

12. Eiskjaer H, Sorensen SS, Danielsen H, Pedersen EB: Glomerular and tubular antinatriuretic actions of low-dose angiotensin –II infusion in man. J Hypertens 10:1033–1040, 1992.

13. Matsusaka T, Hymes J, Ichikawa I: Angiotensin in progressive renal disease: theory and practice J Am Soc Nephrol 7:2025–2043, 1996.

14. Dubey RK, Jackson EK, Rupprecht HD, Sterzel RB: Factors controlling growth and matrix production in vascular smooth muscle and glomerular mesangial cells. Curr Opin Nephrol Hypertens 6:88–105, 1997.

15. Wolf G, Ziyadeh FN: The role of angiotensin II in diabetic nephropathy: Emphasis on non-hemodynamic mechanisms. Am J Kidney Dis 29:153–163, 1997.

16. Klahr S, Morrissey J: Angiotensin II and gene expression in the kidney. Am J Kidney Dis 31:171–176, 1998.

17. Anderson S, Rennke HG, Brenner BM: Therapeutic advantage of converting enzyme inhibitors in arresting progressive renal disease associated with systemic hypertension in the rat. J Clin Invest 77:1993–2000, 1986.

18. Gansevoort RT, Sluiter WJ, Hemmelder MH, et al: Antiproteinuric effect of blood pressure lowering agents: a meta-analysis of comparative trials. Nephrol Dial Transplant 10:1963–1974, 1995.

19. Keilani T, Schlueter WA, Levin ML, Gatlle DC: Improvement of lipid abnormalities associated with proteinuria using fosinopril, an angiotensin converting enzyme inhibitor. Ann Intern Med 118:246–254, 1993.

20. Dullaart RPF, Gansevoort RT, Dikkeschei BD, et al: Role of elevated LCAT and CETP activities in abnormal lipoproteins from proteinuric patients. Kidney Int 44:91–97, 1993.

21. Lewis EJ, Hunsicker LG, Bain RP, Rohde RD: The effect of angiotensin-converting-enzyme inhibition on diabetic nephropathy. The Collaborative Study Group. N Engl J Med 329:1456–1462, 1993.

22. Giatras I, Lau J, Levey AS: Effect of angiotensin-converting-enzyme inhibitors on the progression of nondiabetic renal disease: A meta-analysis of randomized trials. Angiotensin-Converting-Enzyme Inhibition and Progressive Renal Disease Study Group. Ann Intern Med 127:337–345, 1997.

23. Heeg JE, de Jong PE, van der Hem GK, de Zeeuw D: Efficacy and variability of the antiproteinuric effect of ACE inhibition by lisinopril. Ey Int 36:272–279, 1989.

24. Cambien F, Poirier O, Lecerf L, et al: Deletion polymorphism in the gene for angiotensin-converting enzyme is a potent risk factor for myocardial infarction. Nature 359:641–644, 1992.

25. Ueda S, Meredith PA, Morton JJ, et al: The insertion/deletion (I/D) polymorphism of the human ACE gene differentiates the response to enalaprilat in normotensive males. J Hypertens 14(Suppl 1):S6, 1996.

26. Van der Kleij FG, Schmidt A, Navis GJ, et al: Angiotensin converting enzyme insertion/deletion polymorphism and short-term renal response to ACE inhibition: Role of sodium status. Kidney Int 63(Suppl):S23–S26, 1997.

27. Parving HH, Jacobsen P, Tarnow L, et al: Effect of deletion polymorphism of angiotensin converting enzyme gene on progression of diabetic nephropathy during inhibition of angiotensin converting enzyme: Observational follow up study. BMJ 313:591–594, 1996.

28. Essen, van GG, Rensma PL, de Zeeuw D, et al: Association between angiotensin-converting-enzyme gene polymorphism and failure of renoprotective therapy. Lancet 347:94–95, 1996.

29. Matsubara H: Pathophysiological role of angiotensin II type 2 receptor in cardiovascular and renal diseases. Circ Res 83:1182–1191, 1998.

30. De Gasparo M, Siragy HM: The AT₂ receptor: Fact, fancy and fantasy. Regul Pept 81:11–24, 1999.

31. Morrissey JJ, Klahr S: Effect of AT₂ receptor blockade on the pathogenesis of renal fibrosis. Am J Physiol 276:F39–F45, 1999.

32. Ma J, Hidcki H, Fogo A, et al: Accelerated fibrosis and collagen disposition develop in the renal interstitium of angiotensin type 2 (AT₂) receptor null mutant mice during ureteral obstruction. Kidney Int 53:937–944, 1998.

33. Arima S, et al: Possible role of P-450 metabolite of arachidonic acid in vasodilator mechanism of angiotensin type 2 receptor in the isolated microperfused rabbit afferent arteriole. J Clin Invest 100:2816–2823, 1997.

34. Hutchison FN, Webster SK: Effect of ANG II receptor antagonist on albuminuria and renal function in passive Heymann nephritis. Am J Physiol 263:F311–F319, 1992.

35. Hutchison FN, Martin VI: Effects of modulation of renal kallikrein-kinin system in the nephrotic syndrome. Am J Physiol 258:F1237–F1244, 1990.

36. Gainer JV, Morrow JD, Loveland A, et al: Effects of bradykinin receptor blockade on the response to angiotensin-converting enzyme inhibitor in normotensive and hypertensive subjects. N Eng J Med 339:1285–1292, 1998.

37. Wapstra FH, Navis GJ, de Zeeuw D, de Jong PE: in press.
38. Kakinuma Y, Kawamurra T, Bills T, et al: Blood pressure-independent effect of angiotensin inhibition on vascular lesions of chronic renal failure. Kidney Int 42:46–55, 1992.
39. Kohara K, Mikami H, Okuda N, et al: Angiotensin blockade and the progression of renal damage in the spontaneously hypertensive rat. Hypertension 21:975–979, 1993.
40. Lafayette RA, Mayer G, Park SK, Meyer TW: Angiotensin II receptor blockade limits glomerular injury in rats with reduced renal mass. J Clin Invest 90:766–771, 1992.
41. Burnier M, Rutschmann B, Nussberger J, et al: Salt-dependent renal effects of an angiotensin antagonist in healthy subjects. Hypertension 22:339–347, 1993.
42. Burnier M, Hagman M, Nussberger J, et al: Short-term and sustained renal effects of angiotensin II receptor blockade in healthy subjects. Hypertension 25:602–609, 1995.
43. Doig JK, MacFayden RJ, Sweet CS, Reid JL: Haemodynamic and renal responses to oral losartan potassium during salt depletion or salt repletion in normal human volunteers. J Cardiovasc Pharmacol 25:511–517, 1995.
44. Schmitt F, Natov S, Martinez F, et al: Renal effects of angiotensin I-receptor blockade and angiotensin convertase inhibition in man. Clin Sci 90:205–213, 1996.
45. Price DA, De'Oliveira JM, Fisher NDL, Hollenberg NK: Renal hemodynamic response to an angiotensin II antagonist, eprosartan, in healthy men. Hypertension 30:240–246, 1997.
46. Fumeron C, Schmitt F, Brillet G, et al: Renal effects of valsartan and losartan in healthy volunteers. J Am Soc Hypertens 1998 [abstract].
47. Burnier M, Pechere-Bertschi A, Nussberger J, et al: Studies of the renal effects of angiotensin II receptor blockade: The confounding factor of acute water loading on the action of vasoactive systems. Am J Kidney Dis 26:108–115, 1995.
48. Kawabata M, Takabatake T, Ohta H, et al: Effects of an angiotensin-II receptor antagonist, TCV-116, on renal hemodynamics in essential hypertension. Blood Pressure 3(Suppl 5):S117–S121, 1994.
49. Erley CM, Bader B, Scheu M, et al: Renal hemodynamics in essential hypertensives treated with losartan. Clin Nephrol 43(Suppl 1):S8–S11, 1995.
50. Fauvel JP, Velon S, Berra N, et al: Effects of losartan on renal hemodynamics in patients with essential hypertension. J Cardiovasc Pharmacol 28:259–263, 1996.
51. Nielsen S, Dollerup J, Nielsen B, et al: losartan reduces albuminuria in patients with essential hypertension. An enalapril controlled 3 months study. Nephrol Dial Transplant 12(Suppl 2):S19–S23, 1997.
52. Chan JCN, Critchley JAJH, Tomlinson B, et al: Antihypertensive and anti-albuminuric effects of losartan potassium and felodipine in Chinese elderly with or without non-insulin-dependent diabetes mellitus. Am J Nephrol 17:72–80, 1997.
53. Pechere-Bertschi A, Nussberger J, Decosterd L, et al: Renal response to the angiotensin II receptor subtype 1 antagonist irbesartan versus enalapril in hypertensive patients. J Hypertens 16:385–393, 1998.
54. Gansevoort RT, de Zeeuw D, de Jong PE: Is the antiproteinuric effect of ACE inhibition mediated by interference in the renin angiotensin system? Kidney Int 45:861–867, 1994.
55. Perico N, Spormann D, Peruzzi E et al: Efficacy and tolerability of valsartan compared with lisinopril in patients with hypertension and renal insufficiency. Clin Drug Invest 14:252–259, 1997.
56. Buter H, Navis GJ, de Zeeuw D, de Jong PE : Renal hemodynamic effects of candesartan in normal and impaired renal function in humans. Kidney Int 52(Suppl 63):S185–S187, 1997.
57. Perico N, Remuzzi A, Sangalli F, et al: The antiproteinuric effect of angiotensin antagonism in human IgA nephropathy is potentiated by indomethacin. J Am Soc Nephrol 9:2308–2317, 1998.
58. Plum J, Bunten B, Nemeth R, Grabensee B: Effects of the angiotensin II antagonist valsartan on blood pressure, proteinuria and renal hemodynamics in patients with chronic renal failure and hypertension. J Am Soc Nephrol 9:2223–2234, 1998.
59. Holdaas H, Hartmann A, Berg KJ, et al: Renal effects of losartan and amlodipine in hypertensive patients with non-diabetic nephropathy. Nephrol Dial Transplant 13:3096–3102, 1998.
60. Fernandez-Andrade C, Russo D, Iversen B,et al: Comparison of losartan and amlodipine in renally impaired hypertensive patients. Kidney Int 54(Suppl 68):S120–S124, 1998.
61. Toto R, Shultz P, Raij L, et al: Efficacy and tolerability of losartan in hypertensive patients with renal impairment. Hypertension 31:684–691, 1998.
62. Russo D, Pisani A, Balletta MM, et al: Additive antiproteinuric effect of converting enzyme inhibitor and losartan in normotensive patients with IgA nephropathy. Am J Kidney Dis 33:851–856, 1999.
63. Andersen S, Tarnow L, Rossing P, et al: Renoprotective effects of angiotensin II receptor blockade in type 1 diabetic patients with diabetic nephropathy. Kidney Int 2000 [in press].
64. Nakashima M, Uematsu T, Kosuge K, Kanamaru M: Pilot study of the uricosuric effect of DuP-753, a new angiotensin II receptor antagonist, in healthy subjects. Eur J Clin Pharmacol 42:333–335, 1992.

65. Tsunoda K, Abe K, Hagino T, et al: Hypotensive effect of losartan, a nonpeptide angiotensin II receptor antagonist, in essential hypertension. Am J Hypertens 6:28–32, 1993.

66. Gansevoort RT, de Zeeuw D, Shahinfar S, et al: Effects of the angiotensin II antagonist losartan in hypertensive patients with renal disease. J Hypertens 12(Suppl):S37–S42, 1994.

67. Wong PC, Price WA, Chiu AT, et al: Nonpeptide angiotensin II receptor antagonists. XI: Pharmacology of EXP 3174: an active metabolite of DuP 753, an orally active antihypertensive agent. J Pharmacol Exp Therapeut 255:211–217, 1990.

68. Boike S, Ilson B, Audet P, et al: The angiotensin II receptor antagonist SK&F 108566 does not increase uric acid excretion in healthy men. J Am Soc Nephrol 4:530, 1993.

69. Mimran A, Ruilope L, Kerwin L, et al: A randomised, double-blind comparison of the angiotensin II receptor antagonist, irbesartan, with the full dose range of enalapril for the treatment of mild-to-moderate hypertension. J Hum Hypertens 12:203–208, 1998.

70. Puig JG, Mateos F, Buno A, et al: Effect of eprosartan and losartan on uric acid metabolism in patients with essential hypertension. J Hypertens 17:1033–1099, 1999.

71. Tikkanen I, Omvik P, Jensen HA: Comparison of the angiotensin II receptor antagonist losartan with the angiotensin converting enzyme inhibitor enalapril in patients with essential hypertension. J Hypertens 13:1343–1351, 1995.

72. Edwards RM, Trizna W, Stack EJ, Weinstock J: Interaction of nonpeptide angiotensin II receptor antagonist with the urate transporter in rat renal brush-border membranes. J Pharmacol Exp Ther 276:125–129, 1996.

73. Burnier M, Roch-Ramel F, Brunner HR: Renal effects of angiotensin II receptor blockade in normotensive subjects. Kidney Int 49:1787–1790, 1996.

74. Trenkwalder P, Dahl K, Letovirta M, Mulder H: Antihypertensive treatment with candesartan cilexetil does not effect glucose homeostasis or serum lipid profile in patients with mild hypertension and type II diabetes. Blood Pressure 7:170–175, 1998.

75. Laakso M, Karjalainen L, Lempiainen-Kuosa P: Effects of losartan on insulin sensitivity in hypertensive subjects. Hypertension 28:392–396, 1996.

76. Joven J, Villabona C, Vilella E, et al: Abnormalities of lipoprotein metabolism in patients with the nephritic syndrome. N Eng J Med 323:579–584, 1990.

77. Thomas ME, Freestone A, Varghese Z, et al: Lipoprotein (a) in patients with proteinuria. Nephrol Dial Transplant 30:21–25, 1992.

78. Kanno H, Saito E, Fujioka T, Yasugi T: Lipoprotein (a) levels in the nephrotic syndrome. Intern Med 31:1004–1008, 1992.

79. Gansevoort RT, Heeg JE, Dikkeschei BD, et al: Symptomatic antiproteinuric treatment decreases serum lipoprotein (a) concentration in patients with glomerular proteinuria. Nephrol Dial Transplant 9:244–250, 1994.

80. Allen TJ, Cao Z, Youssef S,et al: Role of angiotensin II and bradykinin in experimental diabetic nephropathy. Functional and structural studies. Diabetes 46:1612–1618, 1997.

81. Bos H, de Boer E, Henning RH, et al: No improvement of antiproteinuric efficacy of ACE inhibition by co-treatment with AT1 receptor blockade in established adriamycin nephrosis. Submitted.

82. Erley CM, Rebmann S, Strobel U, et al: Effects of antihypertensive therapy on blood pressure and renal function in rats with hypertension due to chronic blockade of nitric oxide synthesis. Exp Nephrol 3:293–299, 1995.

83. Hirawa N, Uehara Y, Kawabata Y, et al: Mechanistic analysis of renal protection by angiotensin converting enzyme inhibitor in Dahl salt-sensitive rats. J Hypertens 12:909–918, 1994.

84. Imamura A, MacKenzie HS, Lacy ER, et al: Effects of chronic treatment with angiotensin converting enzyme inhibitor or an angiotensin receptor antagonist in two-kidney, one-clip hypertensive rats. Kidney Int 47:1394–1402, 1995.

85. Inada Y, Wada T, Ojima M, et al: Protective effects of candesartan cilexetil (TCV-116) against stroke, kidney dysfunction and cardiac hyperthrophy in stroke-prone spontaneously hypertensive rats. Clin Exp Hypertens 19:1079–1099, 1997.

86. Kim S, Ohta K, Hamaguchi A, et al: Contribution of renal angiotensin II type I receptor to gene expressions in hypertension-induced renal injury. Kidney Int 46:1346–1358, 1994.

87. Klahr S, Ishidoya S, Morrissey J: Role of angiotensin II in the tubulointerstitial fibrosis of obstructive nephropathy. Am J Kidney Dis 26:141–146, 1995.

88. Kohzuki M, Kanazawa M, Fu Liu P, et al: Kinin and angiotensin II receptor antagonists in rats with chronic renal failure: Chronic effects on cardio- and renoprotection of angiotensin converting enzyme inhibitors. J Hypertens 13:1785–1790, 1995.

89. Kohzuki M, Yasujima M, Kanawaza M, et al: Antihypertensive and renal-protective effects of losartan in streptozotocin diabetic rats. J Hypertens 13:97–103, 1995.

90. Larivière R, Lebel M, Kingma I, et al: Effects of losartan and captopril on endothelin-1 production in blood vessels and glomeruli of rats with reduced renal mass. Am J Hypertens 11:989–997, 1998.

91. Nakamura T, Obata J, Kimura H, et al: Blocking angiotensin II ameliorates proteinuria and glomerular lesions in progressive mesangioproliferative glomerulonephritis. Kidney Int 55:877–889, 1999.

92. Noda M, Fukuda R, Matsuo T, et al: Effects of candesartan cilexetil (tcv-116) and enalapril in 5/6 nephrectomized rats. Kidney Int 52:S136–S139, 1997.

93. Okada H, Suzuki H, Kanno Y, et al: Renal responses to angiotensin receptor antagonist and angiotensin-converting enzyme inhibitor in partially nephrectomized spontaneously hypertensive rats. J Cardiovasc Pharmacol 26:564–569, 1995.

94. Ots M, MacKenzie HS, Troy JL, et al: Effects of combination therapy with enalapril and losartan on the rate of progression of renal injury in rats with 5/6 renal mass ablation. J Am Soc Nephrol 9:224–230, 1998.

95. Otsuka F, Yamauchi T, Kataoka H, et al: Effects of chronic inhibition of ACE and AT1 receptors on glomerular injury in Dahl salt-sensitive rats. Am J Physiol 274:1797–1806, 1998.

96. Pollock DM, Divish BJ, Polakowski JS, Opgenorth TJ: Angiotensin II receptor blockade improves renal function in rats with reduced renal mass. J Pharmacol 267:656–663, 1993.

97. Remuzzi A, Fassi A, Sangalli F, et al: Prevention of renal injury in diabetic MWF rats by angiotensin II antagonism. Exp Nephrol 6:28–38, 1998.

98. Shibouta M, Chatani F, Ishimura Y, et al: TCV-116 inhibits renal interstitial and glomerular injury in glomerulosclerotic rats. Kidney Int 49:S115–S118, 1996.

99. Sugimoto K, Tsuruoka S, Matsushita K, Fujimara A: Effects of candesartan cilexetil on oxidative state and renal function in 5/6 nephrectomized rats. J Human Hypertens 13(Suppl 1):S63–S70, 1999.

100. Tanaka R, Kon V, Yoshioka T, et al: Angiotensin converting enzyme inhibitor modulates glomerular function and structure by distinct mechanisms. Kidney Int 45:537–543, 1994.

101. Wagner J, Drab M, Bohlender J, et al: Effects of AT1 receptor blockade on blood pressure and the renin-angiotensin system in spontaneously hypertensive rats of the stroke prone strain. Clin Exper Hypertens 20:205–221, 1998.

102. Webb RL, Barclay BW, Navarette AE, et al: Protective effects of valsartan and benazeprilat in salt-loaded stroke-prone spontaneously hypertensive rats. Clin Exp Hypertens 20:775–793, 1998.

103. Yo Y, Moriguchi A, Higaki J, et al: Renal effects of an angiotensin II antagonist in stroke-prone spontaneously hypertensive rat. Nephron 76:466–471, 1997.

104. Ziai F, Ots M, Provoost AP, et al: The angiotensin receptor antagonist, irbesartan, reduces renal injury in experimental chronic renal failure. Kidney Int 50(Suppl 57):S132–S136, 1996.

105. Zoja C, Donadelli R, Corna D, et al: The renoprotective properties of angiotensin-converting enzyme inhibitors in a chronic model of membranous nephropathy are solely due to the inhibition of angiotensin II: Evidence based on comparative studies with a receptor antagonist. Am J Kidney Dis 29:254–264, 1997.

106. Dorer FE, Kahn JR, Lentz KE, et al: Hydrolysis of bradykinin by angiotensin-converting enzyme. Circ Res 34:824–827, 1974.

107. Hebert LA, Falkenhain ME, Stanley Nahman NS, et al: Combination ACE inhibitor and angiotensin II receptor antagonist therapy in diabetic nephropathy. Am J Nephrol 19:1–6, 1999.

CHAPTER 21

Evolving Role of Angiotensin II Receptor Antagonists in Diabetes Mellitus

MARK COOPER, M.D., Ph.D., FRACP
MURRAY EPSTEIN, M.D., FACP

Recent interest has focused on the worldwide growth in prevalence of non–insulin-dependent diabetes mellitus (NIDDM) and its related consequence, end-stage renal disease. The costs of end-stage renal disease programs have grown enormously and have given a major impetus to prevention strategies. Prominent among these strategies is pharmacologic blockade of the renin-angiotensin system. Rodby et al. published a detailed examination of the financial considerations of end-stage renal disease treatment and concluded that angiotensin-converting enzyme (ACE) inhibitor therapy provides significant cost savings in patients with insulin-dependent diabetes mellitus (IDDM).[1]

■ Prevalence and Pathogenesis of Diabetic Nephropathy

Diabetes is now the major cause of end-stage renal disease in the Western world.[2] Patients with IDDM and NIDDM account for a similar proportion of patients entering end-stage renal failure programs. Diabetic nephropathy is characterized by the development of hypertension, proteinuria, and ultimately renal impairment.[3] Preceding this overt phase is a phase of incipient nephropathy, characterized by the presence of microalbuminuria, rising blood pressure, and evidence of glomerular ultrastructural injury.[4] With increasing evidence that blood pressure is a major determinant of the rate of progression of diabetic renal disease, a large number of international organizations have published guidelines for the management of hypertension in diabetes.[5,6] Aggressive targets for blood pressure reduction have been suggested, particularly in the context of diabetic renal disease.[5,6]

The cause of diabetic nephropathy remains unknown, but most likely it is multifactorial, involving an interaction between metabolic and hemodynamic factors.[7] It is now thought that angiotensin II (Ang II) plays a pivotal role in mediating various forms of renal injury, including diabetic nephropathy. Ang II has multiple actions (Table 1) relevant to the pathogenesis and progression

Table 1.   Postulated Mode of Action of ACE Inhibitors as Renoprotective Agents

1. Reduction in systemic blood pressure
2. Reduction of intraglomerular pressure
3. Inhibition of growth factor expression leading to reduced collagen deposition
4. Inhibition of Ang II-induced solute transport across the proximal tubule
5. Inhibition of macrophage proliferation and migration

of diabetic nephropathy. It not only is a potent vasoconstrictor but also has potent trophic properties. In vitro Ang II promotes collagen expression in both vascular smooth muscle cells and mesangial cells, primarily via activation of the prosclerotic cytokine, transforming growth factor beta (TGFβ).[8] Experimental studies in various animal models of renal injury, including diabetes, have explored in vivo the relationship between Ang II and cytokine and matrix protein expression. In the model of subtotal nephrectomy, which has many functional and structural similarities to diabetic nephropathy,[9] ACE inhibition and AT_1 receptor antagonism prevent overexpression of TGFβ and type IV collagen.[10] Similar findings have been observed in experimental diabetes with ACE inhibitor treatment in association with reduced tubulointerstitial injury.[11] Although this chapter focuses on the role of Ang II in diabetic nephropathy, other factors, including metabolic pathways such as advanced glycation, polyol accumulation, and activation of protein kinase C, also play a major role in the genesis of this disease[12] (Fig. 1).

■ *Evolution of ACE Inhibitor Therapy in the Management of Diabetes*

A seminal event in the development of ACE inhibitor therapy for renal protection was the 1985 report by Taguma et al.[13] of the striking and consistent effect of captopril in reducing heavy proteinuria in azotemic patients with diabetes mellitus. Because it contradicted the conventional wisdom that ACE inhibitors should be avoided in patients with proteinuria, this report created widespread interest.

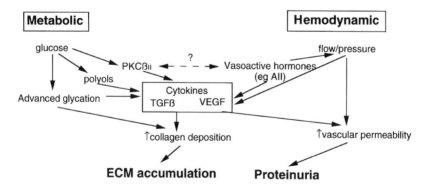

Figure 1.   Potential interactions among metabolic and hemodynamic factors in the pathogenesis of diabetic nephropathy. AII = angiotensin II, TGFβ = transforming growth factor beta, VEGF = vascular endothelial growth factor, PCK = protein kinase C, ECM = extracellular matrix. (Adapted from Cooper ME, Gilbert RE, Epstein M: Pathophysiology of diabetic nephropathy. Metab Clin Exp 47(Suppl1):3–6, 1998, with permission.)

The timing was propitious because a few months later the first meeting was convened to discuss the possibility of an ambitious therapeutic trial to assess whether captopril would influence the natural history of renal injury in diabetes (i.e., the Collaborative Study Trial).[14]

During the next few years an enormous literature accrued. By 1993 Kasiske et al. reported a meta-analysis of 100 clinical studies performed over a relatively brief interval.[15] The major study that focused attention on ACE inhibitor therapy in diabetic renal disease was the report by Lewis et al. from the Collaborative Group.[14] The investigators reported a greater than 50% reduction not only in doubling of serum creatinine, the primary study endpoint, but also in crucial clinical endpoints, including death from end-stage renal disease. The authors concluded that ACE inhibition provided renal protection beyond that which could be expected by blood pressure control alone, because blood pressure control was not statistically different in the two study groups. These results led regulatory agencies to recommend for the first time a specific drug, captopril, for the treatment of renal injury in patients with IDDM.

Studies in Patients with NIDDM

Despite clearcut differences between IDDM and NIDDM, increasing evidence suggests that pharmacologic interruption of the renin-angiotensin system may help to prevent nephropathy in patients with NIDDM. Ravid et al. reported a 7-year follow-up to a previously reported 5-year study of normotensive, microalbuminuric patients with NIDDM randomized to enalapril or no treatment.[16] Treatment with enalapril stabilized renal function and prevented progression of proteinuria over the 5 years of double-blind treatment. This improvement was sustained in the additional 2 years of treatment in the open study but lost in patients in whom ACE inhibitor treatment was discontinued.[16] The beneficial effect of ACE inhibition in normotensive patients with NIDDM also has been reported in placebo-controlled trials in Japanese and Indian patients with NIDDM.[17,18] In a recent study in which ACE inhibitor treatment was used as a preventative strategy, fewer patients with NIDDM who received enalapril therapy developed microalbuminuria and possibly showed a slower decline in renal function.[19]

A large number of studies have used ACE inhibitors in hypertensive patients with NIDDM and either overt nephropathy or microalbuminuria, mostly versus conventional antihypertensive agents that do not directly inhibit the renin-angiotensin system.[20] Tables 2 and 3 summarize studies in which treatment with an ACE inhibitor was continued for at least 12 months. Parving's group reported a disparity in effects on albuminuria and renal function in hypertensive patients with NIDDM.[21] Whereas lisinopril was more effective than atenolol in reducing albuminuria, both agents showed similar efficacy in terms of rate of decline in glomerular filtration rate (GFR). Several studies have confirmed that ACE inhibitors are superior to other antihypertensive agents, including the dihydropyridine calcium channel blocker (CCB), nifedipine,[22,23] and the vasodilator, hydralazine,[24] in reducing albuminuria in hypertensive patients with NIDDM and macroproteinuria.

Significant differences in the effect on albuminuria obtained with various CCBs have been attributed by Bakris and coworkers to the particular class of CCB.[25-27] Slataper et al. reported a randomized parallel group study comparing diltiazem, lisinopril, and conventional therapy (atenolol and furosemide) in hypertensive patients

Table 2. Effect of ACE Inhibition in Hypertensive Patients with NIDDM and Overt Nephropathy

Agent	Duration	n	AER (%)*	GFR	BP	Reference
Lisinopril	18 mo	10	↓ (– 42)	→	↓	Slataper et al.[26]
Diltiazem		10	↓ (– 45)	→	↓	
Furosemide + atenolol		10	↓	↓	↓	
Lisinopril	12 mo	16	↓ (– 45)	↓	↓	Nielsen et al.[21]
Atenolol		19	→	↓	↓	
Enalapril	12 mo	18	↓ (– 87)	→	↓	Ferder et al.[23]
Nifedipine		12	→	→	↓	
Enalapril	52 wk	7	↓ (– 71)	→	↓	Chan et al.[22]
Nifedipine		10	→		↓	
Captopril	12 mo	24	↓ (– 27)	→	↓	Liou et al.[24]
Hydralazine		18	→		↓	
Lisinopril	12 mo	8	↓ (– 59)	↓	↓	Bakris et al.[25]
Verapamil		8	↓ (– 50)	↓	↓	
Lisinopril + verapamil		8	↓ (– 78)	↓	↓	
Guanfacine + hydralazine		6	→	↓	↓	
Lisinopril	5 yr	18	↓ (– 25)	↓	↓	Bakris et al.[28]
Atenolol		16	→	↓↓	↓	
Verapamil or diltiazem		16	↓ (– 18)	↓	↓	

AER = albumin excretion rate, GFR = glomerular filtration rate, BP = blood pressure.
* In some studies total proteinuria was measured.

Table 3. Effect of ACE Inhibition in Hypertensive Patients with NIDDM and Microalbuminuria

Agent	Duration	n	AER (%)*	GFR	BP	Reference
Captopril	36 mo	9	↓ (– 65)	→	↓	Lacourcière et al.[29]
Metoprolol or hydro-chlorothiazide		12	→	→	↓	
Enalapril	12 mo	16	↓ (– 70)	→	↓	Chan et al.[22]
Nifedipine		15	→	→	↓	
Enalapril + nifedipine	48 mo	11	↓ (– 42)	→	↓	Sano et al.[17]
Nifedipine		13	↑ (+ 29)	→	↓	
Nifedipine	12 mo	13	→	→	→	MDNSG[34]
Perindopril		11	→	→	→	
Enalapril	12 mo	8	↓ (– 28)	↑	↓	Ruggenenti et al.[31]
Nitrendipine		8	↓ (– 17)	↑	↓	
Lisinopril	12 mo	156	↓ (– 37)	→	↓	Agardh et al.[33]
Nifedipine		158	→	→	↓	
Cilazapril	36 mo	9	↓ (– 27)	↓	↓	Velussi et al.[32]
Amlodipine		9	↓ (– 31)	↓	↓	
Ramipril ± felodipine	12 mo	46	→	→	↓	Schnack et al.[30]
Atenolol ± hydro-chlorothiazide		45	↑	↓	↓	

AER = albumin excretion rate, GFR = glomerular filtration rate, BP = blood pressure.
* In some studies total proteinuria was measured.

with NIDDM, marked albuminuria (> 2.5 gm/24 hr), and renal insufficiency (creatinine clearance < 70 ml/min/1.73 m^2).[26] After 18 months of therapy the rate of decline in GFR was attenuated with either diltiazem or lisinopril compared with conventional therapy, despite comparable blood pressure reduction.[26] Recently Bakris et al. reported that in hypertensive patients with NIDDM and macroproteinuria followed for over 4 years, the beta blocker atenolol was associated with a more rapid decline in GFR and less efficacy in reducing albuminuria than the ACE inhibitor, lisinopril.[28]

The use of antihypertensive therapy in hypertensive patients with NIDDM and microalbuminuria has been evaluated by an increasing number of investigators over the past decade.[20] A double-blind study compared captopril with conventional therapy (metoprolol and hydrochlorothiazide) in microalbuminuric, hypertensive patients with NIDDM over a 3-year period.[29] Despite a comparable reduction in blood pressure with both treatments, only captopril induced a persistent decline in albuminuria during the 36 months of therapy. Schnack et al. reported that ramipril with or without felodipine stabilized albuminuria. By contrast, atenolol with or without diuretic treatment was associated with an increase in urinary albumin excretion.[30] Furthermore, the ramipril-treated group had stable renal function, whereas the group receiving beta blockers had a decline in GFR.

A reduction in albuminuria by ACE inhibition also has been observed by several other investigators.[22,31–33] In the Melbourne Diabetic Nephropathy Study, nifedipine produced a similar response to perindopril in decreasing albuminuria over 12 months in patients with NIDDM and microalbuminuria.[34] Chan et al. reported that the ACE inhibitor, enalapril, was more effective than nifedipine in reducing albuminuria in a group of hypertensive microalbuminuric patients.[22] Recent studies have compared calcium channel blockade with ACE inhibition in hypertensive, microalbuminuric patients with NIDDM.[31–33] In a 3-year study with a relatively small number of subjects, amlodipine was as effective as the ACE inhibitor, cilazapril, in reducing albuminuria; both treatment groups had similar declines in renal function.[32] However, in a much larger multicenter study of over 300 subjects, the ACE inhibitor, lisinopril, reduced albuminuria over 12 months, whereas nifedipine failed to influence urinary albumin excretion significantly.[33] Therefore, the status of ACE inhibitors as the treatment of choice for patients with NIDDM and any evidence of nephropathy remains controversial. Most studies suggest the superiority of ACE inhibitors, primarily in terms of reducing albuminuria. No meaningful data about Ang II antagonists in this population are yet available.

■ *Advantages of ACE Inhibitors vs. Angiotensin II Blockers: Theoretical Considerations*

Theoretical considerations suggest that it is far better to block the system either at the rate-limiting step, which involves the interaction between renin and its substrate, or at the level of the Ang II receptor (see Hollenberg chapter). The second approach has the distinct advantage of blocking the actions of Ang II,[35] whatever the pathways for its generation, which in some cases may involve neither renin nor ACE. The past several years have witnessed publication of many articles arguing for and against the view that the pharmacologic differences between ACE inhibitors and Ang II receptor antagonists are clinically important. As an example, some authors emphasize that Ang II levels tend to rise during ACE inhibition, reflecting incomplete blockade. In contrast, proponents of the view that there are no clinical advantages to either agent argue that much of the protective action of ACE inhibitors involves mechanisms other than Ang II.[36]

In acute studies, ACE inhibitors have been compared with Ang II antagonists.[37] In various models of experimental renal disease, including diabetes, differences in renal hemodynamics were observed between the two treatments.[37,38] A possible role for bradykinin was suggested by the ability of the beta$_2$ receptor blocker, icatibant (Hoe 140), to attenuate the effects of the ACE inhibitor, ramipril, and to reproduce the effects of the Ang II antagonist, valsartan.[38] However, more recent studies evaluating the long-term effects of both agents suggest that ACE inhibitors and Ang II antagonists have similar efficacy.[39] For example, our group compared the ACE inhibitor, ramipril, with the Ang II antagonist, valsartan, in experimental diabetes.[40] Both treatments retarded the increase in urinary albumin excretion and prevented glomerular basement membrane thickening and glomerular hypertrophy. Furthermore, concomitant administration of the bradykinin receptor blocker, icatibant, failed to reverse the renoprotective effect of the ACE inhibitor (Fig. 2). This finding is consistent with the view that the major long-term effects of ACE inhibition are via suppression of Ang II-dependent pathways.

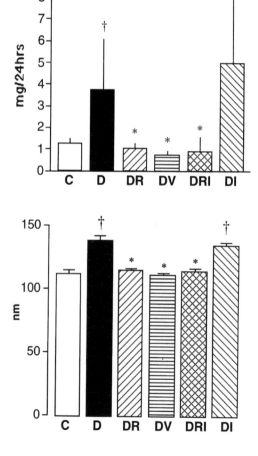

Figure 2. Data are shown for albuminuria as geometric means (upper panel) and glomerular basement membrane thickness (lower panel) in control (C), untreated diabetic (D), and diabetic rats treated with ramipril (R), valsartan (V), ramipril + the bradykinin receptor blocker, icatibant (RI), or icatibant alone. $^{\dagger}p < 0.01$ vs. C, $^{*}p < 0.01$ vs. D. (Adapted from Allen TJ, Cao Z, Youssef S, et al: The role of angiotensin II and bradykinin in experimental diabetic nephropathy: Functional and structural studies. Diabetes 46:1612–1618, 1997, with permission.)

The pivotal question is whether the alternatives to ACE inhibition for blocking the renin-angiotensin system are in fact more effective. In the case of blood pressure and reversal of hypertension, the answer appears to be no. ACE inhibitors and Ang II receptor antagonists have induced similar reductions in blood pressure.[35] In contrast, Hollenberg proposed that Ang II receptor blockade may have a more profound effect on the renal circulation than ACE inhibitors.[41] A series of studies using both renin inhibitors and Ang II receptor antagonists in healthy humans on a low-salt diet concluded that the renal hemodynamic response to ACE inhibition has underestimated, systemically, the contribution of Ang II to renal vascular tone in humans.[41] The effectiveness of renin inhibition suggests that this response represents interruption of primarily renin-dependent but non–ACE-dependent pathways.

A recent report by Price et al.[42] emphasizes the complexities of the renin-angiotensin cascade in diabetes mellitus and suggests future therapeutic niches for intervention with Ang II antagonists. Early studies of plasma renin activity (PRA) in diabetes frequently found renin suppression rather than elevated PRA levels, which might have accounted for the hypertension. The low renin state generally has been attributed to sclerotic renal arterioles and glomeruli, possibly amplified by functional factors such as autonomic neuropathy and sodium retention. On the other hand, a disassociation between reduced PRA and evidence suggesting well-maintained or even increased renin levels in renal tissue has been described in animal models of diabetes.

The authors hypothesized that circulating renin might not reflect intrarenal tissue levels in type 2 diabetes, as suggested by many, but not all, studies in rat models. According to their hypothesis, Ang II antagonists should raise PRA levels substantially in diabetic patients, if reduced PRA reflected, at least in part, intrarenal Ang II-mediated suppression. PRA and renal vascular responses (inulin and paraaminohippurate clearance) to graded doses of irbesartan, an Ang II antagonist, were assessed in 8 healthy volunteers and 12 patients with type 2 diabetes mellitus and nephropathy who ingested 10 mmol of sodium to activate the renin system. Serial measurements of PRA were made over the 48 hours after each irbesartan dose, with subjects on a constant diet and in recumbency. Despite the low basal PRA levels, renal perfusion rose more in response to irbesartan in patients with type 2 diabetes mellitus than in normal volunteers. The authors found a striking dose- and time-related renal vasodilator response and rise in PRA after administration of the Ang II antagonist in diabetic patients.

In interpreting their findings, Price et al. proposed that increased intrarenal Ang II production in type 2 diabetes mellitus may account for the apparent paradox of heightened renal hemodynamic response to an Ang II antagonist in the face of low PRA and the rise in PRA after administration of the Ang II antagonist. This increase may account for suppressed circulating renin, the exaggerated renal vasodilator response to irbesartan, and the therapeutic effectiveness of interrupting the renin-angiotensin system in diabetic nephropathy. Thus, all of their findings support the original hypothesis: PRA and the state of the intrarenal renin-angiotensin system are disparate in type 2 diabetic patients.

Because Ang II antagonists are selective AT_1 receptor antagonists, one cannot assume that they block all Ang II receptors. There are at least two Ang II receptor subtypes. This is not a major problem in the kidney, in which the

AT_1 receptor subtype predominates. At other sites, however, particularly in the context of injury, there are a significant number of AT_2 receptors.[43] The role of the AT_2 receptor has not been fully clarified, but it is not believed to mediate most of the classic actions of Ang II, such as vasoconstriction and tubular sodium reabsorption.[44] Indeed, the AT_2 receptor may be antitrophic and in fact beneficial. AT_1 receptor blockade is associated with an increase in plasma levels of Ang II and theoretically leads to unopposed and presumably increased Ang II action on the AT_2 receptor. However, these concepts remain theoretical, and several groups have suggested an opposite action for the AT_2 receptor[45] (see chapter by Douglas and Feng).

■ *Clinical Studies with Angiotensin II Receptor Antagonists*

The role of Ang II antagonists in the management of hypertension has been well described. A similar beneficial role in heart failure also has been reported. However, data about their role in progressive renal disease are limited. Gansevoort et al. reported that losartan and ACE inhibitors have a similar effect in reducing blood pressure and proteinuria in nondiabetic renal disease.[46] Such studies have been performed over weeks to months and therefore did not explore the long-term renoprotective effects potentially afforded by Ang II antagonists. In a small study of 29 elderly Chinese hypertensive patients, 12 of whom had diabetes, losartan was compared with felodipine.[47] After 12 weeks, despite similar effects on blood pressure, urinary albumin excretion was reduced by 27% with losartan, whereas no change was observed with felodipine. Subgroup analysis of the diabetic patients revealed a similar pattern. Losartan reduced albuminuria by 24%, whereas felodipine was less potent, reducing albuminuria by only 11%. The authors concluded that for comparable reductions in blood pressure, a greater reduction in albuminuria was seen with Ang II receptor antagonism than with calcium channel blockade.[47]

Several as yet unpublished studies suggest that Ang II antagonists reproduce the antiproteinuric effects of ACE inhibitors in diabetic patients.[48,49] In a recent comparison of amlodipine and irbesartan, reduction in urinary albumin excretion appeared to be greater with the Ang II receptor antagonist.[48] Similar findings have been suggested in a multicenter European study using losartan.[49] Two large multicenter studies exploring the role of Ang II antagonists in patients with NIDDM, hypertension, impaired renal function, and macroproteinuria should assist in delineating the role of these agents in overt diabetic nephropathy[50,51] (Table 4). One study compares the Ang II antagonist, irbesartan, with amlodipine,[50a] whereas the RENAAL study compares the Ang II antagonist, losartan, with conventional antihypertensive agents such as beta blockers, CCBs, diuretics, and alpha blockers.[55]

In addition, preliminary reports from several small studies of relatively short duration support the efficacy of Ang II antagonists in both IDDM and NIDDM.[52-55] In a study comparing enalapril with losartan in both IDDM and NIDDM patients with persistent microalbuminuria, losartan and enalapril were associated with a similar decrease in urinary albumin excretion.[54] Losartan and ACE inhibitors had a similar effect on albuminuria in a small group of Japanese patients with NIDDM and albuminuria.[53] In a 4-week study of patients with IDDM and low-range albuminuria, losartan was associated with an approximately 50% decrease in urinary albumin excretion as well as a reduction in atherogenic apo-B-containing

Table 4. **Summary of Trials in Progress Exploring the Effects of Ang II Receptor Antagonists in Patients with NIDDM and Macroproteinuria**

Study	Inclusion Criteria	Design	n	Follow-up	Funding	Reference	Primary Endpoint	Secondary Outcomes
IDNT	NIDDM Hypertension Macroproteinuria	Irbesartan Placebo Amlodipine	1650	Minimum: 2 yr	Bristol-Myers Squibb	http://www.cardiosource.com/trials[49]	Doubling serum creatinine, renal transplantation, dialysis, and all-cause death	Heart failure, hospitalization, above-ankle amputation
RENAAL	NIDDM Macroproteinuria (urinary ablumin/ creatinine > 300 mg/gm)	Losartan vs. placebo (all agents except ACE inhibitor or Ang II receptor antagonist)	1500	Mean duration: 4.5 yr	Merck Research Laboratories	Brenner et al.[55]	Doubling serum creatinine, renal transplantation, dailysis, and all-cause death	Cardiovascular mortality and morbidity

lipoproteins.[55] Finally, in a randomized, double-blind, crossover trial Parving's group recently compared 2 months of treatment with varying doses of losartan and enalapril in patients with IDDM and overt nephropathy.[52] A similar reduction in albuminuria was observed with both drugs, suggesting that agents which interrupt the renin-angiotensin system either at the level of Ang II formation or at the AT_1 receptor are effective in reducing albuminuria. Whether these relatively short-term effects on urinary albumin excretion ultimately translate to long-term renoprotection remains to be ascertained.

■ *Conclusion*

Ang II receptor antagonists appear to be an exciting new class of antihypertensive agents for the prevention and treatment of diabetic nephropathy. We await with interest the results of a number of studies in progress in diabetic patients with either incipient or overt nephropathy.

References

1. Rodby RA, Firth LM, Lewis EJ: An economic analysis of captopril in the treatment of diabetic nephropathy. The Collaborative Study Group. Diabetes Care 19:1051–1061, 1996.
2. Held PJ, Port FK, Webb RL, et al: The United States Renal Data System's 1991 annual data report: An introduction. Am J Kidney Dis 18:1–16, 1991.
3. Mogensen CE: How to protect the kidney in diabetic patients: With special reference to IDDM. Diabetes 46(Suppl 2):S104–S111, 1997.
4. Mogensen CE, Keane WF, Bennett PH, et al: Prevention of diabetic renal disease with special reference to microalbuminuria. Lancet 346:1080–1084, 1995.
5. Joint National Committee on Prevention, Detection, Evaluation, and Treatment of High Blood Pressure: The sixth report of the Joint National Committee on Prevention, Detection, Evaluation, and Treatment of High Blood Pressure. Arch Intern Med 157:2413–2445, 1997.
6. Guidelines Subcommittee: 1999 World Health Organization–International Society of Hypertension guidelines for the management of hypertension. J Hypertens 17:151–183, 1999.
7. Cooper ME: Pathogenesis, prevention and treatment of diabetic nephropathy. Lancet 352: 213–219, 1998.
8. Wolf G, Ziyadeh FN: The role of angiotensin II in diabetic nephropathy: Emphasis on nonhemodynamic mechanisms. Am J Kidney Dis 29:153–163, 1997.
9. Hostetter T, Rennke H, Brenner B: The case for intrarenal hypertension in the initiation and progression of diabetic and other glomerulopathies. Am J Med 72:375–380, 1982.
10. Wu L, Cox A, Roe C, et al: Transforming growth factor β1 and renal injury following subtotal nephrectomy in the rat: Role of the renin-angiotensin system. Kidney Int 51:1553–1567, 1997.
11. Gilbert RE, Cox A, Wu LL, et al: Expression of transforming growth factor-β1 and type IV collagen in the renal tubulointerstitium in experimental diabetes: Effects of angiotensin converting enzyme inhibition. Diabetes 47:414–422, 1998.
12. Cooper ME, Gilbert RE, Epstein M: Pathophysiology of diabetic nephropathy. Metab Clin Exp 47(Suppl 1):3–6, 1998.
13. Taguma Y, Kitamoto Y, Futaki G, et al: Effect of captopril on heavy proteinuria in azotemic diabetics. N Engl J Med 313:1617–1620, 1985.
14. Lewis EJ, Hunsicker LG, Bain RP, Rohde RD: The effect of angiotensin converting enzyme inhibition on diabetic nephropathy. N Engl J Med 329:1456–1462, 1993.
15. Kasiske BL, Kalil RS, Ma JZ, et al: Effect of antihypertensive therapy on the kidney in patients with diabetes: A meta-regression analysis. Ann Intern Med 118:129–138, 1993.
16. Ravid M, Lang R, Rachmani R, Lishner M: Long-term renoprotective effect of angiotensin-converting enzyme inhibition in non-insulin-dependent diabetes mellitus. A 7-year follow-up study. Arch Intern Med 156:286–289, 1996.
17. Sano T, Kawamura T, Matsumae H, et al: Effects of long-term enalapril treatment on persistent micro-albuminuria in well-controlled hypertensive and normotensive NIDDM patients. Diabetes Care 17:420–424, 1994.
18. Ahmad J, Siddiqui MA, Ahmad H: Effective postponement of diabetic nephropathy with enalapril in normotensive type 2 diabetic patients with microalbuminuria. Diabetes Care 20:1576–1581, 1997.

19. Ravid M, Brosh D, Levi Z, et al: Use of enalapril to attenuate decline in renal function in normotensive, normoalbuminuric patients with type 2 diabetes mellitus: A randomized, controlled trial. Ann Intern Med 128:982–988, 1998.

20. Cooper ME, McNally PG: Antihypertensive treatment in NIDDM, with special reference to abnormal albuminuria. In Mogensen CE (ed): The Kidney and Hypertension in Diabetes Mellitus, 4th ed. Norwell, MA, Kluwer Academic Publications, 1998, pp 427–440.

21. Nielsen FS, Rossing P, Gall MA, et al: Impact of lisinopril and atenolol on kidney function in hypertensive NIDDM subjects with diabetic nephropathy. Diabetes 43:1108–1113, 1994.

22. Chan JC, Cockram CS, Nicholls MG, et al: Comparison of enalapril and nifedipine in treating non-insulin-dependent diabetes associated with hypertension: One-year analysis. BMJ 305: 981–985, 1992.

23. Ferder L, Daccordi H, Martello M, et al: Angiotensin-converting enzyme inhibitors versus calcium antagonists in the treatment of diabetic hypertensive patients. Hypertension 19:II237–II242, 1992.

24. Liou HH, Huang TP, Campese VM: Effect of long-term therapy with captopril on proteinuria and renal function in patients with non-insulin-dependent diabetes and with nondiabetic renal diseases. Nephron 69:41–48, 1995.

25. Bakris GL, Barnhill BW, Sadler R: Treatment of arterial hypertension in diabetic humans: Importance of therapeutic selection. Kidney Int 41:912–919, 1992.

26. Slataper R, Vicknair N, Sadler R, Bakris GL: Comparative effects of different antihypertensive treatments on progression of diabetic renal disease. Arch Intern Med 153:973–980, 1993.

27. Epstein M, Cooper ME: Diabetic nephropathy: Focus on ACE inhibition and calcium channel blockade. In Epstein M (ed): Calcium Antagonists in Clinical Medicine, 2nd ed. Philadelphia, Hanley & Belfus, 1998, pp 243—271.

28. Bakris GL, Copley JB, Vicknair N, et al: Calcium channel blockers versus other antihypertensive therapies on progression of NIDDM associated nephropathy. Kidney Int 50:1641–1650, 1996.

29. Lacourciere Y, Nadeau A, Poirier L, Tancrede G: Captopril or conventional therapy in hypertensive type II diabetics. Three year analysis. Hypertension 21:786–794, 1993.

30. Schnack C, Hoffmann W, Hopmeier P, Schernthaner G: Renal and metabolic effects of 1-year treatment with ramipril or atenolol in NIDDM patients with microalbuminuria. Diabetologia 39:1611–1616, 1996.

31. Ruggenenti P, Mosconi L, Bianchi L, et al: Long-term treatment with either enalparil or nitrendipine stabilizes albuminuria and increases glomerular filtration rate in non-insulin-dependent diabetic patients. Am J Kidney Dis 24:753–761, 1994.

32. Velussi M, Brocco E, Frogato F, et al: Effects of cilazapril and amlodipine on kidney function in hypertensive NIDDM patients. Diabetes 45:216–222, 1996.

33. Agardh CD, Garcia Puig J, Charbonnel B, et al: Greater reduction of urinary albumin excretion in hypertensive type II diabetic patients with incipient nephropathy by lisinopril than by nifedipine. J Hum Hypertens 10:185–192, 1996.

34. Melbourne Diabetic Nephropathy Study Group: Comparison between perindopril and nifedipine in hypertensive and normotensive diabetic patients with microalbuminuria. BMJ 302:210–216, 1991.

35. Johnston CI: Angiotensin receptor antagonists: Focus on losartan. Lancet 346:1403–1407, 1995.

36. Ichikawa I, Madias NE, Harrington JT, et al: Will angiotensin II receptor antagonists be renoprotective in humans? Kidney Int 50:684–692, 1996.

37. Kon V, Fogo A, Ichikawa I: Bradykinin causes selective efferent arteriolar dilatation during angiotensin I converting enzyme inhibition. Kidney Int 44:545–550, 1993.

38. Komers R, Cooper ME: Acute renal haemodynamic effects of angiotensin converting enzyme inhibition in diabetic hyperfiltration: The role of kinins. Am J Physiol 268:F588–F594, 1995.

39. Mackenzie HS, Ziai F, Omer SA, et al: Angiotensin receptor blockers in chronic renal disease: The promise of a bright clinical future. J Am Soc Nephrol 10:S283–S286, 1999.

40. Allen TJ, Cao Z, Youssef S, et al: The role of angiotensin II and bradykinin in experimental diabetic nephropathy: Functional and structural studies. Diabetes 46:1612–1618, 1997.

41. Hollenberg NK: Non-insulin-dependent diabetes mellitus, nephropathy, and the renin system. J Hypertens 15:S7–S13, 1997.

42. Price DA, Porter LE, Gordon M, et al: The paradox of the low-renin state in diabetic nephropathy. J Am Soc Nephrol 10:2382–2391, 1999.

43. Masakai H, Kurihara T, Yamaki A, et al: Cardiac-specific overexpression of angiotensin II AT2 receptor causes attenuated response to AT1 receptor-mediated pressor and chronotropic effects. J Clin Invest 101:527–535, 1998.

44. Dzau VJ, Mukoyama M, Pratt RE: Molecular biology of angiotensin receptors—Target for drug research. J Hypertens 12:S1–S5, 1994.

45. Levy BI, Benessiano J, Henrion D, et al: Chronic blockade of AT2-subtype receptors prevents the effect of angiotensin II on the rat vascular structure. J Clin Invest 98:418–425, 1996.

46. Gansevoort RT, DeZeeuw D, Shahinfar S, et al: Effects of the angiotensin II antagonist losartan in hypertensive patients with renal disease. J Hypertens 12:S37–S42, 1994.
47. Chan JCN, Critchley J, Tomlinson B, et al: Antihypertensive and anti-albuminuric effects of losartan potassium and felodipine in Chinese elderly hypertensive patients with or without non-insulin-dependent diabetes mellitus. Am J Nephrol 17:72–80, 1997.
48. Ruilope LM: Renoprotection and renin-angiotensin system blockade in diabetes mellitus. Am J Hypertens 10:S325–S331, 1997.
49. Losartan vs. amlodipine in hypertensive patients with NIDDM. Proceedings of the 15th International Congress of Nephrology Symposium, 1997.
50. Rodby RA: Antihypertensive treatment in nephropathy of type II diabetes: Role of the pharmacological blockade of the renin-angiotensin system. Nephrol Dial Transplant 12:1095–1096, 1997.
50a. Rodby RA, Rohde RD, Clarke WR, et al. for the Collaborative Study Study Group: The Irbesartan Type II Diabetic Nephropathy Trial: Study design and baseline patient characteristics. Nephrol Dial Transplant 15:487–497, 2000.
51. Burnier M, Brunner HR: Angiotensin II receptor antagonists: Clinical development and future perspectives. Therapie 53:279–284, 1998.
52. Andersen S, Tarnow L, Rossing P, et al: Renoprotective effects of angiotensin II receptor blockade in type 1 diabetic patients with diabetic nephropathy. Kidney Int 57:601–606, 2000.
53. Yokota C, Okuda Y, Odawara M, et al: The effect of losartan on urinary albumin excretion in type 2 diabetic patients. Diabetologia 42(Suppl 1):A274, 1999.
54. Açbay O, Mazlum A, Kural E, Gündogdu S: Losartan reduces albuminuria in normotensive type 1 and type 2 diabetic patients. Diabetologia 42(Suppl 1):A274, 1999.
55. Buter H, van Tol A, Navis GJ, et al: AT(1) receptor antagonism lowers plasma total and VLDL + LDL cholesterol in type I diabetic patients with albuminuria. Diabetologia 42(Suppl 1):A289, 1999.
56. Brenner B, Shahinfar S, for the RENAAL Investigators: Reduction of endpoints in NIDDM with angiotensin II antagonist losartan. Proceedings of the XVth International Congress of Nephrology, 1999 [abstract 648].

CHAPTER 22

AT₁ Receptor Antagonists in Combination with Other Antihypertensive Agents

BERNARD WAEBER, M.D.
HANS R. BRUNNER, M.D.

Essential hypertension is a common disease and major health problem in industrialized countries. Despite worldwide efforts at diagnosis and treatment because of increased cardiovascular risk, blood pressure in the community is still poorly controlled, even in countries in which access to medical care is reputed to be easy. In the United States, for example, 68% of people with high blood pressure are aware of their condition, and 54% of hypertensive patients receive antihypertensive treatment.[1] However, in only 27% of hypertensive patients is blood pressure truly normalized (<140/90 mmHg). The situation may be even worse elsewhere. In the United Kingdom, for example, as few as 6% of hypertensive patients have normalized blood pressure.[2] The difficulty in lowering blood pressure of hypertensive patients is also reflected by the results of a recent survey in the north of Italy. No significant difference was observed between blood pressures of treated vs. untreated hypertensive patients,[3] regardless of whether blood pressures were measured at the clinic, at home, or by noninvasive ambulatory monitoring.

■ Monotherapy vs. Combination Therapy

In view of the disappointing results in hypertensive patients, one should wonder whether it is possible to lower blood pressure to recommended targets with currently available medications. Because essential hypertension is a heterogeneous disease, it is not surprising that a drug acting by a given mechanism cannot normalize blood pressure in every patient.[4] Fortunately, physicians can choose among several classes of antihypertensive agents, including diuretics, beta blockers, alpha₁ blockers, calcium antagonists, and blockers of the renin-angiotensin system (angiotensin-converting enzyme [ACE] inhibitors and angiotensin II antagonists [AT₁ receptor antagonists]).[5] Monotherapy with a drug from any of these classes can control blood pressure in roughly one-half of hypertensive patients. But what can be done if blood pressure is not satisfactorily controlled by a given medication?

For many years dosage adjustment was advocated in an attempt to improve antihypertensive efficacy. This approach is no longer popular because most antihypertensive agents show a dose-dependent increase in the incidence of side-effects (Fig. 1).[6] In this respect AT_1 receptor antagonists have a tremendous advantage because characteristically they are well tolerated independently of dosage.[7-9] With AT_1 receptor antagnoists, therefore, it is possible to achieve full inhibition of the renin-angiotensin system without triggering more side-effects. One must realize, however, that even optimal blockade of AT_1 receptors does not normalize blood pressure in patients with a non–renin-dependent form of hypertension.

If a medication is not sufficiently effective, a rational option is to switch to another drug belonging to a different class of antihypertensive agents.[4] This approach, known as sequential monotherapy, was evaluated recently in a trial in which each patient received for 4-week periods a diuretic, a beta blocker, a calcium antagonist, and an ACE inhibitor.[10] During the initial treatment phase blood pressure was normalized in 39% of the patients. Considering the results of subsequent rotations, blood pressure normalization was achieved with at least one of the tested medications in 73% of patients. This study, therefore, confirms that it is possible to control blood pressure in most hypertensive patients through successive exposure to several monotherapies. This approach, however, is time-consuming, and patients may become discouraged and interrupt the treatment.

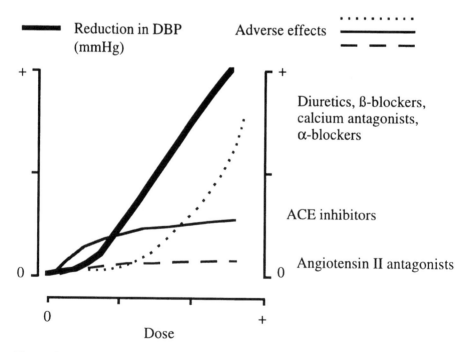

Figure 1. Relationship between the antihypertensive efficacy (ordinate on the left part of the graph) and the dose (abcissa) of the medication. The dose-dependency of side effects is illustrated in the same way; the incidence of side effects is shown on the ordinate on the right part of the graph.

Another way to improve antihypertertensive efficacy is to combine drugs acting by different mechanisms.[11–14] Multiple effects on the cardiovascular system increase the likelihood of normalizing blood pressure. The enhanced antihypertensive efficacy is also due to the fact that the blood pressure-lowering effect induced by a given drug may be attenuated by compensatory cardiovascular or renal responses, an undesirable phenomenon that can be largely prevented by coadministering another type of antihypertensive agent. By increasing urinary sodium excretion, for example, diuretics trigger the release of renin from juxtaglomerular cells. This stimulation of the renin-angiotensin system limits blood pressure response to a diuretic-induced decrease in total body sodium. It is possible, however, to neutralize compensatory hyperreninemia with simultaneous blockade of the renin-angiotensin system.[15] Understanding of the close interplay between the activity of the renin-angiotensin system and sodium balance led to the development of a number of fixed-dose combinations containing an ACE inhibitor and thiazide diuretic. Such combinations are widely accepted because they are highly effective and well tolerated. One reason for the good tolerability is the fact that low doses of diuretics are generally sufficient when given with an ACE inhibitor, and the major metabolic side effects of diuretics are dose-dependent. Other rational fixed-dose regimens combine an ACE inhibitor with a calcium antagonist or a beta blocker with either a diuretic or a calcium antagonist.[5]

Low-dose combinations of antihypertensive drugs are becoming more and more attractive to initiate treatment because they enhance efficacy without impairing tolerability. A few fixed-dose combinations have been or are in the process of being approved as potential first-line therapy by the U.S. Food and Drug Administration. The usefulness of these combinations also was recognized by the most recent World Health Organization/International Society of Hypertension Guidelines for the Management of Hypertension.[5]

■ Combinations of AT₁ Receptor Antagonists and Diuretics

Antihypertensive Efficacy

The compensatory rise in renin secretion induced by sodium depletion may become the predominant factor sustaining high blood pressure during diuretic therapy. Simultaneous blockade of the renin-angiotensin system makes this reactive hyperreninemia ineffective and allows maximal benefit from sodium depletion. Not surprisingly, efforts were quickly made to develop fixed-dose combinations of an AT₁ receptor antagonist and a diuretic.

The efficacy of losartan, the first orally active AT₁ receptor antagonist, combined with the diuretic hydrochlorothiazide (HCTZ) has been compared with the efficacy of losartan alone, HCTZ alone, and placebo.[16] A total of 703 patients with mild-to-moderate hypertension (diastolic blood pressure of 95–105 mmHg) were randomized to 12 weeks of once-daily treatment with 50 mg losartan + 6.25 mg HCTZ, 50 mg losartan + 12.5 mg HCTZ, 50 mg losartan only, 12.5 mg HCTZ only, or placebo. There was no significant difference in baseline blood pressure among the study groups (around 152/101 mmHg). Figure 2 shows the mean changes in trough blood pressure for the five treatment groups. The reduction in both systolic and diastolic blood pressure was

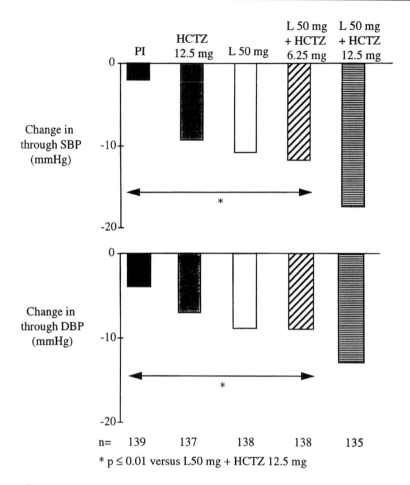

Figure 2.   Mean changes in trough systolic (SBP) and diastolic (DBP) blood pressure induced by 12-week, once-daily treatment with either placebo (PI), 12.5 mg hydrochlorothiazide (HCTZ 12.5 mg), 50 mg losartan (L 50mg), L 50 mg + HCTZ 6.25 mg, or L 50 mg + HCTZ 12.5 mg. (Adapted from Schoenberger JA: Losartan with hydrochlorothiazide in the treatment of hypertension. J Hypertens 13(Suppl 1):S43–S47, 1995.)

significantly more pronounced with 50 mg losartan +12.5 mg HCTZ than with the other four treatments. The combination of 50 mg losartan with 6.25 mg HCTZ was equally as effective as 50 mg losartan only, but significantly more effective than 12.5 mg HCTZ only and placebo. The control rate, as defined by a trough diastolic blood pressure < 90 mmHg, was 20.9% for placebo, 34.3% for HCTZ alone, 40.6% for losartan alone, and 43.5 % and 57.8% for losartan combined with 6.25 and 12.5 mg HCTZ, respectively.

HCTZ also enhances the blood pressure-lowering effect of the newer AT_1 receptor antagonists. In a double-blind trial 1096 patients with mild-to-moderate hypertension (sitting diastolic blood pressure of 95–110 mmHg) were randomly allocated to once-daily treatment for 8 weeks with either candesartan (2, 4, 8, or 16 mg), HCTZ (12.5 or 25 mg), combination therapy with both agents at the respective doses, or placebo.[17] Figure 3 depicts the mean reductions in blood

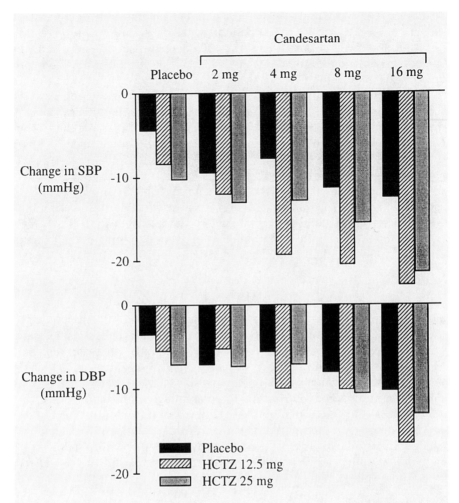

Figure 3. Mean changes in systolic (SBP) and diastolic (DBP) blood pressure induced by a 8-week treatment with candesartan, 2–16 mg; hydrochlorothiazide (HCTZ), 12.5 or 25 mg; a combination of both; or placebo. (Adapted from Philip T, Letzel H, Arens HJ: Dose-finding study of candesartan cilexetil plus hydrochlorothiazide in patients with mild to moderate hypertension. J Hum Hypertens 11(Suppl 2):67–68, 1997.)

pressure during the course of the trial. The greatest blood pressure decrease was observed with 16 mg candesartan combined with 12.5 mg HCTZ. This study is of particular interest becaues it found no real advantage to increasing the dose of HCTZ beyond 12.5 mg when it was given with candesartan.

In another trial candesartan was administered to 234 patients with hypertension unresponsive (sitting diastolic blood pressure ≥ 90 mmHg) to 6 weeks of treatment with HCTZ, 12.5 mg once daily.[8] The patients were randomized to receive for 8 weeks either 4 mg candesartan, 8 mg candesartan, or placebo, each in addition to 12.5 mg HCTZ. The combined treatments with candesartan and HCTZ lowered blood pressure significantly more (–13.4/–7.9 mmHg with 8 mg candesartan and –11.0/–7.0 mmHg with 4 mg candesartan) than HCTZ given with placebo (–3/–3 mmHg).

Another interesting trial was performed in 432 patients with a diastolic blood pressure of 95–115 mmHg.[19] The patients were randomized to receive either irbesartan, 150 mg once daily, or losartan, 50 mg once daily. The dose of the two AT_1 receptor antagonists could be doubled after 4 weeks if diastolic blood pressure was still $\geq$ 90 mmHg. After 8 weeks of monotherapy, HCTZ (12.5 mg once daily) was combined with the AT_1 receptor antagonist for 4 additional weeks if diastolic blood pressure was $\geq$ 90 mmHg. An 8-week treatment with irbesartan was significantly more effective in lowering diastolic blood pressure than a corresponding treatment with losartan (–10.2 vs. –7.9 mmHg, respectively, p < 0.05). At the end of the study (week 12), reductions in diastolic blood pressure were significantly greater in irbesartan-treated patients (–13.8 mmHg) than in losartan-treated patients (–10.8 mmHg). These data suggest that an AT_1 receptor antagonist with longer duration of action is more effective in lowering blood pressure when given alone or in combination with a diuretic than an AT_1 receptor antagonist with a shorter duration of action, although some of the difference certainly can be attributed to the respective doses chosen for the study.

Tolerability

The tolerability of AT_1 receptor antagonists is quite good—almost the same as that of placebo.[7–9] This class effect is well established and much appreciated. Another classic advantage of AT_1 receptor antagonists is the lack of a dose-dependent increase in the incidence of side effects. Thus, the physician can choose the dosage large enough to provide sustained blockade of the renin-angiotensin system without worrying about troublesome side effects. This advantage may be of particular importance when an AT_1 receptor antagonist is combined with a diuretic. In a salt-depleted condition, circulating Ang II levels are expected to be high, and doses of AT_1 receptor antagonists capable of optimal blockade may be required. In fact, the experience to date clearly shows that adding a dose of 12.5 mg hydrochlorothiazide to an AT_1 receptor antagonist has no adverse effect in terms of tolerability.

Metabolic Effects

AT_1 receptor antagonists have no deleterious effects on glucose homeostasis and lipid metabolism in hypertensive patients, whether they are administered alone or in combination with a diuretic. Of note, the dosage of thiazides added to an AT_1 receptor antagonist can be kept in the lower range, which accounts for the neutral metabolic effects of combination therapy.

Thiazides are known to induce a dose-dependent decrease in serum potassium and a dose-dependent increase in serum uric acid. Because of the low doses of thiazides used in combination with AT_1 receptor antagonists, generally there are no consistent changes in these parameters. Diuretic-induced salt depletion normally leads to secondary hyperaldosteronism, which in turn enhances urinary potassium excretion. This aldosterone response is blunted during Ang II blockade because all currently available AT_1 receptor antagonists specifically bind to AT_1 receptors (i. e., the receptors involved in the angiotensin-mediated release of aldosterone). Table 1 summarizes the effects of the AT_1 receptor antagonist losartan on serum potassium when it was administered with HCTZ.[20] In this trial 304 patients with a diastolic blood pessure of 93–120 mmHg received HCTZ, 25

Table 1. Effect of Losartan on Serum Potassium Levels*

	Baseline	After 4 Weeks of HCTZ (25 mg/day)	Ater 8 Weeks of Combined Therapy
Placebo	4.26 ± 0.3	3.92 ± 0.4	3.88 ± 0.4
Losartan, 25 mg/day	4.30 ± 0.4	4.03 ± 0.4	4.10 ± 0.4[†]
Losartan, 50 mg/day	4.35 ± 0.3	4.00 ± 0.4	4.05 ± 0.4[†]
Losartan, 100 mg/day	4.26 ± 0.4	4.00 ± 0.4	4.10 ± 0.4[†]

* Levels given in mmol/L (mean ± standard deviation).
[†] p < 0.05 vs. HCTZ
From Soffer BA, Wright JT, Pratt JH, et al: Effects of losartan on a background of hydrochlorothiazide in patients with hypertension. Hypertension 26:112–117, 1995, with permission.

mg daily, for 4 weeks. Then, in addition to the HCTZ, they were randomly allocated to receive 25, 50, or 100 mg losartan once daily or placebo. HCTZ administered alone induced a clear-cut decrease in serum potassium concentrations. Cotreatment with losartan prevented the decrease to a large extent.

Recently increasing attention has been paid to the effect of diuretics on uricemia because of indications that elevated serum uric acid may be an independent risk factor for cardiovascular diseases.[21] An interesting feature of losartan is its uricosuric action, which is unique among Ang II antagonists and results in a dose-dependent decrease in uric acid concentration.[22] The ability of losartan to increase uric acid excretion is a property of the mother compound and is not observed with the active metabolite, E-3174. Losartan enhances urate elimination and reduces serum uric acid by inhibiting an anion-proton exchanger in the proximal tubules of the nephron. Addition of losartan to HCTZ prevents diuretic-induced hyperuricemia[20] (Table 2), as demonstrated by the study described above of hypertensive patients who received different doses of losartan in addition to HCTZ.

■ *Combination of AT₁ Receptor Antagonists and ACE Inhibitors*

Theoretically the combination of an AT₁ receptor antagonist with an ACE inhibitor may be of clinical benefit in the treatment of hypertension. Some Ang II can still be formed during effective ACE inhibition through alternative enzymes, such as chymase, cathepsin G, and trypsin,[23] or through less-than-complete ACE inhibition in the face of stimulated renin secretion and high Ang I levels.[24] Combination with an AT₁ receptor antagonist, therefore, seems

Table 2. Effect of Losartan on Serum Uric Acid Concentrations*

	Baseline	After 4 Weeks of HCTZ (25 mg/day)	Ater 8 Weeks of Combined Therapy
Placebo	395 ± 89	463 ± 107	472 ± 107
Losartan, 25 mg/day	393 ± 77	462 ± 95	447 ± 95[†]
Losartan, 50 mg/day	385 ± 95	453 ± 113	437 ± 101[†]
Losartan, 100 mg/day	378 ± 95	435 ± 101	410 ± 101[†]

* Concentrations given in µmol/L (mean ± standard deviation).
[†] p < 0.001 vs. HCTZ
From Soffer BA, Wright JT, Pratt JH, et al: Effects of losartan on a background of hydrochlorothiazide in patients with hypertension. Hypertension 26:112–117, 1995, with permission.

appealing because direct action at the AT_1 receptor is expected to provide complete Ang II blockade. Furthermore, ACE is involved not only in Ang I processing but also in bradykinin metabolism. ACE inhibition, therefore, may lead to some accumulation of bradykinin,[25] a potent vasodilating peptide that releases nitric oxide (NO) and prostacyclin from the endothelium. The ACE inhibition-induced decrease in breakdown of bradykinin may have positive effects on the vasculature in addition to enhanced vasorelaxation. For example, NO has an inhibitory effect on mitogenesis and proliferation of vascular smooth muscle cells, and both NO and prostacyclin decrease platelet aggregation. Thus, ACE inhibition seems appealing to block the renin-angiotensin system.

On the other hand, blocking the renin-angiotensin system with an AT_1 receptor antagonist alone causes overstimulation of AT_2 receptors. Indeed, activation of AT_1 receptors on juxtaglomerular cells exerts negative feedback for renin release, with an ensuing increase in circulating levels of Ang II. The exact impact of unopposed overstimulation of AT_2 receptors is still unclear. Simultaneous stimulation of both AT_1 and AT_2 receptors may have a "yin-yang" effect: AT_1 receptors may enhance vascular smooth muscle growth, whereas AT_2 receptors may have the opposite effect. Chronic AT_1 blockade, therefore, would lead to enhanced antiproliferative activity.[26] Whether such a salutary effect really occurs during chronic AT_1 receptor blockade remains unknown. Potentially sustained stimulation of AT_2 receptors also may have unrecognized harmful effects, even if current experience with AT_1 receptor antagonists does not support such a concern. The combination of an ACE inhibitor and an Ang II antagonist may reduce the conversion of Ang I to Ang II and consequently attenuate the stimulation of AT_2 receptors. Whether this effect has any clinically relevant advantage, however, is speculative.

AT_1 receptor antagonists and ACE inhibitors are equally effective in lowering blood pressure in hypertensive patients.[27,28] When given together, possibly because of maximal blockade of the renin-angiotensin system or—less likely—the presence of an underlying bradykinin-induced vasodilation, the blood pressure-lowering effect seems to be increased, as suggested by a study in salt-depleted normotensive humans.[29] This finding also seems to apply to hypertensive patients. For example, 30 patients with diastolic blood pressure > 90 mmHg despite 2 weeks of treatment with the ACE inhibitor, lisinopril (20 mg once daily), were randomly allocated to receive in addition for 4 weeks either losartan, 50 mg once daily, or placebo.[30] Blood pressure was assessed both conventionally at the doctor's office and by ambulatory monitoring. The combination treatment was significantly more effective in lowering blood pressure than the ACE inhibitor alone (Fig. 4). This finding was true in all conditions of blood pressure measurement. However, more studies combining an ACE inhibitor with an AT_1 receptor antagonist should explore the full dose-response relationship for each component to assess whether a similar effect may be achieved with higher doses. Currently no published information is available about the tolerability of the combination of an ACE inhibitor and an AT_1 receptor antagonist. The combination is expected to be less well tolerated than monotherapy with an AT_1 receptor antagonist, mainly because of the cough associated with ACE inhibition.

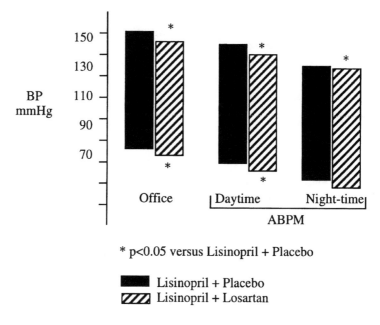

* p<0.05 versus Lisinopril + Placebo

▓▓ Lisinopril + Placebo
▨▨ Lisinopril + Losartan

Figure 4.   Effect of losartan, 50 mg once daily, or placebo on office and ambulatory blood pressure of hypertensive patients taking lisinopril, 20 mg once daily after 4 weeks of combined treatment. (Adapted from Fogari R, Corradi L, Preti P, et al: Effects of losartan addition to lisinopril in hypertensives:A 24-hour ABPM study. J Hypertens 16(Suppl 2):S24, 1998.)

■ Other Possible Combinations with AT₁ Receptor Antagonists

A logical combination is an AT_1 receptor antagonist and a calcium antagonist. Based on current experience with an existing ACE inhibitor-calcium antagonist fixed-dose combination, such a combination is expected to be efficacious and well tolerated.[31] Combinations involving other classes of antihypertensive agents appear less promising in terms of efficacy. Nonetheless, for whatever indication, AT_1 receptor antagonists can be safely administered with any other cardiovascular drug. Caution should be used only when they are combined with potassium-sparing diuretics in patients with reduced renal function

■ Conclusion

The most rational combination of an AT_1 receptor blocker is with a low-dose thiazide diuretic. Fixed-dose combinations containing these agents are now available and have the advantage of being both efficacious and well tolerated, which is expected to improve long-term compliance with treatment. They may be useful not only as second-line therapy but also as initial treatment in hypertensive patients.

References

1. Joint National Committee on Prevention, Detection, Evaluation, and Treatment of High Blood Pressure: The sixth report of the Joint National Committee on Prevention, Detection, Evaluation, and Treatment of High Blood Pressure. Arch Intern Med 57:2413–2446, 1997.
2. Colhoun HM, Dong W, Poulter NR: Blood pressure screening, management and control in England: Results from the health survey for England 1994. J Hypertens 16:747–752, 1998.
3. Mancia G, Sega R, Milesi C, et al: Blood-pressure control in the hypertensive population. Lancet 349:454–457, 1997.

4. Brunner HR, Menard J, Waeber B, et al: Treating the individual hypertensive patient: considerations on dose, sequential monotherapy and drug combinations. J Hypertens 8:3–11, 1990.

5. World Health Organization-International Society of Hypertension: 1999 Guidelines for the Management of Hypertension. J Hypertens 17:905–918, 1999.

6. Fagan TC: Remembering the lessons of basic pharmacology. Arch Intern Med 154:1430–1431, 1994.

7. Goldberg AI, Dunlay MC, Sweet CS: Safety and tolerability of losartan potassium, an angiotensin II receptor antagonist, compared with hydrochlorothiazide, atenolol, felodipine ER, and angiotensin-converting enzyme inhibitors for the treatment of systemic hypertension. Am J Cardiol 75:793–795, 1995.

8. Sever P: Candesartan cilexetil: A new, long-acting, effective angiotensin II type 1 receptor blocker. J Hum Hypertens 11(Suppl 2):91–95, 1997.

9. Man in't Veld A: Clinical overview of irbesartan: Expanding the therapeutic window in hypertension. J Hypertens 15(Suppl 7):27–33, 1997.

10. Dickerson CJE, Hingorani AD, Ashby MJ, et al: Optimisation of antihypertensive treatment by crossover rotation of four major classes. Lancet 353:2008–2013, 1999.

11. Oster JR, Epstein M: Fixed-dose combination medications for treatment of hypertension: A critical review. J Clin Hypertens 3:278–293, 1987.

12. Waeber B, Brunner HR: Main objectives and new aspects of combination treatment of hypertension. J Hypertens 13(Suppl):S15–S19, 1995.

13. Epstein M, Bakris G: Newer approaches to antihypertensive therapy. Use of fixed-dose combination therapy. Arch Intern Med 156:1969–1978, 1996.

14. Waeber B, Brunner HR: Low-dose combinations versus monotherapies in the treatment of hypertension. J Hypertens 15(Suppl):S17–S20, 1997.

15. Brunner HR, Gavras H, Waeber B: Enhancement by diuretics of the antihypertensive action of long-term angiotensin converting enzyme blockade. Clin Exp Hypertens 2:639–657, 1980.

16. Schoenberger JA: Losartan with hydrochlorothiazide in the treatment of hypertension. J Hypertens 13(Suppl 1):S43–S47, 1995.

17. Philip T, Letzel H, Arens HJ: Dose-finding study of candesartan cilexetil plus hydrochlorothiazide in patients with mild to moderate hypertension. J Hum Hypertens 11(Suppl 2):67–68, 1997.

18. Plouin PF: Combination therapy with candesartan cilexetil plus hydrochlorothiazide in patients unresponsive to low-dose hydrochlorothiazide. J Hum Hypertens 11(Suppl 2):65–66, 1997.

19. Oparil S, Guthrie R, Lewin AJ, et al: On behalf of the Irbesartan/Losartan Study Investigators. Clin Ther 20:398–409, 1998.

20. Soffer BA, Wright JT, Pratt JH, et al: Effects of losartan on a background of hydrochlorothiazide in patients with hypertension. Hypertension 26:112–117, 1995.

21. Burnier M, Waeber B, Brunner HR: Clinical pharmacology of the angiotensin II receptor antagonist losartan potassium in healthy subjects. J Hypertens 13:S23–S28, 1995.

22. Burnier M, Brunner HR: Is hyperuricemia a predictor of cardiovascular risk? Curr Opinion Nephrol Hypertens 8:167–172, 1999.

23. Urata H, Nishimura H, Ganten D, Arakawa K: Angiotensin-converting enzyme-independent pathways of angiotensin II formation in human tissues and cardiovascular diseases. Blood Pressure 5(Suppl 2):22–28, 1996.

24. Juillerat L, Nussberger J, Rénard J, et al: Determinants of angiotensin II generation during converting enzyme inhibition. Hypertension 16:564–572, 1990.

25. Pellacani A, Brunner HR, Nussberger J: Plasma kinins increase after angiotensin-converting enzyme inhibition in human subjects. Clin Sci 87:567–574, 1994.

26. Chung O, Stoll M, Unger T: Physiologic and pharmacologic implications of AT1 versus AT2 receptors. Blood Pressure Suppl 2:47–52, 1996.

27. Gradman AH, Arcuri KE, Goldberg AI, et al: A randomized, placebo-controlled, double-blind, parallel study of various doses of losartan potassium compared with enalapril maleate in patients with essential hypertension. Hypertension 25:1345–1350, 1995.

28. Tikkanen I, Omvik P, Jensen HA: Comparison of the angiotensin II antagonist losartan with the angiotensin converting enzyme inhibitor enalapril in patients with essential hypertension. J Hypertens 13:1343–1351, 1995.

29. Azizi M, Chatellier G, Guyene TT, et al: Additive effects of combined angiotensin-converting enzyme inhibition and angiotensin II antagonism on blood pressure and renin release in sodium-depleted normotensives. Circulation 92:825–834, 1995.

30. Fogari R, Corradi L, Preti P, et al: Effects of losartan addition to lisinopril in hypertensives:A 24-hour ABPM study. J Hypertens 16(Suppl 2):S24, 1998.

31. deLeeuw P, Kroon A: Fixed low-dose combination of an angiotensin converting enzyme inhibitor and a calcium channel blocker drug in the treatment of essential hypertension. J Hypertens 15(Suppl 2):39–42, 1997.

CHAPTER 23

Angiotensin II Receptor Antagonists: Safety and Tolerability Profile

LUCIA MAZZOLAI, M.D.
MICHEL BURNIER, M.D.

Angiotensin-converting enzyme (ACE) inhibitors, which interfere with the renin-angiotensin system by blocking the conversion of angiotensin I into angiotensin II (Ang II) are highly effective for the treatment of essential hypertension and congestive heart failure. In addition, ACE inhibitors are useful in retarding the progression of chronic renal failure in diabetic and nondiabetic patients. Despite their recognized benefits, ACE inhibitors often are underused or underdosed, particularly in heart failure; this observation is sometimes attributed to side-effects. Compared with other antihypertensive agents, such as diuretics or beta blockers, ACE inhibitors have a relatively favorable side-effect profile. Nonetheless, their administration is associated with cough in about 10% of patients, and many physicians fear that in some clinical conditions ACE inhibition may cause acute renal failure.

The side-effect profile of ACE inhibitors can be attributed in part to the nonspecificity of ACE, which also interferes with the metabolism of other peptides, and in part to the changes in plasma Ang II and blood pressure. The recent development of nonpeptide Ang II receptor antagonists, which block the renin-angiotensin system (RAS) more specifically without interfering with other systems, should improve the safety and tolerability profile while preserving an effective blockade of the RAS. Information about safety and tolerability of Ang II receptor antagonists has been acquired in several thousands of hypertensive patients in various clinical trials performed for registration purposes and follow-up studies. Most of our knowledge derives from studies conducted with losartan, the first Ang II antagonist to be commercialized, but important information also has been gathered with the other five antagonists available on the market: valsartan, irbesartan, candesartan, telmisartan, and eprosartan.

■ Overall Incidence of Side Effects and Withdrawal from Studies

The main characteristic of Ang II antagonists appears to be their favorable side-effect profile. Thus, data derived from clinical studies indicate that the overall incidence of any clinically relevant adverse effect is 15.3% in patients treated with losartan compared with 15.5% in patients receiving placebo.[1] Similar results were obtained with candesartan, valsartan, irbesartan, telmisartan, and eprosartan.[2-8] None of the compounds induced a clear, specific, dose-dependent drug-related side-effect.

With all Ang II antagonists, the withdrawal rate in clinical studies is relatively low and comparable to placebo (Table 1). Thus, of more than 2000 patients, 2.3% discontinued losartan because of possible side effects compared with 3.7% who discontinued placebo and 2.5–9.3% who discontinued other comparative antihypertensive drugs.[9] Comparable figures were reported with other antagonists, such as candesartan, irbesartan, and eprosartan.[2,4,6]

■ *Clinically Relevant Adverse Events*

Headache, Dizziness, and Fatigue

In terms of side effects, patients treated with losartan did not differ from those treated with a placebo. The most frequent drug-related side-effects were headache (14.1%), dizziness (2.4%), and asthenia/fatigue (2.0%).[1,10] However, only dizziness occurred with a frequency greater than that observed in placebo-treated patients (2.4% vs. 1.3%). With candesartan, valsartan, and irbesartan, headache was also a commonly reported adverse effect. However, it was less frequent than in placebo recipients. In a recent study, which compared telmisartan with enalapril, the incidence of dizziness was 2.9% in the telmisartan-treated group compared with 15.8% in the enalapril-treated group; the incidence of headache was similar with the two compounds (2.2% vs 2.9%, respectively).[11] Compared with placebo, the most common side effects of both telmisartan and eprosartan were headache, dizziness, and fatigue, which occurred at a rate statistically lower than that observed with placebo.[6,12]

Cutaneous Reactions

The incidence of rash in patients undergoing treatment with AT_1 antagonists was less than that observed in patients receiving a placebo. Among patients who developed cutaneous reactions, only one patient developed a rash upon rechallenge with losartan.[13]

Another report describes the onset of Henoch-Schönlein purpura in a patient treated with losartan. Purpura disappeared upon discontinuation of the treatment and rapidly reappeared when losartan was reintroduced.[14] Two patients developed an atypical cutaneous lymphoid hyperplasia while receiving losar-

Table 1.   Comparative Patient Withdrawal Rate from Clinical Studies

Compound	Angiotensin II Antagonist (%)	Placebo (%)
Losartan	2.3	3.7
Irbesartan	3.3	4.5
Candesartan	2.4	2.6
Eprosartan	3.9	6.5

No figures were found for valsartan and telmisartan.

tan.[15] The skin disorder disappeared upon drug withdrawal. Drug hypersensitivity reactions may induce atypical lymphoid hyperplasia, a phenomenon already observed with ACE inhibitors.[16]

Cough

Cough is the most frequent side effect observed with ACE inhibitors. It is considered a class effect related to the nonspecificity of ACE.[17] Cough occurs in around 10% of patients treated with an ACE inhibitor, but this incidence appears to be greater with different racial and ethnic backgrounds. Thus, cough may occur more frequently in Black and Asian patients.[18,19] Because Ang II antagonists do not interfere with the metabolism of kinins and other peptides, the absence of cough is the major clinical advantage of Ang II receptor antagonists. Losartan caused a low level of spontaneous reports of cough in hypertensive patients (ranging from 2.3–4.1%). Patients on ACE inhibitors experienced cough more often (8.8%).[20] In various comparative studies, cough was more frequent in patients treated with ACE inhibitors than in patients treated with irbesartan, eprosartan, telmisartan, candesartan, or valsartan, in whom the incidence of cough was not different from placebo.[5,6,21–23]

Double-blind studies have addressed specifically the issue of cough in patients complaining of cough on ACE inhibitors. In the first study, after a positive challenge with lisinopril, patients were randomized in three parallel groups to receive lisinopril, losartan, and hydrochlorothiazide.[24] After 8 weeks of treatment, the incidence of cough was comparable in the losartan and hydrochlorothiazide groups but significantly lower than in the lisinopril group. A similar study design was used to demonstrate that the occurrence of cough with valsartan is comparable to that observed with diuretic therapy but significantly lower than that observed with lisinopril.[25] More recently, the incidence of cough also was studied in 88 patients with a history of ACE inhibitor cough randomized to receive telmisartan, lisinopril, or a placebo. Cough was significantly less frequent with telmisartan (16%) than with lisinopril (60%, p = 0.001) and comparable to placebo (10%).[23] In an Asian population, losartan also was associated with a decrease in the incidence of cough in patients with previous ACE inhibitor-induced cough.[26]

Angioedema

Angioedema is another adverse event related to the use of ACE inhibitors. Its development appears to involve the accumulation of bradykinin, but whether this is the only mechanism remains to be demonstrated.[17,27,28] To date, available data do not allow a firm conclusion that Ang II receptor antagonists cause angioedema. Indeed, the literature contains several reports of angioedema during losartan therapy, and several other cases may not have been reported.[29–31] Because angioedema may occur with many substances, including drugs and some foods, whether these episodes truly represent a losartan-induced side effect is difficult to ascertain. With eprosartan cases of facial edema have been reported.[6]

Others

Ageusia is a rare complication of ACE inhibitors, reported only when higher doses were used.[32] Two reports describe patients with progressive dysgeusia or ageusia during treatment with losartan; symptoms were reversed after drug withdrawal.[33,34] One report described migraine in a patient with no history of migraine. Symptoms developed after losartan administration and were confirmed on rechallenge.[35] Another report describes a patient who developed reversible psychosis on losartan therapy, a reaction that reversed completely after drug discontinuation.[36] Few studies have investigated the effect of Ang II antagonists on impotence. Telmisartan induced significantly less impotence than the beta blocker atenolol.[5]

■ Laboratory Adverse Events

Effect on Hematologic Parameters

Hematologic parameters do not appear to be routinely altered in patients undergoing treatment with Ang II antagonists.[37] However, a recent report describes a case of anemia in a patient treated with losartan.[38,39] In the hypertensive population, only minor, clinically nonsignificant decreases in serum hemoglobin (1–2%) have been reported. To date, there have been no reported cases of leucopenia or thrombopenia. In posttransplant erythrocytosis, ACE inhibitors suppress erythropoiesis. Several case reports and studies in renal transplant patients suggest that losartan also lowers hematocrit effectively in this setting.[40–43]

Effect on Potassium

Long-term treatment with losartan was associated with slight increases in serum potassium levels.[44] This effect is expected and has been attributed to the transient decrease in plasma aldosterone levels. However, the increase in potassium did not lead to discontinuation of antihypertensive treatment. In hypertensive patients with normal renal function, the changes in serum potassium induced by valsartan, candesartan cilexetil, and irbesartan were negligible. With losartan, the incidence of hyperkalemia (1.5%) was similar to that observed with ACE inhibitors (1.3%) and placebo. As with ACE inhibitors, hyperkalemia is more likely to develop in patients with renal insufficiency, diabetics, or patients taking potassium-sparing diuretics or potassium supplementations.

Effect on Liver Enzymes

Elevation of transaminases (2–3 times above baseline level) occurred rarely and usually resolved with or without discontinuation of therapy.[44] In only one case was it necessary to discontinue losartan.[29] Among patients treated with candesartan cilexetil, occasional minor increases in plasma liver enzymes (particularly alanine aminotransferase) have been observed; usually they were transient despite continued therapy. Significant increases in transaminases have been reported with the administration of tasosartan, a long-acting Ang II receptor antagonist that has not been made available for clinical use. Whether this effect on liver enzymes is specific to tasosartan or associated with its longer duration of action is not known.

Effect on Uric Acid Excretion

Losartan increases urinary uric acid excretion and hence lowers plasma uric acid in normotensive people.[45–47] The uricosuric effect of losartan is due to its specific effect on urate transport in the renal proximal tubule and is independent of Ang II receptor blockade.[46,47] EXP3174, the active metabolite of losartan, has no effect on uric acid excretion.[48] A decrease in serum uric acid levels has been found consistently in hypertensive patients treated with losartan. In diuretic-treated patients, the addition of losartan prevents the diuretic-induced increase in serum uric acid.[49] The uricosuric effect of losartan is not associated with an increased incidence of urate stone formation. This finding may be due to the fact that losartan simultaneously increases urinary pH by decreasing the proximal reabsorption of bicarbonate.[46,50] Losartan also reduces serum uric acid levels in cyclosporine-treated, hyperuricemic heart transplant patients.[51] As with other hypouricemic agents, the losartan-induced decrease in uric acid occasionally may trigger an episode of gout.[51] The other nonpeptide AT_1 antagonists have no effect on uric acid excretion.[52,53]

Other Effects

AT_1 antagonists showed no effect on serum cholesterol or plasma lipoprotein in hypertensive patients.[54] A preliminary study suggests that losartan may improve the lipid profile of patients with nephrotic syndrome.[55] This effect on plasma lipids in nephrotic patients may be linked to the ability of losartan to lower proteinuria. No adverse effect of Ang II antagonists was observed on serum glucose, and preliminary studies suggest that losartan has a neutral effect on insulin sensitivity and glucose and lipid metabolism.[56,57] Similarly, telmisartan has no clinically relevant effect on glucose or lipid metabolism.[58]

Two cases of pancreatitis in patients treated with losartan have been reported recently.[59,60]

■ *First-Dose Hypotension and Rebound Hypertension*

First-dose hypotension is a common problem when ACE inhibitors are administered to salt-depleted or hypovolemic hypertensive patients. Thus, adverse effects that suggest first-dose hypotension also have been analyzed in patients newly treated with Ang II receptor antagonists. In diuretic-treated patients, the addition of increasing doses of losartan caused no first-dose hypotension.[44,49] In another study, the incidence of orthostatic hypotension in candesartan-treated hypertensive patients did not differ from that observed in the placebo group.[61] Even in elderly patients who are more susceptible to first-dose hypotension, candesartan cilexetil did not induce orthostatic hypotension.[62]

Rebound hypertension is a potential problem with drugs acting directly on a receptor, such as beta blockers or clonidine. During Ang II receptor blockade, plasma Ang II levels increase significantly and theoretically might cause rebound hypertension upon withdrawal.[63] Studies conducted with losartan and candesartan cilexetil have clearly demonstrated that rebound hypertension is not a problem with Ang II receptor antagonists.[44,62–65] The short half-life of Ang II in plasma and the pharmacokinetics of Ang II antagonists, in particular their slow dissociation rate from the receptor, may account for the absence of rebound.

■ *Safety and Tolerability in Special Populations*

Safety and tolerability of Ang II receptor antagonists have been evaluated in terms of gender, age, and race. None of these factors influences the incidence of drug-related adverse events. In particular, Ang II receptor antagonists are equally well tolerated by elderly (> 65 years), younger (< 65 years), and very old patients (> 75 years).[2–6,62,66–67]

Patients with Renal Impairment

The clearance of losartan is primarily nonrenal, whereas its active metabolite is cleared through both renal and nonrenal routes.[68] Renal excretion of irbesartan, eprosartan, and telmisartan is less than 5%, whereas the renal contribution to systemic clearance of valsartan and candesartan is 30% and 60%, respectively.[5,67–74] In patients with mild-to-moderate hypertension included in clinical trials, adverse effects on parameters of renal function have not been reported with any Ang II antagonist. The tolerability of losartan has been examined in 112 hypertensive patients with different degrees of renal impairment.[72] Losartan was well tolerated in all groups of patients. No significant change in creatinine clearance was observed during the 12 weeks of administration. When eprosartan was investigated in 9 hemodialysis patients, results showed that it was safe and well tolerated.[74] However, its pharmacokinetics showed a greater variability in patients undergoing dialysis than in volunteers; in patients undergoing dialysis, therefore, eprosartan therapy should be individualized based on tolerability and response.

In normotensive subjects and hypertensive patients with or without renal diseases, Ang II receptor antagonists generally increase renal plasma flow, decrease renal resistance, and have no significant effect on glomerular filtration rate.[47,52,75,76] In patients with renal artery stenosis, mainly those with bilateral disease or a single functioning kidney, blockade of the RAS may cause a deterioration of renal function. So far, few studies have evaluated the safety of Ang II receptor antagonists in patients with renal artery stenosis. In a preliminary report, renal hemodynamics were measured in 17 patients with atheromatous renal artery stenosis and mild-to-moderate renal failure who received a single dose of losartan, 200 mg, and captopril, 50 mg.[77] Both losartan and captopril had a deleterious effect on renal hemodynamics; transient anuria occurred after both agents in one patient with bilateral renal artery stenosis. Another report describes an alteration of renal function parameters in a woman treated with losartan.[78] Of note, the patient was diabetic and had diffuse vascular disease; therefore, she was at risk for developing renal dysfunction. Taken together, preliminary results suggest that, as with ACE inhibitors, acute renal failure may occur with Ang II receptor antagonists when they are administered to patients with severe renal artery stenosis or diffuse intrarenal vascular sclerosis.[79–82]

Patients with Hepatic Impairment

Although most Ang II receptor antagonists are partly cleared by the liver and bile, few studies have examined safety and tolerability in patients with hepatic impairment. Several studies have shown that the pharmacokinetics of losartan, valsartan, and candesartan are not significantly altered in patients with mild-to-moderate liver dysfunction.[70,71,83,84] A recent study reported the effect of hepatic disease on the pharmacokinetic and plasma protein binding of eprosartan.[85] The drug was safe and well tolerated. However, because of an increase in area under the curve in patients with hepatic disease compared with patients with normal hepatic function, the dosage of eprosartan in patients with hepatic disorders should be individualized based on tolerability and response.

Patients with Congestive Heart Failure

ACE inhibitors reduce mortality and morbidity in patients with heart failure, and their use is now recommended in clinical guidelines. Ang II receptor blockade also may be advantageous for this indication. Several preliminary studies have demonstrated that Ang II antagonists have favorable hemodynamic effects in heart failure.[86–88] The ELITE study was designed to compare the safety and tolerability of losartan and captopril in 722 elderly patients with heart failure.[89] In addition, the incidence of renal dysfunction, hypotension-related symptoms, hyperkalemia, and cough was analyzed. A persistent increase in serum creatinine (> 0.3 mg/dl) was observed in 10.5% of losartan-treated patients and 10.5% of captopril-treated patients. The incidence of cough was significantly lower in the losartan-treated group (6.5% vs. 17.8%, p < 0.001). Persistent increases in serum potassium (≥ 0.5 mEq/L) were found in 18.8% of patients treated with losartan and 22.7% of those treated with captopril (p = 0.069). Significantly fewer discontinuations were observed in the losartan-treated group (43 vs. 77 in the placebo group, p < 0.002). The RESOLVD study, which compared candesartan alone or in combination with enalapril to enalapril alone, showed that candesartan alone was as effective and safe as enalapril in preventing left ventricular remodeling.[90] However, because mortality was slightly but not significantly higher in candesartan-treated patients, the study was prematurely stopped. Two large trials in patients with heart failure are now ongoing with different Ang II receptor antagonists (CHARM and Val-Heft studies). These studies will provide further insights into the safety and tolerability profile of Ang II receptor antagonists given alone or in combination with ACE inhibitors in patients with heart failure.

Safety in Pregnancy and Fetal Toxicity

The administration of ACE inhibitors during pregnancy may lead to severe hypotension and renal failure in the newborn.[91] Developmental and fetal toxicologic studies suggest that Ang II antagonists also should be discontinued during pregnancy. Losartan administered to animals had no effect on fetal development in early pregnancy. However, when administered in the second half of gestation, it was associated with serious fetal toxicity. It is unknown whether Ang II antagonists are excreted in human milk. In rats, however, losartan and its active metabolite were detected in milk. Therefore, the risk of using angiotensin antagonists in a breast-feeding mother should be taken into account.

■ Drug Interactions

Published data about drug interactions show that AT_1 antagonists can be administered safely with hydrochlorothiazide, warfarin, cimetidine, phenobarbital, and ketoconazole.[4,67,92–94] Only telmisartan appeared to cause a slight increase in digoxin serum levels.[5] Therefore, plasma serum digoxin levels should be monitored in patients taking the two drugs concomitantly. A study conducted in normotensive subjects suggests that the administration of nonsteroidal antiinflammatory drugs (NSAIDs) abolishes the natriuretic response to Ang II receptor blockade.[95] Hence, the concomitant use of NSAIDs may blunt the antihypertensive efficacy of Ang II receptor antagonists, as they do with ACE inhibitors and diuretics.

Table 2. Comparative Side-effect Profile of ACE Inhibition and Specific Angiotensin II
Receptor Blockade

Mechanism	Angiotensin II Receptor Blockade	ACE Inhibition
Inhibition of ACE		
Cough	—	+
Angioedema	—(?)	+
Inhibition of angiotensin II effect		
Acute renal failure (renal artery stenosis or severe heart failure)	+	+
Decreased hematocrit in post-transplant erythrocytosis	+	+
Fetal toxicity	+	+
Rebound hypertension	—	—
Decrease in aldosterone effect		
Hyperkalemia	±	+
Decrease in blood pressure		
First-dose hypotension	—	±
Dizziness	±	±
Drug interaction		
Sodium retention with NSAIDs	+	+

ACE, angiotensin-converting enzyme; NSAIDs, nonsteroidal antiinflammatory drugs.

■ *Conclusion*

Information gathered from clinical trials shows that Ang II antagonists are effective antihypertensive agents with an excellent safety and tolerability profile. Compared with beta blockers, diuretics, or calcium channel blockers, they seem to be free of side effects that impair long-term compliance to antihypertensive therapy. The development of Ang II receptor antagonists also demonstrates that targeting a more specific site in the RAS improves the side-effect profile and avoids cough, the most frequent untoward effect of ACE inhibitors. However, the increased specificity of Ang II receptor antagonists does not reduce the occurrence of side effects linked to a decrease in Ang II or to the reduction in blood pressure (Table 2). Thus, Ang II antagonists should be used cautiously in patients with renal artery stenosis or severe heart failure. Because of their excellent safety and tolerability profile, Ang II antagonists represent a good alternative for the treatment of hypertension. Several large trials are now under way to demonstrate that they are effective not only in lowering blood pressure but also in preventing end-organ damage and that they reduce cardiovascular morbidity and mortality in patients with hypertension, congestive heart failure, and chronic renal failure.

References

1. Mallion JM, Goldberg AI: Global efficacy and tolerability of losartan, an angiotensin II subtype 1-receptor antagonist in the treatment of hypertension. Blood Press 5(Suppl 2):82–86, 1996.
2. McClellan JK, Goa KL: Candesartan cilexetil: A review of its use in essential hypertension. Drugs 56:847–869, 1998.
3. Markham A, Goa KL: Valsartan: A review of its pharmacology and therapeutic use in essential hypertension. Drugs 54:299–311, 1997.
4. Gillis JC, Markham A: Irbesartan: A review of its pharmacodynamic and pharmacokinetic properties and therapeutic use in the management of hypertension. Drugs 54:885–902, 1997.
5. McClellan KJ, Markham A: Telmisartan. Drugs 56:1039–1044, 1998.

6. McClellan KJ, Balfour JA: Eprosartan. Drugs 55:713–718, 1998.

7. Gavras I, Gavras H: Safety and tolerability of eprosartan. Pharmacotherapy 19(4 Pt 2):102S–107S, 1999.

8. Shusterman NH: Safety and efficacy of eprosartan, a new angiotensin II receptor blocker. Am Heart J 138(3 Pt 2):238–245, 1999.

9. McIntyre M, Coffe SE, Michalok RA, et al: Losartan, an orally active angiotensin (AT1) receptor antagonist: A review of its efficacy and safety in essential hypertension. Pharmacol Ther 74:181–194, 1997.

10. Weber M: Clinical safety and tolerability of losartan. Clin Ther 19:604–616, 1997.

11. Karlberg BE, Lins L-E, Hermansson K, et al, for the TEES Study Group: Efficacy and safety of telmisartan, a selective AT1 receptor antagonist, compared with enalapril in elderly patients with primary hypertension. Hypertension 17:293–302, 1999.

12. Neutel JM, Smith DHG: Dose response and antihypertensive efficacy of the AT1 receptor antagonist telmisartan in patients with mild to moderate hypertension. Adv Ther 15:206–217, 1998.

13. Haddad AM, Scholer G: Possible losartan-induced rash. Am J Health Syst Pharm 54:1333–1334, 1997.

14. Bosch X: Henoch-Schönlein purpura induced by losartan therapy. Arch Intern Med 158:191–192, 1998.

15. Viraben R, Lamant L, Brousset P: Losartan-associated atypical cutaneous lymphoid hyperplasia. Lancet 350:1366, 1997.

16. Magro C, Crowson A: Drug-induced immune dysregulation as a cause of atypical cutaneous lymphoid infiltrates. Hum Pathol 27:125–132, 1996.

17. Israili ZH, Hall WD: Cough and angioneurotic edema associated with angiotensin-converting enzyme inhibitor therapy. A review of the literature and pathophysiology. Ann Intern Med 117:234–242, 1992.

18. Tomlinson B, Young RP, Chan JC, et al: Pharmacoepidemiology of ACE inhibitor induced cough. Drug Safety 16:150–151, 1997.

19. Elliott WJ: Higher incidence of discontinuation of angiotensin converting enzyme inhibitors due to cough in black subjects. Clin Pharm Ther 60:582–588, 1996.

20. Lacourcière Y, Lefebvre J, Nakhle G, et al: Association between cough and angiotensin converting enzyme inhibitory versus angiotensin II antagonists: The design of a prospective, controlled study. J Hypertens 12:549–553, 1994.

21. Black HR, Graff A, Shute D, et al: Valsartan, a new angiotensin II antagonist for the treatment of essential hypertension: Efficacy, tolerability and safety compared to an angiotensin-converting enzyme inhibitor, lisinopril. J Hum Hypertens 11:483–489, 1997.

22. Belcher G, Hübner R, George M, et al: Candesartan cilexetil: Safety and tolerability in healthy volunteers and patients with hypertension. J Hum Hypertens 11:S85–S89, 1998.

23. Lacourciere Y: The incidence of cough: A comparison of lisinopril, placebo and telmisartan, a novel angiotensin II antagonist. Int J Clin Pract 52:99–103, 1999.

24. Lacourcière Y, Brunner HR, Irwing R, et al, and Losartan Cough Study Group: Effects of modulators of the renin-angiotensin-aldosterone system on cough. J Hypertens 12:1387–1393, 1994.

25. Benz J, Oshrain C, Henry D, et al: Valsartan, a new angiotensin II receptor antagonist: A double-blind study comparing the incidence of cough with lisinopril and hydrochlorothiazide. J Clin Pharmacol 37:101–107, 1997.

26. Chan P, Tomlinson B, Huang TY, et al: Double-blind comparison of losartan, lisinopril, and metolazone in elderly hypertensive patients with previous angiotensin-converting enzyme inhibitor-induced cough. J Clin Pharmacol 37:253–257, 1997.

27. Nussberger J, Cugno M, Amstutz C, et al: Plasma bradykinin in angio-oedema. Lancet 351:1693–1697, 1998.

28. Vleeming W, van Amsterdam JG, Stricker BH, de Wildt DJ: ACE inhibitor-induced angioedema: Incidence, prevention and management. Drug Safety 18:171–188, 1998.

29. Merck & Co., Inc: Losartan Potassium Prescribing Information. West Point, NY, PSA 19486, 1995.

30. Acker G, Greenberg A: Angioedema induced by the angiotensin II blocker losartan. N Engl J Med 333:1572, 1995.

31. van Rijnsoever EW, Kwee-Zuiderwijk WJ, Feenstra J: Angioneurotic edema attributed to the use of losartan. Arch Intern Med 158:2063–2065, 1998.

32. Griffin J: Drug-induced disorders of taste. Adverse Drug React Toxicol 11:229–239, 1992.

33. Schlienger R, Saxer M, Haefli W: Reversible ageusia associated with losartan. Lancet 347:471–472, 1996.

34. Heeringa M, van Puijenbroek EP: Reversible dysgeusia attributed to losartan. Ann Intern Med 129:72, 1998.

35. Ahmad S: Losartan and severe migraine. JAMA 274:1266–1267, 1995.

36. Ahmad S: Losartan and reversible psychosis. Cardiology 87:569–570, 1996.
37. Shand B, Gilchrist N, Nicholls M, Bailey R: Effect of losartan on haematology and haemorheology in elderly patients with essential hypertension: A pilot study. J Hum Hypertens 9:233–235, 1995.
38. Schwarzbeck A, Wittenmeier KW, Hallfritzsch U: Anaemia in dialysis patients as a side-effect of sartanes. Lancet 352:286, 1998.
39. Naeshiro I, Sato K, Chatani F, Sato S: Possible mechanism for the anemia induced by candesartan cilexetil (TCV-116), an angiotensin II receptor antagonist, in rats. Eur J Pharmacol 354:179–187, 1998.
40. Julian BA, Brantley RR Jr, Barker CV, et al: Losartan, an angiotensin II type 1 receptor, lowers hematocrit in posttransplant erythrocytosis. J Am Soc Nephrol 9:1104–1108, 1998.
41. Navarro JF, Garcia J, Macia M, et al: Effects of losartan on the treatment of posttransplant erythrocytosis. Clin Nephrol 49:370–372, 1998. ˜
42. Ducloux D, Fournier V, Bresson-Vautrin C, Chalopin JM: Long-term follow-up of renal transplant recipients treated with losartan for post-transplant erythrosis. Transplant Int 11:312–315, 1998.
43. Hortal L, Fernandez A, Vega N, et al: Losartan versus ramipril in the treatment of postrenal transplant erythrocytosis. Transplant Proc 30:2127–2128, 1998.
44. Goldberg AI, Dunlay MC, Sweet CS: Safety and tolerability of losartan potassium, an angiotensin II receptor antagonist, compared with hydrochlorothiazide, atenolol, felodipine ER, and angiotensin converting enzyme inhibitors for the treatment of systemic hypertension. Am J Cardiol 75:793–795, 1995.
45. Nakashima M, Uematsu T, Kosuge K, Kanamura M: Pilot study of the uricosuric effect of DuP 753, a new angiotensin II receptor antagonist, in healthy subjects. Eur J Clin Pharmacol 42:333–335, 1992.
46. Burnier M, Rutschmann B, Nussberger J, et al: Salt-dependent renal effects of angiotensin II antagonist in healthy subjects. Hypertension 22:339–347, 1993.
47. Burnier M, Roch-Ramel F, Brunner HR: Renal effects of angiotensin II receptor blockade in normotensive subjects. Kidney Int 49:1787–1790, 1996.
48. Sweet CS, Bradstreet DC, Berman RS, et al: Pharmacodynamic activity of intravenous E-3174, an angiotensin II antagonist, in patients with essential hypertension. Am J Hypertens 7:1035–1040, 1994.
49. Soffer BA, Wright JT, Pratt H, et al: Effects of losartan on a background of hydrochlorothiazide in patients with hypertension. Hypertension 26:112–117, 1995.
50. Shahinfar S, Simpson C, Carides A, et al: Safety of losartan in hypertensive patients with thiazide-induced hyperuricemia. Kidney Int 56:1879–1885, 1999.
51. Minghelli G, Seydoux C, Goy J, Burnier M: Uricosuric effect of losartan in cyclosporine-treated heart transplant recipients. Transplantation 66:268–271, 1998.
52. Burnier M, Hagman M, Nussberger J, et al: Short-term and sustained renal effects of angiotensin II receptor blockade in healthy subjects. Hypertension 25(Pt 1):602–609, 1995.
53. Ilson BE, Martin DE, Boike SC, Jorkasky DK: The effects of eprosartan, an angiotensin II AT1 receptor antagonist, on uric acid excretion in patients with mild to moderate essential hypertension. J Clin Pharmacol 38:437–441, 1998.
54. Smith DHG, Neutel JM, Morgenstern P: Once-daily telmisartan compared with enalapril in the treatment of hypertension. Adv Ther 15:229–240, 1998.
55. De Zeeuw D, Gansevoort RT, Dullaart RP, De Jong PE: Angiotensin II antagonism improves the lipoprotein profile in patients with nephrotic syndrome. J Hypertens 13:S53–S58, 1995.
56. Moan A, Hoieggen A, Seljeflot I, et al: The effect of angiotensin II receptor antagonism with losartan on glucose metabolism and insulin sensitivity. J Hypertens 14:1093–1097, 1996.
57. Laakso M, Karjalainen L, Lempiäinen-Kuosa P: Effects of losartan on insulin sensitivity in hypertensive subjects. Hypertension 28:392–396, 1996.
58. Smith DHG, Neutel JM, Morgenstern P: Once-daily telmisartan compared with enalapril in the treatment of hypertension. Adv Ther 15:229–240, 1998.
59. Bosch X: Losartan-induced acute pancreatitis. Ann Intern Med 127:1043–1044, 1997.
60. Birck R, Keim V, Fiedler F, et al: Pancreatitis after losartan. Lancet 351:1178, 1998.
61. Sever P: Candesartan cilexetil: A new, long-acting, effective angiotensin II type 1 receptor blocker. J Hum Hypertens 11:S91–S95, 1997.
62. McInnes GT, O'Kane KPJ, Jonker J, Roth J: The efficacy and tolerability of candesartan cilexetil in an elderly hypertensive population. J Hum Hypertens 11(Suppl 2):S75–S80, 1997.
63. Christen Y, Waeber B, Nussberger J, et al: Oral administration of DuP 753, a specific angiotensin II receptor antagonist, to normal male volunteers. Inhibition of pressor response to exogenous angiotensin I and II. Circulation 83:1333–1342, 1991.
64. Mallion JM, Bradstreet DC, Makris L, et al: Antihypertensive efficacy and tolerability of once daily losartan potassium compared with captopril in patients with mild to moderate essential hypertension. J Hypertens 13(Suppl 1):35–41, 1995.

65. Dahlöf B, Keller S, Makris L, et al: Efficacy and tolerability of losartan potassium and atenolol in patients with mild to moderate essential hypertension. Am J Hypertens 8:578–583, 1995.
66. Burrell LM, Johnston CI: Angiotensin II receptor antagonists. Potential in elderly patients with cardiovascular disease. Drug Ther 10:421–434, 1997.
67. Chioléro A, Burnier M: Pharmacology of valsartan, an angiotensin II receptor antagonist. Exp Opin Invest Drugs 7:1915–1925, 1998.
68. Sica DA, Lo MW, Shaw WC, et al: The pharmacokinetics of losartan in renal insufficiency. J Hypertens 13:S49–S52, 1995.
69. Sica DA, Marino MR, Hammett JL, et al: The pharmacokinetics of irbesartan in renal failure and maintenance hemodialysis. Clin Pharm Ther 62:610–618, 1997.
70. DeZeeuw D, Remuzzi G, Kirch W: Pharmacokinetics of candesartan cilexetil in patients with renal or hepatic impairment. J Hum Hypertens 11(Suppl 2):S37–S42, 1997.
71. Johnston CI: Angiotensin receptor antagonists: Focus on losartan. Lancet 346:1403–1407, 1995.
72. Toto R, Shultz P, Raij L, et al, for the Collaborative Group: Efficacy and tolerability of losartan in hypertensive patients with renal impairment. Hypertension 31:684–691, 1998.
73. Bottorf MB, Tenero DM: Pharmacokinetics of eprosartan in healthy subjects, patients with hypertension, and special populations. Pharmacotherapy 19(4 Pt 2):73S–78S, 1999.
74. Kovacs SJ, Tenero DM, Martin DE, et al: Pharmacokinetics and protein binding of eprosartan in hemodialysis-dependent patients with end-stage renal disease. Pharmacotherapy 19:612–619, 1999.
75. Gansevoort RT, DeZeeuw D, deJong PE: Is the antiproteinuric effect of ACE inhibition mediated by interference in the renin-angiotensin system? Kidney Int 45:861–867, 1994.
76. Pechère-Bertschi A, Nussberger J, Decosterd L, et al: Renal response to the AT$_1$ antagonist irbesartan vs enalapril in hypertensive patients. J Hypertens 16:385–393, 1998.
77. Mimran A, Ribstein J, DuCailar G: Comparison of the acute renal effect of losartan and captopril in atheromatous renovascular disease. Am J Hypertens 11:47A, 1998.
78. Saine D, Ahrens E: Renal impairment associated with losartan. Ann Intern Med 124:775, 1996.
79. Faulhaber HD, Mann JF, et al: Effect of valsartan on renal function in patients with hypertension and stable renal insufficiency. Curr Ther Res 60:170–183, 1999.
80. Holm EA, Randlov A, Strandgard S: Acute renal failure after losartan treatment in a patient with bilateral renal artery stenosis. Blood Pressure 5:360–362, 1996.
81. Missouris CG, Ward DE, Eastwood JB, MacGregor GA: Deterioration in renal function with enalapril but not losartan in a patient with renal artery stenosis in a solitary kidney. Heart 77:391–392, 1997.
82. Ostermann M, Goldsmith DJA, Doyle T, et al: Reversible acute renal failure induced by losartan in a renal transplant recipient. Postgrad Med J 73:105–107, 1997.
83. Marino MR, Langenbacher KM, Raymond RH, Ford NF, Lasseter KC: Pharmacokinetics and pharmacodynamics of irbesartan in patients with hepatic cirrhosis. J Clin Pharmacol 38:347–356, 1998.
84. Brookman LJ, Rolan PE, Benjamin IS, et al: Pharmacokinetics of valsartan in patients with liver disease. Clin Pharm Ther 62:272–278, 1997.
85. Tenero D, Martin D, Chapelsky M, et al: Effect of hepatic disease on the pharmacokinetics and plasma protein binding of eprosartan. Pharmacotherapy 18:42–50, 1998.
86. Gottlieb SS, Dickstein K, Fleck E, et al: Hemodynamic and neurohormonal effects of the angiotensin II antagonist losartan in patients with congestive heart failure. Circulation 8(Pt 1): 1602–1609, 1993.
87. Dickstein K, Chang P, Willenheimer R, et al: Comparison of the effects of losartan and enalapril on clinical status and exercise performance in patients with moderate or severe heart failure. J Am Coll Cardiol 26:438–445, 1995.
88. Crozier I, Ikram H, Awan N, et al, for the Losartan Hemodynamic Study Group: Losartan in heart failure. Hemodynamic effects and tolerability. Circulation 91:691–697, 1995.
89. Pitt B, Segal R, Martinez FA, et al: Randomised trial of losartan versus captopril in patients over 65 with heart failure (Evaluation of Losartan In The Elderly study, ELITE). Lancet 349:747–752, 1997.
90. McKelvie RS, Yusuf S, Pericak D, et al: Comparison of candesartan, enalapril, and their combination in congestive heart failure: Randomized Evaluation of Strategies for Left Ventricular Dysfunction (RESOLVD) pilot study. Circulation 100:1056–1064, 1999.
91. Kreft-Joris C, Plouin PF, Tchobroutsky C: Angiotensin converting enzyme inhibitors during pregnancy. J Hypertension 5(Suppl 5):553–554, 1987.
92. Kong AN, Tomasko L, Waldman SA, et al: Losartan does not affect the pharmacokinetics and pharmacodynamics of warfarin. J Clin Pharmacol 35:1008–1015, 1995.
93. Martin DE, Tompson D, Boike SC, et al: Lack of effect of eprosartan on the single dose pharmacokinetics of orally administered digoxin in healthy male volunteers. Br J Clin Pharmacol 43:661–664, 1997.

94. Kazierad DJ, Martin DE, Ilson B, et al: Eprosartan does not affect the pharmacodynamics of warfarin. J Clin Pharmacol 38:649–653, 1998.
95. Fricker A, Nussberger J, Meilenbrock S, et al: Effect of indomethacin on the renal response to angiotensin II receptor blockade in healthy subjects. Kidney Int 54:2089–2097, 1998.

CHAPTER 24

Morbidity and Mortality Trials with Angiotensin Receptor Antagonists in Hypertensive Patients

ALBERTO ZANCHETTI, M.D.

Antihypertensive treatment has been widely investigated since the 1960s by morbidity and mortality trials.[1,2] Although they are not the only source of evidence in favor of antihypertensive therapy,[3,4] they are of paramount importance for therapeutic decision-making. Most of the trials initiated in the 1960s to 1980s were based on diuretics and beta blockers[5–13] and were designed as comparisons of active and placebo treatments.[5,6,8–13] More recent trials have compared calcium antagonists with placebo.[14–16] Trials comparing two different classes of antihypertensive agents began in the 1980s[9,17,18]; recently their number has increased significantly because of the obvious difficulties in doing placebo-controlled trials after demonstration of the overwhelming benefits of antihypertensive therapy.[19] Many comparative trials are under way[20]; two recently have been completed.[21,22]

Angiotensin II (Ang II) receptor antagonists also became the object of investigation by morbidity and mortality trials, which were planned and initiated much earlier in the development of this new class of agents than with any previous class of antihypertensive agents. Major trials are ongoing using three different molecules within the class of Ang II receptor antagonists: the Losartan Intervention for End-point Reduction in Hypertension Study (LIFE),[23] the Valsartan Antihypertensive Long-term Use Evaluation (VALUE),[24] and the Study on Cognition and Prognosis in the Elderly (SCOPE).[25] The first two trials compare active treatment with an Ang II antagonist (losartan in LIFE and valsartan in VALUE) with another active treatment (the beta blocker atenolol in LIFE and the calcium antagonist amlodipine in VALUE). SCOPE[25] is a placebo-controlled study that compares the Ang II antagonist candesartan with less active antihypertensive treatment to which placebo is added. All three trials involve hypertensive patients at high risk, which is defined as the presence of left ventricular hypertrophy in the LIFE study,[23] as the presence of various risk factors in the VALUE study,[24] and as old age (70–89 years) in the SCOPE study.[25]

■ *Losartan Intervention for End-point Reduction in Hypertension Study*

Rationale and Study Design

The rationale of the study is based on the evidence that left ventricular hypertrophy (LVH) is an independent risk factor for cardiovascular disease[26,27] and that interference with the renin-angiotensin system (e.g., with an angiotensin-converting enzyme [ACE] inhibitor) appears to be more effective than other mechanisms of blood pressure reduction in inducing regression of LVH.[28–30] The LIFE study is a prospective, multinational, multicenter, double-blind, double-dummy, randomized, active-controlled study with two parallel groups.

Study Objectives

The primary objective is to compare the long-term effects ($\geq$ 4 years) of losartan and atenolol in hypertensive patients with LVH on the combined incidence of cardiovascular mortality (sudden death or death due to myocardial infarction, stroke, progressive heart failure, or other cardiovascular causes) and morbidity (nonfatal, clinically evident acute myocardial infarction and nonfatal stroke). Secondary objectives include the effects of the two treatments on LVH, independently of mortality and morbidity, and softer cardiovascular end-points.

Patient Population

Eligible patients were men and women 55–80 years old with sitting diastolic blood pressure (DBP) of 95–115 mmHg or sitting systolic blood pressure (SBP) of 160–200 mmHg after 1–2 weeks of single-blind placebo treatment. Eligible patients also should have electrocardiographically documented LVH, as diagnosed before randomization according to Cornell criteria: (RaVL + SV_3) voltage (+ 0 mm in men, + 6 mm in women) $\times$ QRS duration > 2.440 mm $\times$ msec. The usual exclusion criteria for antihypertensive treatment trials were applied. Patients were recruited by approximately 830 centers in the United States, United Kingdom, and Scandinavia.

Study Procedures

After 1–2 weeks of single-blind placebo treatment, eligible patients were randomized to either losartan or atenolol once daily. Throughout the on-treatment follow-up period, blood pressure is taken at trough (22–26 hours after dosing). Antihypertensive therapy is adjusted, according to a given time schedule, to achieve a goal blood pressure of 140/90 mmHg or lower (Fig. 1). Patients initially receive 50 mg losartan plus atenolol placebo or 50 mg atenolol plus losartan placebo. After 2 months, 12.5 mg hydrochlorothiazide is added to either treatment regimen if the target blood pressure has not been reached. At month 4, if goal blood pressure is not achieved, the dose of double-blind medication is doubled (either 100 mg losartan or 100 mg atenolol plus 12.5 mg hydrochlorothiazide). At month 6, additional open-label antihypertensive medications (except Ang II receptor antagonists, beta blockers, or ACE inhibitors) can be added for patients not achieving goal blood pressure. The duration of treatment (see below) is not based on an absolute time frame, but on the number of observed events. The investigation will continue until all patients have completed a minimum of 4 years of study treatment.

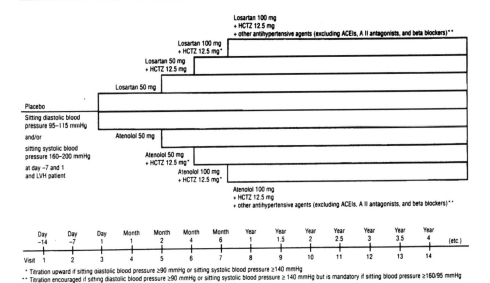

Figure 1. Flow chart and titration schedule for the LIFE Study. (From Dalhöf B, Devereux R, deFaire V, et al: The Losartan Intervention for Endpoint Reduction (LIFE) in Hypertension Study: Rationale, design and methods. Am J Hypertens 10:705–713, 1997, with permission.)

Power of the Study

From available evidence the 5-year event rate for the primary end-point of combined cardiovascular death and nonfatal myocardial infarction and stroke in the atenolol group has been estimated at 15%. With a sample size of 8,300 patients, the study will have 80% power to detect at least a 15% further reduction of the primary end-points in the losartan group. Therefore, it is planned to terminate the study when 1040 patients have experienced a primary end-point, provided no patient is treated for less than 4 years. At the end of the randomization period (April 30, 1997), 9218 patients (that is, 10% more than the planned minimum) had been randomized.

Statistical Analysis

The intent-to-treat approach will be used for all efficacy and safety analyses. The main conclusion of the trial will be based on the single primary variable. No conclusions will be drawn from the secondary/tertiary end-points unless the primary end-point is statistically significant. In the case of a nonconclusive main result, secondary/tertiary variables will be used mainly for hypothesis generation.

Organizational Structure

As usual in major trials, the LIFE study is governed by an independent, blinded international steering committee with two coordinators, one in Scandinavia and one in the United States. A central electrocardiographic (EKG) laboratory is responsible for LVH diagnosis and other EKG changes. End-points are validated by a double-blind end-point committee. Finally, the data and safety monitoring board advises the steering committee at regular intervals about ethical aspects of study continuation. The organizational structure of LIFE is illustrated in Figure 2. The

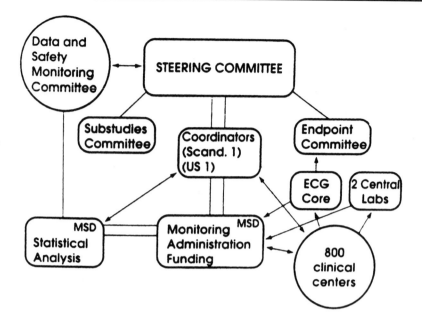

Figure 2.   Organizational structure for the LIFE Study. (From Dalhöf B, Devereux R, deFaire V, et al: The Losartan Intervention for Endpoint Reduction (LIFE) in Hypertension Study: Rationale, design and methods. Am J Hypertens 10:705–713, 1997, with permission.)

investigation is sponsored by Merck & Co.; its central administration and monitoring office is located at Merck Research Laboratories, Scandinavia, which handles blinded data for the duration of the study.

■ *Valsartan Antihypertensive Long-term Use Evaluation Study*

Rationale and Study Design

The rationale for the VALUE Study is the increasing recognition that antihypertensive treatment has a better effect on cardiovascular morbidity and mortality due to strokes and congestive heart failure than to coronary events.[31] This divergence in the benefits of antihypertensive therapy suggests a classification of hypertensive complications into two categories: pressure-related (strokes and congestive heart failure) and atherosclerosis-related (coronary events). An extension of this concept is that factors other than blood pressure elevation may be involved in coronary morbidity. Of particular interest to the hypothesis tested in the VALUE Study is evidence that in the setting of elevated blood pressure the renin-angiotensin system may have important cardiovascular effects.[32] The VALUE Study is a prospective, multinational, multicenter, double-blind, randomized, active-controlled study with two parallel groups.

Study Objectives

The primary objective is to investigate whether, for the same level of blood pressure control, valsartan is more effective in reducing cardiac end-points (acute myocardial infarction, congestive heart failure, and cardiac mortality) than the calcium antagonist amlodipine. Secondary objectives are to test whether valsartan is more effective than amlodipine in reducing all causes of death, cerebrovascular mortality and morbidity, and coronary events other than acute myocardial infarction.

Patient Population

Eligible patients are men and women of any racial background, 50 years of age or older, with a known diagnosis of systolic and/or diastolic essential hypertension. For previously untreated patients, mean sitting SBP must be between 160 and 210 mmHg and mean sitting DBP ≤ 115 mmHg or mean DBP between 95 and 115 mmHg and sitting SBP ≤ 210 mmHg before randomization. For patients already under antihypertensive treatment there is no lower limit of mean sitting SBP or DBP, but the upper limit must not exceed 210 and 115 mmHg, respectively. Therefore, a noticeable feature of the VALUE Study is that no placebo run-in is required. The blood pressure effects of the two treatments to be compared are the achieved blood pressures rather than the reductions in blood pressure.

Because the VALUE Study intends to recruit only high-risk hypertensive patients, the following characteristics must be present to make patients eligible for randomization:

1. Men aged 50–59 years with at least three risk factors (diabetes mellitus; current smoking of at least 10 cigarettes/day; total serum cholesterol > 240 mg/dl; LVH verified by central EKG reading; proteinuria defined as 1+ or more; serum creatinine > 1.7 mg/dl) or one disease (documented coronary heart disease, peripheral arterial disease, documented stroke or transient ischemic attack, LVH with strain pattern).

2. Women aged 50–59 years with at least two risk factors and one disease or at least two diseases.

3. Men and women aged 60–69 years with at least two risk factors or one disease or aged 70 and older with at least one risk factor or one disease.

The usual exclusion criteria for antihypertensive treatment trials are applied. Patients are being recruited in 31 countries in North and Latin America, Europe, and Asia.

Study Procedures

The flow chart of the VALUE Study is summarized in Figure 3. Patients already under antihypertensive treatment directly enter the double-blind treatment period and are rolled over to double-blind medication without a preceding run-in period. Tapering of previous medication is left to the investigator's discretion. Throughout the on-treatment follow-up period, blood pressure must be measured on the same arm (the arm with the higher blood pressure values) at approximately the same time of the day. At the various visits antihypertensive therapy must be adjusted to achieve goal blood pressure, which is defined as sitting values < 140/90 mmHg, unless DBP < 90 mmHg and SBP has fallen ≥ 20 mmHg from baseline and, in the judgment of the investigator, a further decrease may not be in the best interest of the patient. The five titration steps are as follows:

1. Valsartan, 80 mg/day, or amlodipine, 5 mg/day

2. Valsartan, 160 mg/day, or amlodipine, 10 mg/day

3. Valsartan, 160 mg/day, + hydrochlorothiazide (HCTZ), 12.5 mg/day, or amlodipine, 10 mg/day, + HCTZ, 12.5 mg/day

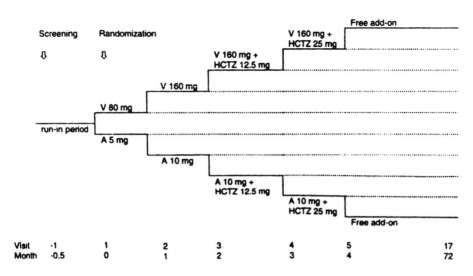

Figure 3. Flow chart and titration schedule for the VALUE Trial. (From Mann J, Julius S: The Valsartan Antihypertensive Long-term Use Evaluation (VALUE) Trial of cardiovascular events in hypertension: Rationale and design. Blood Pressure 7:176–183, 1998.

4. Valsartan, 160 mg/day, + HCTZ, 25 mg/day, or amlodipine, 10 mg/day, + HCTZ, 25 mg/day

5. Valsartan, 160 mg/day, + HCTZ, 25 mg/day, + free add-on or amlodipine, 10 mg/day, + HCTZ, 25 mg/day, + free add-on (e.g., alpha blockers, centrally acting hypertensives, peripheral vasodilators, beta blockers)

The on-treatment follow-up period is planned to be up to 6 years (72 months).

Power of the Study

A total of 1,450 patients with primary end-point occurrences is required to give 90% power for detecting a 15% reduction in the primary end-point (cardiac event) rate for patients randomized to the valsartan arm (10.63% during 5 years vs. 12.5% in the amlodipine arm), using a two-sided 0.05 significance level. According to this calculation, a total of 14,400 patients, equally allocated to each of the two treatment arms, is required. This calculation assumes 2 years of patient accrual and a total trial length (including the accrual period) of 6 years.

Statistical Analysis

Efficacy is established by achieving a statistically significant difference with respect to the primary end-point, time to cardiac mortality or morbidity event, in favor of valsartan over amlodipine, either at the defined end of the trial or at one of the two planned interim analyses if a predefined efficacy boundary has been crossed. To conclude superior efficacy for valsartan versus amlodipine, a preliminary assessment should first establish noninferiority of valsartan vs. amlodipine in relation to the combined end-point of cardiac mortality and morbidity plus stroke.

Organizational Structure

The VALUE Study is governed by an executive committee and steering committee; the latter is formed by representatives of all participant countries. As usual in most mortality and morbidity trials, events are adjudicated by an independent event committee, blind to the randomized medication to which each patient is assigned. The data and safety monitoring board is responsible for monitoring progress of patient safety and demonstration of efficacy based on two interim analyses performed in a semiblind fashion. Blinded data are handled at a central location by Novartis, the sponsor of the trial.

■ Study on Cognition and Prognosis in Elderly

Rationale and Study Design

Although treatment of hypertension in the elderly has been shown to have conspicuous beneficial effects,[10-16] the value of antihypertensive treatment in elderly hypertensive patients with DBP in the range 90–99 mmHg is still an open issue. It has not been proved that antihypertensive treatment in this range provides protection against stroke. Furthermore, old age, especially very old age, is associated with an increased risk of dementia,[33] in the development of which hypertension recently was shown to have a role.[34,35] Ang II recently was shown to impair learning and memory paradigms, whereas treatment with Ang II receptor antagonists improved cognitive performance in animal experiments.[36,37] The SCOPE rationale is to test whether blood pressure reduction by the Ang II receptor antagonist candesartan cilexetil reduces cardiovascular events in elderly hypertensives and favorably affects their cognitive function. SCOPE is a prospective, multinational, multicenter, randomized, double-blind, placebo-controlled study with two parallel groups (candesartan cilexetil vs. placebo) in elderly patients with mild hypertension.

Study Objectives

The primary objective is to assess the effect of candesartan cilexetil on major cardiovascular events (cardiovascular deaths, nonfatal myocardial infarction, and nonfatal stroke) in elderly patients with mild hypertension. Secondary objectives are to assess the effects of treatment on (1) cognitive function, as measured by the Mini Mental State Examination (MMSE); (2) total mortality; (3) several separate types of cardiovascular events, considered together as primary end-points; (4) impaired renal function; and (5) hospitalization.

Patient Population

Eligible patients are men and women, aged 70–89 years, with or without antihypertensive treatment. When patients are already under antihypertensive treatment, the antihypertensive medication is standardized to HCTZ, 12.5 mg/day. With this treatment or with no treatment, SBP at randomization should be between 160 and 179 mmHg or DBP between 90 and 99 mmHg (mean of two measurements) after 5–10 minutes of rest in the sitting position on two consecutive occasions, separated by at least 14 days. To be eligible, patients should undergo an MMSE test with a score of 24 or above on two consecutive occasions, separated by at least 14 days. The usual exclusion criteria for trials of antihypertensive therapy were applied.

Study Procedures

Figure 4 summarizes the SCOPE flow chart. During the run-in period previously untreated patients, if blood pressure is within the range of inclusion criteria,

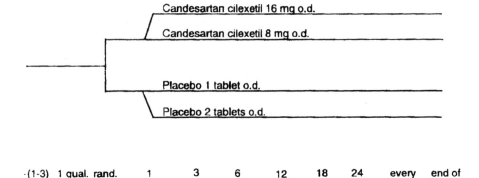

·(1-3)	1 qual.	rand.	1	3	6	12	18	24	every	end of
mths	visit	visit	month	mths	mths	mths	mths	mths	6 mths	study

Figure 4. Overall design of the SCOPE Study. (From Hansson L, Lithell H, Skoog I, et al: Study on Cognition and Prognosis in the Elderly (SCOPE). Blood Pressure 8:177–183, 1999.

are left untreated, whereas in previously treated patients a standardized therapy of HCTZ, 12.5 mg/day, is given as baseline therapy (to be continued during double-blind randomized treatment). The run-in period should be between 1 and 3 months. During the double-blind treatment period candesartan cilexetil, 8 mg, or placebo is given initially as 1 tablet once daily in the morning. During subsequent visits, if SBP remains above 160 mmHg or the decrease in SBP is less than 10 mmHg compared with the randomization visit, or if DBP is above 85 mmHg, the dose of the study medication should be doubled to two tablets once daily, which is the maximal dose of double-blind medication. If at any time during the study a mean sitting SBP $\geq$ 160 mmHg or a mean sitting DBP $\geq$ 90 mmHg is observed and confirmed within 2 weeks, despite study medication, initiation of additional antihypertensive medication is recommended, preferably HCTZ, 12.5 mg. Ang II antagonists and ACE inhibitors are not allowed. Blood pressure is measured at all visits, and an MMSE test is performed at all visits except after 1 and 3 months. The follow-up under double-blind treatment is planned for a mean period of at least 2.5 years; no patient will be treated for less than 2 years.

Power of the Study

Calculation of the sample size was based on an estimated risk for a major cardiovascular event derived from data from the STOP-Hypertension 1 Study,[12] using achieved DBP as the blood pressure risk. Assuming an initial mean DBP of 95 mmHg and a decrease to 92 mmHg with placebo treatment, the yearly incidence rate for a major cardiovascular event during placebo treatment was estimated at 44 per 1000 patient years. If 4000 patients are randomized and followed for an average of 2.5 years, the result is a total of 10,000 patient years of treatment. With this number of patient years, the SCOPE Study will have a power of 80%, using significance level of 0.05, to detect a reduction of at least 23% in the yearly incidence rate of major cardiovascular events during active treatment. With 2000 patients in each treatment arm, approximately 220 major cardiovascular events can be expected in the placebo group and approximately 170 in the active group. If the event rate is lower than anticipated, the study may be prolonged. At the end of the randomization phase 20 January 1999, 4964 patients had been randomized, exceeding the original target of 4000.

Statistical Analysis

To study the primary objective of the trial (effect on major cardiovascular events), the time from start of treatment to such an event is considered the primary variable. Life-table techniques will be used to construct survival functions. The primary statistical comparisons of the two survival functions (candesartan and placebo groups) will be made using a one-sided log-rank test, with the significance level set to 0.05. The secondary objective of the effect on cognitive function will be studied using the change in MMSE score from baseline to the final visit. The mean difference in the change of the MMSE score between the candesartan group and the placebo group will be analyzed in a linear model with factors for treatment and center. An analysis of covariance with these factors and the baseline as covariates will be performed to estimate the residual variance for the MMSE score.

Organizational Structure

The SCOPE Study is governed by an executive committee responsible for the planning and conduct of the study and by a steering committee with two representatives from each of the 15 participating countries. Events are adjudicated by an independent clinical event committee, blind to the study group to which the patients have been randomized. An independent safety committee supervises the evolution of the study, especially with respect to the occurrence of clinical events in the different study groups. The independent safety committee is empowered to advise the steering committee about study termination. Central handling of double-blind data is done by AstraZeneca, the sponsor of the study, at AstraZeneca Research and Development, Mölndal, Sweden.

References

1. Zanchetti A: What have we learned and what haven't we from clinical trials on hypertension? In Laragh JH, Brenner BM (eds): Hypertension: Pathophysiology, Diagnosis and Management, 2nd ed. New York, Raven Press, 1995, pp 2509–2529.
2. Zanchetti A: Antihypertensive therapy: Pride and prejudice [presidential lecture]. J Hypertens 13:1522–1528, 1995.
3. Mancia G, Zanchetti A: Evidence-based medicine: An educational instrument or a standard for implementation? J Hypertens 17:1509–1510, 1999.
4. Swales JD: Evidence-based medicine and hypertension. J Hypertens 17:1511–1516, 1999.
5. Veterans Administration Cooperative Study Group on Antihypertensive Agents: Effects of treatment on morbidity in hypertension: Results in patients with diastolic blood pressure averaging 115 through 129 mmHg. JAMA 202:1028–1034, 1967.
6. Veterans Administration Cooperative Study Group on Antihypertensive Agents: Effects of treatment on morbidity in hypertension. II: Results in patients with diastolic blood pressure averaging 90 mmHg through 114 mmHg. JAMA 213:1143–1152, 1970.
7. Hypertension Detection and Follow-up Program Cooperative Group: Five-year findings of the Hypertension Detection and Follow-up Program. I: Reduction in mortality in persons with high blood pressure, including mild hypertension. JAMA 242:2562–2571, 1979.
8. Australian National Blood Pressure Management Committee: The Australian therapeutic trial in mild hypertension. Lancet 1:1261–1267, 1980.
9. Medical Research Council Working Party: MRC trial of treatment of mild hypertension: Principal results. BMJ 291:97–104, 1985.
10. Amery A, Birkenhäger W, Brixko P, et al: Mortality and morbidity results from the European Working Party on High Blood Pressure in the Elderly trial. Lancet 1:1349–1354, 1985.
11. Coope J, Warrender TS: Randomized trial of treatment with hypertension in the elderly in primary care. BMJ 293:1145–1151, 1986.

12. Dahlöf B, Lindholm LH, Hansson L, et al: Morbidity and mortality in the Swedish Trial in Old Patients with Hypertension (STOP-Hypertension). Lancet 338:1281–1285, 1991.

13. SHEP Cooperative Research Council: Prevention of stroke by antihypertensive drug treatment in older persons with isolated systolic hypertension: Final results of the Systolic Hypertension in the Elderly Program (SHEP). JAMA 265:3255–3264, 1991.

14. Gong L, Zhang W, Zhu Y, et al: 11 collaborating centres in the Shanghai area: Shanghai Trial Of Nifedipine in the Elderly (STONE). J Hypertens 14:1237–1245, 1996.

15. Staessen JA, Fagard R, Thijs L, et al for the Systolic Hypertension in Europe (Sys-Eur) Trial Investigators: Randomised double-blind comparison of placebo and active treatment for older patients with isolated systolic hypertension. Lancet 350:757–764, 1997.

16. Liu L, Wang JG, Gong L, et al, for the Systolic Hypertension in China (SYST-China) Collaborative Group: Comparison of active treatment and placebo for older Chinese patients with isolated systolic hypertension. J Hypertens 16:1823–1829, 1998.

17. IPPSH Collaborative Group: Cardiovascular risk and risk factors in a randomised trial of treatment based on the beta-blocker oxyprenolol: The International Prospective Primary Study in Hypertension (IPPSH). J Hypertens 3:379–392, 1985.

18. Wilhelmsen L, Berglund G, Elmfeldt D, et al: Beta-blockers versus diuretics in hypertensive men. Main results from the HAPPHY Trial. J Hypertens 5:561–572, 1987.

19. Guidelines Subcommittee: 1999 World Health Organization–International Society of Hypertension guidelines for the management of hypertension. J Hypertens 17:151–183, 1999.

20. World Health Organization–International Society of Hypertension Blood Pressure Lowering Treatment Trialists' Collaboration: Protocol for prospective collaborative overviews of major randomized trials of blood pressure lowering treatments. J Hypertens 16:127–137, 1998.

21. Hansson L, Lindholm LH, Niskanen L, et al, for the Captopril Prevention Project (CAPP) study group: Effect of angiotensin-converting-enzyme inhibition compared with conventional therapy on cardiovascular morbidity and mortality in hypertension. Lancet 353:611–616, 1999.

22. Hansson L, Lindholm LH, Ekbom T, et al: Randomized trial of old and new antihypertensive drugs in elderly patients: Cardiovascular mortality and morbidity in the Swedish Trial in Old Patients with Hypertension-2 study. Lancet 354:1751–1756, 1999.

23. Dalhöf B, Devereux R, deFaire V, et al: The Losartan Intervention For Endpoint Reduction (LIFE) in Hypertension Study: Rationale, design and methods. Am J Hypertens 10:705–713, 1997.

24. Mann J, Julius S: The Valsartan Antihypertensive Long-term Use Evaluation (VALUE) Trial of cardiovascular events in hypertension: Rationale and design. Blood Pressure 7:176–183, 1998.

25. Hansson L, Lithell H, Skoog I, et al: Study on Cognition and Prognosis in the Elderly (SCOPE). Blood Pressure 8:177–183, 1999.

26. Levy D: Left ventricular hypertrophy: Epidemiological insights from the Framingham Heart Study. Drugs 35(Suppl 5):1–5, 1988.

27. Koren MJ, Devereux RB, Casale PN, et al: Relation of left ventricular mass and geometry to morbidity and mortality in uncomplicated essential hypertension. Ann Intern Med 114:345–352, 1991.

28. Dalhöf B, Pennert K, Hansson L: Reversal of left ventricular hypertrophy in hypertensive patients—a meta-analysis of 109 treatment studies. Am J Hypertens 5:95–110, 1992.

29. Schmieder RE, Martus P, Klingbeil A: Reversal of left ventricular hypertrophy in essential hypertension. Meta-analysis of randomized double-blind studies. JAMA 275:1507–1513, 1996.

30. Agabiti-Rosei E, Ambrosioni E, Dal Palú C, et al, on behalf of the RACE Study Group: ACE inhibitor ramipril is more effective than the beta-blocker atenolol in reducing left ventricular mass in hypertension. Results of the RACE (Ramipril Cardioprotective Evaluation) study. J Hypertens 11:1325–1334, 1995.

31. Collins R, Peto R, MacMahon S, et al: Blood pressure, stroke and coronary heart disease. II: Short-term reductions in blood pressure. Overview of randomized drug trials in their epidemiological context. Lancet 335:827–838, 1990.

32. Brunner HR, Laragh JH, Baer L, et al: Essential hypertension: Renin and aldosterone, heart attack and stroke. N Engl J Med 286:441–449, 1972.

33. Jorn AF: The Epidemiology of Alzheimer's Disease and Related Disorders. London, Chapman & Hall, 1990.

34. Kilander L, Nyman H, Andrén B, et al: Hypertension and associated metabolic disturbances are related to cognitive impairment: A 20-year follow-up of 999 men. Hypertension 31:780–786, 1998.

35. Skoog I, Hernfelt B, Landahl S, et al: 15-year longitudinal study of blood pressure and dementia. Lancet 347:1141–1145, 1996.

36. Barnes JM, Barnes NM, Costall B, et al: Angiotensin II inhibits the release of [^{3}H] acetylcholine from rat entorhinal cortex in vitro. Brain Res 492:136–143, 1989.

37. Barnes JM, Champaneria S, Costall B, et al: Cognitive enhancing actions of DUP 753 detected in a mouse habituation paradigm. Neuroreport 1:239–242, 1990.

CHAPTER 25

Evolving Perspectives and Future Challenges

HANS R. BRUNNER, M.D.
MURRAY EPSTEIN, M.D., F.A.C.P.

The discovery of renin 100 years ago became much more clinically relevant with the development of angiotensin-converting enzyme (ACE) inhibitors and AT_1 receptor antagonists as therapeutic tools. The AT_1 receptor antagonists are highly effective at reducing blood pressure and devoid of known side effects. In addition, when AT_1 receptor antagonists are combined with hydrochlorothiazides, which greatly enhance their efficacy, the side-effect profile still does not differ from that of placebo. With this combination, blood pressure can be controlled in 70–80% of all hypertensive patients. At present, depending on the country, control rates are at unacceptable levels of less than 30 or even 20% of all patients diagnosed with elevated blood pressure. The absence of side effects with AT_1 receptor antagonists opens new avenues for primary prevention of cardiovascular diseases. If the problem of adherence to therapy can be solved, cardiovascular diseases such as congestive heart failure, stroke, myocardial infarction, and renal failure may be prevented with AT_1 receptor antagonists before symptoms become apparent.

Nonetheless, many questions about AT_1 receptor antagonists remain to be answered in the areas of (1) mechanisms of action, (2) practical use, and (3) clinical outcome. Obviously, these questions are interconnected.

■ Mechanisms of Action

The development of AT_1 receptor antagonists has led to the discovery of a whole family of angiotensin (Ang) receptors and, in particular, to the characterization and cloning of AT_1 and AT_2 receptors, both of which are present in human tissue. The AT_2 receptor has been associated with a wide array of cellular and tissue functions, such as apoptosis, antigrowth, tissue repair, and vasodilation. Many of these effects have been well documented in carefully designed experiments. Nevertheless, in integrative physiology, pathophysiology, and clinical medicine, it is important to delineate the quantitative contribution of each potential mechanism. To what extent,

361

for example, does stimulation of AT_2 receptors contribute to the clinical therapeutic effect of AT_1 receptors? At present this question is unanswerable; indeed, it is not even clear to what extent AT_2 receptors at critical sites are stimulated by enhanced levels of Ang II. In a recent mouse study during which Ang II levels were carefully measured in plasma and various tissues, AT_1 receptor blockade raised plasma Ang II levels, as expected, but did not increase Ang II concentration in the heart, liver, or kidney.[1] Thus, even if stimulation of AT_2 receptors has all of the potentially beneficial effects outlined in this book, the crucial question remains: to what extent are AT_2 receptors stimulated during treatment with an AT_1 receptor antagonist?

Similarly, the existence of alternative pathways of Ang II synthesis that do not involve the conversion of Ang I to Ang II by ACE (see chapter by Hollenberg) is often proposed as an important mechanism in favor of AT_1 receptor antagonists over ACE inhibitors. AT_1 receptor antagonists should provide more complete blockade of the renin-angiotensin system by blocking alternative pathways of Ang II synthesis. Again, the quantitative contribution of alternative pathways is difficult to determine. To date, no clear superiority of AT_1 receptor antagonists over ACE inhibitors in blocking the renin-angiotensin system has been demonstrated. Yet this comparison is confounded by the possible contribution of enhanced bradykinin levels to the effect of ACE inhibitors. Crucial questions include whether ACE inhibitors and AT_1 receptor blockers exert their therapeutic effect mainly or exclusively by blocking the synthesis of Ang II or inhibiting stimulation of AT_1 receptors or whether other Ang-independent actions play a role.

Despite these open questions, ACE inhibitors and AT_1 receptor blockers seem to exhibit similar efficacy in a large variety of experimental and clinical situations, strongly suggesting that blockade of the renin-angiotensin system is a predominant mechanism of both classes of drugs. The similarity ends when side effects, particularly cough and angioedema, are taken into consideration.

■ Practical Use

Like ACE inhibitors, AT_1 receptor antagonists are best combined with diuretics, but combination with any other class of antihypertensive drugs may prove useful. Whether the combination of an AT_1 receptor antagonist with an ACE inhibitor provides additive or even synergistic efficacy remains an open question. This combination may be theoretically beneficial, especially if there is concern that AT_1 receptor blockade alone will not secure the positive effects of ACE inhibition due to decreased breakdown of bradykinin. It is also possible, however, that combined therapy is less effective than AT_1 receptor blockade alone, because combined therapy may lead to formation of less Ang II and thus less stimulation of AT_2 receptors. A combination of doses that block submaxilly should provide at least an additive effect, considering that the two types of drugs block at different levels of the enzymatic cascade. More to the point is whether a combination of maximally blocking doses provides additive efficacy. This question, which to date has no satisfactory answer, has obvious clinical relevance, because the combination of an AT_1 receptor antagonist with an ACE inhibitor inevitably adds potential side effects not present with monotherapy.

A somewhat related question is whether vasopeptidase inhibitors (e.g., omapatrilat),[2] which with a single molecule simultaneously inhibit two key enzymes (neutral endopeptidase [EC 24.11; NEP] and ACE) involved in the regulation of cardiovascular function, provide any advantage over the combination of an AT_1 receptor antagonist with 12.5 mg of hydrochlorothiazide. Unfortunately, direct comparison of these two therapeutic principles has not been carried out. Whatever the efficacy of the NEP–ACE inhibitors, however, the combination of an AT_1 receptor antagonist and a diuretic will always have the advantage of no demonstrable side effects.

■ Outcome

We treat patients with hypertension, congestive heart failure, or diabetic nephropathy with the clear goals of reducing morbidity and mortality and improving overall quality of life. The achievement of these goals provides the major advantage to blockade of the renin-angiotensin system with ACE inhibitors. The many outcome trials conducted with ACE inhibitors have provided strong evidence that their use makes a difference in the outcome of cardiovascular diseases, mainly congestive heart failure and coronary heart disease. Because the class of AT_1 receptor antagonists is at least 15 years younger, comparable evidence is not yet available. However, many outcome trials with AT_1 receptor antagonists are currently under way. The results of these trials are important, not only to determine what we can anticipate with long-term treatment, but also to answer such "proof-of-principle" questions as what bradykinin contributes to the cardio- or vasculoprotective actions of ACE inhibitors. We need to know whether we can routinely substitute an AT_1 receptor antagonist for an ACE inhibitor when side effects are induced and expect the same long-term protection.

Currently we have access to the results of a single trial, ELITE II. Unfortunately, interpretation of this study is confounded: it was not designed to demonstrate equal efficacy of losartan and captopril but rather to show the superiority of losartan, which in fact was not demonstrated. Furthermore, losartan was administered at 50 mg/day, a dose that provides less than maximal blockade. Fortunately, two ongoing double-blind, randomized, multinational trials, the Losartan Intervention for End-point Reduction in Hypertension Study[3] (LIFE) and the Valsartan Antihypertensive Long-term Use Evaluation Study[4] (VALUE), are designed to detect differential outcomes between an AT_1 receptor blocker and a conventional antihypertensive drug. The LIFE Study enrolled more than 8000 patients aged 55–88 years with hypertension and left ventricular hypertrophy, as documented by electrocardiography. The purpose is to compare over a period of 5 years the effects of losartan and atenolol on cardiovascular morbidity and mortality. The VALUE Study involves 14,400 patients in over 30 countries. Patients will be followed for 4–6 years or until 1450 patients experience a primary cardiac endpoint.

Because outcome data for AT_1 receptor antagonists are not yet available, it is reasonable to favor ACE inhibitors for the treatment of diabetic nephropathy, congestive heart failure, and coronary heart disease. Whether a switch to AT_1 receptor antagonists should be recommended when ACE inhibitor-related side effects are encountered must be left to the treating physician. The decision depends on whether the physician adheres strictly to evidence-based medicine or is willing to extrapolate clinical outcome from preliminary data, as progressive medicine has done in the past.

■ *Conclusions*

AT$_1$ receptor antagonists are an exciting new complement to the therapeutic armamentarium for cardiovascular diseases. An important attribute is their use as pharmacologic probes to enhance understanding of the mechanisms underlying the progression to cardiovascular diseases. Other desirable features are their unquestionable efficacy and lack of recognizable side effects. Despite an impressive amount of data about these agents, questions about mechanism of action and comparison with ACE inhibitors remain unanswered. As more results become available in the coming years, new therapeutic applications will be explored. The results of several ongoing studies of long-term outcome should help to establish the therapeutic role of AT$_1$ receptor antagonists in the treatment of hypertensive and cardiovascular disease.

References

1. Mazzolai L, Pedrazzini P, Nicoud F, et al: Increased cardiac angiotensin II levels induce right and left ventricular hypertrophy in normotensive mice. Hypertension [in press].
2. Weber M: Emerging treatments for hypertension: Potential role for vasopeptidase inhibition. Am J Hypertens 12(11 Pt 2):139S–147S, 1999.
3. Dahlof B, Devereux R, de Faire U, et al: The Losartan Intervention For Endpoint Reduction (LIFE) in Hypertension Study: Rationale, design, and methods. The LIFE Study Group. Am J Hypertens 10(7 Pt 1):705–713, 1997.
4. Mann J, Julius S: The Valsartan Antihypertensive Long-term Use Evaluation (VALUE) trial of cardiovascular events in hypertension: Rationale and design. Blood Pressure 7(3):176–183, 1998.

Index

Page numbers in **boldface** type indicate complete chapters.